Julien's
Primer of Drug Action

Julien's Primer of Drug Action

A Comprehensive Guide to the Actions, Uses, and Side Effects of Psychoactive Drugs

Fifteenth Edition

Robert M. Julien, M.D., Ph.D.
Portland, Oregon

with

Claire D. Advokat, Ph.D.
Louisiana State University

Joseph E. Comaty, Ph.D., M.P.
Baton Rouge, Louisiana

worth publishers
Macmillan Learning
New York

Executive Vice President and General Manager: Charles Linsmeier
Vice President, Social Sciences and High School: Shani Fisher
Senior Executive Program Manager: Christine Cardone
Assistant Editor: Olivia Madigan
Development Editor: Len Neufeld
Marketing Manager: Kate Nurre
Marketing Assistant: Claudia Cruz
Director of Media Editorial: Noel Hohnstine
Media Editor: Clarah Grossman
Media Project Manager: Joe Tomasso
Director, Content Management Enhancement: Tracey Kuehn
Senior Managing Editor: Lisa Kinne
Senior Project Manager: Vanavan Jayaraman, Lumina Datamatics, Inc.
Senior Workflow Project Manager: Paul Rohloff
Senior Permissions Manager: Jennifer MacMillan
Director of Design, Content Management: Diana Blume
Senior Design Services Manager: Natasha Wolfe
Interior Designer: Rick Korab
Senior Cover Design Manager: John Callahan
Art Manager: Matthew McAdams
Composition: Lumina Datamatics, Inc.
Printing and Binding: Transcontinental

Library of Congress Control Number: 2022933844

Student Edition:
ISBN-13: 978-1-319-24486-6
ISBN-10: 1-319-24486-6

International Edition:
ISBN-13: 978-1-319-49854-2
ISBN-10: 1-319-49854-1

Printed in Canada.
1 2 3 4 5 6 28 27 26 25 24 23

Worth Publishers
120 Broadway
New York, NY 10271
www.macmillanlearning.com

ABOUT THE AUTHORS

Robert M. Julien received his Ph.D. in pharmacology from the University of Washington and his M.D. from the University of California at Irvine. His many research articles focus on the psychopharmacology of sedative and antiepileptic drugs. Formerly an associate professor of pharmacology and anesthesiology at Oregon Health Sciences University, Dr. Julien is retired as staff anesthesiologist at St. Vincent Hospital and Medical Center in Portland, Oregon. For almost five decades, Dr. Julien has been taking on and bringing to completion the herculean task of revising each edition of *Julien's Primer of Drug Action* to maintain its succinct yet comprehensive and clear presentation of the most up-to-date advances in psychopharmacology. He remains active as a psychopharmacology consultant.

Claire Advokat, Ph.D., is a professor emerita in the Department of Psychology at Louisiana State University. **Joseph Comaty, Ph.D.**, formerly served as chief psychologist in the division of quality management of the Louisiana State Office of Behavioral Health and adjunct professor of psychology at Louisiana State University. He is licensed to prescribe psychotherapeutic drugs in the state of Louisiana. Both Dr. Advokat and Dr. Comaty remain on the faculty of the Postdoctoral Master of Science program in Clinical Psychopharmacology at Alliant International University, in San Francisco. They currently reside in Highland Park, Illinois.

Contact information
Dr. Julien: drsjulien@comcast.net

BRIEF CONTENTS

CONTENTS

PREFACE

As a youth I spent considerable time in my father's pharmacy in Seattle. I remember being fascinated by the question of why someone would purchase aspirin to treat a headache or obtain a prescription for Dilantin in order to prevent seizures. Understanding the mechanism of "why" a drug might effectively do something was a childhood fantasy, but it became a deeply engrained ambition. Eventually, I obtained a Ph.D. in pharmacology at the University of Washington. I became a professor at the University of California at Irvine and directed a psychopharmacology laboratory, studying epilepsy, antiepileptic drugs, and hypnotic drugs. In 1977, I completed my M.D. at UC Irvine and then became a professor of pharmacology and anesthesiology at Oregon Health Sciences University, followed by a 25-year clinical practice as an anesthesiologist at a large community hospital in Portland. Through all this I wrote extensively, taught pharmacology and anesthesiology, and eventually traveled extensively teaching psychopharmacology.

The story of the origin of this book actually began on November 13, 1971. At that time, I was a young professor at UC Irvine teaching and conducting psychopharmacology research. Tragically, a plane crash took the lives of three football coaches from a neighboring college, California State College, Fullerton, along with the pilot of the plane. As a result of the crash, that college was left without teachers for their winter classes. They asked UC Irvine for assistance. I agreed to teach one of their scheduled courses in drug education, starting in January 1972. Following the course, I complained to a senior colleague that I had no materials from which to teach. I naively stated that someone ought to write a book on psychopharmacology. A few weeks later I received in the mail a contract from his publisher. I signed the contract and wrote what turned out to be the first edition of this book. Since then, updated and expanded editions have appeared about every three years.

Thus, counting my boyhood experiences in my father's pharmacy, I have been a witness to the evolution of psychopharmacology for 70 years, from its earliest days in the 1950s to the present. This lifelong passion for psychopharmacology is what led me to embark on this 15th edition of *Julien's Primer of Drug Action*.

As in each of the prior editions, I strive in this 15th edition to present the latest developments in psychopharmacology as clearly and concisely as I can, describing the general principles of structure and mechanisms of action of each class of psychoactive drugs, as well as providing specific information about the individual agents. Also like prior editions, this edition is divided into four parts: (1) Chapters 1–3 provide an introduction to the basics of psychopharmacology; (2) Chapters 4–10 cover the concept of addiction and the various kinds of drugs of abuse; (3) Chapters 11–14 cover the different classes of psychotherapeutic drugs; and (4) Chapters 15–18 cover the uses and effects of psychoactive drugs in special populations (pregnant women, children and adolescents, and older adults), ending in Chapter 18 with a review of psychopharmacology in the context of the COVID-19 pandemic and with a look into the future of the field.

The chapters on drugs of abuse provide historical context and epidemiological updates, discussions of the classic agents, and descriptions of the most recent drugs of concern, as well as the latest developments in regard to pharmacological treatments of the disorders associated with abuse of these drugs. Each chapter on psychotherapeutic drugs includes an overview of the disorders for which the drugs are indicated, discussion of the mechanisms of action of the drugs, and discussion of the rationales for drug treatment.

Certainly, there is overlap between the therapeutic and addictive effects of drugs. Many types of therapeutic drugs, such as the stimulants, benzodiazepines, and opiates, are involved in the ongoing epidemic of abuse and overdose deaths. Extraordinary efforts are being made to develop products that are resistant to misuse and to diversion into illicit channels of distribution. At the same time, research on substances primarily considered to be drugs of abuse (such as the psychedelic drugs and cannabis) is exploring new therapeutic possibilities. As always, we psychopharmacologists are optimistic that scientific investigation will result in new insights into the etiology of mental illness and addiction and that the future will bring more effective treatments for these devastating disorders.

In the years since the 14th edition, societal interest in psychopharmacology has continued to increase. New features and focuses that characterize this 15th edition reflect the following factors involved in this increasing interest:

- The opioid crisis has resulted in hundreds of thousands of deaths, a majority of which followed from the adulteration of opioid products with fentanyl and potent fentanyl derivatives.
- Rapid-acting opioid antagonists are now widely available.
- Increasing public acceptance of medical and recreational marijuana, cannabidiol (CBD), and other cannabis products has accompanied changes in their legal status.
- Pharmacological management of opioid and alcohol dependence has gained increasing interest.
- New antipsychotic medications with off-label uses continue to appear commercially.
- New products for the treatment of bipolar depression have also continued to appear.
- Psychedelic psychopharmacology has expanded widely, including with an increasing therapeutic use of psychedelic drugs for treatment of pain and depression.
- Psychotherapeutic drugs for treatment-resistant depression have become an expanding focus of research.

- Medications to treat personality and other disorders have also gained increasing interest.
- The treatment of cognitive dysfunction in Alzheimer's disease—both its promises and its failures—continues to be a focus of research.
- Off-label uses of psychoactive medications continue to expand.
- The COVID-19 pandemic has had profound effects on our society, including effects on mental health and long-term effects of having been infected with the virus.

Finally, a word about a new feature in this edition, **Dr. J's Musings**: it is my privilege to share some of my "musings" about events that have occurred during my long career in psychopharmacology. I hope that the reader will find them interesting, informative, and perhaps even entertaining.

Acknowledgments

The editorial work of Len Neufeld and Stephanie Ventura on this 15th edition has been marvelous, as has the support of Senior Executive Program Manager and Editor Christine Cardone, reflecting her commitment to this project. I am also indebted to Drs. Joe Comaty and Claire Advokat, who authored the 13th and 14th editions of this text; without their work, this new edition would not have been possible.

Finally, I am indebted to the instructors who have provided insightful feedback for this 15th edition, especially Michael Hylin of Southern Illinois University, who provided excellent feedback on the *Did You Know* boxes. Reviewers included:

Rachel Branco, *University of Notre Dame*
Carol DeVolder, *Saint Ambrose University*
Christopher Montoya, *Thompson Rivers University*
Anthony H. Risser, *Adler School of Professional Psychology*
John Rossi III, *Florida Gulf Coast University*
Fred Shaffer, *Truman State University*
Patti M. Simone, *Santa Clara University*
Emese Vitalis, *National Louis University*
Lawrence J. Wichlinski, *Carleton College*

Julien's
Primer of Drug Action

PART 1

Introduction to Psychopharmacology: The Biological Basis of Drug Action

A **drug** is a chemical substance used for its effects on bodily processes. **Pharmacology** is the science of *how* drugs affect living organisms; **psychopharmacology**, more specifically, is the study of how drugs affect the brain and behavior. To understand the actions, behavioral uses, therapeutic uses, and abuse potentials of **psychoactive drugs**—chemical substances that alter mood or behavior as a result of alterations in the functioning of the brain—it is helpful to know how the body responds to the presence of such drugs. This understanding involves the basic principles of drug absorption, distribution, metabolism, and elimination as well as the interactions of drugs with their receptors, the interactions that produce the effects of drugs.

As an introduction to psychopharmacology, this book presents not only drugs useful in treating psychological disorders, but also drugs prone to compulsive use and abuse. Before discussing specific drugs or classes of drugs, it is necessary to discuss fundamentals of drug action common to all drugs.

Chapter 1 explores **pharmacokinetics**, the movement of drug molecules into, through, and out of the body. It addresses such questions as these: What are the ways by which drugs get into the body and how does that relate to their actions? Once in the body, how do drugs get to the sites at which they produce their effects? Once a drug exerts its effect, how is that action terminated? Finally, how does the body eventually get rid of the drug?

For readers without a background in neuroscience, Chapter 2 introduces the structure and function of the nervous system and the neuron, because this is where psychoactive drugs produce their effects. We focus on the synapse (the connection between two different neurons) and on neurotransmitters, the chemical substances through which neurons communicate. By studying the process of synaptic transmission, we begin to understand the mode of action of psychoactive drugs. The phenomenon of synaptic transmission is not static; rather, neurons have the ability to remodel themselves continually, a process called **synaptic plasticity**, which mediates learning and memory as well as such disorders as anxiety, depression, and addiction. A healthy, functioning brain is one that through this process of synaptic plasticity is continually remodeling itself in response to the environment. Healthy neurons continually form new synaptic contacts, maintaining the beautiful architecture built through normal interactions with millions of other neurons.

Chapter 3 explores **pharmacodynamics**. It examines the interaction between drugs and the **receptors** to which the drugs attach and through which they produce their effects. We describe receptors both structurally and functionally, and we discuss how drugs alter receptor structure and function. Finally, we summarize the ways in which such actions underlie the therapeutic effects and the side effects of drugs. These three chapters provide the basic foundation for understanding the more specific information in subsequent chapters.

CHAPTER 1

Pharmacokinetics: How the Body Handles Drugs

CHAPTER OUTLINE

When we have a headache, we take it for granted that after taking some aspirin our headache will probably disappear within 15 to 30 minutes. We also take it for granted that, unless we take more aspirin later, the headache may recur within 3–4 hours. This aspirin scenario illustrates the four basic processes in pharmacokinetics (collectively referred to as ADME):

1. *Absorption* of the aspirin into the body from the swallowed tablet
2. *Distribution* of the aspirin throughout the body and the brain, including into the fetus if a pregnant female has taken the drug
3. *Metabolism* as the aspirin that has exerted its analgesic effect is broken down into metabolites (by-products or waste products) that no longer exert any effect
4. *Elimination* of the metabolic waste products, usually in the urine

DR. J'S MUSINGS 1.1

Can I Have Dessert Without Eating My Vegetables?

Beginning in the 1960s, the continuing explosion in drug development, clinical research, and medication approvals for mental health disorders has made this the most exciting period in the history of pharmacology. How to share this excitement has always been a challenge. Many educators immediately delve into marijuana, opioids, hallucinogens, and stimulants. However, I have long been convinced that understanding the basics makes it easier to understand the actions of *all* drugs, including psychoactive drugs—hence this opening chapter on pharmacokinetics. It is a bit like eating your vegetables before eating dessert—not fun, but necessary for good nutrition. In other words, it's useful to learn the basics of how drugs work in general before delving into the actions of specific drugs.

In concert, these four processes determine the **bioavailability** of a drug at its receptors—that is, how much of the drug that is administered actually reaches its target and how long it persists there.

The goal of this chapter is to introduce these pharmacokinetic processes. Because many drugs need to be taken chronically and for various periods of time, the chapter also explores the steady-state maintenance of therapeutic blood levels of drugs in the body and the usefulness of therapeutic drug monitoring. Finally, the chapter introduces the concepts of drug tolerance and drug dependence, concepts that become very important as certain classes of drugs (e.g., opioids) are discussed later in the book.

Usually, the time course of a particular drug's actions—the time to onset and the duration of effect—simply reflects the amount of time required for the rise and fall of the drug's concentration at the target site. Figure 1.1 summarizes drug movement through the body to its site of action, where it produces a pharmacological response, and then to the kidneys where the drug and its metabolites are excreted in urine.

The root *kinetics* in the word *pharmacokinetics* implies both movement and time. Knowledge of movement and time offers significant insight into the action of a drug. At the very least, it helps distinguish a particular drug from related drugs. For example, the main difference between the two benzodiazepine sedatives lorazepam (Ativan)[1]

[1]Most drugs used in medicine are known by two or even three names. The most detailed name for a drug is its structural name, which accurately describes its chemical structure in words. In this book, the structural names for drugs are not used. The second name for a drug is its **generic name** (e.g., lorazepam), often an abbreviated form derived from the structural name, given to the drug by its discoverer or original manufacturer. After a drug's patent protection runs out (usually 17 years after the date of its patent registration by the manufacturer), any other generic drug manufacturer may legitimately sell the drug under the generic name. The third name is the drug's trade name, a unique name given to the drug by its original patent holder. Only that manufacturer can ever sell the drug under that name, even after the patent runs out and others sell the drug under its generic name. For example, many companies sell aspirin, a generic name for acetylsalicylic acid, the structural name. But only Bayer Pharmaceuticals, the original company that patented acetylsalicylic acid, can call it "Bayer Aspirin." In this book, when a drug is introduced, the generic name is given first and is not capitalized. The trade name follows in parentheses, is capitalized, and usually is not given again.

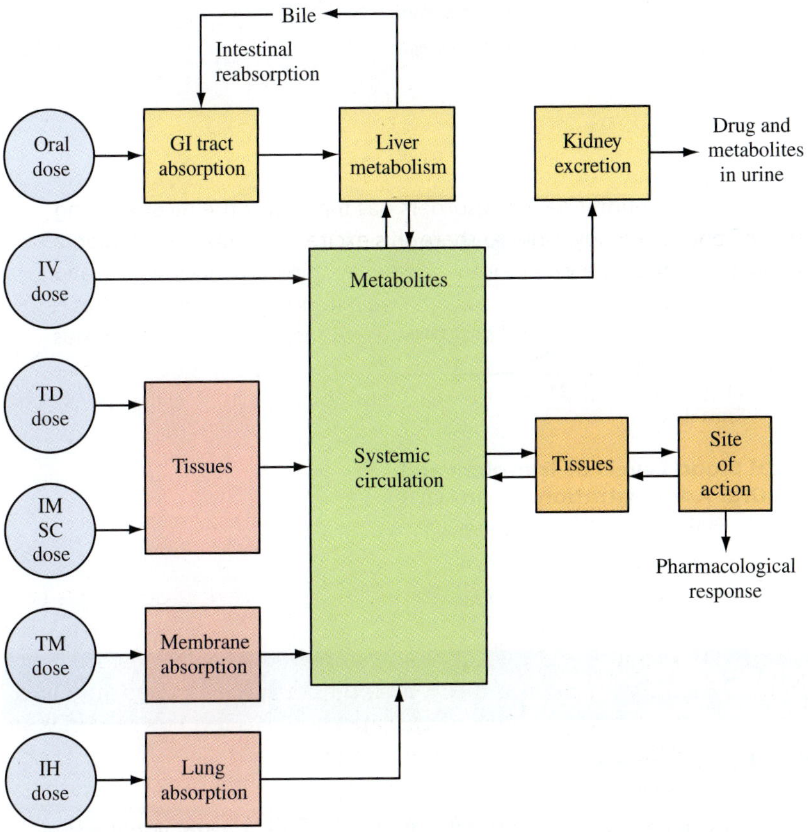

FIGURE 1.1 The Fate of a Drug in the Body.
IV = intravenous; TD = transdermal; IM = intramuscular; SC = subcutaneous; TM = transmembrane; IH = inhalational.

and triazolam (Halcion) is in their pharmacokinetics. Both of these drugs have sedative and antianxiety effects. Lorazepam, however, persists in the body for at least 24 hours, while triazolam persists for only about 6–8 hours. If lorazepam is taken at bedtime for treatment of insomnia, daytime sedation the next day can be a problem because lorazepam persists in the body through the next day. But for treating anxiety, where a longer, steady action might be useful, lorazepam would work better than triazolam.

The kinetic differences between lorazepam and triazolam are illustrated in Figure 1.2, which shows three ranges in the blood plasma: an ineffective range (where not enough drug is present to produce either sedative or antianxiety effect), a therapeutic range, and a toxic range (where sedation becomes excessive). Triazolam reaches peak blood level rapidly and stays in the therapeutic range for only a short time. Lorazepam, in contrast, reaches peak blood level more slowly and persists longer in the therapeutic range. In essence, pharmacokinetic differences between the two drugs account for these results and allow two similar drugs to be used to achieve different therapeutic goals.

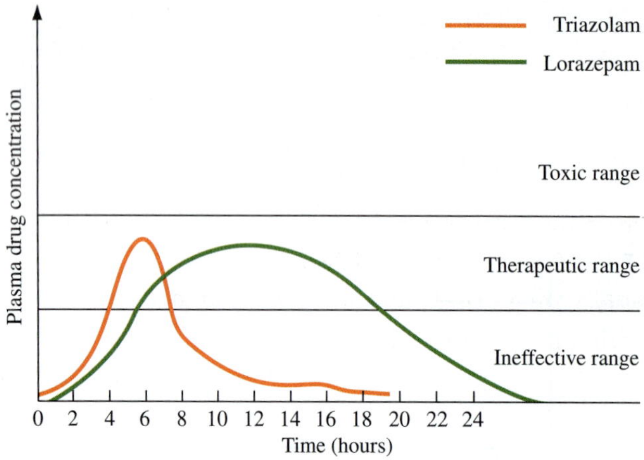

FIGURE 1.2 Theoretical Blood Levels of Triazolam and Lorazepam Following Oral Administration. Triazolam is a short-acting benzodiazepine, and lorazepam is a longer-acting benzodiazepine.

DR. J'S MUSINGS 1.2

How ADME Can Work for You

If you remember to consider the acronym ADME when you study a drug, you'll get a brief overview of how the drug is handled by the body:

- *Absorption* is usually oral, unless the drug must be given as an injection
- *Distribution* of most psychoactive drugs is in the blood, to reach the brain
- *Metabolism* breaks the drug down, usually into inactive by-products
- *Elimination* is the excretion of these by-products in urine

DRUG ABSORPTION

The term **drug absorption** refers to processes and mechanisms by which drugs pass into the bloodstream (usually from the stomach and intestine). For any drug, a route of administration, a dose of the drug, and a dosage form (liquid, tablet, capsule, injection, patch, spray, or gum) must be selected that will both place the drug at its site of action in a pharmacologically effective concentration and maintain the concentration for an adequate period of time. **Drug administration** is most often oral (the drug is swallowed when taken by mouth) and the drug then passes into the blood through absorption from the stomach and GI tract. A drug can also be administered for absorption through the membranes of the GI tract by embedding the drug in a suppository, which is placed in the rectum. Drugs can also be administered by the following routes, which bypass the GI tract:

- Inhalation (breathed in through the lungs as gases, vapors, or particles carried in smoke or in an aerosol)
- Absorption through mucous membranes (from "snorting," or sniffing, the drug, with the drug being deposited on the oral or nasal mucosa)
- Absorption through the skin (usually via a drug-containing skin patch)
- Injection (given in liquid form with a needle and syringe)

Oral Administration

To be effective when administered orally, a drug must be soluble (able to dissolve) and stable in stomach fluid (not destroyed by gastric acids), must penetrate the lining of the stomach or enter the intestine and penetrate the intestinal lining, and must then pass into the bloodstream. Because they are already in solution, drugs that are administered in liquid form tend to be absorbed more rapidly than those given in solid form in a tablet or capsule. When a drug is taken in solid form, both the rate at which it dissolves and its chemistry limit the rate of absorption. Food in the stomach usually tends to slow the rate of absorption. Rarely, an oral formulation contains a precursor of a drug, called a **prodrug**, rather than the active drug itself. A prodrug must undergo chemical conversion by metabolic processes in order to become an active pharmacological agent. One example of this type of medication is the drug lisdexamfetamine (Vyvanse), approved for the treatment of attention deficit/hyperactivity disorder (ADHD) (discussed in Chapter 16).

After a tablet dissolves, the drug molecules contained within it are carried into the upper intestine, where they are absorbed across the intestinal mucosa by a process of passive diffusion—that is, passing from an area of high concentration into an area of lower concentration. This process necessitates that the drug molecules, at least to some degree, be lipid soluble (soluble in fat). In reality, even a small amount of **lipid solubility** allows for absorption after oral administration; drugs that are more lipid soluble are merely absorbed faster than those that are less lipid soluble. Most psychoactive drugs have good solubility in the lipid linings of the stomach and intestine; typically, about 75% (or more) of the amount of an orally administered psychoactive drug is absorbed into the bloodstream within 1–3 hours after administration.

As illustrated in Figure 1.3, nutrients (and orally administered drugs) absorbed from the small intestine flow into veins for fairly even distribution throughout the body. As part of this distribution process, venous blood (containing drugs that were absorbed) passes in the portal vein to the liver, where most drug metabolism takes place. Unmetabolized drug then passes through the liver and into the general circulation and into all body compartments, including the brain.

There are some exceptions to this general rule. One involves buspirone (BuSpar), an antianxiety drug that has limited clinical efficacy, primarily because an enzyme called CYP-3A4, located in the walls of the stomach lining, rapidly metabolizes most of

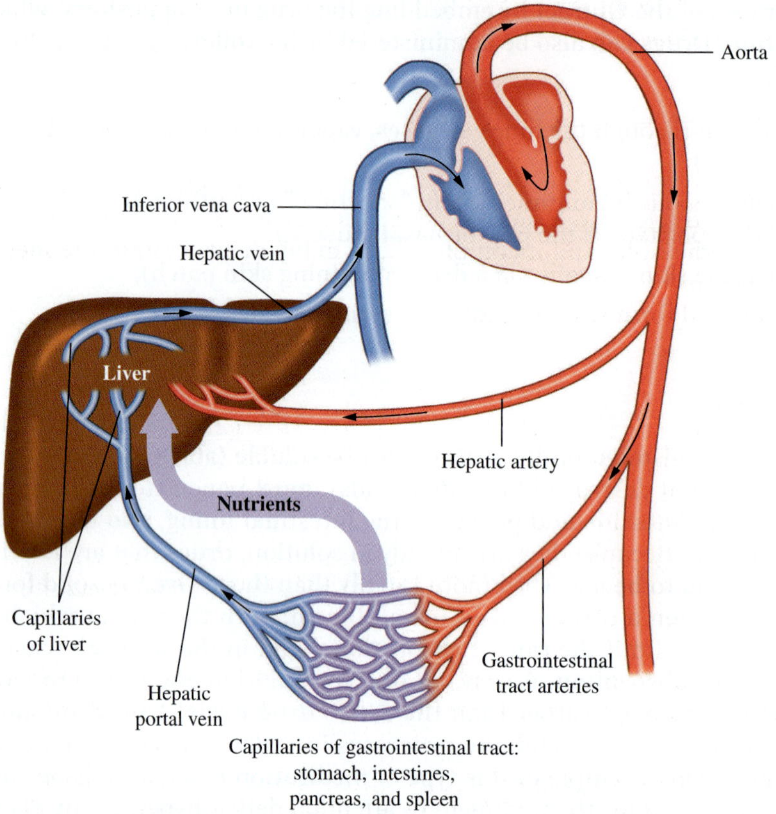

FIGURE 1.3 The Hepatic Portal Connection Between the Gastrointestinal Tract and the Liver.

it, reducing the oral absorption of buspirone by over 90%. Should buspirone be taken with grapefruit juice, however, a component in the juice (furanocoumarin) inhibits the CYP-3A4 enzyme, allowing the buspirone to be more completely absorbed, which increases its blood concentration and thus affects both its therapeutic utility and its toxicity.

More broadly, grapefruit and other juices taken with certain medications increase drug absorption and may increase the toxicity of those drugs. A review of multiple clinical studies on such interactions identified 22 juice-drug combinations of clinical relevance (Chen et al., 2018).

Although oral administration of drugs is common, it does have disadvantages. First, it may occasionally lead to vomiting and stomach distress. Second, although the amount of a drug that is put into a tablet or capsule can be calculated, how much of it will be absorbed into the bloodstream cannot always be accurately predicted because of genetic differences among people (in the amount and composition of the enzymes they have that metabolize the drugs) and because of differences in the manufacture of the drugs. Finally, the acid in the stomach destroys some orally administered drugs, such as local anesthetics and insulin, before they can be absorbed. To be effective, those drugs must be administered by injection.

Rectal Administration

Drugs are administered rectally (usually in suppository form) if the patient is vomiting, unconscious, or unable to swallow. However, absorption after rectal administration is often irregular, unpredictable, and incomplete, and many drugs irritate the membranes that line the rectum.

Administration by Inhalation

Inhalation is a popular method of administration of recreational drugs such as nicotine in tobacco cigarettes and vapors, tetrahydrocannabinol (THC) in marijuana, heroin when smoked, crack cocaine, ice methamphetamine, and the various inhalants of abuse, all of which are discussed later in this book. In addition, certain therapeutic drugs are effectively administered by inhalation, such as bronchodilators (used to treat asthma) and certain general anesthetics. The use of inhalation as a route of administration follows from two observations:

1. Lung tissues have a large surface area through which large amounts of blood flow, allowing for rapid absorption of drugs from the lungs into the blood (often within seconds).
2. Drugs absorbed into pulmonary (lung) capillaries are carried in the pulmonary veins directly to the left side of the heart (the arterial side, as shown in Figure 1.4) and from there directly into the aorta and the arteries carrying blood to the brain. As a result, drugs administered by inhalation may have an even faster onset of effect than drugs administered intravenously, with an intense effect that may promote compulsive use.

Administration Through Mucous Membranes

Occasionally, drugs are administered through the mucous membranes of the mouth or nose. Here are a few examples:

- Cocaine powder, when sniffed, adheres to the membranes on the inside of the nose and is absorbed directly into the bloodstream. (Cocaine is discussed in Chapter 7.)
- Nicotine in snuff, nasal spray, and chewing gum formulations is absorbed through the mucosal membranes directly into the bloodstream. (Nicotine is discussed in Chapter 6.)
- Since 1998, the opioid narcotic fentanyl (Sublimaze) has been available in lollipop form for use before and after surgery on children. This allows this pain-relieving drug to be provided without subjecting children to a painful injection. As the lollipop is sucked, the drug is released and absorbed through the mucous membranes of the

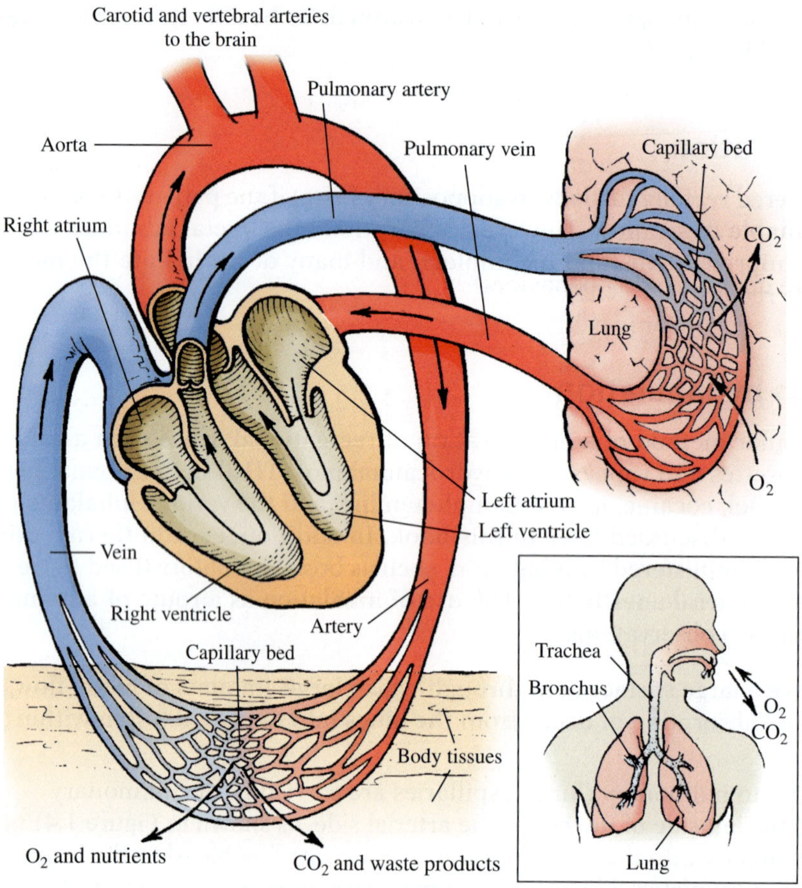

FIGURE 1.4 Heart and Circulatory System. Blood returning from the systemic venous circulation to the heart enters the right atrium and flows into the right ventricle. With contraction of the heart, this blood is pumped into the pulmonary arteries leading to the lungs. Once the blood is in the pulmonary capillaries, carbon dioxide (CO_2) is lost and replaced by oxygen. The oxygenated blood returns to the heart in the pulmonary veins, which empty into the left atrium, from which the blood flows into the left ventricle. With heart contraction, the oxygenated blood is pumped from the left ventricle into the aorta and is carried throughout the body. In the systemic capillary beds, oxygen and nutrients are supplied to the body tissues and brain through the walls of the capillaries, while CO_2 and other waste products are returned to the blood. The CO_2 is eliminated through the lungs, and the other waste products are metabolized in the liver and excreted in the urine.

mouth. This form of administering fentanyl has also become popular for patients with disabling pain when orally administered pain relievers are insufficient and injection of opioid narcotics is too painful. (Fentanyl is discussed in Chapter 10.)

- A sublingual (placed under the tongue) combination of buprenorphine (an opioid narcotic) and naloxone (an opioid antagonist) is available for the office-based treatment of opioid dependency. (This is also discussed in Chapter 10.)

Administration Through the Skin

Over the past several years, several medications have been incorporated into **transdermal patches** that adhere to the skin. A transdermal patch is a bandage-like therapeutic system that provides continuous, controlled release of a drug from a reservoir through a semipermeable membrane. The drug is slowly absorbed into the bloodstream at the area of contact. Here are some examples of drugs that can be administered in this way:

- Nicotine (used to deter smoking behaviors)
- Fentanyl (used to treat chronic pain)
- Clonidine (used to treat hypertension)
- Estrogen or other hormones (used to replace reduced hormones in postmenopausal women or for contraception)
- Scopolamine (used to prevent motion sickness)
- Buprenorphine (Butrans, used to treat opioid dependence)
- Selegiline (Emsam, used to treat depression)
- Methylphenidate (Daytrana, used to treat ADHD in children)
- Rivastigmine (used to treat Alzheimer's disease)

All these transdermal skin patches allow for slow, continuous absorption of the drug over hours or even days, potentially minimizing side effects associated with rapid rises and falls in plasma concentrations of the drug.

Administration by Injection

Administration of drugs by injection can be done by **intravenous injection** (directly into a vein), **intramuscular injection** (directly into a muscle), or **subcutaneous injection** (just under the skin). Each of these routes of administration has its advantages and disadvantages (see Table 1.1).

Perhaps the greatest advantage is that the rate of absorption can be controlled, from immediate absorption in intravenous injection to rapid absorption or slow and sustained absorption in both intramuscular and subcutaneous injection. Also, injection by any route permits a more accurate dosage than does oral administration because injection avoids the unpredictable processes of absorption through the stomach and intestine.

Administration of drugs by injection, however, has several drawbacks. First, the rapid rise of blood concentrations after intravenous injection leaves little time to respond to an unexpected reaction or overdose (the epidemic of deaths following opioid injection is discussed in Chapter 10). Second, administration by injection requires the use of sterile techniques in order to avoid transmission of diseases such as hepatitis and AIDS. Third, once a drug is administered by injection, it cannot be recalled. There are few antidotes for drug overdoses, with the exception of naloxone for opioid overdoses and flumazenil for benzodiazepine overdoses (as discussed in Chapters 10 and 13, respectively).

TABLE 1.1 Some Characteristics of Drug Administration by Injection

Route	Absorption Pattern	Special Utility	Limitations and Precautions
Intravenous	Immediate absorption Avoids unpredictability of absorption after oral administration	Valuable for emergency use Permits extremely precise dosage Permits dilution of drug for administration of large volumes or irritating substances	Increased risk of adverse effects Solutions must usually be injected slowly Not suitable for oily solutions or insoluble substances
Intramuscular	Fairly rapid absorption from aqueous solution Slow and sustained absorption from oily solution (depot administration)	Suitable for moderate volumes, oily solutions, and some irritating substances	Precluded when patient is on anticoagulant medication May interfere with interpretation of certain diagnostic tests (e.g., creatinine phosphokinase)
Subcutaneous	Rapid absorption Slow and sustained absorption from oily solution (depot administration)	Suitable for some insoluble suspensions and for implantation of solid pellets	Not suitable for large volumes Possible pain or necrosis from irritating substances

Intravenous Administration

In an intravenous injection, a drug is introduced directly into the bloodstream. This technique avoids all the variables related to oral absorption. Intravenous injection can be done slowly, and it can be stopped instantaneously if untoward effects develop. In addition, the dosage can be extremely precise, and the practitioner can dilute and administer in large volumes drugs that at higher concentrations would be irritants to the blood vessels.

The intravenous route is one of the most dangerous of all routes of administration because of the rapid onset of pharmacological action. Too-rapid injection can be catastrophic, producing life-threatening reactions (such as collapse of respiration). Also, allergic reactions, should they occur, may be extremely severe. Finally, drugs that are not completely solubilized before injection usually cannot be given intravenously because of the danger of blood clots or emboli forming.

Intramuscular Administration

Drugs that are injected into skeletal muscle (usually in the arm, thigh, or buttock) are generally absorbed fairly rapidly. Absorption of a drug from muscle is more rapid than absorption of the same drug from the stomach but slower than intravenous absorption. The absolute rate of absorption of a drug from muscle varies, depending on the rate of blood flow to the muscle, the solubility of the drug, the volume of the injection, and the solution in which the drug is dissolved and injected.

Intramuscular injections are of two types: (1) fairly rapid onset and short duration of action and (2) slow onset and prolonged action. In the first type, the drug is dissolved in an aqueous (water) solution. Following injection, the water and dissolved drug are quite rapidly absorbed, with complete absorption occurring over a few hours. In the second type, known as *depot administration*, the drug typically is suspended in an oily solution that is only slowly absorbed, with complete absorption taking days or weeks. Modern manufacturing techniques have enabled another form of depot administration in which the drug is placed in bioabsorbable polymer microspheres that release a constant amount of drug each day for a period of a week or more (as with the antipsychotic Risperdal, discussed in Chapter 11). Similarly, injected microcapsules containing the opioid narcotic antagonist naltrexone (discussed in Chapter 10) release a constant amount of drug into blood over a period of several weeks (see Chapter 5 for discussion of naltrexone—under the trade name Vivitrol—used for the treatment of alcohol dependence).

Subcutaneous Administration

Absorption of drugs that have been injected under the skin (subcutaneously) is quite rapid. The exact rate depends mainly on how easy it is for the drug to penetrate the blood vessels in the skin and the rate of blood flow through the skin. Irritating drugs should not be injected subcutaneously because they may cause severe pain and may damage local tissue.

DRUG DISTRIBUTION

Once absorbed into the bloodstream, a drug is distributed throughout the body by the circulating blood, passing across various barriers to reach its target, that is, its site of action (its receptors). At any given time during this process of **drug distribution**, only a very small portion of the total amount of a drug that is in the body is actually in contact with its receptors. For example, in the case of a psychoactive drug, most of the drug circulates outside the brain and therefore does not contribute directly to its pharmacological effect. This wide distribution often accounts for many of the **side effects** of a drug, the effects that accompany the primary, or therapeutic, effect for which a drug is taken.

Distribution in the Bloodstream

Every minute, in an average-size adult, the heart pumps a volume of blood that is roughly equal to the total amount of blood in the circulatory system. That is, the entire blood volume circulates in the body about once every minute. Once absorbed into the bloodstream, a drug is rapidly (usually within the 1-minute circulation time) distributed throughout the circulatory system.

As shown in Figure 1.4, blood returning to the heart through the veins is first pumped into the pulmonary (lung) circulation system, where carbon dioxide is removed and replaced by oxygen. The oxygenated blood then returns to the heart and is pumped into the great artery (the aorta). From there, blood flows into the smaller arteries and finally into capillaries. At that point, nutrients (and drugs) are exchanged between the blood and the cells of the body. After blood passes through the capillaries, it is collected by the veins and returned to the heart to circulate again. Psychoactive drugs quite quickly become evenly distributed throughout the bloodstream, diluted not only by blood but also by the total amount of water in the body.

If a drug is taken orally, it passes through the cells lining the GI tract and then through the liver; from there, the drug enters central circulation and is carried to the heart to be distributed throughout the body (see Figure 1.3).

Occasionally, in a process called **first-pass metabolism**, drug-metabolizing enzymes in the cells of either the GI tract or the liver can markedly reduce the amount of drug that reaches the bloodstream. For example, as discussed in Chapter 5, the enzyme alcohol dehydrogenase, which metabolizes alcohol, is found in the cells lining the GI tract and in cells of the liver. Women have less of this enzyme in the GI tract cells than men do, which means that women exhibit higher blood alcohol levels for a given amount of alcohol ingested (corrected for body weight).

Body Membranes That Affect Drug Distribution

Four types of membranes in the body affect drug distribution: (1) cell membranes, (2) walls of the capillary vessels in the circulatory system, (3) the blood-brain barrier, and (4) the placental barrier.

Cell Membranes

The structure and properties of cell membranes determine their permeability to drugs. As shown in Figure 1.5, a cell membrane is made up of two layers of complex lipid molecules called *phospholipids*. The phospholipid heads form a nearly continuous layer on both the inside and outside of the membrane. The tails of the phospholipids are lipid chains. Therefore, for our present purposes, the interior of the cell membrane can be considered to consist of a sea of lipid in which large proteins are suspended.

Cell membranes provide a physical barrier that is permeable to small, lipid-soluble drug molecules but is impermeable to large, lipid-insoluble drug molecules. They are important for the passage of drugs (1) from the stomach and intestine into the bloodstream, (2) from the fluid that closely surrounds tissue cells into the interior of cells, (3) from the interior of cells back into the body water, and (4) from the kidneys back into the bloodstream.

Capillaries

Within a minute or so of entering the bloodstream, a drug is distributed fairly evenly throughout the entire blood volume. From there, the drug leaves the bloodstream and

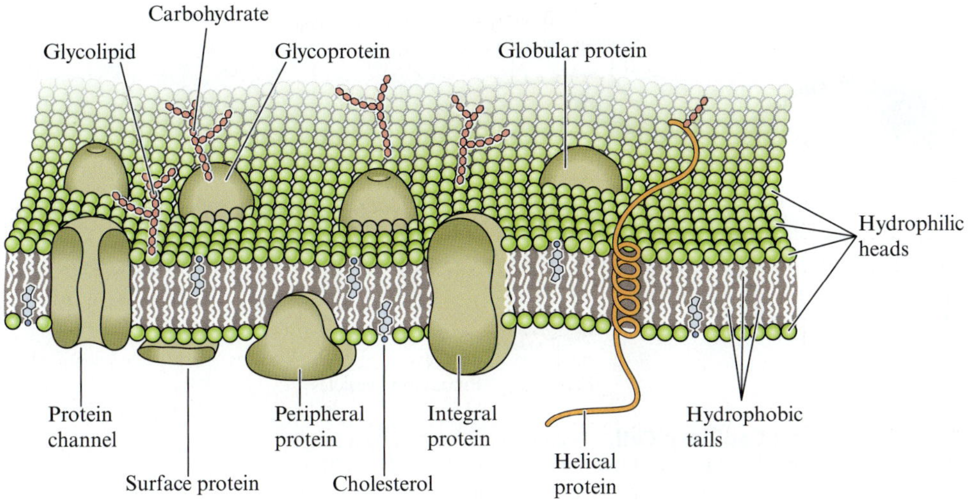

FIGURE 1.5 A Cell Membrane. The membrane is a phospholipid bilayer in which the phospholipids have hydrophilic heads and hydrophobic tails. Cholesterol molecules and protein molecules are embedded in the bilayer, and both globular and helical proteins traverse the bilayer. Cholesterol molecules tend to keep the tails of the phospholipids relatively fixed and orderly in the regions closest to the hydrophilic heads; the parts of the tails closer to the core of the membrane move about freely.

is exchanged (in equilibrium) between blood capillaries and body tissues. Capillaries are tiny, cylindrical blood vessels with walls that are formed by a single thin layer of cells packed tightly together. As shown in Figure 1.6, between the cells are small pores (clefts or fenestra) that allow passage of small molecules between blood and the body tissues. The diameter of these pores is between 90 and 150 angstroms (Å), which is larger than most drug molecules. Thus, most drugs freely leave the blood through these pores in the capillary membranes, moving along their concentration gradient until equilibrium is established between the concentrations of drug in the blood, body tissues, and the surrounding water. (Figure 1.6 also shows that substances can enter capillary cells in small vesicles formed by invagination of the cell wall.)

The transport of drug molecules between blood plasma and body tissues is independent of lipid solubility because the membrane pores are large enough for even fat-insoluble drug molecules. These pores, however, are not large enough to permit red blood cells and plasma proteins to leave the bloodstream. Thus, the only drugs that do not readily pass through capillary pores are drugs that bind to plasma proteins. The rate at which drug molecules enter specific body tissues depends on two factors: the rate of blood flow through the tissue and the ease with which drug molecules pass through the capillary membranes.

Because blood flow is greatest to the brain and much less to the bones, joints, and fat deposits, drug distribution generally follows a similar pattern. For example, when marijuana is smoked, the active drug, tetrahydrocannabinol (THC) (discussed in Chapter 9), achieves plasma concentrations in the brain of about 10–20 nanograms of

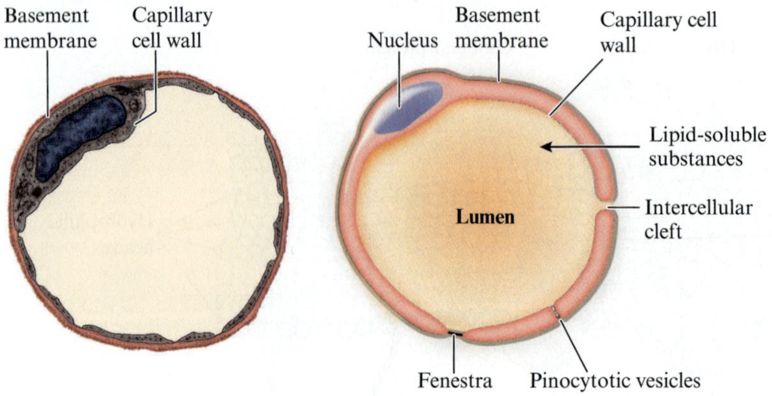

FIGURE 1.6 A Typical Capillary Cell. A capillary is formed by a single thin layer of flattened cells like the one shown here in a micrograph at left and schematically at right. Fenestrae and intracellular clefts allow small molecules to pass into and out of the interior of the capillary (the lumen), while other substances can enter the lumen in pinocytotic vesicles. Lipid-soluble substances can pass through the cell wall into the lumen.

drug per milliliter (ng/mL) of plasma soon after initiation of smoking. Within about 30 minutes, it achieves levels of about 50–100 ng/mL, which fall off within 1 hour to less than 5–10 ng/mL because the drug is rapidly taken up into body fat. From there, it slowly returns to plasma and is metabolized to an inactive metabolite (carboxy-THC) that is excreted in the urine.

Blood-Brain Barrier

The brain requires a protected environment to function normally. A specialized structural barrier, called the **blood-brain barrier**, plays a key role in maintaining this environment (see Figure 1.7). A number of factors combine to create this barrier. First, in contrast to capillaries in most of the body, the capillary walls in the brain do not have pores. In addition, the endothelial cells that make up the capillary wall are tightly joined together, without intercellular clefts. Finally, the capillary is covered on the outside by the glial sheath, a fatty layer that arises from nearby astrocyte glial cells.

Thus, to reach the neurons in the brain, a drug in a brain capillary has to traverse both the wall of the capillary itself (because there are no pores to pass through) and the glial sheath. Therefore, the rate of passage of a drug into the brain is generally determined by two factors: the size of the drug molecule and its lipid solubility. Large drugs penetrate poorly, while small, fat-soluble drugs penetrate rapidly. Most psychoactive drugs are both small enough and sufficiently lipid soluble to cross the blood-brain barrier. Drugs that cannot cross the blood-brain barrier are restricted to structures outside the central nervous system. Penicillin, for example, does not cross the blood-brain barrier, so its use as an antibiotic is restricted to infections located outside the brain. In addition, some lipid-soluble drugs, such as steroids, antitumor drugs, and beta blockers, are unable to pass through capillary walls and reach the brain because their transport

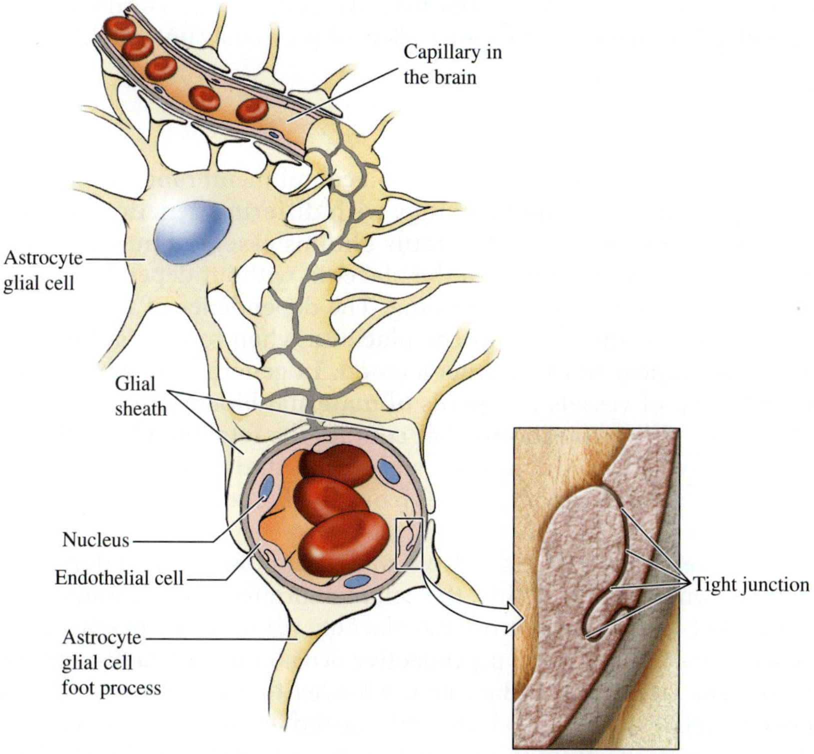

FIGURE 1.7 The Blood-Brain Barrier. The enlarged view of the brain capillary at bottom left shows that the blood inside the capillary and the surrounding brain tissue are separated in three main ways that, taken together, constitute the blood-brain barrier. First, the capillary is covered by the glial sheath, a fatty layer made up of extensions (foot processes) from nearby astrocyte glial cells. Second, the cells of the capillary are packed tightly together, as shown in the enlarged electron micrograph at bottom right. Third, there are no pores like the fenestrae and intracellular clefts shown in Figure 1.6. Thus, in order to diffuse from blood to brain, drug molecules must move through the capillary wall and then must move through the fatty glial sheath.

is blocked by glycoproteins that protect the brain (as well as a number of other sensitive tissues) from toxins (Finch and Pillians, 2014).

Large molecules such as glucose, insulin, amino acids, and vitamins can enter the brain because they are carried out of the capillaries by special transport systems in a process called *transcytosis*. In this process, the molecules attach to a receptor in the cell wall membrane, and a small segment of this membrane forms a vesicle containing the molecule and its receptor. The vesicle then crosses over to and fuses with the membrane on the opposite side of the capillary wall, after which the receptor releases the substance into the brain (Pulgar, 2019).

All this makes it clear that both passive and active mechanisms prevent molecules from entering the brain or assist them in doing so. Obviously, these mechanisms provide potential targets for drug therapies that may overcome the constraints of the blood-brain barrier and deliver medications for a variety of previously untreatable brain disorders.

Placental Barrier

Among all the membrane systems of the body, the placental membranes are unique because they separate two distinct human beings with differing genetic compositions and differing sensitivities to drugs. The fetus obtains essential nutrients and eliminates metabolic waste products through the placenta without depending on its own organs, many of which are not yet functioning. The dependence of the fetus on the mother places the fetus at the mercy of the placenta when foreign substances (such as drugs or toxins) appear in the mother's blood. In general, the mature placenta consists of a network of vessels and pools of maternal blood into which protrude treelike or fingerlike villi (projections) that contain the fetal blood capillaries. Oxygen and nutrients travel from the mother's blood to that of the fetus, while carbon dioxide and other waste products travel from the blood of the fetus to the mother's blood.

The membranes that separate fetal blood from maternal blood in the intervillous space resemble, in their general permeability, the cell membranes that are found elsewhere in the body. In other words, drugs cross the placenta primarily by passive diffusion. Fat-soluble substances (including all psychoactive drugs) diffuse readily, rapidly, and without limitation. The view that the placenta is a barrier to drugs is inaccurate. As a general rule, all psychoactive drugs (and all those discussed in this book) will be present in the fetus at concentrations quite similar to the concentrations in the mother's bloodstream. Many psychoactive medicines pose relatively little risk to fetal growth and development; however, some drugs certainly are detrimental (e.g., ethyl alcohol), and women who are or might become pregnant should avoid using them. Throughout this text, we will discuss the effects of specific psychoactive drugs on the fetus.

TERMINATION OF DRUG ACTION

Drugs can exit the body via the kidneys, lungs, bile, and skin. Excretion through the lungs is unusual, occurring only with highly volatile or gaseous agents, such as the general anesthetics and, in small amounts, alcohol (as "alcohol breath"). Similarly, few drugs exit the body through the bile or the skin (small amounts can be excreted in sweat, perhaps 10–15% of the total amount of a drug). As a general principal, *most drugs leave the body in urine, either as the unchanged molecule or as a broken-down metabolite of the original drug.*[2]

[2]Another, more correct, way of stating this principle is as follows: *The major route of drug elimination from the body is renal (urinary) excretion of drug metabolites produced by the metabolic biodegradation of the drug in the liver.* Regarding the evaluation of urine for the presence of drugs of abuse: given that the inactive drug metabolites are in the urine, rather than the active drug, it is often unclear whether the presence of the metabolite in urine means that there was active drug in plasma at the time the urine sample was taken.

Biotransformation (Drug Metabolism)

Biotransformation refers to the processes whereby active drug molecules are metabolized to molecules that are more readily eliminated from the body. It consists of two phases:

1. Initial reactions involving cytochrome P450 enzymes to break apart the drug molecules.
2. Conjugation reactions primarily involving glucuronidation, where a large sugar molecule is bound to the drug to make it larger, bulkier, less able to pass back into the brain, and, once filtered by the kidneys, less able to be reabsorbed and thus excreted in urine.

Psychoactive drugs are usually too lipid soluble to be excreted passively with the excretion of urine. They have to be transformed (generally, by enzymes located in the liver) into metabolites that are more water soluble, bulkier, less lipid soluble, and (usually) less biologically active (even inactive) when compared with the parent molecule (the molecule that was originally ingested and absorbed).[3] For example, THC (the active drug in marijuana) is metabolized by liver enzymes to carboxy-THC, which is totally inactive and slowly excreted in urine. Indeed, this metabolite may be detected in urine for days or even weeks following cessation of smoking. Thus, the presence of carboxy-THC in urine only indicates that marijuana was smoked, but does not indicate when the drug was used or whether the person was intoxicated at the time the urine sample was taken. This issue can be critically important in legal situations—for example, when a charge of driving under the influence might be incorrectly based on the presence of carboxy-THC in a urine sample.

The Cytochrome P450 System

The enzymes required for drug metabolism are in liver cells called *hepatocytes*, on smooth endoplasmic reticulum membranes within the hepatocytes. There are several categories of these enzymes, which are collectively referred to as the **cytochrome P450 enzyme family** (or simply *P450 enzymes* or *CYP enzymes*). The main function of P450 enzymes is to turn lipophilic fat-soluble drugs into more water-soluble compounds. This process involves changing the drug molecule into a polar compound, a molecule that is positively charged on one end and negatively charged on the other. Polar molecules are attracted to water because water is also a

[3]As a general rule, most metabolites excreted in urine are either inactive or much less active than the parent drug. However, some parent drugs are exceptions, being metabolized into an "active" metabolite that is at least as active as the parent drug and may even be more active and may have a longer duration of action. Two examples in psychopharmacology are diazepam (Valium, discussed in Chapter 13), which is metabolized to nordiazepam, and fluoxetine (Prozac, discussed in Chapter 12), which is metabolized to norfluoxetine. In both cases, the parent drug has an effect that lasts for two or three days, while the metabolite is active for over a week until it is eventually biotransformed to an inactive compound that can be excreted.

polar substance. Our kidneys are designed to excrete polar compounds and to reabsorb, and thus conserve, lipophilic compounds. Remember that most psychoactive drugs are lipid soluble and therefore, unless metabolized, are readily reabsorbed from the kidney to return to the bloodstream. Unless metabolized, such drugs may persist indefinitely in the body.

In the first phase of biotransformation of psychoactive drugs, three primary chemical reactions are catalyzed by P450 enzymes: oxidation, reduction, and hydrolysis. Oxidation means removing electrons, which have a negative charge, thereby creating a polar compound with a net positive charge. Most psychotropic medications are metabolized through this mechanism. A few drugs are biotransformed by reduction (adding electrons by adding a hydrogen atom, thereby creating a polar compound with a net negative charge), and still others are biotransformed by hydrolysis (adding H_2O—i.e., water—which causes the drug molecule to split up into two polar water-soluble molecules).

The cytochrome P450 enzyme family is the major system involved in drug metabolism. The genes that encode this family originated more than 3.5 billion years ago and have since evolved to enable the metabolism (detoxification) of a chemically diverse group of environmental chemicals, food toxins, and drugs. About 50 different types of CYP enzymes are functionally active in humans, and members of several P450 enzyme groups can be found within any given hepatocyte.

The enzymes involved in most drug biotransformations are members of just a few of these P450 enzyme groups, particularly those designated *CYP-1*, *CYP-2*, and *CYP-3*. The enzymes in these three groups each promote the breakdown of numerous drugs and toxins—that is, enzyme specificity is low. In particular, as shown in Figure 1.8, the enzymes in the CYP-3 subgroup CYP-3A4/5 catalyze about 50% of drug biotransformations, and those in the CYP-2 subgroups CYP-2D6 and CYP-2C each catalyze about 20% of drugs. Other CYP enzyme variants are responsible for metabolizing the remaining 10% of drugs.

Conjugation Reactions

As described at the beginning of this section, the second phase of drug biotransformation consists of conjugation reactions, which involve combining a drug with another molecule. The most common conjugation reaction is glucuronidation, in which glucuronic acid ($C_6H_{10}O_7$) is bound to the drug. Glucuronidation is common partly because glucuronic acid is made from glucose, which is plentiful in the body. Many psychotropic drugs are metabolized mainly by glucuronidation, including benzodiazepines, such as lorazepam and temazepam (Restoril), and drugs used to treat bipolar disorder (see Chapter 14), such as lamotrigine (Lamictal) and valproate (Depakote). This can result in drug interactions:

> Since both Lamictal and Depakote are metabolized by glucuronidation, there's a drug interaction between them. As it turns out, Depakote latches onto the glucuronidation enzyme more strongly than Lamictal, shoving Lamictal aside, preventing it from being metabolized, and thereby increasing its levels to about double what they are otherwise. (Carlat, 2015, p. 51)

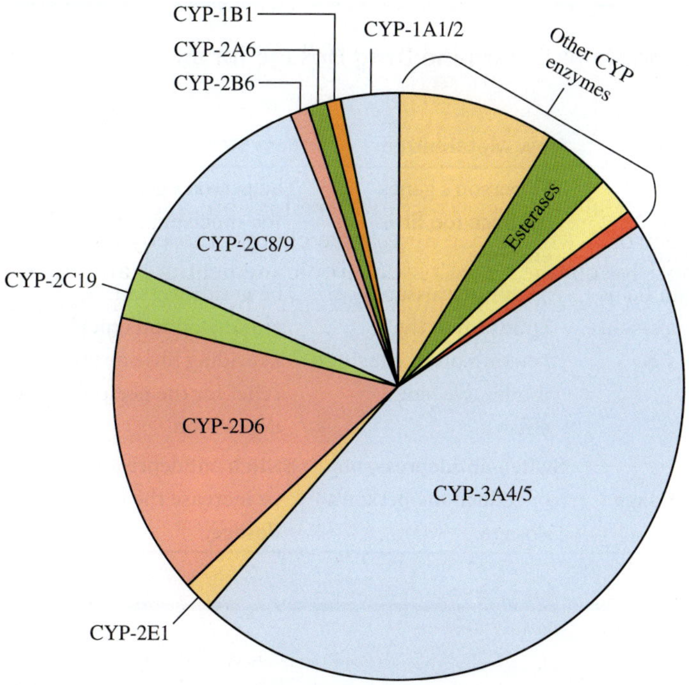

FIGURE 1.8 Drug Metabolism by the Major Hepatic CYP Enzymes. The pie sections indicate the estimated contribution of each CYP enzyme group to the metabolism of drugs. "Other CYP enzymes" includes enzymes such as acetylcholine esterase and alcohol dehydrogenase that are discussed later in this book.

Factors Affecting Drug Biotransformation

Several different factors can alter the rate at which drugs are metabolized, either increasing or decreasing the rate of drug elimination from the body. Such factors can profoundly alter the amount of drug in the bloodstream and therefore greatly affect the body's response to a given dose of drug.

First, it is now becoming apparent that genetic variations may affect how different people respond to medications. DNA testing using a simple mouth swab can indicate whether a person is a normal, slow, or fast metabolizer of specific drugs, including drugs of different therapeutic classes, such as antidepressants, analgesics, and antipsychotics (the Mayo Clinic, for example, offers a pharmacogenomics program for such testing). Results provide a scientific basis for understanding why a person might have an unexpectedly toxic reaction after the usual therapeutic doses of a drug or, in contrast, why the person might fail to respond to the usual dose. Table 1.2 indicates how genetic differences between normal, slow, and fast metabolizers might affect patients and their treatment options.

Second, if more than one drug is present in the body, the drugs may interact with one another, either increasing or decreasing the blood levels of either medication. For

TABLE 1.2 How Genetic Testing Helps Determine Drug Dosage for an Antidepressant

	Normal Metabolizer	Slow Metabolizer	Fast Metabolizer
Genetic variation	The person's genes produce a typical amount of enzyme.	The person's genes produce too little enzyme.	The person's genes produce too much enzyme.
Effects on the person	The antidepressant helps the person's depression and causes few side effects.	The antidepressant builds up in the person's body, causing intolerable side effects.	The antidepressant is eliminated too quickly, providing little or no relief for the person's depression.
Treatment options	Follow the recommended dosage.	Switch antidepressants or reduce the person's dosage.	Switch antidepressants or increase the person's dosage.

example, carbamazepine (Tegretol) (discussed in Chapter 14) is particularly effective in stimulating the production of the drug-metabolizing enzymes in the CYP-3 group in the liver (a process called **enzyme induction**). Thus, in the presence of carbamazepine, the rate at which all drugs are metabolized by CYP-3 enzymes increases, which means that the blood level of a drug taken along with carbamazepine will fall more rapidly than would be otherwise expected (this is an example of metabolic tolerance, discussed more fully later in this chapter). In essence, the second drug becomes less effective because it is metabolized more rapidly as a result of the increased amount of metabolic enzyme.

In contrast to carbamazepine (which increases the amount of drug-metabolizing enzymes in the liver), some psychoactive drugs *depress* the activity or *decrease* the amount of CYP enzymes. This process *increases* the blood level of other drugs that might be present and thus unexpectedly increases their toxicity. For example, antidepressants that are selective serotonin reuptake inhibitors (SSRIs), such as fluoxetine (discussed in Chapter 12), inhibit several metabolic enzymes, increasing the toxicity of several other drugs that are metabolized by the same enzyme system. As an interesting aside, the pain-relieving drug codeine (discussed in Chapter 10) is metabolized by enzymes in the CYP-2D6 group into morphine, which is codeine's active metabolite responsible for its analgesic effect. Some SSRIs (e.g., fluoxetine and paroxetine) block this metabolic conversion of codeine to morphine, so for patients taking SSRIs, codeine is ineffective as a pain-relieving agent.

As shown in Table 1.3 (Andrade, 2012), not all psychoactive medications are metabolized by CYP enzymes, and such drugs can be useful in patients who have liver disease, patients who are rapid metabolizers, or patients who have induced enzymes (such as heavy cigarette smokers).

TABLE 1.3 Some Psychoactive Drugs That Are Not Metabolized or Are Minimally Metabolized by CYP Enzymes in the Liver

Category	Drugs
Anxiolytics	Pregabalin Lorazepam
Antidepressants	Milnacipran Desvenlafaxine Low doses of amisulpride, sulpiride, and levosulpiride
Antipsychotics	Paliperidone High doses of amisulpride, sulpiride, and levosulpiride
Anticonvulsants and mood stabilizers	Gabapentin Levetiracetam Lithium Lamotrigine
Dementia treatment	Memantine

SOURCE: C. Andrade, "Drugs That Escape Hepatic Metabolism," *Journal of Clinical Psychiatry* 73 (2012): e889–e890.

The vast increase in the number of new psychotropic and other drugs during the last two decades has increased the number of combinations that patients take and thus increased the likelihood of drug-drug interactions. In addition to combinations involving just prescription drugs, combinations of prescription drugs with herbs and dietary supplements can also increase the risk of adverse reactions. It has been estimated that more than 50% of patients with chronic disorders use herbal supplements and that nearly 20% of those patients take these products together with prescription medications (Tsai et al., 2012).

Role of the Kidneys and Liver in Drug Elimination

Our two kidneys perform two major physiological functions. First, they excrete most of the metabolites formed in the liver; second, they closely regulate the levels of most of the substances found in body fluids. The kidneys are a pair of bean-shaped organs that lie at the rear of the abdominal cavity at the level of the lower ribs. The outer portion of the kidney is made up of more than a million functional units called *nephrons.* As shown in Figure 1.9, each nephron has a knot of capillaries (the glomerulus), through which blood flows from the renal artery to the renal vein. Fluid (essentially, blood plasma) filters out of these capillaries due to the pressure of the blood in the glomerulus, and this fluid then flows into Bowman's capsule, which surrounds the glomerulus. From Bowman's capsule, the fluid flows through the proximal tubule, through the

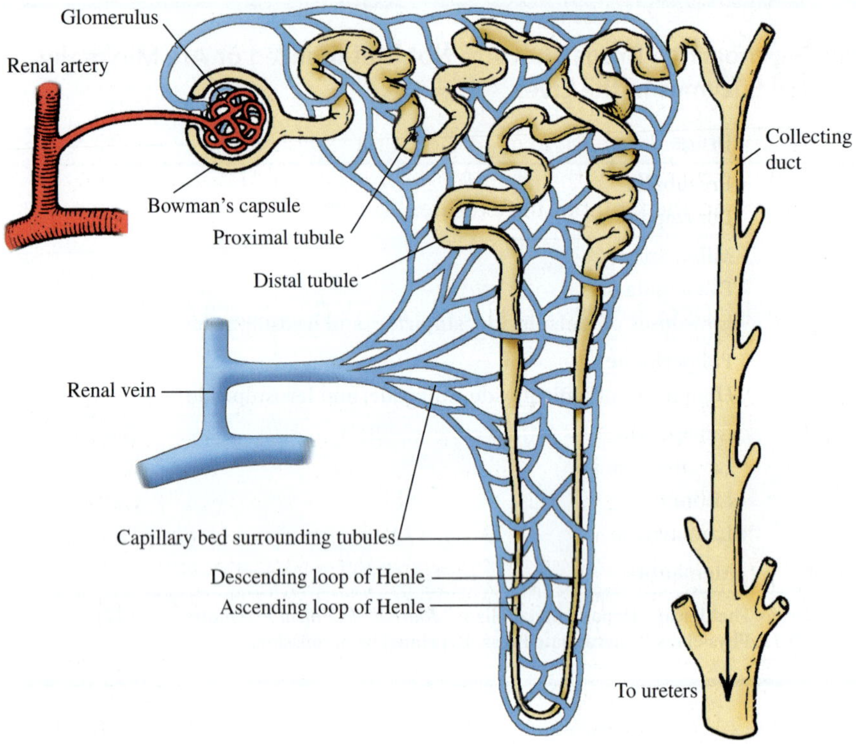

FIGURE 1.9 A Nephron. Note the complexity of the structure and the intimate relation between the blood supply and the nephron. Each kidney is composed of more than a million nephrons.

descending and ascending portions of the loop of Henle into the distal tubule, and then into a duct that collects fluid from several nephrons. The fluid from the collecting duct is eventually passed through the ureters and into the urinary bladder, which is emptied periodically.

In an adult, about 1 liter (1000 cubic centimeters) of plasma is filtered through the nephrons of the kidneys each minute. Left behind in the bloodstream are blood cells, plasma proteins, and the remaining plasma. As the filtered fluid (largely water) flows through the nephrons, most of it is reabsorbed by the surrounding capillaries into the plasma. By the time fluid (now urine) reaches the collecting ducts and bladder, only 0.1%, or 1 cubic centimeter of the original volume of 1000 cubic centimeters, remains to be excreted, which means that 99.9% of filtered fluid is reabsorbed.

Lipid-soluble drugs, which easily cross the membranes of renal tubular cells, are reabsorbed along with the 99.9% of reabsorbed water. Drug reabsorption occurs passively, along a developing concentration gradient—the drug becomes concentrated inside the nephrons (as a result of water reabsorption), and the drugs are themselves reabsorbed with water back into plasma. Thus, the kidneys alone are not capable of eliminating most psychoactive drugs from the body; some other mechanism must overcome this process of passive renal reabsorption of drugs. This mechanism involves the liver. The reabsorbed (still pharmacologically active) drug molecules circulate in the blood and are picked up by liver cells and enzymatically biotransformed (as discussed above) into metabolites that are less lipid soluble and thus less capable of being reabsorbed, and that will therefore be excreted in urine. Indeed, a drug will repeatedly circulate in blood through both the liver and the kidneys until it is eventually fully metabolized in the liver and the metabolites excreted in urine.

TIME COURSE OF DRUG DISTRIBUTION AND ELIMINATION: THE CONCEPT OF DRUG HALF-LIFE

Knowledge about the relationship between the time course of drug action in the body and its pharmacological effects is essential for (1) predicting the optimal dosages and dose intervals needed to reach a therapeutic effect; (2) maintaining a therapeutic drug level for the desired period of time; and (3) determining the time needed to eliminate the drug. The relationship between the pharmacological response to a drug and its concentration in blood is fundamental to pharmacology. With psychoactive drugs, the level of drug in the blood closely approximates the level of drug at the drug's site of action in the brain.

Figure 1.10 illustrates the concept of a drug's **half-life**, the time it takes for the concentration of the drug in blood to fall by half—that is, the time needed for half of the amount of the drug in the blood to be eliminated. The figure shows the time-concentration relationship for a drug that is injected intravenously and therefore reaches peak plasma concentration immediately (using intravenous injection for this example avoids the variability involved with oral absorption and the slow attainment of peak blood levels). Note that the plasma concentration falls very rapidly after the immediate peak, followed by a slower decline. The rapid fall reflects the rapid **redistribution** of the drug out of the bloodstream into body tissues (more generally, redistribution can be defined as the movement of a drug from more perfused organs to less perfused organs).[4] This process of redistribution (also illustrated in Figure 1.10) takes only minutes to spread a drug nearly equally throughout the major tissues of the body. The shallower part of the curve after redistribution represents a slower, prolonged decrease in the level of drug in the blood as the body eliminates the drug by hepatic metabolism. The half-life, which is a measure of this process of elimination, allows the time course of drug action to be determined.

---

[4]Organs such as the heart, liver, kidneys, and brain receive most of the drug and become highly perfused during the first few minutes after absorption (these organs may be referred to as the *central compartment*). Other tissues, such as skeletal muscle and adipose (fat) tissue (which may be referred to as the *peripheral compartment*), are less perfused and equilibrate with drugs less rapidly. Compartmental drug redistribution can alter the duration of effect at the target tissue. Consider, for example, the barbiturate thiopental, which produces anesthesia within seconds because of its high lipid solubility and rapid blood-brain equilibration. However, the duration of anesthesia is brief (even though the metabolism of thiopental is slow) because the drug is redistributed from the brain and stored in adipose tissue, which acts as a reservoir. The same principle applies to the redistribution of THC following the smoking of marijuana.

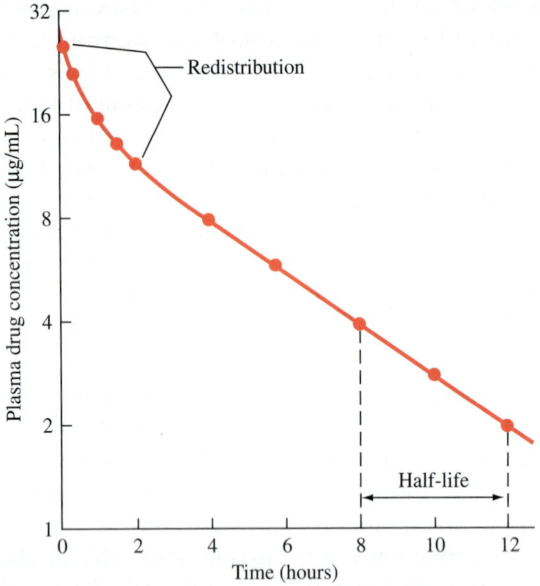

FIGURE 1.10 Redistribution and Half-Life of a Drug. After intravenous injection, the plasma concentration of the drug rises rapidly to about 31 micrograms/milliliter (μg/mL). The concentration is measured every 30 minutes for the first 2 hours and every 2 hours thereafter until 12 hours after injection. Redistribution occurs over the first 2 hours, as the drug leaves plasma, enters body tissues, and equilibrates with those tissues. After redistribution, the fall in plasma concentration is linear, decreasing by half every 4 hours. Thus, the half-life of the drug is 4 hours.

DR. J'S MUSINGS 1.3

Does Ethyl Alcohol Have a Half-Life?

The principles of ADME are important for understanding drug travel into and out of the body (see Dr. J's Musings 1.2), but ultimately for drug administration, the half-life of a drug is perhaps most important. Intuitively, however, the concept of half-life can be difficult to understand: Why is more drug metabolized per unit time when drug levels are high and relatively little when levels are low? Shouldn't the rate be constant until the drug is gone? As we will see, it doesn't work that way except with one drug, ethyl alcohol (discussed in Chapter 5). Alcohol is eliminated at a constant rate regardless of its concentration in blood (this rate of elimination of ethyl alcohol is 0.015 grams of alcohol per 100 cubic centimeters of blood per hour). Thus, the concept of half-life is irrelevant to alcohol metabolism.

The half-life of a drug remains constant over time. In Figure 1.10, for example, it takes the same amount of time for the blood level to fall from 8 to 4 micrograms per milliliter as it does to fall from 4 to 2 micrograms per milliliter or from 2 to 1 micrograms per milliliter. Clearly, this constant time interval means that a different absolute amount of drug is metabolized within each half-life.

Knowledge of a drug's half-life is vitally important because it tells us how long a drug remains in the body. As shown in Table 1.4, it takes four half-lives for 94% of a drug to be eliminated by the body and six half-lives for 98% of the drug to be eliminated, at which point a person is, for most practical purposes, drug-free. It is important to remember that even though the blood level of a drug is reduced by 75% after two half-lives, the drug persists in the body at low levels for at least six half-lives, resulting in a so-called drug hangover.

Throughout this book, drug half-lives are cited to describe the duration of action of psychoactive drugs in the body and allow comparisons between drugs with similar actions but differing half-lives. Most drug half-lives are measured in hours; others are measured in days, with recovery from the drug possibly taking a week or more. For example, the half-life of diazepam (discussed in Chapter 13) is about 30 hours in a healthy young adult, and the half-life of its active metabolite, nordiazepam, is even longer, on the order of several days to a week. In older adults, the half-lives of both diazepam and nordiazepam are even more prolonged: the duration of action can be four weeks or longer.

Given that a drug's half-life is independent of the absolute level of the drug in blood, the metabolism rate of the drug is a constant fraction of the drug remaining in the body, rather than a constant amount of drug per hour. Therefore, a varying amount of the drug is metabolized with each half-life (fewer actual molecules are metabolized per half-life as the plasma level of the drug falls).

TABLE 1.4 Half-Life Calculations

	Amount of Drug in the Body	
Number of Half-Lives	**% Eliminated**	**% Remaining**
0	0	100
1	50	50
2	75	25
3	87.5	12.5
4	93.8	6.2
5	96.9	3.1
6	98.4	1.6

DRUG ACCUMULATION AND STEADY-STATE CONCENTRATION

If only a single dose of a drug is administered, its concentration in blood reaches a peak and then falls according to its half-life, as shown in Figure 1.10. However, if a second dose of the drug is administered before the body has eliminated the first dose, the total amount of drug in the body and the peak level of the drug in the blood will be greater than the total amount and peak level produced by the first dose, because the second dose is added on to whatever remains of the first dose. If doses continue to be administered at regular intervals, the drug will accumulate in the body until its concentration in blood reaches a plateau, or **steady-state concentration**. This concentration (where the amount administered per unit time equals the amount eliminated per unit time) will be reached after about five to six half-lives, as shown in Figure 1.11.

Note that the time needed to reach the steady-state concentration (about five to six half-lives) is independent of the actual dosage of the drug. Consider, for example, what happens if a dose is given after each half-life:

- At one half-life after the first dose, the amount of drug in the body will be 50% of the dose, at which point the second dose is given.
- After two half-lives, the amount of drug in the body will be 75% of the dose (25% of the first dose + 50% of the second dose), at which point the third dose is given.

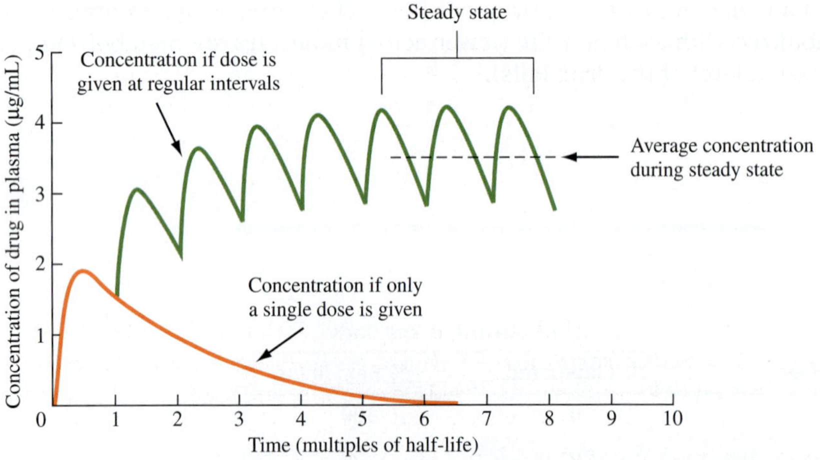

FIGURE 1.11 Steady-State Concentration. If only a single dose of a drug is given, the concentration peaks rapidly and then falls according to the drug's half-life (as shown in Figure 1.10 and by the smoothly declining bottom curve here). In contrast, the wavy top curve shows that if a dosage of the drug is given at regular intervals (here, at intervals equal to the half-life), the concentration rises after each dose, then falls as the drug is metabolized, and then, after the next dose, rises to a higher level, until a steady-state concentration is reached after five to six half-lives. The peaks and valleys in this curve show the maximal and minimal drug concentrations at the beginning and end of each dosage interval, respectively.

- After three half-lives, the amount of drug in the body will be 87.5% of the dose (12.5% of the first dose + 25% of the second dose + 50% of the third dose), at which point the fourth dose is given.
- Continuing in this way, after six half-lives, the amount of drug in the body will be about 98.4% of the dose and will essentially remain at this level thereafter—that is, the drug will have reached a steady-state concentration, regardless of the actual dosage. (But note that the dosage, along with the dosage interval and the drug's half-life, *does* determine the ultimate concentration level at steady state.)

In summary, steady dosing at regular-intervals leads to a predictable accumulation with a steady-state concentration reached after about six half-lives, a concentration that is proportional to the dose and the dosage interval. Clinically, these factors guide drug therapy when blood levels of the drug are monitored and correlated with therapeutic results.

DR. J'S MUSINGS 1.4

Can Half-Life Help Determine Dosage?

It is obvious that a drug does not accumulate in the body until more is taken per unit time than is metabolized during that same time. But now consider that the same point can be stated in terms of the drug's half-life—that is, levels increase until more is metabolized per half-life than is ingested per half-life. However, this steady-state concentration may be below, at, or above the required therapeutic level of the drug. The drug half-life can often guide the dosage necessary to achieve a therapeutic blood level.

THERAPEUTIC DRUG MONITORING

Therapeutic drug monitoring (TDM)—the process of correlating the plasma level of a drug with the therapeutic response—can aid a clinician in making critical decisions in therapeutic applications. The basic principle underlying TDM is that a threshold plasma concentration of a drug is needed at the receptor site to initiate and maintain a pharmacological response. Critically important is that plasma concentrations of psychoactive drugs correlate well with tissue or receptor concentrations. Therefore, TDM is an indirect, although usually quite accurate, measurement of drug concentration at the receptor site. To make the correlation between TDM, dosage, and therapeutic response, large-scale clinical trials are performed, with blood samples being drawn at several time periods during both acute (short-term) and chronic (long-term) therapy. Statistical correlation is made between the level of drug in plasma and the degree of therapeutic response. A dosage regimen can then be designed to achieve the appropriate steady-state blood level of a drug. A well-defined range of blood levels associated with optimal clinical response is called the **therapeutic window**. The important point is that levels either below *or above* that range are associated with a poor response.

One goal of TDM is to assess whether a patient is taking medication as prescribed: if the patient has not been taking the required medication, the plasma levels of the drug will be below the therapeutic level and the therapeutic results will be poor. Another goal is to avoid toxicity: if plasma levels of the drug are above the therapeutic level, the dosage can be lowered, effectiveness maintained, and toxicity minimized. A third goal is to enhance the therapeutic response by focusing not on the amount of drug taken, but on the measured amount of drug in the plasma. Other goals include possible reductions in the cost of therapy (if the patient's illness is better controlled) and substantiation of the need for unusually high doses (some patients require a higher-than-normal intake of prescribed medication to maintain a therapeutic blood level of a drug).

In addition, TDM can be involved when assessing drug concentrations in legal matters. For example, in determining whether a person was driving under the influence of a drug, blood is drawn and drug concentrations are measured in the blood sample, which are then correlated with published values based on TDM for therapeutic and impairing (toxic) concentrations (Schulz et al., 2012).

DRUG TOLERANCE AND DRUG DEPENDENCE

Drug tolerance is a progressively decreasing responsiveness to a drug, meaning that progressively increasing doses of the drug are needed to produce the same effect. Drug tolerance that develops as a result of pharmacological mechanisms includes metabolic tolerance and cellular-adaptive tolerance. Tolerance can also develop as a result of behavioral conditioning processes.

In metabolic tolerance, an increased amount of enzyme becomes available to metabolize a drug as a result of enzyme induction (discussed above). In cellular-adaptive tolerance (also called *pharmacodynamic tolerance*), neurons adapt to the accumulation of a drug either by reducing the number of receptors available to the drug or by reducing the receptors' sensitivity to the drug (receptors are discussed in detail in Chapter 3). Such reduction in numbers or sensitivity is termed *down regulation*. Both the increase in drug metabolism due to enzyme induction and the receptor effects of down regulation mean that more drug must be administered to maintain the same concentration in the body and achieve the same therapeutic response.

Neither enzyme induction nor receptor down regulation can account for the substantial degree of apparent tolerance that many people acquire to opioids, ethyl alcohol, and other drugs. Rather, this type of tolerance is the result of behavioral conditioning processes. For example, a novice drinker might be terribly impaired at a blood alcohol concentration level of twice the legal limit for driving, whereas a chronic drinker might appear to be much less intoxicated at the same level. In such cases, diagnosis of impairment in the chronic drinker may necessitate additional testing.

Tolerance can also take the form of **cross-tolerance**, in which tolerance of one drug results in tolerance of one or more other drugs. An example of this was discussed above in the section on factors affecting drug biotransformation, where we saw that enzyme induction due to the administration of carbamazepine results in tolerance of carbamazepine and all other drugs metabolized by CYP-3 enzymes.

Drug dependence—a state in which the use of a drug is necessary for either physical or psychological well-being—is an entirely different phenomenon from drug tolerance, even though the two are often seen together. In **physical dependence**, the drug is needed for normal physical functioning, including to avoid physical withdrawal (symptoms that occur if the drug is not taken). In **psychological dependence**, there is a compulsion to use the drug for its pleasurable effects. Dependence is revealed by withdrawing the drug (either completely or by a rapid decrease in dosage) and noting the occurrence of physical and/or psychological withdrawal symptoms that are collectively referred to as a **withdrawal syndrome** (also termed an *abstinence syndrome*). Readministering the drug can relieve the withdrawal symptoms.

Because physical dependence is often revealed after abstinence from drugs of abuse such as alcohol and heroin, the term *dependence* has been linked with *addiction*, implying that withdrawal symptoms are "bad" and observed only with drugs of abuse (see Chapter 4 for further discussion of addiction). This conclusion is incorrect; withdrawal symptoms can also follow cessation of therapeutic drugs, such as the SSRI type of clinical antidepressants (see the discussion of SSRI discontinuation syndrome in Chapter 12). Regardless of whether a drug is considered "good" (a therapeutic drug) or "bad" (a drug of abuse), withdrawal symptoms may occur after the drug is discontinued if the person has become dependent on the drug. Dependence and withdrawal symptoms indicate that brain and body functions were altered by the presence of the drug and that the brain and the body need time (typically, from a few days to about two weeks) to adapt and find a new state of equilibrium without the drug.

DR. J'S MUSINGS 1.5

What Does "Addiction" Mean?

In my early days of training, *addiction* was defined as the combination of tolerance and dependence, and the term was applied mainly to drugs of abuse. Today, we recognize that many therapeutic drugs, even when used properly, can result in tolerance and dependence, although these drugs are not generally considered addicting. This has led to a more specific definition of addiction: tolerance and dependence *plus* drug-seeking behaviors that interfere with a normal healthy life.

CHAPTER REVIEW

1. Define *pharmacokinetics*.
2. Summarize the advantages and disadvantages of the various methods of administering drugs.

3. Compare the roles of these body membranes in drug distribution: cell membranes, capillaries, blood-brain barrier, and placental barrier.
4. Why must a psychoactive drug be altered metabolically in the body before it can be excreted?
5. Describe the roles of the hepatic enzyme system, kidneys, and liver in drug metabolism.
6. What is the half-life of a drug? How is half-life involved in reaching a steady-state concentration of a drug in plasma? If a drug has a half-life of 6 hours, how long does it take for the drug to be essentially eliminated from the body after administration of a single dose?
7. What is meant by the terms *therapeutic drug monitoring* and *therapeutic window*? How are these concepts used in clinical and legal situations?
8. What is drug tolerance and why does it occur? What is drug dependence?
9. What was relatively easy for you to understand in this chapter and what was more difficult? Explain why.

KEY TERMS

bioavailability
blood-brain barrier
cross-tolerance
cytochrome p450 enzyme family
drug
drug absorption
drug administration
drug dependence
drug distribution
drug tolerance
enzyme induction
first-pass metabolism
generic name
half-life
intramuscular injection
intravenous injection
lipid solubility
pharmacodynamics
pharmacokinetics
pharmacology
physical dependence
prodrug
psychoactive drugs
psychological dependence
psychopharmacology
receptor
redistribution
side effects
steady-state concentration
subcutaneous injection
synaptic plasticity
therapeutic drug monitoring (TDM)
therapeutic window
transdermal patches
withdrawal syndrome

CHAPTER 2

Brain, Neurons, Synaptic Transmission, and Neurotransmitters

CHAPTER OUTLINE

The brain is the most complex part of the human body. This 3-pound organ is responsible for our intelligence, memory, sensations, perceptions, emotions, and nearly all our behaviors. All these functions of the brain are carried out via biochemical interactions that take place in and between neurons. The brain is also the site of action of psychoactive drugs (i.e., drugs that alter the normal biochemical interactions of neurons). Therefore, to understand the actions of psychoactive drugs, it is necessary to have some idea of how the brain is organized, what a neuron is, and how neurons interact.

CENTRAL NERVOUS SYSTEM AND PERIPHERAL NERVOUS SYSTEM

The human nervous system consists of two divisions, the **central nervous system (CNS)** and the **peripheral nervous system (PNS)**. The CNS includes the brain and the spinal cord; the PNS includes the nerves that originate in the spinal cord and that connect the spinal cord to the rest of the body. The drugs discussed in this book exert their primary actions within the CNS, while many of their side effects are expressed via the PNS—that is, at various organ systems, such as the digestive system and the cardiovascular system.

BRAIN AND SPINAL CORD

The **spinal cord**—the large group of nerves that run through the center of the spine and carry messages between the brain and the rest of the body—is essentially the body's "information highway," transmitting signals with information about the external and internal environment and signals telling muscles to move. Extending from the bottom of the brain to the lower part of the spine, the spinal cord is made up of neurons and nerve fiber tracts that

- Carry sensory information from the skin, muscles, joints, and internal body organs to the brain
- Modulate sensory input (including pain impulses)
- Organize and modulate signals to the muscles (to produce coordinated movement)
- Provide autonomic (involuntary) control of vital body functions

Divisions, Structures, and Functions of the Brain

The human brain consists of perhaps 90 billion individual neurons and about an equal number of supporting cells called *glial cells*. Figure 2.1A shows how the brain is organized into three major divisions—the **forebrain**, the **midbrain**, and the **hindbrain**—and five subdivisions. Figure 2.1B shows the locations of these divisions and subdivisions within the brain.

Brain Stem, Cerebellum, and Midbrain

The **brain stem**—the part of the brain attached to the top of the spinal cord—consists of the medulla, the pons, and the midbrain (see Figure 2.2). All nerve impulses in either direction between the spinal cord and the brain pass through these structures. Different portions of the brain stem regulate respiration, blood pressure, heart rate, gastrointestinal functioning, and the states of sleep and wakefulness. The brain stem is also involved in alerting, attentional, and arousal responses. Multiple psychoactive drugs affect the functioning of neurons within the brain stem, either as the drugs' primary actions or as side effects.

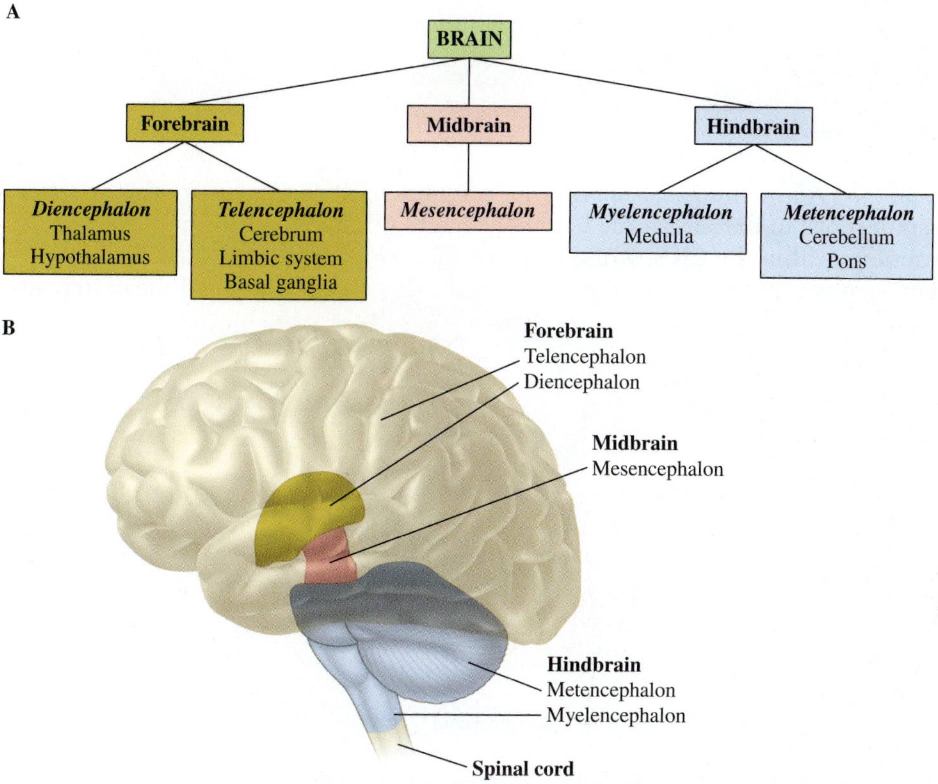

FIGURE 2.1 The Human Brain. **A.** The brain has three major divisions (forebrain, midbrain, and hindbrain) and five subdivisions (diencephalon, telencephalon, mesencephalon, myelencephalon, and metencephalon). The subdivisions of the forebrain and hindbrain contain a variety of important brain structures including those listed here. **B.** The hindbrain is the lower part of the brain attached to the spinal cord. The midbrain is the smallest division of the brain, lying between the hindbrain and the largest and uppermost division, the forebrain.

Figure 2.2 also shows the **cerebellum**, a large, bulbous structure located behind the brain stem. The cerebellum is necessary for the proper integration of movement and posture. The staggering gait that is associated with drunkenness, termed **ataxia** (loss of coordination and balance), is caused largely by an alcohol-induced depression of cerebellar function.

An important part of the brain stem, even though it is only about 2 centimeters long, is the midbrain. The upper half (the tectum, or "roof") contains nerve pathways that carry sensory information, while the bottom half (the tegmentum, or "floor") contains two important nuclei (the substantia nigra and the ventral tegmental area, both discussed below) connected to structures in the forebrain.

Hypothalamus and Thalamus

As shown in Figure 2.1, the diencephalon is the forebrain subdivision located immediately above the midbrain and below the cerebrum. It consists primarily of the

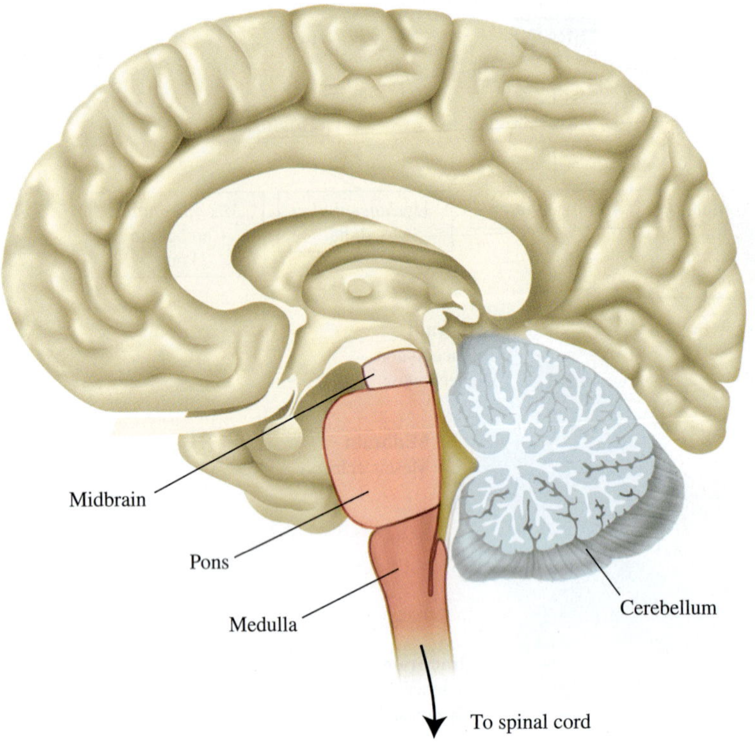

FIGURE 2.2 Brain Stem and Cerebellum. The brain stem connects the spinal cord to the forebrain. It consists of two hindbrain structures (medulla and pons) and the midbrain. The cerebellum, while also a hindbrain structure, is not part of the brain stem.

hypothalamus and the thalamus (see Figure 2.3). The **hypothalamus** is a collection of neuronal structures near the junction of the midbrain and the thalamus just above the pituitary gland (whose function it modulates). By regulating the hormonal output of the pituitary gland, the hypothalamus is involved in the integration of our autonomic nervous system, which controls such functions as eating and drinking, sleeping, regulation of body temperature, and sexual behavior. Like the brain stem, the hypothalamus is a site of action for many psychoactive drugs, either for the drugs' primary effects or for their side effects.

The **thalamus**, located above the hypothalamus, relays information between multiple subcortical areas and the cerebral cortex. Nerve fibers carrying information from most sensory systems pass through the thalamus, which sends the information to the appropriate cortical areas for processing and integration.

Basal Ganglia and Limbic System

The telencephalon, the largest major subdivision of the brain (see Figure 2.1), includes three important structures: the basal ganglia, the limbic system, and the cerebrum (which itself includes the cerebral cortex). As shown in Figure 2.4, the **basal ganglia**

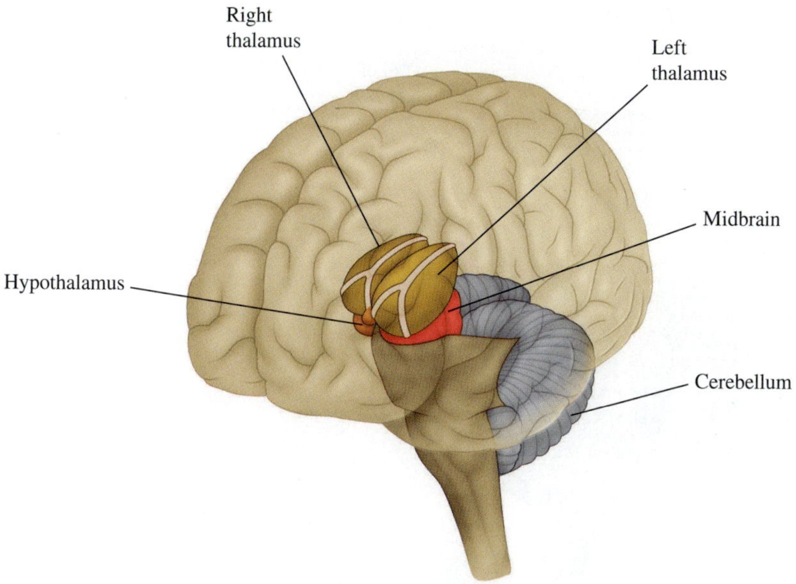

FIGURE 2.3 Thalamus and Hypothalamus. The thalamus is an important relay station for signals containing sensory information. The hypothalamus is involved in the regulation of body temperature, certain metabolic processes, and other autonomic activities.

include various structures located near the thalamus. One major function of the basal ganglia is the integration of movement. Disorders of the basal ganglia include Parkinson's disease and Huntington's disease.

The **limbic system** includes the **amygdala** (involved in emotion), the **hippocampus** (involved in memory), and the **cingulate cortex** (involved in integrating sensory, motor, visceral, motivational, and emotional information), as well as a number of other brain structures (see Figure 2.5A). The limbic system and the hypothalamus interact to regulate emotion and emotional expression, which means that these structures are the site of therapeutic action, as well as the site of side effects, of many psychoactive drugs (as discussed in subsequent chapters). In addition, the limbic system includes the **ventral tegmental area**, a midbrain structure that is an important component of the **reward circuit** of the brain, sending signals to other brain structures such as the amygdala, the medial forebrain bundle, the nucleus accumbens, the septum, and the prefrontal cortex (see Figure 2.5B). The reward circuit is believed to be responsible for the feelings of pleasure that we experience in response to activities that we enjoy, such as eating and drinking. Because such activities include the recreational use of abused drugs, the reward circuit is considered to be the substrate for drug addiction (see Chapter 4).

Cerebrum and Cerebral Cortex

The **cerebrum** is the largest part of the brain, almost completely covering the brain stem and the diencephalon. It is separated into two distinct hemispheres, left and right, with numerous fiber tracts connecting the two. The outer layer of the cerebrum,

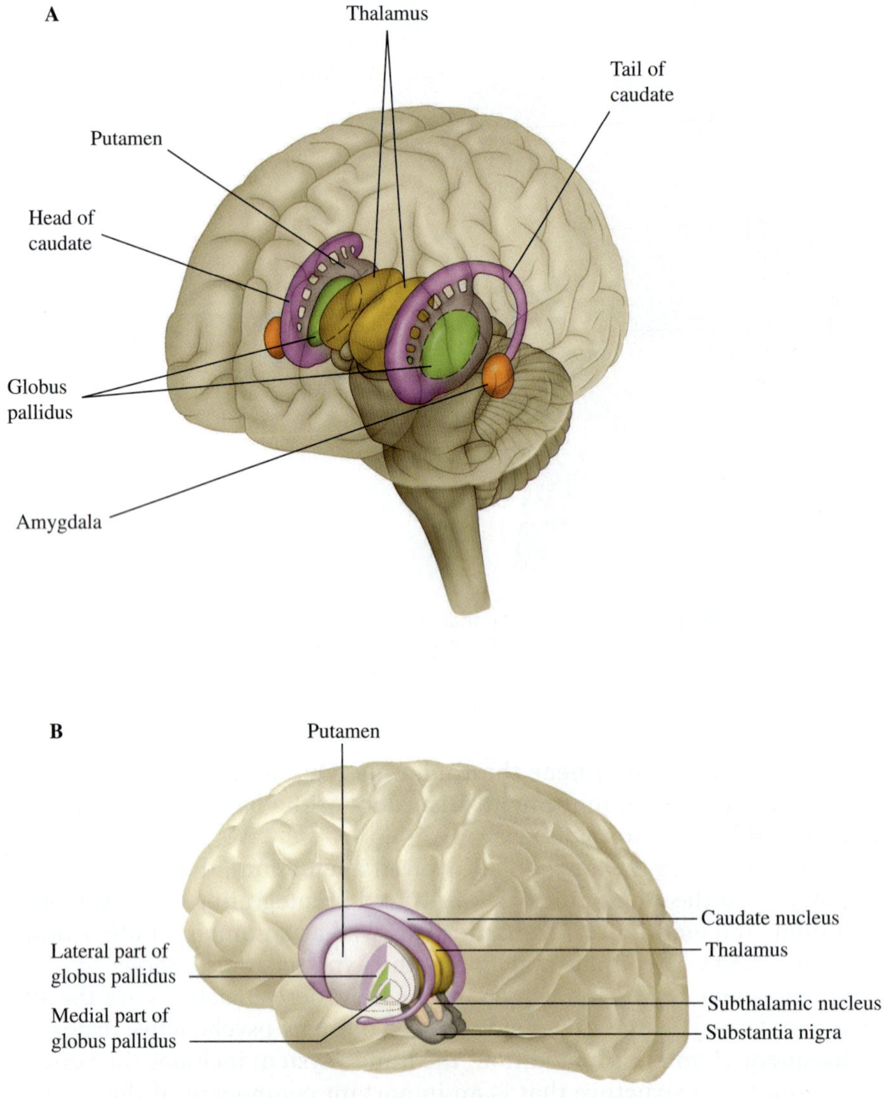

FIGURE 2.4 Basal Ganglia. **A.** The basal ganglia include the caudate nucleus, putamen, and globus pallidus. **B.** The subthalamic nucleus and the substantia nigra are two important structures associated with the basal ganglia.

the **cerebral cortex**, is deeply convoluted and fissured, giving it a much larger surface area than would otherwise fit within the skull. Like the rest of the cerebrum, the cerebral cortex is divided into left and right hemispheres, and the cortex in each hemisphere is divided into the four lobes shown in Figure 2.6. Each lobe includes areas that are responsible for specific functions, such as vision (occipital lobe), hearing (temporal lobe), somatosensory perception (parietal lobe), and higher-level cognitive functions (frontal lobe).

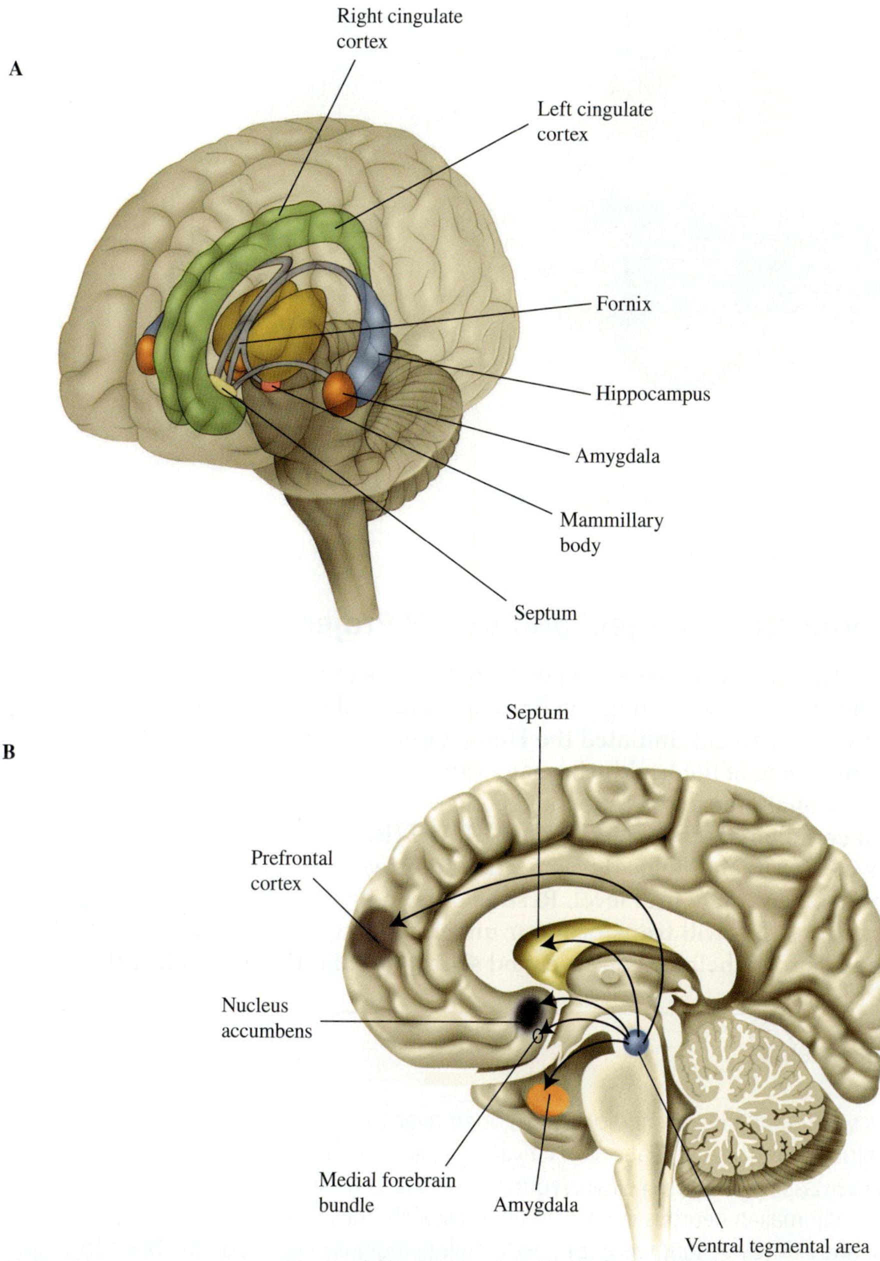

FIGURE 2.5 Limbic System and Reward Circuit. **A.** The major structures of the limbic system include the cingulate cortex, fornix, hippocampus, amygdala, mammillary body, and septum. **B.** The limbic system also includes the ventral tegmental area (VTA), which is part of the reward circuit of the brain. Signals from the VTA travel to other structures both within and outside the limbic system.

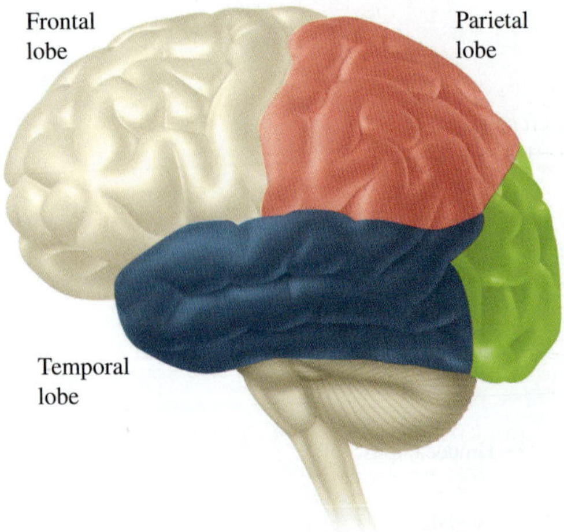

FIGURE 2.6 Cerebral Cortex. The cerebral cortex is the outer layer of the cerebrum. In each hemisphere, the cerebral cortex is divided into four lobes.

Human Connectome Project and BRAIN Project

A nagging problem in neuroscience is figuring out how neurons and nerve tracts connect with each other within and among the brain structures discussed above. In 2010, the National Institutes of Health initiated the Human Connectome Project[1] with the goal of building a connectome of the healthy human brain—that is, a "network map" that would shed light on the anatomical and functional connectivity within the (see Figure 2.7).

In 2013 a complementary project called BRAIN (Brain Research Through Advancing Innovative Neurotechnologies) was funded to provide insights into how we think, learn, and remember at a neural level. Results of both projects are expected to provide revolutionary ideas that will transform our understanding of how to treat brain disorders such as autism, Alzheimer's disease, and schizophrenia (Ramos et al., 2019).

Did You Know?

Optogenetics

Optogenetics, a remarkable technology developed over the past two decades, permits scientists to actually control—activate or inactivate—specific neurons to see what happens. In early experiments, the technology involved inserting the gene for an opsin (a light-sensitive protein) into mammalian neurons in vitro; in later research, these genes were inserted into living animals, and flashes of light were used to stimulate regions deep inside the brain through a fiber-optic wire. With this technique, researchers identified new pathways that control anxiety in mice, and they used the technique to turn depression on and off in rats and mice as well as to create false memories in laboratory animals (Berglund et al., 2021; Biselli et al., 2021; Muir et al., 2019).

[1]www.humanconnectomeproject.org

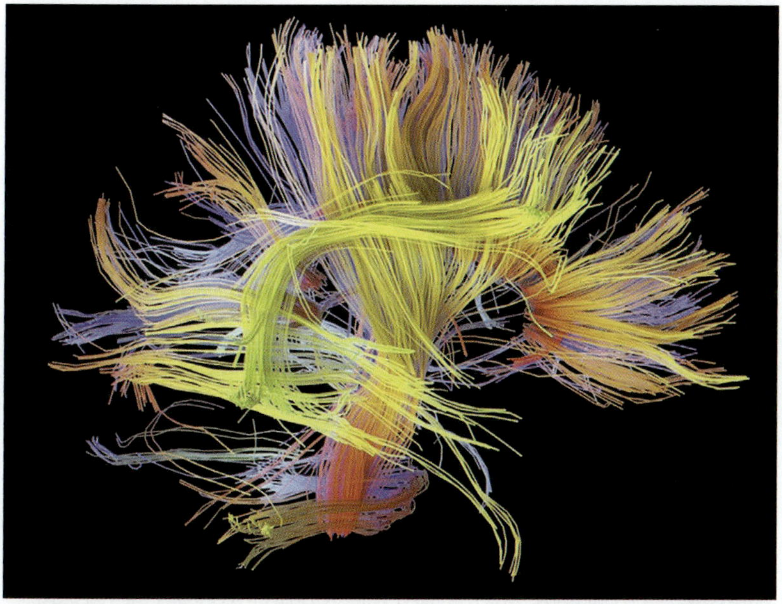

Pasieka/Science Source

FIGURE 2.7 A Connectome of the Brain. Network maps like this one have been developed by the Human Connectome Project to show active connections between neurons when the brain is relatively quiet—that is, connections that keep the brain ready to perform various functions.

NEURONS AND SYNAPSES

The neuron is the basic functional unit of the CNS. As shown in Figure 2.8, a typical neuron has a soma (cell body), which contains the nucleus (including the genetic material of the cell) and several other structures, called *organelles*, that perform vital functions. Examples of organelles include mitochondria, which produce energy from nutrients, and Golgi bodies, which package substances (such as neurotransmitters) into vesicles for storage.

Dendrites (short fibers that extend from the soma) receive signals from other neurons and respond by sending a signal to the soma, which then sends the signal down the axon for transmission to the dendrites of other neurons, which may continue the process of signal reception and transmission with still other neurons, or may transmit signals directly to muscles, organs, or glands in order to stimulate their activity. Each neuron has just a single axon, which transmits signals through an electrochemical process known as an *action potential*. Axons can vary in length from a few millimeters up to a meter or more. Longer axons are usually covered with a myelin sheath, produced by specialized types of glial cells, which increases the speed of the signal.

Signals flow from an axon to the next neuron or other cell by way of a specialized structure called a **synapse**. As the following passage makes dramatically clear, the human brain contains an unimaginably large number of synapses, creating a system of almost limitless interconnections:

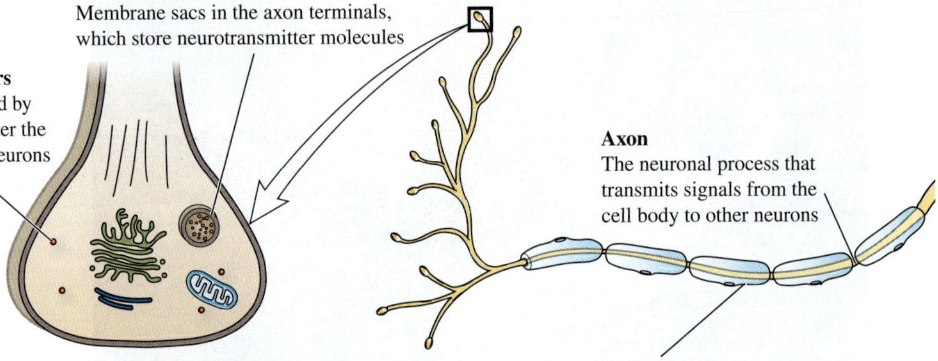

FIGURE 2.8 A Typical Neuron. The cell body, which is filled with cytoplasm, contains the nucleus, which contains the genetic material (DNA). Within the cytoplasm are various organelles, each of which performs specific functions. The endoplasmic reticulum (a network of flattened sacs and branching tubules that extends throughout the cytoplasm) provides a platform for ribosomes and a transport mechanism for movement of cellular products. Ribosomes synthesize proteins according to the genetic code, mitochondria produce energy for cell functions, and the Golgi body combines simple molecules into more complex structures and packages them into vesicles. Axons transmit and dendrites receive neural signals. A myelin sheath speeds the transmission of signals by certain axons. Axon branches end in terminal buttons, which contain vesicles filled with neurotransmitter molecules.

> A given neuron in the brain may receive several thousand synaptic connections from other neurons. . . . The number of possible different combinations of synaptic connections among the neurons in a single human brain is larger than the total number of atomic particles that make up the known universe. (Thompson, 2000)

It was once thought that the brain has its maximal number of neurons at birth and that once a neuron dies, it cannot be replaced. However, we now know that new neurons form every day (a process called *neurogenesis*). In addition, synaptic plasticity (first discussed in the introduction to Part 1) involves a continual reshaping of synaptic connections among neurons, with axon terminals and dendrites forming new synaptic connections and with old connections being eliminated. This remodeling probably begins before birth and continues throughout our lives.

As shown in Figure 2.9, a synapse consists of the presynaptic membrane of the transmitting neuron (typically, the membrane of an axon terminal button), the postsynaptic membrane of the receiving neuron (typically, the membrane of a dendrite), and a minute space between them (the **synaptic cleft**). Synaptic vesicles within the axon terminal each contain several thousand **neurotransmitter** molecules. These vesicles both store the neurotransmitter and protect it from being destroyed by metabolic enzymes. When an action potential reaches the axon terminal, it triggers a series of biochemical actions that cause the vesicles to fuse with the presynaptic membrane and release the

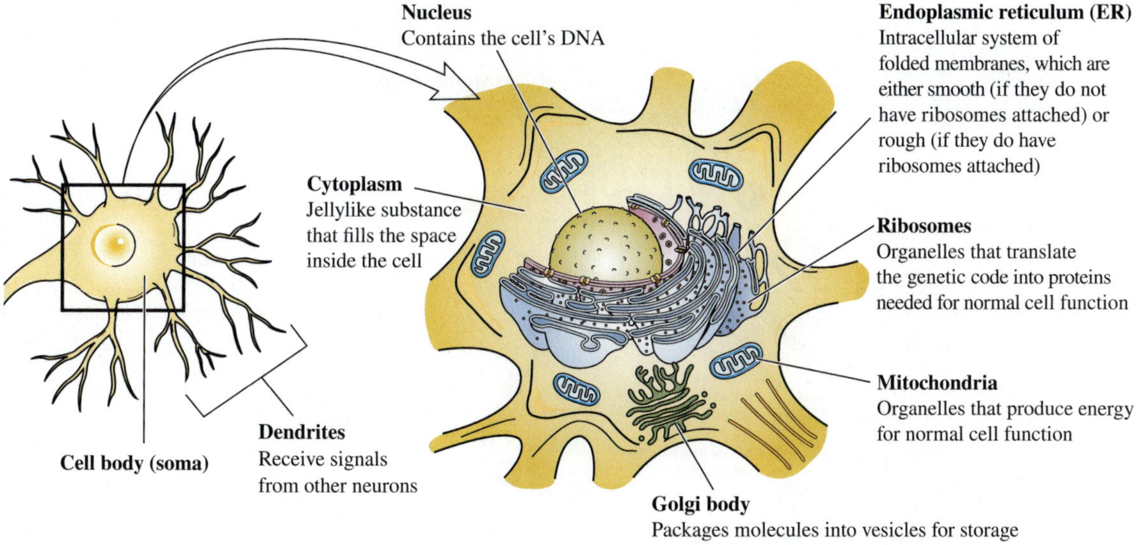

neurotransmitter into the synaptic cleft, a process called **exocytosis**. The neurotransmitter molecules diffuse across the synaptic cleft and attach to receptors on the postsynaptic membrane of the receiving neuron. It is important to note two aspects of this process of synaptic transmission (which is discussed in more detail in the next section): (1) the transmitting and receiving neurons do not physically touch each other, and (2) synaptic transmission is a chemical rather than an electrical process.

DR. J'S MUSINGS 2.1

Neural Communication: The Excitement of Discovery

As I was starting my career in psychopharmacology in 1966, the controversy about how neurons communicated with each other was being settled: the old concept of "tight junctions" between neurons and connectivity via an electrical "spark" was replaced by the newer concept of "gap" synapses with a chemical liberated from one neuron affecting the function of a second neuron. The development of the electron microscope enabled the visualization of synaptic architecture, revealing distinct presynaptic and postsynaptic elements, a synaptic cleft, and presynaptic vesicles. The study of synaptic transmission flourished, perhaps culminating in the seminal work *The Physiology of Synapses*, by John Eccles (1964). Thereafter, study of specific chemical transmitters and the effects of drugs on synaptic transmission came to the fore. For a pharmacologist, it was a terribly exciting era to be part of, with, for example, the identification of cannabinoid receptors in the mid-1980s followed by the identification of an endogenous neurotransmitter at the cannabinoid receptor in the early 1990s (Pertwee, 2006). The discovery of new receptors and how they function as targets of drug action continues.

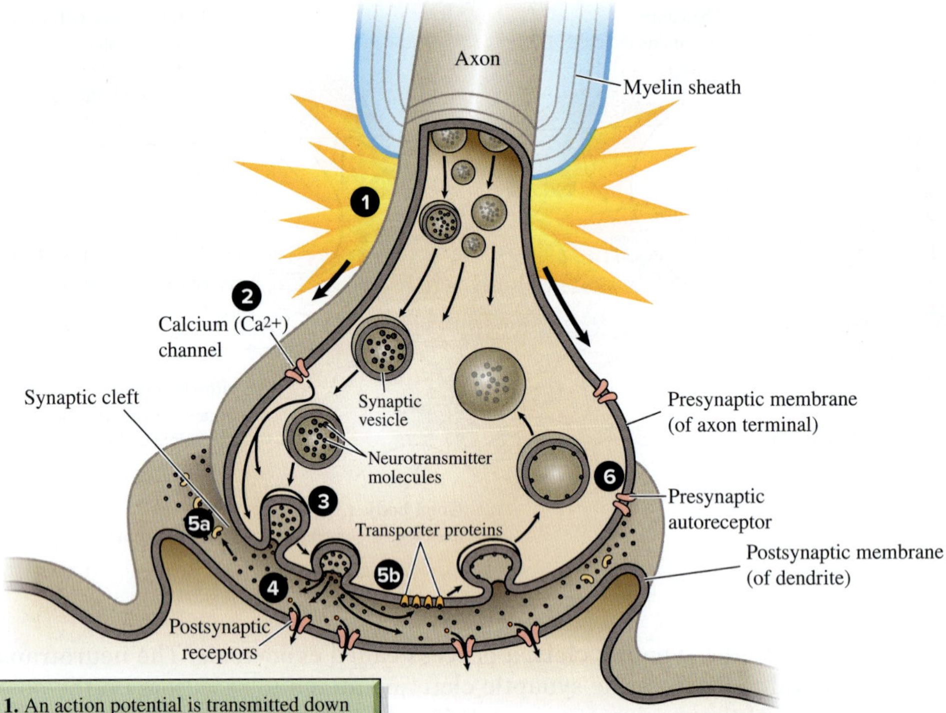

1. An action potential is transmitted down the axon to the presynaptic membrane.

2. When the action potential reaches the presynaptic membrane, it opens ion channels for calcium to enter the axon terminal.

3. Calcium causes synaptic vesicles to fuse with the terminal membrane, open, and release neurotransmitter molecules.

4. Neurotransmitter molecules attach to and activate receptors on the postsynaptic membrane.

5a. Enzymes in the synaptic cleft may break down neurotransmitter molecules.

5b. Transporter proteins take up some neurotransmitter molecules for release again in the future.

6. Neurotransmitter molecules may bind to autoreceptors to regulate the presynaptic neuron's activity.

FIGURE 2.9 A Typical Synapse. Neurotransmitter molecules are synthesized and stored in vesicles within the axon terminal. An action potential causes channels to open in the presynaptic membrane, allowing calcium ions to enter the axon terminal and initiate exocytosis (the release of neurotransmitter molecules into the synaptic cleft). After release, neurotransmitter molecules bind to and activate receptors on the postsynaptic membrane; excess neurotransmitter molecules may be taken back up by transporter proteins to be recycled for later release or may bind to autoreceptors on the presynaptic membrane to modulate the release of additional neurotransmitter molecules into the synaptic cleft.

SYNAPTIC TRANSMISSION AND NEUROTRANSMITTERS

Synaptic transmission is remarkably fast; the entire process may occur over a time span as short as a millisecond, from neurotransmitter release from presynaptic vesicles, to diffusion across the synaptic cleft, to receptor attachment and activation. Depending on the characteristics of the receptor, activation may begin and end within a few milliseconds after neurotransmitter attachment or may last hundreds of milliseconds.

Once release has occurred, there must be a way to get rid of excess neurotransmitter molecules in the synaptic cleft, which otherwise would continue to bind to and activate receptors. In most cases, neurotransmitter removal occurs through one of two general types of mechanisms:

- An enzyme in the synaptic cleft breaks down neurotransmitter molecules there, yielding metabolites that are then taken back up into the presynaptic neuron to be resynthesized into neurotransmitter molecules and repackaged for release (this is how the effect of the neurotransmitter acetylcholine is terminated).
- **Transporter proteins** in the presynaptic membrane take neurotransmitter molecules back into the presynaptic neuron to be repackaged for later release. As discussed below, the action of the neurotransmitters dopamine, norepinephrine, and serotonin is terminated by this mechanism. (Chapter 12 discusses a class of antidepressant medications that work by blocking this reuptake process.) In an alternative version of this process, neurotransmitter molecules are taken up into an adjacent glial cell and broken down into metabolites that are then recycled back into the presynaptic neuron where they are resynthesized into neurotransmitter molecules and repackaged for release (the effect of the neurotransmitter glutamate is terminated by this method).

The release of neurotransmitter may be modulated by presynaptic **autoreceptors** (see Figure 2.9) that bind neurotransmitter molecules released by the presynaptic neuron. These autoreceptors serve as a negative feedback mechanism: stimulation by excess neurotransmitter or by certain drugs reduces the synthesis and further release of neurotransmitter. Conversely, if an antagonist blocks an autoreceptor, synthesis and release of neurotransmitter increases.

Neurotransmitter Families

Neurons release specific neurotransmitters from their axon terminals, and these neurotransmitters can be classified into a few major families, such as amines, amino acids, peptides, and lipids. The amines acetylcholine and norepinephrine were the earliest identified CNS neurotransmitters (in the first half of the twentieth century), largely because of their established roles in the peripheral nervous system. In the 1960s, serotonin, epinephrine, and dopamine (also amines) were recognized as neurotransmitters. The amino acids gamma aminobutyric acid (GABA), glycine, and glutamate were identified in the 1970s, as were the endorphins, which are peptides. In the late 1980s, the lipid anandamide was identified as the neurotransmitter for the tetrahydrocannabinol (THC) receptor, and many other neurotransmitters have been identified in the years since. The remaining sections of this chapter provide an overview of some of the most important neurotransmitters involved in the actions of psychoactive drugs.

Acetylcholine

The neurotransmitter **acetylcholine** activates two different types of cholinergic receptors: **nicotinic receptors** and **muscarinic receptors** (the term *cholinergic* means "involving acetylcholine"). These two types of receptors are named for nicotine and muscarine, substances that specifically stimulate each type. Muscarine is found in certain poisonous mushrooms (it was first isolated in *Amanita muscaria*), and muscarinic receptors are involved in various complex CNS functions, such as memory, arousal, heart rate, attention, and analgesia. Nicotinic receptors are found on skeletal muscles, in the nervous system, and in the adrenal glands (see Chapter 6 for detailed discussion of the psychopharmacology of nicotine). Recently, a muscarinic receptor agonist (xanomeline) was successfully combined with a peripherally acting muscarinic antagonist (trospium) for the treatment of schizophrenia (Brannan et al., 2021).

Acetylcholine is distributed widely in the brain. As shown in Figure 2.10, the neurons that release acetylcholine have cell bodies in two main regions, in the forebrain

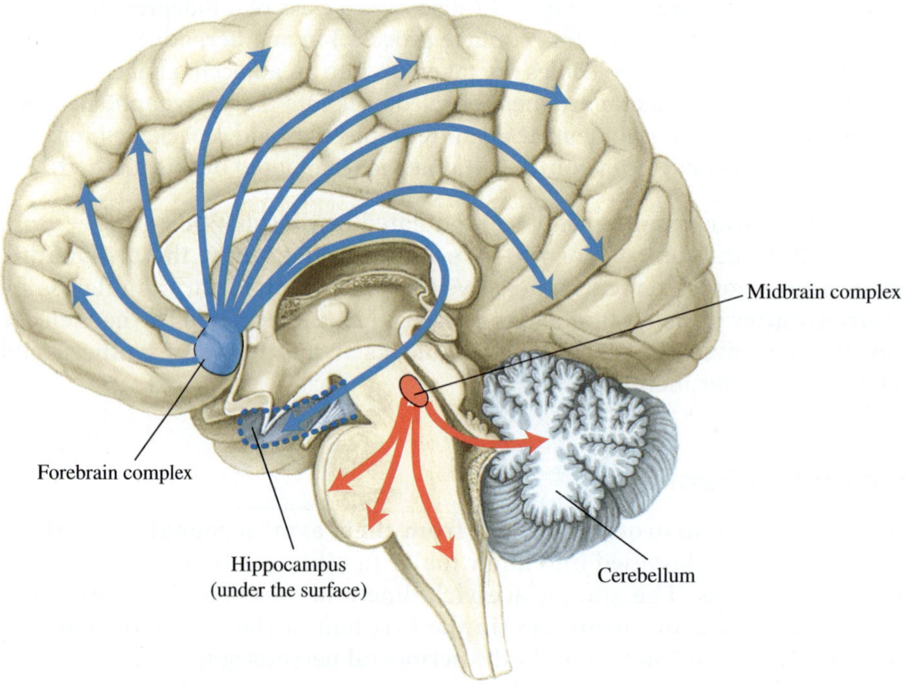

FIGURE 2.10 Acetylcholine in the Brain. Acetylcholine-releasing neurons in the forebrain complex project to the hippocampus and to many other parts of the forebrain. Acetylcholine-releasing neurons in the midbrain complex have descending projections to the pons, medulla, and cerebellum (not shown are ascending projections from the midbrain complex to the thalamus, basal ganglia, and other parts of the diencephalon).

and in the midbrain, with projections from these regions to many other parts of the brain. Acetylcholine is generally recognized as playing important roles in learning and memory. In addition, the diffuse distribution of acetylcholine is consistent with suggestions that it is involved in circuits that modulate sensory reception; in mechanisms related to behavioral arousal, attention, energy conservation, and mood; and in REM (rapid eye movement) activity during dreaming sleep.

Figure 2.11 shows how acetylcholine is synthesized from choline and acetyl coenzyme A within axon terminals and then stored in synaptic vesicles for later release into the synaptic cleft, where it rapidly diffuses across the cleft and binds to postsynaptic cholinergic receptors. Once acetylcholine has exerted its effect on postsynaptic receptors, its action is terminated by the enzyme acetylcholinesterase (AChE) (Chapter 17 discusses how drugs used in the treatment of Alzheimer's disease act by blocking this process, thereby increasing the amount of acetylcholine in the synapse).

Drugs that block the action of AChE, referred to as **AChE inhibitors**, include both "irreversible" and "reversible" compounds. Irreversible AChE inhibitors form a permanent covalent bond with AChE and totally inhibit the enzyme's function. Some of these toxic drugs (such as malathion and parathion) have been used as insecticides because

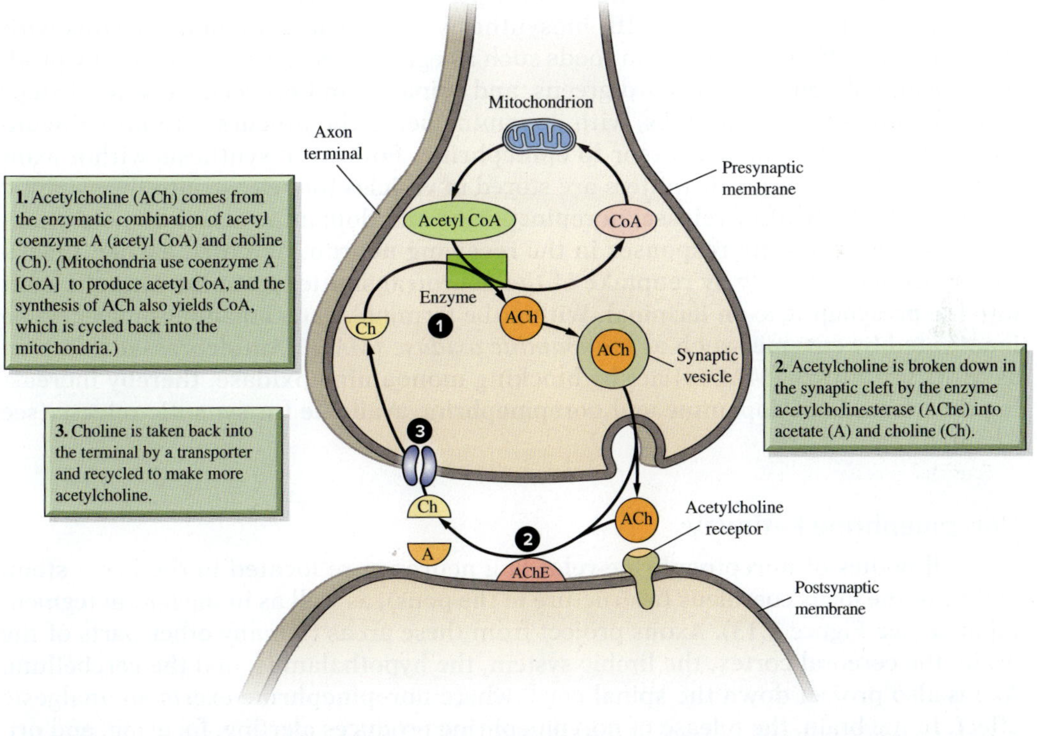

FIGURE 2.11 An Acetylcholine Synapse. Acetylcholine is made in the axon terminal from acetyl coenzyme A (acetyl CoA) and choline and stored in vesicles for release. After release, acetylcholine binds to its receptors and is immediately broken down at the receptors by acetylcholinesterase (AChE) into choline and acetate.

they kill insects on contact. Others (such as sarin and soman) have been used as lethal nerve gases in military operations and by terrorists.

The reversible AChE inhibitors, which are less toxic and shorter acting, are used clinically to delay memory decline in patients with Alzheimer's disease (as discussed in detail in Chapter 17, deficiencies in acetylcholine-releasing neurons have classically been associated with the dysfunctions seen in Alzheimer's disease). Certainly drugs that either inhibit or promote the central action of acetylcholine exert profound effects on memory. Thus, drugs that block central cholinergic receptors (e.g., scopolamine) may produce amnesia, whereas drugs that increase the amount of acetylcholine in the brain appear to improve memory function.

Catecholamines: Norepinephrine and Dopamine

A **catecholamine** is a neurotransmitter that consists of a catechol nucleus (a benzene ring with two attached hydroxyl groups) with an attached amine group (see Figure 2.12A). The CNS catecholamines are **dopamine** and **norepinephrine**. A large number of psychoactive drugs (both licit and illicit, therapeutic and abused) exert their effects by altering the synaptic action of these catecholamines in the brain. (A third catecholamine, epinephrine, functions in the peripheral nervous system.)

As illustrated in Figure 2.12B, biosynthesis of the catecholamines begins with the amino acid tyrosine (found in foods such as egg whites, cottage cheese, soy products, meat, fish, poultry, mustard greens, and spinach) and proceeds in several steps controlled by specific enzymes, with dopamine being the precursor to norepinephrine, which then is the precursor to epinephrine. Following synthesis within axon terminals, these neurotransmitters are stored in vesicles for release into the synaptic space. In the CNS, after release, norepinephrine and dopamine attach to postsynaptic receptors to initiate responses in the receiving neuron. As noted earlier, inactivation occurs primarily by reuptake of the neurotransmitter from the synaptic cleft into the presynaptic axon terminal. Within the terminal, catecholamines may also be inactivated by enzymes such as *monoamine oxidase (MAO)*. Antidepressants known as **MAO inhibitors (MAOIs)** act by blocking monoamine oxidase, thereby increasing the amounts of dopamine and norepinephrine available for synaptic release (see Chapter 12).

Norepinephrine Pathways

The cell bodies of norepinephrine-releasing neurons are located in the brain stem, mainly in the locus coeruleus (a structure in the pons), as well as in the lateral tegmental area (see Figure 2.13). Axons project from these areas to many other parts of the brain: the cerebral cortex, the limbic system, the hypothalamus, and the cerebellum. Axons also project down the spinal cord, where norepinephrine exerts an analgesic effect. In the brain, the release of norepinephrine produces alerting, focusing, and orienting responses, as well as positive feelings of reward.

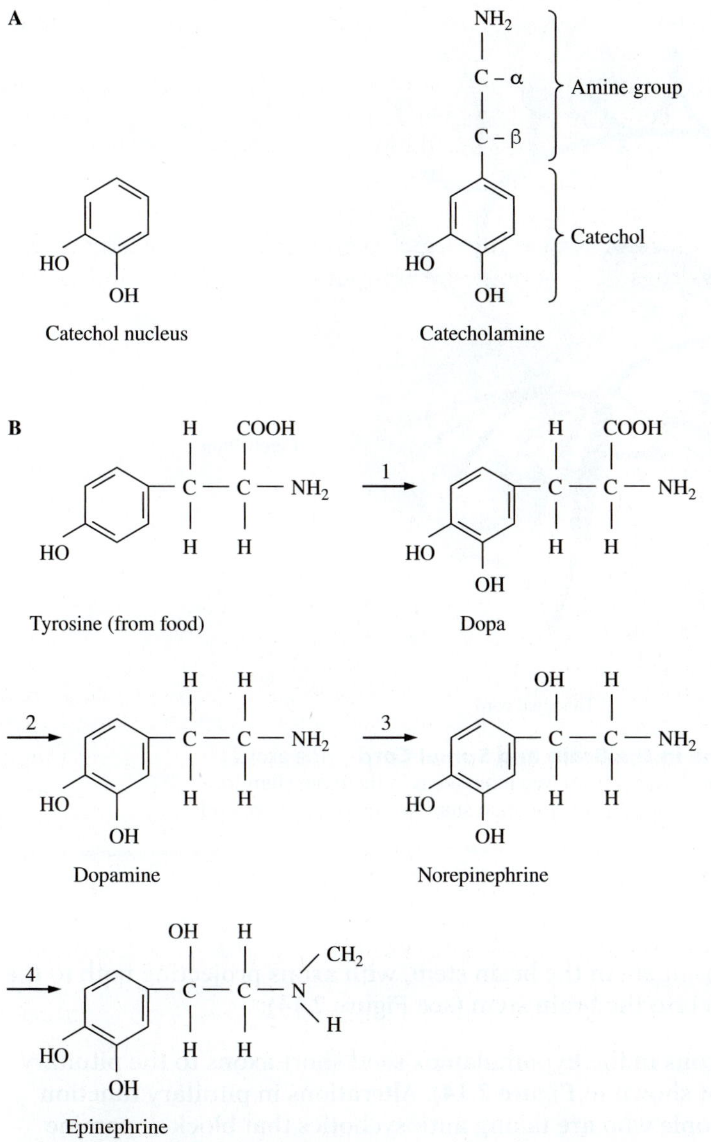

FIGURE 2.12 Catecholamines: Structure and Biosynthesis.
A. Every catecholamine consists of a catechol nucleus (a benzene ring with two adjacent hydroxyl [OH] groups) with an attached amine group.
B. Catecholamine biosynthesis begins with tyrosine (an amino acid found in foods), which is converted into dopa, which is then converted into dopamine. Dopamine is converted into norepinephrine, and norepinephrine into epinephrine (in the peripheral nervous system). Each of these reactions depends on the presence of a particular enzyme in the cell (represented by the arrows labeled 1–4): 1 = tyrosine hydroxylase; 2 = aromatic amino acid decarboxylase; 3 = dopamine-β-oxidase; 4 = phenylethanolamine-*N*-methyltransferase.

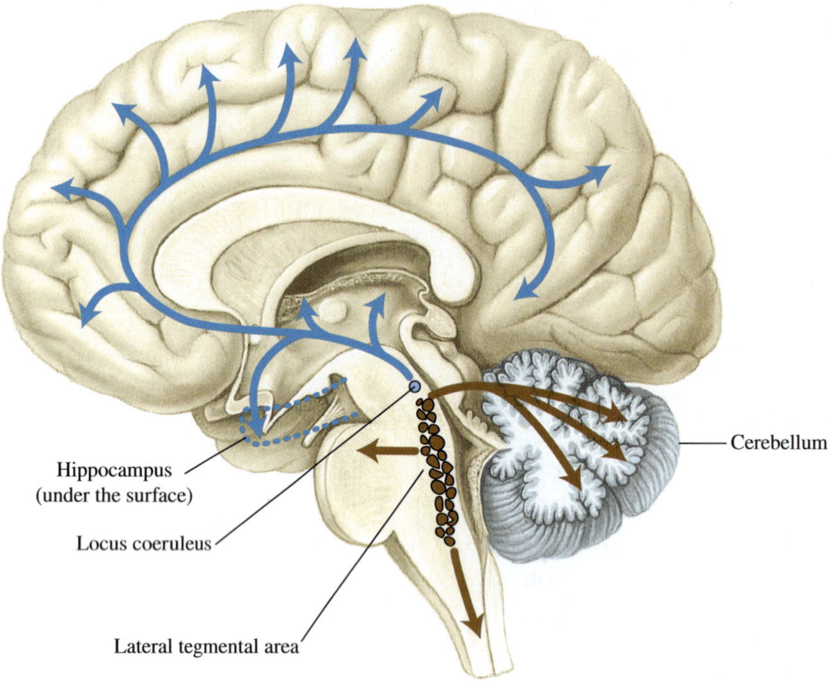

FIGURE 2.13 Norepinephrine in the Brain and Spinal Cord. The axons of norepinephrine-releasing neurons project from two main areas in the brain stem to areas throughout the forebrain, to other parts of the brain stem, to the cerebellum, and into the spinal cord.

Dopamine Pathways

Dopamine pathways also originate in the brain stem, with axons projecting both to the forebrain and farther down into the brain stem (see Figure 2.14):

- Dopamine-releasing neurons in the hypothalamus send short axons to the pituitary gland (this pathway is not shown in Figure 2.14). Alterations in pituitary function are commonly seen in people who are taking antipsychotics that block dopamine receptors in the pituitary (see Chapter 11).
- Dopamine-releasing neurons in the substantia nigra project farther down into the brain stem and to the basal ganglia, where they play a major role in the regulation of movement. Parkinsonism can result from physical loss of these neurons and from antipsychotic drugs that block dopamine receptors in the basal ganglia.
- Dopamine-releasing neurons in the ventral tegmental area project to the frontal cortex and the limbic system, two pathways that are extremely important in psychopharmacology. Alterations in the development of these pathways may be involved both in the pathogenesis of schizophrenia and in its amelioration by antipsychotic drugs. In addition, these pathways include structures that are activated by drugs

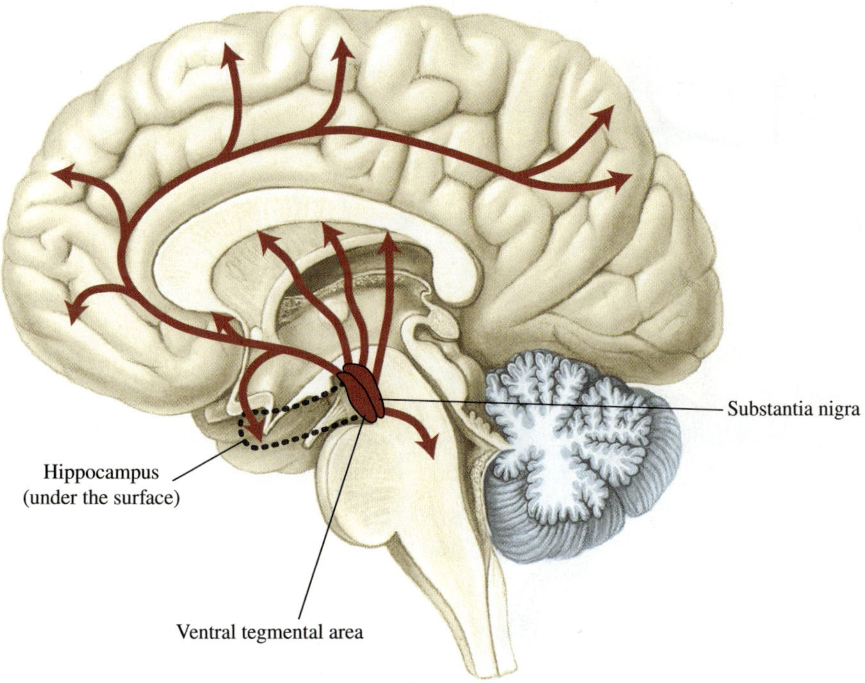

FIGURE 2.14 Dopamine in the Brain. Axons project in two directions from dopamine-releasing neurons in the substantia nigra: farther down into the brain stem and up to the basal ganglia, where dopamine is involved in motor functions (including in Parkinson's disease). Axons from dopamine-releasing neurons in the ventral tegmental area project widely into the forebrain, including to the cerebral cortex and the limbic system.

(and other stimuli) that produce sensations of pleasure; these structures constitute our reward circuit (shown in Figure 2.5), which is involved in addiction to most drugs of abuse (see Chapter 4).

Serotonin

Serotonin (5-hydroxytryptamine, 5-HT) was first investigated as a CNS neurotransmitter in the 1950s when lysergic acid diethylamide (LSD) was found both to resemble serotonin structurally and to block the contractile effect of serotonin on the gastrointestinal tract. At that time, it was hypothesized that LSD-induced hallucinations might be caused by alterations in the functioning of serotonin neurons and that serotonin might be involved in abnormal behavioral functioning. How prescient was that hypothesis!

Today, we know that serotonin plays a role in depression, anxiety, and obsessive-compulsive disorder, as well as in panic, phobias, sleep, sex, cardiovascular function, and the regulation of body temperature. Drugs that potentiate the synaptic actions of serotonin are widely used as antidepressants and as antianxiety agents, and

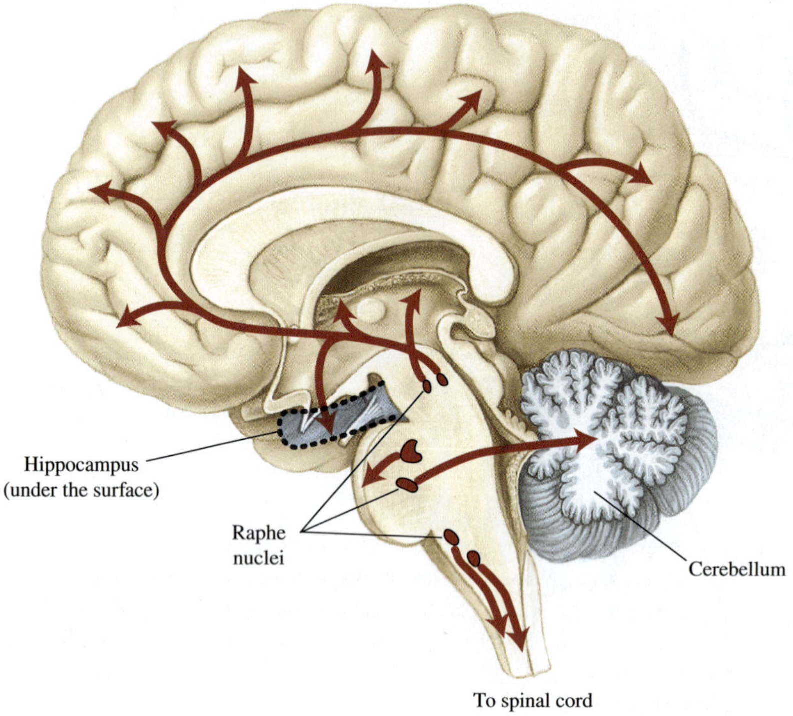

FIGURE 2.15 Serotonin in the Brain. Serotonin-releasing neurons in the raphe nuclei project to the cerebral cortex, hippocampus, hypothalamus, limbic system, cerebellum, and spinal cord.

use of these drugs can be associated with side effects such as insomnia, anxiety, and loss of libido (see Chapter 12).

Serotonin-releasing neurons are found in structures collectively called the *raphe nuclei* in the upper brain stem, particularly in the pons and the medulla. As shown in Figure 2.15, axons from these neurons project widely to the cerebral cortex, hippocampus, hypothalamus, and limbic system, to the cerebellum, and to the spinal cord, where serotonin may be involved in the modulation of both pain and spinal reflexes.

Serotonin-releasing neurons in the brain synthesize serotonin from the amino acid tryptophan. Because the human body cannot make tryptophan, we must get it from foods such as poultry, bananas, tomatoes, and walnuts. Fourteen different serotonin receptors (5-HT receptors) have been identified and have been classified in families and as subtypes within families (see Figure 2.16). Some of these 5-HT receptors are important in drug action, as we will see as in later chapters.

Amino Acid Neurotransmitters

Two amino acid neurotransmitters are widely distributed in the brain: glutamate and gamma aminobutyric acid. Both activate a number of different receptors, maintaining

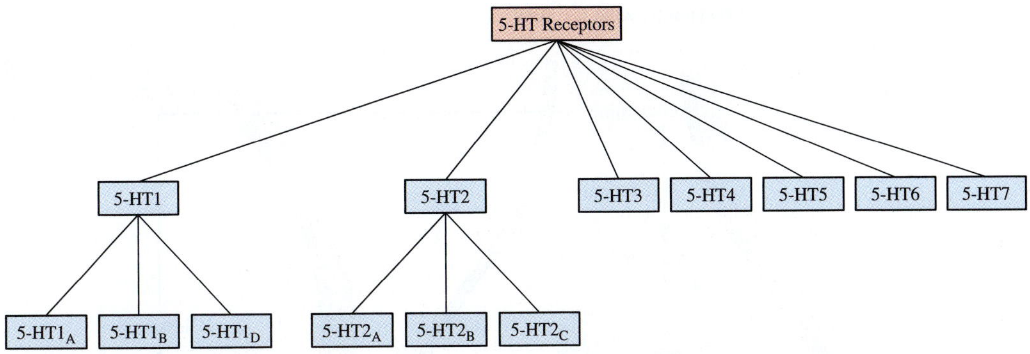

FIGURE 2.16 Serotonin (5-HT) Receptors. The 5-HT1 and 5-HT2 families of receptors each come in three different subtypes.

a balance between excitation and inhibition in the brain, and both are involved in the actions of several psychoactive drugs, including the benzodiazepine antianxiety agents (discussed in Chapter 13) and the mood stabilizers (discussed in Chapter 14). Most other amino acids in the brain are not neurotransmitters but are precursors for the biosynthesis of neurotransmitters (e.g., as discussed above, tyrosine is a precursor for the catecholamines, and tryptophan for serotonin).

Glutamate

Glutamate (or *glutamic acid*), the major excitatory neurotransmitter in the brain, is a nonessential amino acid, meaning that it is not required in the diet. Rather, it is synthesized within glutamate-releasing neurons, both by the normal breakdown of glucose and by a number of other chemical reactions, including the important reaction illustrated in Figure 2.17. In this reaction, after glutamate has been released from a neuron and has exerted its excitatory effect on glutamate receptors, it is transported into adjacent glial cells and converted to the amino acid glutamine, which then eventually diffuses out of the glial cells and into the presynaptic axon terminals, where it is converted back to glutamate. (Figure 2.17 also illustrates the reuptake of glutamate into the presynaptic axon terminal via transporter proteins.)

There are two families of glutamate receptors, fast and slow. As shown in Figure 2.17, the fast (ionotropic) receptors, which include NMDA and AMPA receptors, are found on the postsynaptic membrane, while the slow (metabotropic) receptors are found on both the postsynaptic and presynaptic membranes (ionotropic and metabotropic receptors are discussed in Chapter 3). NMDA and AMPA receptors, which mediate rapid excitation of postsynaptic neurons, have especially high concentrations in the cerebral cortex, hippocampus, basal ganglia, septum, and amygdala (these structures are shown in Figures 2.4 and 2.5).

NMDA receptors in particular are pharmacologically important because they are blocked by the psychedelic drugs phencyclidine (PCP) and ketamine, which likely explains why these drugs block memory formation and induce delusions and

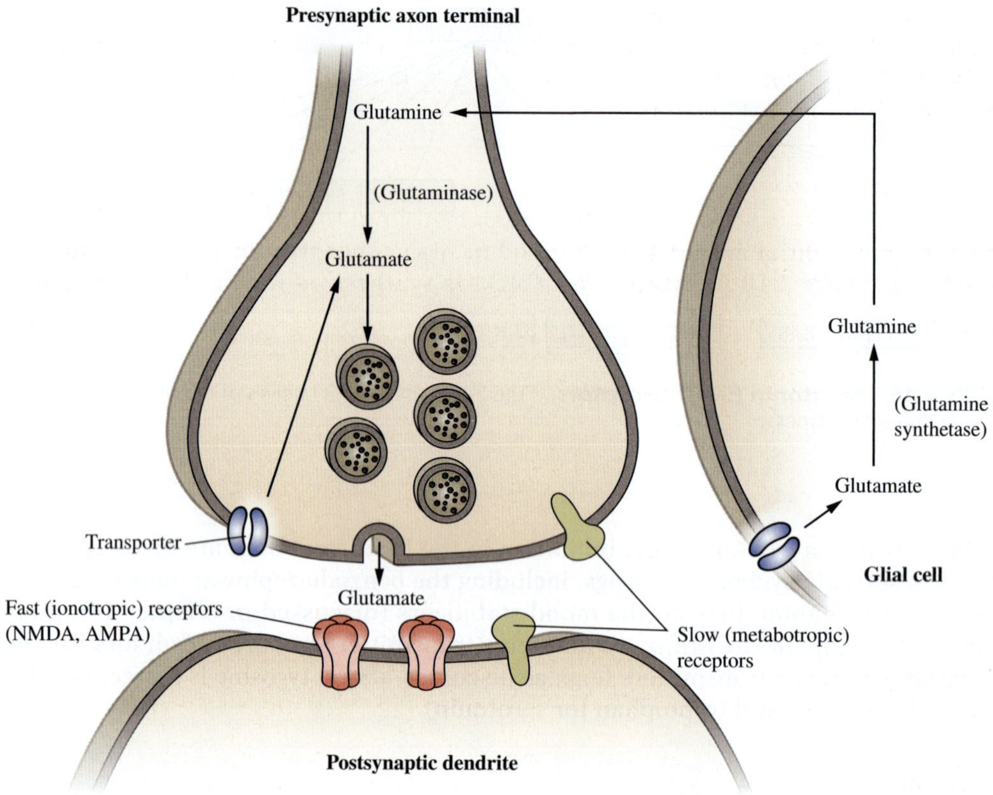

FIGURE 2.17 A Glutamate Synapse. Glutamate is released into the synapse, where it excites fast and slow postsynaptic receptors, as well as slow presynaptic receptors (thereby modulating the release of glutamate from the presynaptic axon terminal). Transporters on the presynaptic membrane take excess glutamate back up into the axon terminal for later release, and transporters on adjacent glial cells take up excess glutamate for conversion into glutamine by the enzyme glutamine synthetase. Glutamine then diffuses out of the glial cells and into the axon terminal, where it is converted back into glutamate by the enzyme glutaminase and stored in vesicles for later release.

hallucinations (psychedelic drugs are discussed in detail in Chapter 8). Reverse thinking then postulates a role for glutamate in learning and memory formation (Bazzari and Parri, 2019), in thought disorders (Tamminga et al., 2012), and in Alzheimer's disease (Liu et al., 2019), which would imply that glutamate receptors are potential targets for therapies for Alzheimer's and other dementias (memantine, the first anti-Alzheimer's drug that acts on NMDA receptors, became available for clinical use in 2004—see Chapter 17). NMDA receptors also play a critical role in regulating synaptic plasticity (Franchini et al., 2020; Lodge et al., 2019).

Overactivity of NMDA receptors, which allows high amounts of calcium ions to enter the neuron, can lead to neuronal damage or destruction (excess calcium activates enzymes that cause damage to cell structures and to DNA). For example, traumatic head injury can result in a massive release of glutamate, and attempts to provide "brain protection" after head injury are aimed at preventing this overactivity. (See Chapter 5 for discussion of alcohol use and glutamate activity, and see Chapter 11 for discussion of possible glutamate dysfunction in the pathogenesis of schizophrenia.)

Gamma Aminobutyric Acid

Gamma aminobutyric acid (GABA), the major inhibitory transmitter and, like glutamate, a nonessential amino acid, is found in high concentrations in the brain and spinal cord. Figure 2.18 illustrates how GABA is synthesized within GABA-releasing

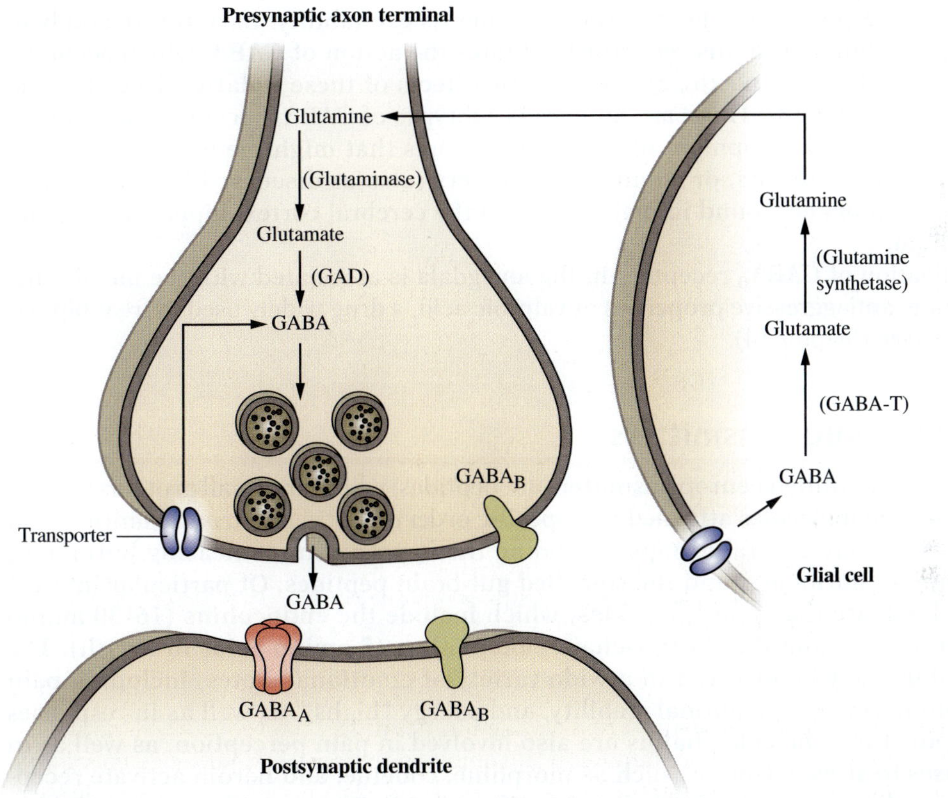

FIGURE 2.18 A GABA Synapse. GABA is released into the synapse, where it inhibits fast and slow postsynaptic receptors, as well as slow presynaptic receptors (thereby modulating the release of GABA from the presynaptic axon terminal). Transporter proteins on the presynaptic membrane take excess GABA back up into the axon terminal for later release, and transporter proteins on adjacent glial cells take up excess GABA for conversion into glutamate by the enzyme GABA-T (GABA-transaminase), which is then converted into glutamine by the enzyme glutamine synthetase. Glutamine then diffuses out of the glial cells and into the axon terminal, where it is converted back into glutamate by the enzyme glutaminase, then back into GABA by the enzyme glutamic acid decarboxylase (GAD); GABA is then stored in vesicles for later release.

neurons (note the similarity with glutamate synthesis, illustrated in Figure 2.17). After GABA has been released from a neuron and has exerted its inhibitory effect on GABA receptors, it is transported into adjacent glial cells and converted to glutamate, which is then converted to the amino acid glutamine, which then eventually diffuses out of the glial cells and into the presynaptic axon terminals, where it is converted back to glutamate and then back to GABA. (Figure 2.18 also illustrates the reuptake of GABA into the presynaptic axon terminal via transporter proteins.)

The two types of GABA receptors are fast and slow (again, like the two families of glutamate receptors). As shown in Figure 2.18, the fast (ionotropic) $GABA_A$ receptors are found on the postsynaptic membrane, while the slow (metabotropic) $GABA_B$ receptors are found on both the postsynaptic and presynaptic membranes. Activation of $GABA_A$ receptors opens an ion channel and leads to an influx of chloride into the cell, hyperpolarizing the cell and reducing its excitability. Barbiturate and benzodiazepine binding to this receptor facilitates the action of GABA, which accounts for the anxiolytic, amnestic, and anesthetic effects of these sedative drugs (as discussed in Chapter 13). There are numerous subtypes of $GABA_A$ receptors, potentially allowing for the development of a variety of drugs that might be novel antianxiety agents, anticonvulsants, or cognitive enhancers (also as discussed in Chapter 13). $GABA_A$ receptors are found in high density in the cerebral cortex, hippocampus, and cerebellum.

Activation of $GABA_B$ receptors in the amygdala is associated with the membrane-stabilizing, antiaggressive properties of valproic acid, a drug widely used to treat bipolar disorder (see Chapter 14).

Peptide Neurotransmitters

Many newly identified neurotransmitters are peptides, which are small proteins (chains of amino acid molecules attached in a specific order). **Peptide neurotransmitters** can be classified into several groups, including the hypothalamic-releasing hormones, the pituitary hormones, and the so-called gut-brain peptides. Of particular interest in this book are the **opioid peptides**, which include the **endorphins** (16–30 amino acids in length) and the shorter-chain **enkephalins** (5 amino acids in length). The endorphins may be involved in a wide variety of emotional states, including pain perception, reward, emotional stability, and energy "highs," as well as in responses to acupuncture (the enkephalins are also involved in pain perception, as well as in responses to stress). Opiates such as morphine, codeine, and heroin activate receptors for endorphins and enkephalins (see Chapter 10). There are three types of these opioid receptors—mu, kappa, and delta—with the mu receptor mediating the analgesic and reinforcing properties of morphine and other opiates.

Another peptide neurotransmitter of interest is **substance P**, a gut-brain peptide (11 amino acids in length) that plays an important role in transmitting sensory information, especially for pain impulses that enter the spinal cord and brain from a peripheral site of tissue injury. Opioids, serotonin agonists, and norepinephrine agonists exert much of their analgesic effect by acting on substance P nerve terminals to limit the release of this pain-inducing peptide.

DR. J'S MUSINGS 2.2

When Is a Fact a Fact?

All my training in psychopharmacology has reinforced my conviction that there are fairly few unchangeable pharmacological "facts." Consider, for example, the "one neuron, one transmitter" hypothesis: the idea that each neuron releases only a single neurotransmitter. Indeed, most of the discussion of neurotransmitters in this chapter presumes that principle. However, research over the last decade has demonstrated that certain neurons throughout the brain are capable of releasing two or maybe even more neurotransmitters (Avalos & Sprecher, 2021). The neurotransmitters released by these neurons, referred to as *dual neurotransmitter neurons*, may be rapid acting (e.g., acetylcholine) or slow acting (e.g., neuropeptides). In some of these neurons, the different neurotransmitters may be packaged within the same synaptic vesicles, while in others they may be in distinct vesicles. At this point, we do not know how these "facts" relate to disease states or to the actions or development of psychoactive drugs. This new concept of dual-transmitter neurons is both unsettling and terribly exciting!

Clearly, pharmacological "facts" are not unchangeable as science advances. Rather—as I learned early in my career—facts are based on observation and interpretation, and as observations change, so do the interpretations of those observations. And as interpretations change, so do the "facts" inherent in those interpretations. As we move forward with new, possibly improved, observations and interpretations, the facts do change. Is the earth flat? We once thought it was!

CHAPTER REVIEW

1. What are the two major parts of the central nervous system and the three major divisions of the brain?
2. Summarize the major structures and functions of the basal ganglia and the limbic system.
3. Match the numbered structures with the lettered descriptions:
   1. brain stem; 2. cerebellum; 3. hypothalamus; 4. thalamus
   A. regulates hormonal output of pituitary gland; B. relays information between subcortical structures and cerebral cortex; C. consists of medulla, pons, and midbrain; D. necessary for proper integration of movement and balance
4. Match the numbered structures with the lettered descriptions:
   1. soma; 2. organelles; 3. dendrites; 4. axon; 5. myelin sheath
   A. transmits signals via action potential; B. cell body; C. increases speed of signals; D. mitochondria, Golgi bodies; E. receive signals

5. Put these steps in the process of synaptic transmission in their correct order: 1. diffusion of neurotransmitter across synaptic cleft; 2. neurotransmitter stored in vesicles; 3. neurotransmitter attachment to postsynaptic receptor; 4. exocytosis
6. What are the two main ways in which neurotransmitter action is terminated?
7. What are the two types of acetylcholine receptors? What are AChE inhibitors and how are they used as drugs?
8. What are the two types of catecholamine neurotransmitters in the brain? What effect does monoamine oxidase have on their activity?
9. Which neurotransmitter is released by neurons in the raphe nuclei?
10. Which two amino acid neurotransmitters are widely distributed in the brain? Which is inhibitory and which is excitatory?
11. Which family of neurotransmitters includes substance P, endorphins, and enkephalins?

KEY TERMS

acetylcholine
AChE inhibitors
amygdala
ataxia
autoreceptors
basal ganglia
brain stem
catecholamine
central nervous system (CNS)
cerebellum
cerebral cortex
cerebrum
cingulate cortex
dopamine
endorphins
enkephalins
exocytosis
forebrain
gamma aminobutyric acid (GABA)
glutamate
hindbrain
hippocampus
hypothalamus
limbic system
MAO inhibitors (MAOIs)
midbrain
muscarinic receptors
neurotransmitter
nicotinic receptors
NMDA receptors
norepinephrine
opioid peptides
peptide neurotransmitters
peripheral nervous system (PNS)
reward circuit
serotonin (5-hydroxytryptamine, 5-HT)
spinal cord
substance P
synapse
synaptic cleft
thalamus
transporter proteins
ventral tegmental area

CHAPTER 3

Pharmacodynamics: How Drugs Act

CHAPTER OUTLINE

Like the neurotransmitters described in Chapter 2, psychoactive drugs exert their effects by attaching to receptors in cells in both the brain and the body. *It is a basic principle of pharmacology that the physiological and behavioral effects induced by a drug result from the drug's interactions with receptors.* The study of these interactions, termed *pharmacodynamics*, involves exploring the mechanisms of drug action that operate at the cellular level. Thus, pharmacokinetics (covered in Chapter 1) is the study of what the body does to drugs, whereas pharmacodynamics is the study of what drugs do to the body.

To produce its intended effect, a drug must bind to and interact with specific receptors that, in the case of psychoactive drugs, are usually located on the surface (i.e., in the outer membrane) of neurons in the brain. **Drug-receptor binding** (the attachment of a drug to a receptor) leads to a change in the functioning of the neuron, which results in the drug's characteristic pharmacological effects. The duration and level of the drug's effects depend partly on the strength of the attachment of the drug to its receptors, which is determined by the fit of the three-dimensional structure of the drug to the three-dimensional site on the receptor, the so-called lock-and-key relationship.

RECEPTORS AND DRUG ACTION

In Chapter 2, we discussed how receptors are involved in synaptic transmission—that is, how neurotransmitters are released into the synaptic cleft where they bind to and activate different types of post- and presynaptic receptors, each of which is specific to a particular type of neurotransmitter. There are dozens of different types of neurotransmitters in humans and literally hundreds of different types of neurotransmitter receptors, each of which is activated by the binding of one specific type of neurotransmitter (e.g., serotonin receptors are activated by the neurotransmitter serotonin only). The difference between the number of neurotransmitters and the much larger number of receptor types is accounted for by the fact that receptor types come in a wide variety of subtypes (e.g., the subtypes of catecholamine, serotonin, and GABA receptors discussed in Chapter 2).

Like neurotransmitters, drugs exert their effects by binding to receptors.[1] To have its intended effect, a drug must exhibit both **specificity** and **affinity** for a given type of receptor—that is, the drug must bind just to that type of receptor (specificity) and must bind well enough to achieve the required strength of effect (affinity). If two drugs given at equal doses produce the same number of molecules at the receptor, then the drug with the greater affinity will produce a greater effect. Apparently minor variations in a drug's chemical structure may greatly alter its affinity for the receptor and therefore its ability to activate the receptor and initiate a neuronal response.

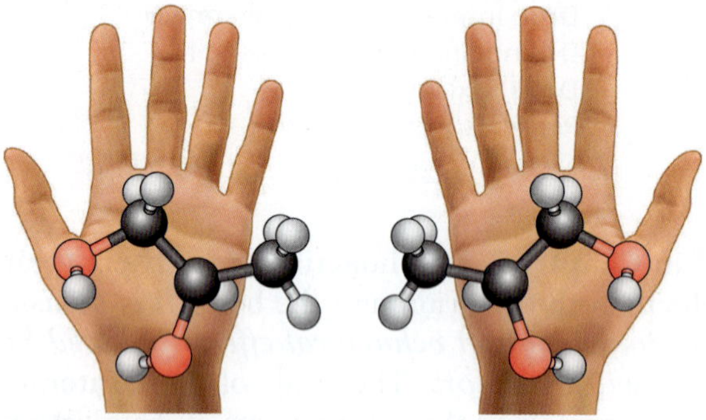

FIGURE 3.1 Optical Isomers. Your left and right hands are mirror images of each other: the two hands can be superimposed only by a rotation in space, as when you rotate one hand palm down to superimpose it on the other hand. Similarly, the molecular structures shown here are mirror images of each other and can be superimposed only by a rotation in space.

One such structural variation involves the concept of **isomers**, molecules that have the same molecular formula—that is, the same number of atoms of each element in the molecule—but have different arrangements of those atoms in space. When two isomers of a molecule are mirror images of each other, they are called *optical isomers* (see Figure 3.1). Optical isomers of drugs differ pharmacologically—that is, even though they have the same chemical structure, they do not act in the same way biologically. One isomer may bind to the drug's receptor and be pharmacologically active, whereas the other may not bind and may thus be

[1]It is a general rule of psychopharmacology that psychoactive drugs do not create any unique effects; they merely modulate normal neuronal functioning by increasing or decreasing the effects of neurotransmitters. For example, a drug might block reuptake of a neurotransmitter, thereby increasing the effect of the neurotransmitter by making more of it available in the synaptic cleft; or a drug might bind to a neurotransmitter's postsynaptic receptor without activating it, thereby decreasing the effect of the neurotransmitter by making those receptors unavailable for activation.

DR. J'S MUSINGS 3.1

Isomers: The Same, Only Different

In 1935, a racemic mixture of amphetamine was marketed under the trade name Benzedrine as an inhaler for nasal congestion. In 1937, dextroamphetamine, an isomer of amphetamine, was marketed under the trade name Dexedrine as a stimulant for the treatment of hyperactivity, depression, and obesity. As patents expired on racemic mixtures of psychiatric drugs, pharmaceutical companies sometimes gained new patent rights by separately marketing the active isomer in the racemic mixture, despite the isomer's having no therapeutic advantage over the racemic mixture. What made this maneuver possible was the fact that the Food and Drug Administration required (and still requires) only demonstrations of safety and efficacy in order to approve a drug for marketing, not necessarily any superiority over the racemic drug. The only advantage claimed is that the drug is "new," with no mention of the fact that it is also more expensive!

pharmacologically inactive; or both may be pharmacologically active but differ in their effects (Andrade, 2017).

When only one isomer of a drug is pharmacologically active, it is typically easier and less costly to synthesize and market the drug as a **racemic mixture** (or *racemate*), a 50/50 mixture of its two isomers, although only one isomer will be biologically active in the body. Occasionally, however, there is financial incentive to go to the effort to separate the isomers, whether in order to market only the active isomer or in order to separately market isomers that differ pharmacologically.[2]

Receptor Structure

The major types of receptor structures were introduced in Chapter 2: **ionotropic receptors** (found on postsynaptic membranes), **metabotropic receptors** (found on both post- and presynaptic membranes), and transporter proteins (found on presynaptic membranes). Activation of ionotropic receptors increases or decreases the activity of postsynaptic neurons—that is, ionotropic receptors have excitatory or

[2]One example of a drug with separately marketed optical isomers is the antidepressant citalopram (discussed in Chapter 12), first marketed as a racemic mixture under the trade name Celexa, until its patent expired and much less expensive generic formulations of the drug became available, at which point the active isomer was separated out, patented, and marketed as escitalopram (Lexapro) and sold at a significantly higher price than generic citalopram. Other drugs with separately marketed isomeric formulations include amphetamine and methylphenidate, used in the treatment of ADHD (see Chapter 16), and modafinil, used in the treatment of narcolepsy (see Chapters 7 and 13). An isomer of amphetamine is marketed separately as Dexedrine; the faster-metabolizing isomer of methylphenidate is marketed separately as Focalin; and the racemic mixture of modafinil is marketed as Provigil while its more water-soluble isomer is marketed as Nuvigil.

inhibitory effects. Activation of metabotropic receptors (more commonly referred to as *G-protein-coupled receptors*) can alter any of a variety of processes in postsynaptic neurons. Transporter proteins take neurotransmitters in the synaptic cleft back up into the presynaptic neuron.

Ionotropic Receptors

As shown in Figure 3.2A, ionotropic receptors (also called *ion channel receptors*) span the membrane of the postsynaptic neuron and form an ion channel, a pore that enlarges when either a neurotransmitter or a drug activates the receptor by binding

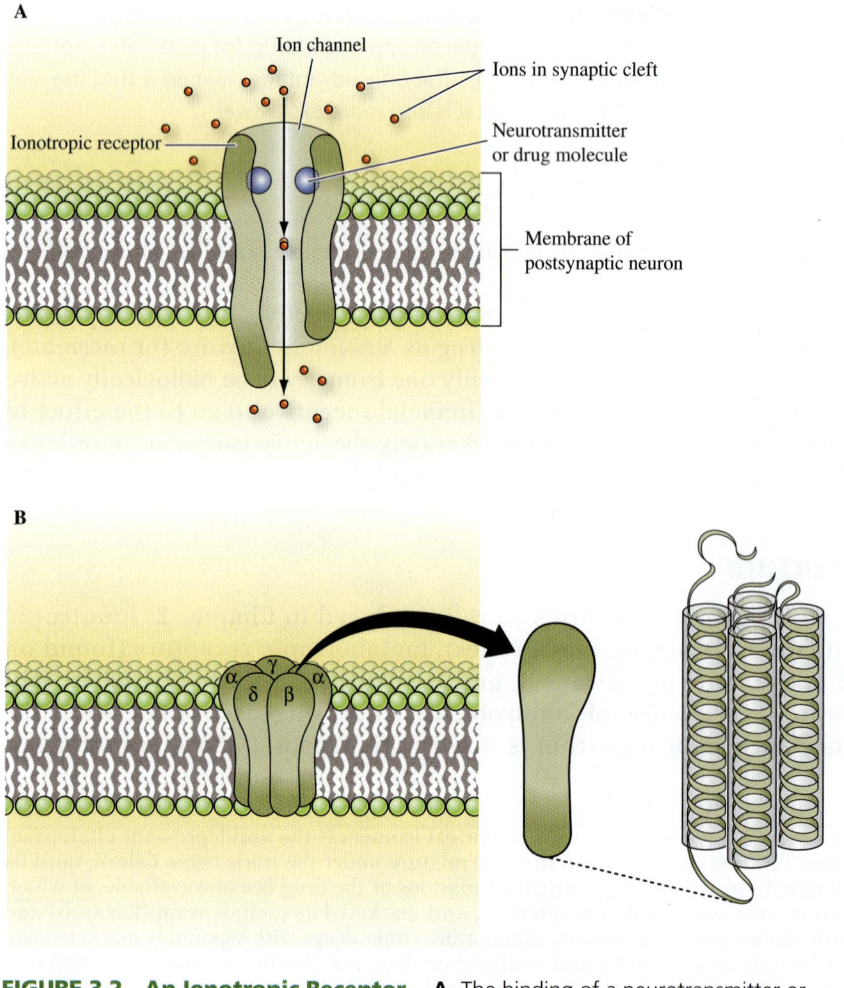

FIGURE 3.2 An Ionotropic Receptor. **A.** The binding of a neurotransmitter or drug molecule activates the receptor, allowing ions to flow through the ion channel and into the postsynaptic neuron. **B.** The receptor is composed of five subunits designated by Greek letters—two alpha (α) subunits, a beta (β) subunit, a gamma (γ) subunit, and a delta (δ) subunit—and each subunit is composed of four helical coils.

to it. The enlarged pore allows specific ions (such as chloride ions) to flow into the neuron (different ionotropic receptors allow the flow of different ions). The influx of ions can result in an action potential in the postsynaptic neuron. Figure 3.2B shows that an ionotropic receptor is composed of five subunits, each of which crosses the cell membrane. Each of these subunits is, in turn, made up of four helical coils, and the entire complex of transmembrane coils forms the receptor's ion channel.

When a drug binds to an ionotropic receptor, the drug does not necessarily bind to the same site on the receptor where a neurotransmitter would bind. This is illustrated in Figure 3.3, which shows that the neurotransmitter gamma aminobutyric acid (GABA) and two drugs (a benzodiazepine and a barbiturate) all bind to different sites on an ionotropic $GABA_A$ receptor ($GABA_A$ receptors and metabotropic $GABA_B$ receptors are described in Chapter 2; the effects of benzodiazepines and barbiturates on $GABA_A$ receptors are discussed in Chapter 13).

Metabotropic Receptors (G-Protein-Coupled Receptors)

Like ionotropic receptors, metabotropic receptors (which we will henceforth refer to as *G-protein-coupled receptors*) span the membrane where they are located (see Figure 3.4). However, unlike ionotropic receptors, G-protein-coupled receptors do not form ion channels. Rather, activation of a G-protein-coupled receptor induces the release of a component of an attached **G protein**. One possible effect of this release is the direct activation of ion channels in nearby ionotropic receptors, as illustrated in Figure 3.5. Other, indirect effects are mediated by enzymes and by molecules known

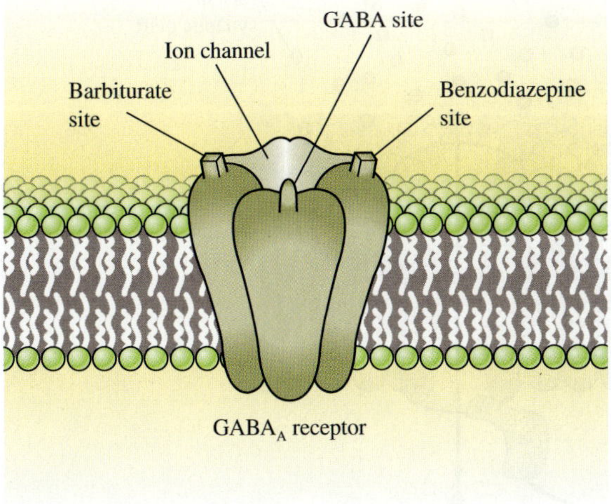

FIGURE 3.3 Drug and Neurotransmitter Binding Sites on an Ionotropic Receptor. GABA, benzodiazepines, and barbiturates bind to different sites on an ionotropic $GABA_A$ receptor. Both drugs enhance the effect of GABA by increasing the flow of ions into the postsynaptic neuron.

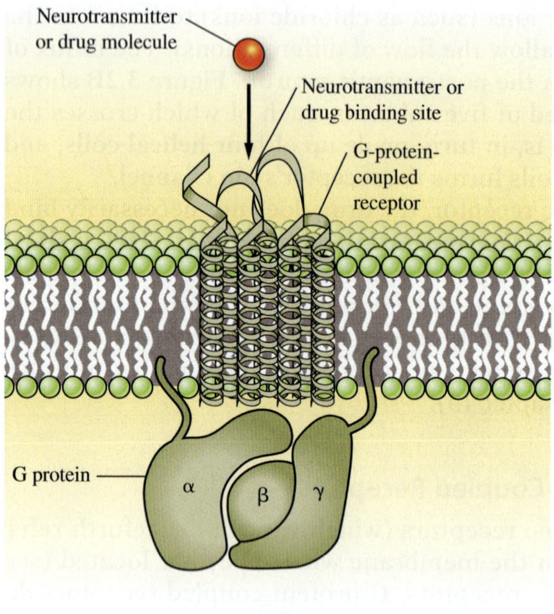

FIGURE 3.4 A G-Protein-Coupled Receptor. The receptor is composed of seven membrane-spanning helical coils and an attached ("coupled") G protein.

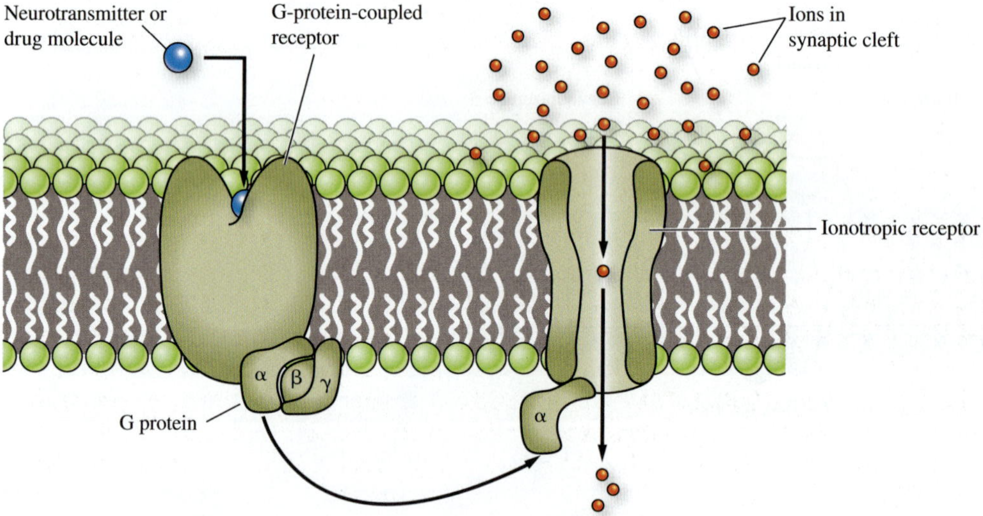

FIGURE 3.5 Activation of an Ionotropic Receptor by a G-Protein-Coupled Receptor. When a neurotransmitter or drug molecule binds to a G-protein-coupled receptor, one of the components (here, the alpha component) of the attached G protein is released and attaches to an ionotropic receptor in the same neural membrane. This activates the ionotropic receptor, which allows ions to flow through its ion channel into the neuron.

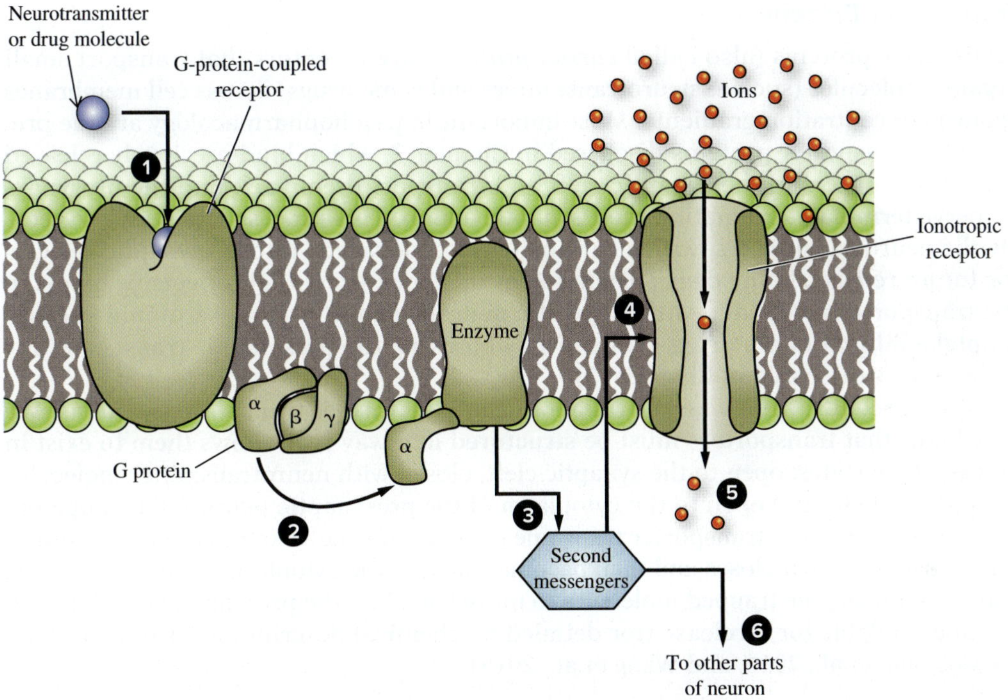

FIGURE 3.6 Second Messengers. Compare the *indirect* process shown here with the *direct* process shown in Figure 3.4. **1.** A neurotransmitter or drug molecule binds to a G-protein-coupled receptor. **2.** The released alpha component of the attached G protein activates an enzyme. **3.** The enzyme produces second messenger molecules. **4.** A second messenger molecule activates an ionotropic receptor. **5.** Ions flow through the channel of the ionotropic receptor into the neuron. **6.** Second messenger molecules initiate other biochemical reactions elsewhere in the neuron.

as **second messengers** (see Figure 3.6; the "first messenger" is the neurotransmitter or drug molecule that binds to the G-protein-coupled receptor).

Second messengers provide the significant benefit of increasing the strength of the original extracellular signal of the first messenger—that is, the first messenger can trigger the synthesis of many second messenger molecules, which can elicit a cascade of effects inside the cell. Thus, G-protein-coupled receptors are essentially intermediaries that facilitate a wide variety of biological responses via the production of second messengers. An example of a second messenger involved in many biological processes is the enzyme cyclic adenosine monophosphate (cyclic AMP, or cAMP), which both activates other intracellular enzymes and affects the activity of specific genes within the nucleus of the neuron.

Most neurotransmitter receptors are G-protein-coupled receptors, a large and diverse family that includes not only the presynaptic autoreceptors discussed in Chapter 2, which provide feedback to prevent excessive neurotransmitter release, but also many of the receptors discussed throughout this book because they mediate the synaptic effects of neurotransmitters involved in the actions of psychoactive drugs.

Transporter Proteins

Transporter proteins (also called *carrier proteins*) are receptors that transport small organic molecules (such as neurotransmitters and some drugs) across cell membranes against concentration gradients. Most important in psychopharmacology are the presynaptic transporter proteins discussed in Chapter 2, which bind previously released neurotransmitters in the synaptic cleft and transport them back into the presynaptic nerve terminal, terminating their synaptic action. This process also serves to recycle the neurotransmitters, which can then be "repackaged" into presynaptic vesicles for future release. Many drugs discussed in this book exert their effects by blocking the transporter associated with a specific neurotransmitter (e.g., serotonin-specific reuptake inhibitors are drugs that work by blocking the presynaptic transporter for serotonin, as discussed in Chapter 12).

Until recently, little was known about the structure of transporter proteins. We now know that transporters must be structured in a way that allows them to exist in at least three states: open to the synaptic cleft, closed with neurotransmitter molecules "trapped" inside, and open to the cytoplasm of the presynaptic neuron. When open to the synaptic cleft, the transporter traps one or more molecules of released transmitter. The transporter then closes and then becomes open to the cytoplasm of the presynaptic neuron, allowing the trapped molecules to move back into the presynaptic terminal and become available for rerelease (for detailed biochemical descriptions of transporters, see Coleman et al., 2016, and Wang et al., 2015).

Acute and Chronic Receptor Effects

When a neurotransmitter or a psychoactive drug binds to a receptor, it has an acute effect—that is, it produces an immediate response. For example, the drugs nicotine, cocaine, and methamphetamine all bind to receptors on dopamine-releasing neurons, producing an immediate release of dopamine from those neurons. Dopamine activates our reward circuit (described in Chapters 2 and 4), and a positively stimulating or pleasurable feeling follows. Many medications also exert acute effects; for example, methylphenidate can rapidly relieve the symptoms of attention deficit/hyperactivity disorder (ADHD), potent opioid analgesics can rapidly relieve severe pain, and certain sedatives can rapidly induce drowsiness, making them useful in the treatment of insomnia. Similarly, many of the side effects of drugs (dry mouth, unwanted sedation, blurred vision, and so on) are acute effects that result from the drugs' binding at other receptors.

In contrast to acute effects, neurotransmitters and psychoactive drugs can also have chronic effects—long-term changes in their receptors and in neuronal functioning—as a result of their presence over a period of time. When a neurotransmitter, an **agonist** (a drug that mimics the neurotransmitter by binding to and activating its receptor), or an **antagonist** (a drug that blocks the action of the neurotransmitter by binding to but not activating its receptor) is continually in contact with receptors, the neurons "adapt," as illustrated in Figure 3.7:

- The left panel of the figure shows the normal situation: neurotransmitter molecules are released intermittently, so the receptors for that neurotransmitter

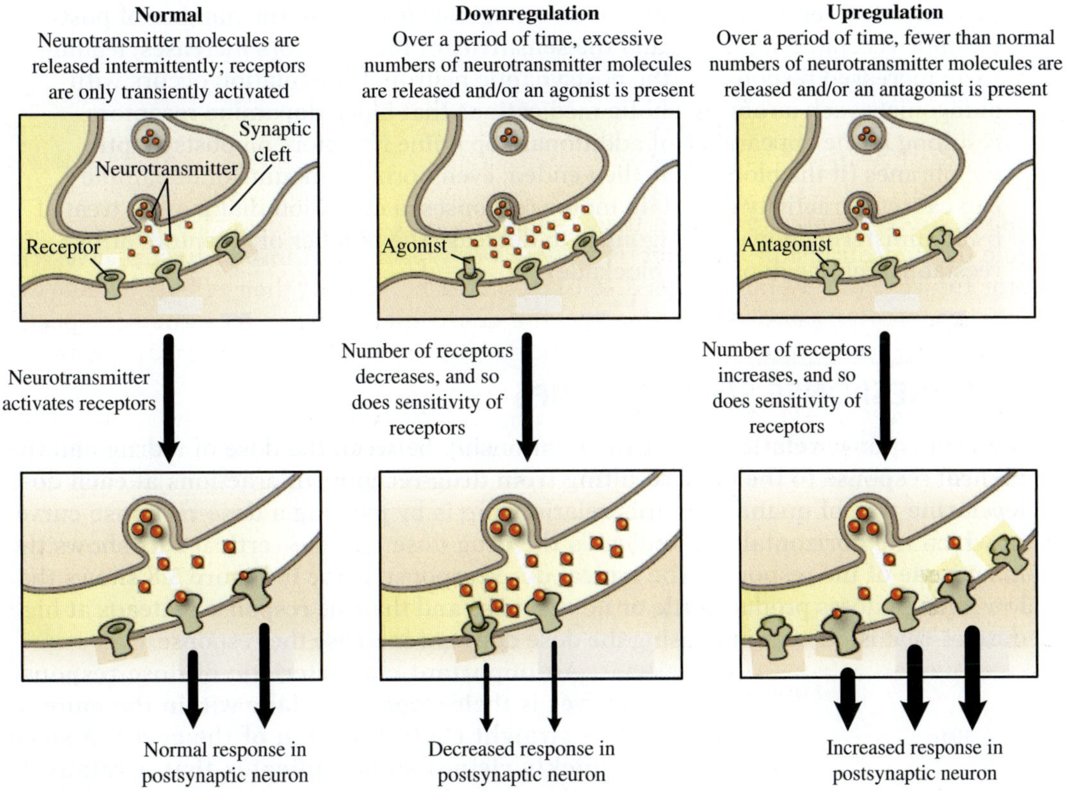

FIGURE 3.7 Downregulation and Upregulation. Downregulation is a decrease in the response of postsynaptic neurons due to the release of excessive numbers of neurotransmitter molecules and/or the presence of an agonist. Upregulation is an increase in the response of postsynaptic neurons due to the release of fewer than normal numbers of neurotransmitter molecules and/or the presence of an antagonist.

are only transiently stimulated, and the action of the neurotransmitter is terminated in the usual way (i.e., by reuptake by transporter proteins and/or by enzymatic breakdown).

- The middle panel of Figure 3.7 shows the chronic effect known as **downregulation** (or *desensitization*): if there are excessive numbers of neurotransmitter molecules and/or an agonist is present, the number of postsynaptic receptors decreases and the sensitivity of the receptors decreases, leading to a decreased response by the postsynaptic neuron. Downregulation may account for some types of tolerance—for example, tolerance to heroin, in which increased amounts of the drug are required to obtain the opioid effect, may develop after a few weeks of continuous exposure to the drug, due to downregulation of the postsynaptic neurons.
- The right panel of Figure 3.7 shows the chronic effect known as **upregulation** (the reverse of downregulation): if there are fewer than normal numbers of

neurotransmitter molecules and/or an antagonist is present, the number of postsynaptic receptors increases and the sensitivity of the receptors increases, leading to an increased response by the postsynaptic neuron. Upregulation occurs with antagonists such as antipsychotic medications that block dopamine receptors, resulting in the appearance of additional dopamine receptors on postsynaptic membranes (if the blockade is then ended, even normal amounts of dopamine can cause overactivity of certain motor responses, a condition that may be treated by administering dopamine agonists to decrease the number of receptors or by reestablishing the dopamine blockade).

DOSE-RESPONSE RELATIONSHIPS

A **dose-response relationship** is the relationship between the dose of a drug and the clinical response to the drug resulting from drug-receptor interactions at each dose level. One way of quantifying this relationship is by plotting a dose-response curve, in which the horizontal axis indicates the drug dose and the vertical axis shows the magnitude of the response. The typical dose-response curve in Figure 3.8 shows that low-enough doses produce little or no response and that the response plateaus at high doses—that is, further increasing the dose does not increase the response.

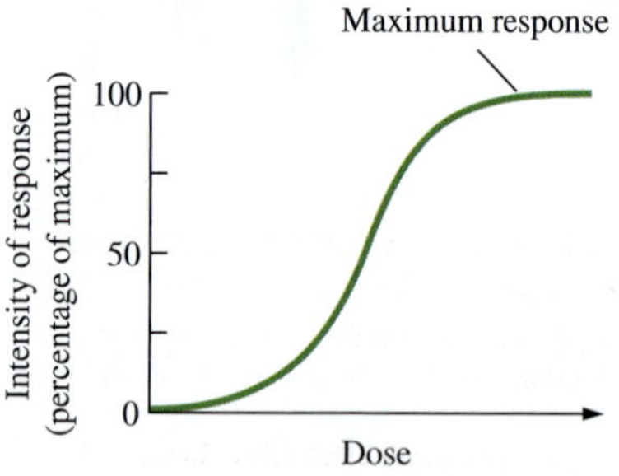

FIGURE 3.8 A Dose-Response Curve. The curve shows the intensity of response to a drug at each dose level. The intensity of response is measured as a percentage of the maximum response.

An important characteristic of dose-response curves is their slope, especially within the more or less straight central portion of the curve. A steep (quickly rising) slope indicates that a relatively small increase in the dose produces a relatively large increase in the response, whereas a flatter (more slowly rising) slope indicates the opposite, that a small increase in the dose produces only a small increase in the response. This is clearly illustrated in Figure 3.9, where the slope of the caffeine curve is much less steep than the slopes of the methamphetamine and dextroamphetamine curves, meaning that small increases in the dose of the latter two drugs would produce much greater responses than a small increase in the dose of caffeine.

Potency and Efficacy

Figure 3.9 also illustrates two other important types of information conveyed by dose-response curves: potency and efficacy. The **potency** of a drug is the amount of the drug required to produce a response of a given intensity. Thus, if two drugs produce responses of equal intensity, but one does so at half the dose level of the other, the former drug is considered to be twice as potent as the latter. In Figure 3.9, the dose-response curves show that methamphetamine is more potent than dextroamphetamine because a lower dose of methamphetamine produces the same level

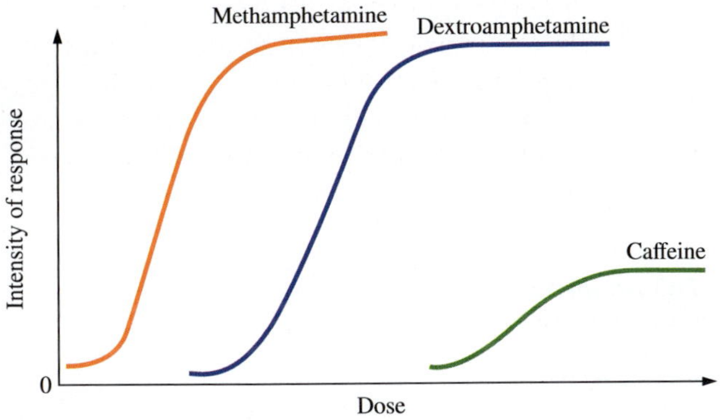

FIGURE 3.9 Dose-Response Curves: Slope, Potency, and Efficacy. *Slope:* Over the steeply sloping portions of the methamphetamine and dextroamphetamine curves, a small increase in the dose is associated with a significant increase in the intensity of response; in contrast, a small increase in the dose of caffeine has much less of an effect on the response. *Potency and efficacy:* The potency of a drug decreases as the dose required to produce a given intensity of response increases. Efficacy is a measure of the maximum intensity of response obtainable from a drug. Thus, methamphetamine has greater potency than dextroamphetamine, while their efficacy is about equal. Caffeine has much less potency and efficacy than either of the other drugs.

of response as a higher dose of dextroamphetamine (and both those drugs are more potent than caffeine). However, for psychoactive medications, potency may be relatively unimportant because it makes little difference whether the dose required to produce the desired response is 1 milligram or 100 milligrams, unless higher doses produce undue toxicity.

Unlike potency, which measures the relationship between changes in dosage and changes in response, **efficacy** simply refers to the maximum response that a drug can produce. Thus, a drug that can produce the maximum possible response has 100% efficacy, whereas a drug that can produce only half the maximum possible response (regardless of dosage) has 50% efficacy. In Figure 3.9, for example, you can see that methamphetamine and dextroamphetamine have about equal efficacy (their maximum responses are about equal) and that caffeine is less efficacious than the amphetamines (caffeine is incapable of achieving the same maximal response as a stimulant). Another example is provided by aspirin, which is much less efficacious than morphine at producing an analgesic effect.

Agonists and Antagonists

Dose-response curves help us understand the relationship between drug-receptor binding and biological responses to drugs that are agonists or antagonists. Agonists have both affinity and efficacy: they bind to their receptors with sufficient strength,

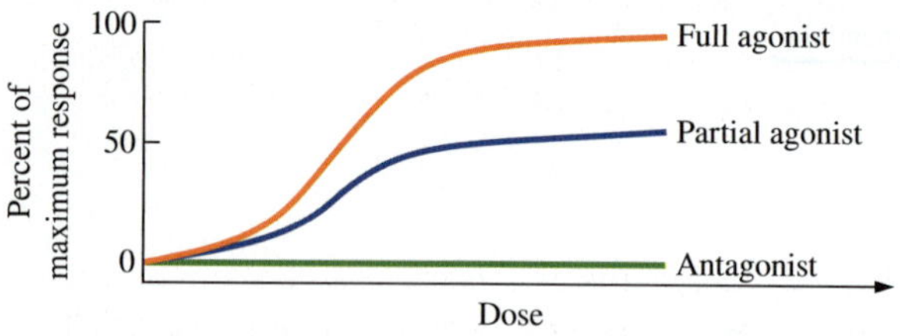

FIGURE 3.10 Dose-Response Curves: Full Agonists, Partial Agonists, and Antagonists. A full agonist can produce the maximum possible effect; a partial agonist is not able to elicit the maximum effect at any dose; an antagonist does not produce any overt effect.

and once bound, they produce the targeted response. A *full agonist* is capable of eliciting the maximum response (which may be much greater than the targeted response), whereas a *partial agonist* is not, regardless of the dose. The dose-response curves in Figure 3.10 illustrate the different efficacies of full and partial agonists versus the zero efficacy of antagonists (drugs that bind to but do not activate their receptors).[3]

Like agonists, antagonists can also be subclassified, on the basis of whether they are competitive or noncompetitive and whether they are reversible or irreversible. *Competitive* means that the antagonist binds to the same site on the receptor as the neurotransmitter or an agonist (i.e., it competes against the neurotransmitter or agonist for access to that site), whereas *noncompetitive* means that the antagonist binds to a different site on the receptor (but still blocks the activation of the receptor). *Reversible* means that the binding of the antagonist can be undone (either naturally over time or due to competition from a neurotransmitter or an agonist), whereas *irreversible* means that the binding cannot be undone (an irreversible antagonist forms a covalent bond with the receptor, and this bond cannot be overcome). The binding of an irreversible antagonist permanently deactivates the receptor and is usually followed by rapid recycling of the now nonfunctional receptor protein.

Figure 3.11 shows how the dose-response curve for an agonist is affected by the presence of a competitive, reversible antagonist versus a noncompetitive, irreversible antagonist. Figure 3.11A shows that the blocking action of the competitive, reversible antagonist can be overcome by increasing the dose of the agonist—in other words, if enough molecules of agonist are added, they will outcompete the antagonist and

[3]Partial agonists include the nicotine replacement medication varenicline (discussed in Chapter 6) and the opioid medications tramadol and buprenorphine (discussed in Chapter 10). When a partial agonist such as buprenorphine is administered to a person who is dependent on a full agonist (e.g., heroin), drug withdrawal symptoms might be expected (this is discussed Chapter 4).

DR. J'S MUSINGS 3.2

From Basic Pharmacology to Therapeutics

The opioid receptor provides a useful pharmacological context for thinking about the uses and effects of agonists and antagonists. Oxycodone and methadone are full agonists at the opioid receptor, buprenorphine is a partial agonist, and naloxone is a competitive antagonist, and each of these drugs has its own place in therapeutics. Oxycodone is a strong opioid analgesic but has a high potential for abuse and dependency. Methadone and buprenorphine are used in medication-assisted therapy for opioid dependence, and naloxone can be a lifesaver in countering opioid agonist overdoses. Consider some statistics confirming the cost effectiveness of these treatments for opioid abuse disorders in a cohort of 100,000 patients over five years (Fairley et al., 2021):

- In the absence of treatment, more than 42,000 overdoses resulting in more than 12,000 deaths were estimated to occur.
- An estimated reduction of 10.7% in the number of overdoses was associated with treatment with methadone, and an estimated reduction of 22.0% was associated with treatment with buprenorphine. When these treatments were combined with nondrug treatments, the estimated reduction in overdoses ranged from 21.0% to 31.4%.
- An estimated reduction of 6.0% in the number of deaths from overdoses was associated with treatment with methadone, and an estimated reduction of 13.9% was associated with treatment with buprenorphine. When these treatments were combined with nondrug treatments, the estimated reduction in deaths from overdoses was 16.9%.
- Combined lifetime savings in health care and criminal justice costs were estimated at $25,000–$105,000 per person.

eventually displace it from the receptor binding sites. That explains why the dose-response curve shifts to the right in the presence of the antagonist and why the height of the curve remains the same: the shift to the right reflects the increased dose of the agonist, and the unchanged height shows that the increased dose achieves the same efficacy as the lesser dose without the antagonist. In Figure 3.11B, we see that the presence of an irreversible antagonist causes a reduction in the height of the dose-response curve (i.e., a reduction in efficacy) but does not cause any shift of the curve to the right or left.

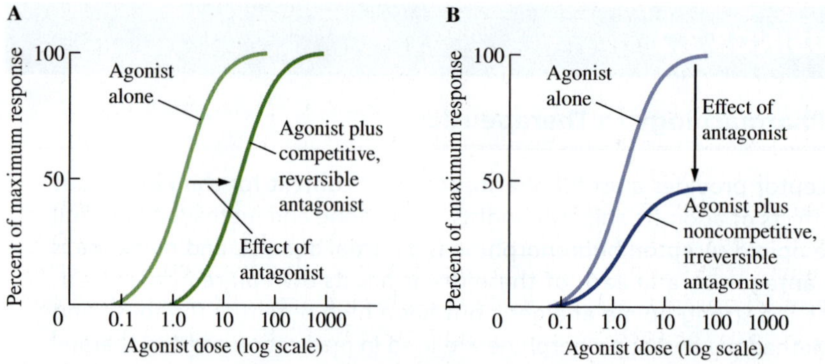

FIGURE 3.11 Dose-Response Curves: Agonists in the Presence of Antagonists. **A.** The dose-response curve for an agonist shifts to the right in the presence of a competitive, reversible antagonist, indicating that a higher dose of the agonist is needed to achieve the same efficacy, but the agonist's maximum efficacy remains the same (here, 100%). **B.** In the presence of a noncompetitive, irreversible antagonist, the agonist's maximum efficacy (represented by the height of the dose-response curve) is much reduced.

RESPONSIVENESS TO DRUGS

The responsiveness of individuals and populations to a particular drug is determined by a number of different factors, the most important of which are discussed in the sections that follow.

Variability

The dose of a drug that produces a specific response varies considerably across individuals. Such variability can result from individual differences in rates of drug absorption and metabolism; previous drug use; various physical, psychological, and emotional states; and other causes. Whatever the cause of the variability, any population will include a few individuals who are remarkably sensitive to a particular drug (i.e., individuals who show large effects and side effects in response to the drug) and a few who are remarkably drug tolerant (i.e., individuals requiring large doses of the drug to produce therapeutic results). The variability usually follows a predictable pattern, the familiar bell-shaped curve; however, specific populations sometimes show unique patterns of responsiveness, usually due to genetic alterations in drug metabolism that are widespread in the population.

The Therapeutic Index

Studies with experimental animals are performed to determine two useful measures of responsiveness to a drug: the ED_{50} and the LD_{50} (ED stands for "effective dose," and LD stands for "lethal dose"). The ED_{50} is the dose of the drug required to elicit the desired effect in 50% of the animals given the drug. Similarly, the LD_{50} is the dose that results in the death of 50% of the animals given the drug. The ratio of the LD_{50} to the ED_{50} (LD_{50}:ED_{50})—called the **therapeutic index** (or *margin of safety*)—is used as a measure of the relative safety of the drug. In humans, for an extra margin of safety, the therapeutic index of a drug is calculated as the ratio of the dose that results in toxicity (not death) in 50% of those given the drug to the ED_{50}.

Figure 3.12 illustrates the concept of the therapeutic index in animal studies. Here, the therapeutic index (LD_{50}:ED_{50}) is 100:10, or 10. Note that, with this particular drug, the ED curve (the sleep curve) and the LD curve (the death curve) overlap (starting at a dose of 10 milligrams), meaning that there is not a dose at which one could expect that 100% of the mice will sleep and none will die. Such a dose would exist only if there were no overlap in the two curves—that is, if the LD curve were all to the right of the dose at which the ED curve plateaus (about 60 milligrams). In other words, given some specific ED_{50}, the higher the LD_{50} (i.e., the greater the therapeutic index), the easier it is to find a dose with a high probability of a good response and a low probability of a toxic or even lethal response. Thus, the benzodiazepine drug diazepam (discussed in Chapter 13), with a therapeutic index of about 100, can be administered with a much greater margin of safety than lithium products (with a therapeutic index of 2 or 3), where it can be difficult to find a dose that is therapeutic but not unduly toxic.

This very simple and basic summary of the therapeutic index concept may be misleading. In actual practice, application of the concept is complicated. Nevertheless, the determination of a drug's therapeutic index is vital in answering important pharmacodynamic questions regarding drug efficacy and safety.

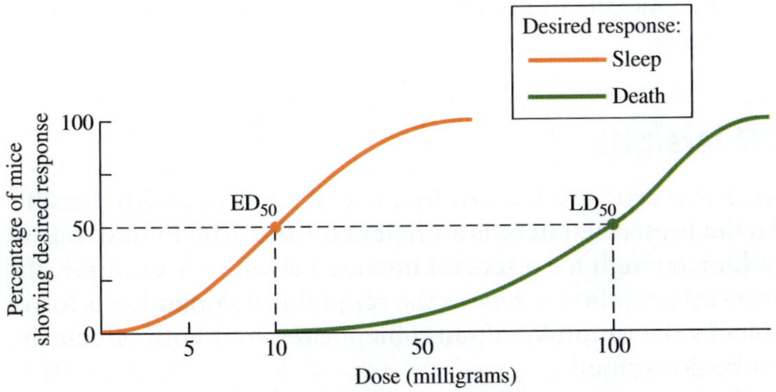

FIGURE 3.12 Therapeutic Index. The therapeutic index of this drug is 10 (LD_{50}:ED_{50} = 100:10 = 10), a low number indicating that it will be difficult to find a dose that will be effective at putting most mice to sleep without killing some mice. If the LD curve (the death curve) began at a dose of 75 milligrams (instead of 10 milligrams), LD_{50} would be much higher than 100 milligrams, the therapeutic index would be greater, and it would not be a problem to find a dose with 100% efficacy and little danger of killing any mice (e.g., a dose of 60 milligrams).

Drug Interactions: Polypharmacy

Combining medications to improve therapeutic outcomes, a practice termed **polypharmacy**, is common in the treatment of mental health disorders—usually because so few patients achieve remission of their illness from a single medication (Zigman and Blier, 2012). However, polypharmacy carries various risks that should be considered in order to reduce the likelihood of inappropriate, or "irrational," polypharmacy (Zigman and Blier, 2012)—that is, in order to avoid exposing patients to unhelpful or even harmful combinations of drugs, including combinations with nonprescription drugs that patients might be using:

- *Pharmacodynamic redundancy.* Two or more drugs are pharmacodynamically redundant when they have the same or overlapping mechanisms of action. For example, benzodiazepine tranquilizers, alcohol, and marijuana are all sedating and also cause loss of coordination. This redundancy of action may have little consequence if the doses of the drugs are low, but combinations of these drugs at higher doses can be dangerous both to the user and to others, as when driving.
- *Pharmacodynamic interactions.* Two or more drugs have undesirable pharmacodynamic interactions when their effects oppose each other—for example, when antipsychotics that block dopamine receptors are combined with ADHD medications that increase dopamine levels.
- *Pharmacokinetic interactions.* When a drug either increases or decreases the rate of hepatic metabolism of one or more other drugs, this pharmacokinetic interaction can have an undesirable effect on the plasma levels of those other drugs. For example (as discussed in Chapter 1), carbamazepine increases the rate of metabolism of certain other medicines, reducing their blood concentration and their effectiveness. Conversely, valproic acid can inhibit the metabolism of other drugs, such as lamotrigine, increasing their blood concentrations and potentially increasing their toxicity or their unwanted side effects.

Dosing and Clinical Oversight

Sometimes, prescribed doses of a drug are too low because of concern about possible side effects, and sometimes the prescribed dose is sufficient for the drug to have one of its intended effects but not high enough for a second intended effect. For example, the dose at which the antidepressant venlafaxine blocks the reuptake of dopamine is lower than the dose at which it blocks the reuptake of norepinephrine, so if both effects are desired, a higher dose must be prescribed.

Drugs started when an illness is severe might need to be reassessed after the patient has stabilized. Or the natural history of a disorder might produce spontaneous remission, allowing dose reduction or even elimination of a drug. Or the appearance of new symptoms might be a result of long-term drug exposure (tolerance or development of a side effect), which might be better treated by reducing the dose or stopping the medication than by adding a new agent (i.e., better than polypharmacy). Ongoing clinical evaluation and oversight is crucial in dealing with all these possibilities.

Drug Toxicity

All drugs can produce harmful side effects as well as beneficial therapeutic effects. It is important to categorize the harmful effects of drugs in terms of their severity in order to recognize and distinguish between effects that cause temporary inconvenience or discomfort and effects that can lead to organ damage, permanent disability, or even death.

Often, some side effects must be tolerated if a drug is to achieve the desired therapeutic effects, but if the side effects are serious, they may be a limiting factor in the use of the drug. The distinction between therapeutic effects and side effects is relative and depends on the purpose for which the drug is administered: one person's side effect may be another person's therapeutic effect. For example, morphine induces constipation, which may be an undesirable side effect that must be tolerated in a patient receiving morphine for pain relief but a therapeutic effect in a patient receiving morphine to treat severe diarrhea.

Severe side effects include blood disorders and abnormalities in fetal development, as well as liver or kidney damage and allergic reactions. Damage to the liver or kidneys results from the role of these organs in concentrating, metabolizing, and excreting drugs. Allergic reactions to drugs may take many different forms, from mild skin rashes to fatal shock, and may be difficult to control. Other types of side effects can often be eliminated or at least made tolerable by a simple reduction in dosage, but dose reduction may have no effect on a drug allergy if exposure to any amount of the drug can cause the reaction.

Placebos

A medical dictionary published in 1811 defined a placebo as "any medicine adopted more to please than to benefit the patient." More recently, **placebo effects** have been defined as positive clinical outcomes attributable to the psychosocial context and individual treatment expectations rather than to the effects of the medication or other treatment (Colloca, 2018; Colloca and Barsky, 2020). As such, placebo effects have been observed across a variety of disorders, including pain, Parkinson's disease, depression, anxiety, sleep disorders, and immunological and endocrinological disorders.

In research studies and in clinical practice, placebos have been found to mimic the actions of nonplacebo treatments and to promote the release of neurotransmitters that contribute to the clinical effectiveness of treatments both in humans and in nonhuman animals. Thus, placebo effects are not merely psychological but, through the release of neurotransmitters, can be measurable physical effects. Indeed, the wise clinician will recognize this and use placebo effects as a part of therapy, both pharmacological and psychotherapeutic (Erick and Zipfel, 2019). The recently formed Society for Interdisciplinary Placebo Studies explores and promotes placebo effect in medical treatment, in psychotherapy, and in complementary and alternative treatments.

In drug development and evaluation studies, placebo effects can profoundly influence research outcomes. For this reason, whenever possible, research studies are "randomized, double-blinded, placebo controlled, crossover" (Micallef et al., 2018) so neither the participants nor the investigators know which participants were given the drug being studied and which were given a placebo. However, even this "gold-standard" research format is not foolproof—for example, if the study drug causes notable side effects while the placebo does not, participants may notice the difference and correctly guess whether they received the drug or the placebo. In the words of a research team, "It should be the goal of therapeutic trials to minimize the placebo effect in clinical trials, while utilizing and maximizing it in clinical routine" (Erick and Klosterhalfen, 2019).

In general, research participants can be divided into three groups: those who sometimes show placebo effects (typically, more than 50% of participants), those who always do (typically, fewer than 20%), and those who never do (typically, around 30%), depending on the severity of the condition and the specific context. Placebo effects are generally greater on subjective "quality of life" measures than on the actual condition being treated, but not always. In a study testing whether a placebo could have real biological effects (Levine et al., 1978), participants recovering from dental surgery were given two doses of drugs that they were told could be morphine, a placebo, or naloxone. Morphine provides pain relief by promoting the release of endorphins, and naloxone is a morphine antagonist—it blocks that action. Of interest in this study were the participants given a placebo for their first dose and naloxone for their second dose. About 40% of those participants were "responders"—they experienced significant pain relief after their first dose, a placebo—and the others were "nonresponders" who experienced little or no pain relief after their first dose. After receiving naloxone for their second dose, responders reported a much greater increase in pain that did nonresponders. This shows that the pain relief produced by placebos in responders was not simply imagined but was the result of the release of endorphins, an effect that was then blocked by the dose of naloxone. In other words, the placebo effect in responders was an actual biological effect.

Three types of factors contribute to placebo effects: the interaction between the practitioner and the patient, the expectations of the patient, and conditioned reactions to drugs (Schedlowski et al., 2015). Evidence suggests that genetics may also play a role in responses to placebos. For example, researchers have found different placebo effects in people with variants of the gene that codes for COMT (catechol-O-methyltransferase), an enzyme that affects synaptic levels of dopamine and thus plays a key role in processes associated with placebo effects, such as reward and pain. In one study, participants with irritable bowel syndrome were divided into three different groups: a control group that received no treatment, an augmented placebo group given fake acupuncture by a *sympathetic* therapist, and a limited placebo group given fake acupuncture by an *unsympathetic* therapist. The participants were assessed for their COMT variant, and results showed that the participants in the two placebo groups who were most likely to report pain relief after the fake acupuncture had a high-dopamine variant of the gene (Hall et al., 2012).

Sometimes, a placebo can have a negative effect, in which case it is termed a *nocebo* (Colloca and Barsky, 2020), or the effect may be less positive than the effect of a placebo given under different conditions. Consider, for example, a study in which 12 participants with Parkinson's disease were told they would each get two injections, one of an expensive drug that cost $1500 per treatment and the other costing only $100 per treatment, although both injections were actually a placebo (saline) (Espay et al., 2015). After an injection of what they were told was the "expensive" drug, participants showed a 7-point improvement on average in a motor test, compared with only a 3-point improvement after an injection of what they were told was the "cheap" drug. This result suggests that participants' lower expectations of what they thought was the cheaper drug had a negative influence on the placebo effect, and this could imply that patients in general might not benefit as much from placebo effects with generic drugs (Andrade, 2015).

Placebos may provide relief, but they rarely cure and they do not alter the pathophysiology of diseases (Kaptchuk and Miller, 2015). Nevertheless, they are not "dummy pills"; they can meaningfully enhance treatment effects. In a study of 42 people undergoing brain stimulation surgery for advanced Parkinsonism, participants were given an injection of saline but were told that it was the antiparkinsonian drug apomorphine (Benedetti et al., 2016). Results showed that the saline injection was followed by signs of improvement (increased neural activity) in participants who had been given one to four daily doses of apomorphine prior to surgery but not in participants who had not previously been given apomorphine. In addition, a neurologist who was "blind" to which participants had been treated with apomorphine determined that the symptoms of the previously treated participants had decreased. In fact, the more previous treatments of apomorphine participants had received, the greater was the improvement after the saline injection. Because it takes only a few hours for apomorphine to be almost completely eliminated from the body, residual amounts of that drug could not account for these effects. Moreover, in participants who had been given four prior doses, the responses to apomorphine and to the placebo were the same. This suggests the possibility of developing effective treatments in which a placebo is paired intermittently with a subtherapeutic drug dose, with the potential to reduce side effects, limit problems with drug dependency and toxicity, and reduce costs.

CHAPTER REVIEW

1. Pick the correct choices in the parentheses: (Pharmacokinetics/Pharmacodynamics) is the study of what drugs do to the body, and (pharmacokinetics/pharmacodynamics) is the study of what the body does to drugs.
2. True or false: To have its intended effect, a drug must exhibit both specificity and affinity for a given type of receptor.
3. True or false: Optical isomers of drugs always have identical pharmacological effects.
4. Which receptor type—ionotropic or metabotropic—fits each characteristic: (a) can be found on postsynaptic and presynaptic membranes; (b) has an attached G protein; (c) contains an ion channel; (d) has effects mediated by second messengers
5. Which type of receptor carries neurotransmitter molecules back into the presynaptic nerve terminal?
6. Drug 1 has greater potency than drug 2, and the two drugs have equal efficacy. Do their dose-response curves rise to the same maximum height? Does the curve for

drug 1 rise to its maximum height at the same dose level as drug 2, at a lower dose level, or at a higher dose level?

7. Arrange these three categories of drugs in order from lowest efficacy to highest efficacy: full agonist, antagonist, partial agonist.
8. Pick the correct choices in the parentheses: Upregulation occurs in the presence of an (agonist/antagonist), and downregulation occurs in the presence of an (agonist/antagonist).
9. What is the difference between a competitive antagonist and noncompetitive antagonist?
10. True or false: The higher a drug's therapeutic index, the harder it is to find a dose with a high probability of a good response and a low probability of a toxic response.
11. Match the numbered factors in responsiveness to drugs with the lettered descriptions:
    1. risks of polypharmacy; 2. causes of variability; 3. placebo effects; 4. effects of drug toxicity
    A. responses to drug treatments that vary with patients' expectations about the treatments; B. previous drug use and individual difference in rates of drug absorption and metabolism; C. responses that range from temporary discomfort to death; D. pharmacodynamic redundancy, pharmacodynamic interactions, and pharmacokinetic interactions

KEY TERMS

affinity
agonist
antagonist
dose-response relationship
downregulation
drug-receptor binding
efficacy
G protein
ionotropic receptors
isomers
metabotropic receptors (G-protein-coupled receptors)
placebo effects
polypharmacy
potency
racemic mixture
second messenger
specificity
therapeutic index
upregulation

PART 2

Pharmacology of Drugs of Abuse

The seven chapters in this part cover the pharmacology of the drugs most associated with compulsive abuse, dependency, and addiction. Chapter 4 presents an overview of the epidemiology and neurobiology of addiction, and the six subsequent chapters present the pharmacology of ethyl alcohol (Chapter 5), caffeine and nicotine (Chapter 6), psychostimulants including cocaine, amphetamines, and nonamphetamines (Chapter 7), psychedelic drugs (Chapter 8), cannabis (Chapter 9), and opioids, including coverage of the socially important effects of the so-called opioid epidemic (Chapter 10).

The therapeutic uses of the drugs covered in this part vary considerably. Ethyl alcohol and nicotine have no therapeutic uses because of their toxicities, and caffeine is limited to occasional use in the treatment of wakefulness and migraine headaches. Other drugs, despite their potential for abuse, have multiple current and potential medical uses. For example:

- Amphetamines and their structural derivatives are used in the treatment of attention deficit/hyperactivity disorder.
- Opioids are irreplaceable for the treatment of severe and otherwise intractable pain.
- Cannabidiol (CBD), an active ingredient in cannabis, may have a range of uses, from treatment of pain and anxiety to treatment of schizophrenia.
- Naturally occurring psychedelics such as psilocybin (found in certain mushrooms) have potential uses in treating depression, anxiety, and posttraumatic stress disorder (PTSD).
- The synthetic psychedelics phencyclidine and ketamine may be useful in treating chronic pain, depression, and substance use disorders including alcohol use disorder.

The fact that these drugs are often abused while also having actual or potential therapeutic uses presents unique challenges for medicine, education, and law enforcement. The federal Controlled Substances Act of 1970 established schedules (categories) of "controlled substances" that classify drugs based upon three criteria: their potential for abuse; their accepted medical uses in the United States, if any; and their safety. The current schedules developed by the Drug Enforcement Administration (DEA)[1] are as follows:

- **Schedule I** drugs are those considered to have a high potential for abuse and no currently accepted medical use and to be unsafe for use even under medical supervision.

  Note: Only Schedule I drugs are considered unsafe for use even under medical supervision. Cannabis (marijuana) is still considered a Schedule I drug by the DEA, even though many U.S. states have legalized marijuana for personal, recreational, and/or medical use. In 2018, the Food and Drug Administration (FDA) and DEA ruled that products including "finished dosage formulations" of CBD, with THC concentrations below 0.1%, will be moved from Schedule 1 to Schedule 5 (THC is tetrahydrocannabinol, the main psychoactive constituent in marijuana). This is the first time the DEA has removed any type of cannabis from Schedule 1.[2]
- **Schedule II** drugs are those considered to have a high potential for abuse that may lead to severe psychological or physical dependence but also to have a currently accepted medical use (in some cases, with severe restrictions).
- **Schedule III** drugs are those considered to have a potential for abuse that may lead to low or moderate physical dependence or high psychological dependence (i.e., less potential for abuse than the drugs in Schedules I and II) and to have a currently accepted medical use.
- **Schedule IV** drugs are those considered to have a lower potential for abuse than the drugs in Schedule III and to have a currently accepted medical use.
- **Schedule V** drugs are those considered to have a lower potential for abuse than the drugs in Schedule IV and to have a currently accepted medical use.

[1]See www.deadiversion.usdoj.gov/schedules/.

[2]Other drugs currently classified in Schedule I are heroin, LSD, mescaline (peyote), MDMA ("ecstasy"), GHB (gamma-hydroxybutyric acid), psilocybin, synthetic marijuana and analogs (Spice, K2), methaqualone (Quaalude), khat (cathinone), and bath salts (MDPV). Certainly, some of these drugs have no known medical use, current or potential; others, however, such as marijuana, mescaline, and psilocybin, may have therapeutic potential.

CHAPTER 4

Addiction: Terminology, Epidemiology, Neurobiology, and Pharmacology

CHAPTER OUTLINE

Drug abuse has probably been a social problem for thousands of years, ever since grain was first fermented (yielding ethyl alcohol with its intoxicating effects) and natural substances were found that produced euphoria (cocaine, from the coca plant), pain relief (opioids, from the opium poppy), or altered states of consciousness (psilocybin, from certain species of mushrooms, and mescaline, from the peyote cactus). Use and abuse of these ancient drugs continue to the present, leading to acute problems such as intoxication and longer-term problems including addiction.

This chapter begins with a section that reviews the continuing debate about the meaning of the term *addiction* and that frames a definition of the term to support the discussions of addiction throughout the book. The chapter then reviews current U.S. trends in drug abuse and addiction, discusses the neurobiological mechanisms believed to be responsible for addiction, and summarizes current approaches to the treatment of addiction. The principles overviewed in this chapter will support our discussions of individual drugs of abuse in later chapters.

TERMINOLOGY AND THE CONCEPT OF ADDICTION

The American Psychiatric Association's *Diagnostic and Statistical Manual of Mental Disorders* (DSM) provides criteria for what constitutes substance use disorders and terminology for describing those disorders. Both the criteria and the terminology have evolved considerably over the course of the DSM's five editions (Schneider, 2019):

- The first through third editions (1952–1993) used the term *addiction* to describe substance use disorders such as opioid addiction.
- The fourth edition (1994) substituted the term *dependence* for *addiction*, which meant, for example, that a person formerly described as addicted to an opioid such as heroin would be described as "opioid dependent."
- The fifth and most recent edition (DSM-5) (American Psychiatric Association, 2022) dropped all use of the term *dependence*, continued to avoid the term *addiction*, and introduced the overarching term **substance use disorder (SUD)** (along with more specific terms such as *opioid use disorder*[3]). In DSM-5, SUDs are defined as mild, moderate, or severe, depending on the number of diagnostic criteria met in each individual case.

Most patients on more than minimal doses of prescribed opioids for more than a couple of weeks will develop a specific set of withdrawal symptoms if they stop the drug suddenly. This reaction is not indicative of addiction, but rather of physical dependence (see Chapter 1), a physiological change in the body in response to ongoing use of certain drugs. This type of change may occur not only with opioids but also with drugs that are not on the schedules of controlled substances, such as some antidepressants (e.g., paroxetine, discussed in Chapter 12). As an unfortunate result of the change from *addiction* to *dependence* in DSM terminology in 1994, the term *opioid dependent* was applied both to patients being treated with opioids for chronic pain and to people who were addicted to an opioid, because individuals in both groups would display withdrawal symptoms if their drug were stopped. That is, the change in terminology obscured the difference between physical dependence and addiction: opioid use may lead to both physical dependence and addiction, but it is perfectly possible to be physically dependent without being "addicted."

In DSM-5, the three elements required to diagnose an SUD indicate clearly that SUDs are now viewed as behavioral disorders:

- Loss of control (also termed *compulsive use*)
- Continuation despite significant adverse consequences

[3]An odd aspect of the discussion of opioid use disorder in DSM-5 is that withdrawal is one of the 11 criteria for diagnosing opioid use disorder but not for individuals taking opioids solely under medical supervision. In other words, DSM-5 says that withdrawal after taking prescribed opioids should not be used as a reason for diagnosing opium use disorder. (See the discussion of withdrawal and physical dependence in Chapter 1.)

- Preoccupation or obsession with obtaining, using, and recovering from the effect of the substance

This view of addiction is not a new concept, as can be seen in this passage defining addiction as

> a behavioral pattern of drug use, characterized by overwhelming involvement with the use of a drug (compulsive use), the securing of its supply and a high tendency to relapse after withdrawal. In addition, it is characterized by craving, withdrawal and tolerance. (Jaffe, 1980, p. 536)

In recent years, the concept of addiction has broadened to encompass not only addiction to substances but also addiction to sociocultural and psychological influences (e.g., addiction to playing video games or to viewing pornography). **Addiction** is best understood as an individual's adjustment to their environment, an adjustment that is often self-destructive and that represents a pattern of coping through habituation.

DR. J'S MUSINGS 4.1

Dependency, Addiction, and Treatments for Pain

In 1994, when DSM-4 mistakenly stopped using the term *addiction* and began using *dependence* instead, the unfortunate implication was that anyone who developed physical dependence was addicted. Then, in 1995, pain was labeled as the "fifth vital sign," meaning that all patients were to be asked about pain, even during routine physical exams in which the patient did not spontaneously report any pain. If the reported pain was serious enough, opioids were to be prescribed to the point of "no pain" (at that time, it was thought that appropriate use of opioids was rarely associated with addiction). In 2000, after Congress passed a resolution establishing the "decade of pain control and research," opioid prescribing skyrocketed, as did the marketing of opioids. In 2001, for example, the maker of OxyContin spent $200 million on marketing the drug, and by 2002 sales of OxyContin had topped the $1.5 billion mark. Between 1991 and 2013, the number of annual opioid prescriptions in the United States increased from 76 million to 207 million, with corresponding increases in the number of cases of addiction, overdose, and death. Eventually, the concept of the "fifth vital sign" was abandoned, and in 2016 the government reversed course and issued strict revised prescribing standards related to the safe and judicious use of opioids. However, this has made it much more difficult for physicians to prescribe opioids needed to treat chronic pain, with the unfortunate result that many patients eventually end up seeking opioids from illicit sources. Further, when illicit sources of commercial opioids became too expensive, many of those patients resorted to heroin, which was much less expensive. Thus, patients who started out looking for medical help to relieve chronic pain ended up addicted to an illegal drug! What a mess we created!

Rather than being thought of as a distinct disease entity, it is better thought of as a continuum of feeling and behavior.

In summary, most patients taking prescribed opioids for an extended period of time do develop a physical dependence on opioids (i.e., they would show withdrawal symptoms if the drug were discontinued). However, DSM-5 specifically says that patients taking opioids solely under appropriate medical supervision should not be considered to have met this criterion for diagnosis of an SUD. In other words, withdrawal symptoms in a patient on prescribed opioids are not considered a sign of addiction. Specifically referring to opioid addiction, DSM-5 introduced the term "opioid use disorder" while entirely deleting any mention of the term "dependence." *Confusion still reigns!*

THE ADDICTION PROBLEM: EXTENT, COMORBIDITIES, AND ATTEMPTS AT SOLUTIONS

The estimated cost of drug use in the United States is more than half a trillion dollars annually, including not only lost productivity but also related costs such as crime and health care (National Institute on Drug Abuse, 2020c). But the cost is more than just monetary: the public health consequences are also staggering, in terms of social dysfunction, unemployment, academic failure, and domestic and other violence. Consider the following:

- Between 1999 and 2017, more than 700,000 Americans died from drug overdoses, contributing to recent reductions in overall life expectancy in the United States (McGinty and Barry, 2020). Most of these deaths are of young healthy males.
- About 8–10% of Americans 12 years of age or older (i.e., 20–22 million people) are addicted to alcohol or other drugs. Of the estimated 20.2 million Americans who met the DSM-5 criteria for an SUD in 2018, nearly 89% did not receive specialized treatment for their condition, and about 90% of those persons felt that they did not need treatment (Volkow et al., 2016a).

Comorbidities

Approximately, one-third of people with a diagnosed SUD have a diagnosed **comorbid disorder**—that is, a *dual diagnosis* (Subodh et al., 2017). The most commonly observed disorder comorbid with an SUD is major depression; across studies, SUDs and depression are found to occur together in 12–80% of cases (Tirado-Muñoz et al., 2018). When they occur together, both of these disorders are more difficult to treat, and treatments are less likely to be successful.

Disorders other than depression are also often comorbid with an SUD, as indicated by the following percentages (which apply equally to males and females): 47% of those who have ever been diagnosed with schizophrenia also have an SUD, as do 23.7% of those with an anxiety disorder, 32.8% of those with obsessive-compulsive disorder, and 50% of those with bipolar disorder (National Institute on Drug Abuse, 2020a). In addition (and not surprisingly), there is an association between SUDs and criminal activity

(Eggink et al., 2019). Clearly, there are powerful influences in both directions between SUDs and other psychiatric disorders.

Attempts at Solutions

To help address the problems of drug abuse and addiction in the United States, a National Drug Control Strategy initiative has been in place for several years, with yearly updates. In 2021, the Biden-Harris administration issued its "Statement of Drug Policy Priorities for Year One,"[4] focusing on seven core goals:

- Expanding access to evidence-based treatment
- Advancing racial equity issues in our approach to drug policy
- Enhancing evidence-based harm reduction efforts
- Supporting evidence-based prevention efforts to reduce youth substance use
- Reducing the supply of illicit substances
- Advancing recovery-ready workplaces and expanding the addiction workforce
- Expanding access to recovery support services

Some of these goals are medical, some are educational, and some are enforcement related. Here, we focus on the medical issues—specifically, on issues where pharmacological treatments are possible. This focus aligns with a 2016 report by the U.S. Surgeon General in which addiction is viewed as a chronic neurological disorder that should be treated as such, rather than as a "moral failing" (U.S. Department of Health & Human Services, 2016).

In addition, the National Institutes of Health supports the HEAL (Helping to End Addiction Long-term) initiative to coordinate and speed government efforts to stem the national opioid crisis, including with improved pain management (Baker et al., 2021; Wandner et al., 2021).

THE BRAIN-DISEASE MODEL OF ADDICTION

The existence of a neural system responsible for experiences of reward (pleasure, satisfaction, etc.) was first suggested by an experiment showing that rats would press a lever "frequently and regularly for long periods of time" in order to receive electrical stimulations in certain areas of the brain (Olds and Milner, 1954). Subsequent research has revealed the anatomical pathways and the neurochemical substances that make up this system, which we have referred to as the *reward circuit* of the brain (see Figure 2.5). This circuit is believed to be the neurobiological basis for the experiences of reward associated not only with natural stimuli, such as food and sex, but also with the use of addictive drugs. However, there are important differences between the

[4]www.whitehouse.gov/wp-content/uploads/2021/03/BidenHarris-Statement-of-Drug-Policy-Priorities-April-1.pdf.

effects of natural stimuli on this circuit and the effects of addictive drugs, differences that are the basis for the **brain-disease model of addiction** (Volkow et al., 2016):

- Addictive drugs can activate the reward circuit more intensely and directly than natural stimuli can.
- Natural stimuli produce satiation, meaning that additional stimulation will no longer activate the reward circuit (e.g., after consuming enough food to feel full, eating more is not rewarding, at least not until hunger sets in again). In contrast, addictive drugs never stop activating the reward circuit.
- Over time, continued use of addictive drugs leads to neurophysiological changes in the reward circuit with consequences such as intense cravings for drugs, loss of control over drug use, and withdrawal symptoms if drug use is stopped—the signs and symptoms of addiction.

According to this model, all addictive drugs, regardless of their specific pharmacological effects, have their initial effects by activating the reward circuit in a way that promotes repeated use, which can lead to addiction. In addicted individuals, withdrawal of the drug produces unpleasant physical and emotional reactions (withdrawal symptoms). Also, even if the drug is stopped until all traces of it are gone from the body (through the process of detoxification), the addicted individual experiences **cravings**—strong urges to use the drug again—and is at risk of relapsing into drug use. The occurrence of cravings, even after long periods of abstinence, implies that *changes have occurred in the brain as a result of long-term drug use, changes that are the basis* for craving and relapse and that constitute the "disease" part of the model.

The sequence from initial use to repeated use to withdrawal symptoms if the drug is stopped, followed by cravings and, often, relapse—a sequence that occurs with all addictive drugs—has prompted increased research into the specific brain mechanisms involved, which can be summarized like this (Volkow and Morales, 2015): initially, the drug triggers surges of dopamine in the nucleus accumbens, activating one pathway in the brain by binding with the D_1 subtype of dopamine receptors and inhibiting another pathway by binding with the D_2 subtype. Continued drug use triggers changes in certain glutamate-releasing neurons and dopamine-releasing neurons, increasing the brain's sensitivity to external stimuli related to drug use, decreasing the brain's sensitivity to non-drug-related rewards, weakening the individual's ability to self-regulate, and increasing the individual's sensitivity to stress and unpleasant feelings.

As noted above, activation of the reward circuit by natural stimuli such as food differs from activation by addictive drugs, because natural stimuli produce satiation—that is, dopamine-releasing neurons eventually stop firing in response to natural stimuli but not in response to addictive drugs. Eventually, however, after repeated exposure to a drug, dopamine-releasing neurons gradually stop firing as much in response to the drug itself and instead begin firing more in response to the various stimuli associated with the drug context (i.e., the environment, persons, and mental states associated with drug taking). In other words, neural responses become conditioned to these contextual cues. Thus, over time, addicted individuals stop experiencing the same intensity of reward in response to the drug as they did initially. They also lose motivation for obtaining rewards from other stimuli and activities that had previously been enjoyable. Furthermore, when the drug effect wears off or the drug is not available, addicted individuals experience an increase in stress and dysphoria as a result of withdrawal, and this unpleasant state motivates further drug use. Rather than taking drugs to feel pleasure, addicted individuals eventually start taking drugs to relieve the discomfort of withdrawal. The relative significance of these two phenomena in the genesis of addiction—drug-induced "high" versus withdrawal-induced dysphoria—still prompts intense discussion (Koob, 2015; Koob and Mason, 2016; Volkow and Morales, 2015; Volkow et al., 2016, 2019; Wise and Koob, 2014).

It is important to note, however, that not everyone who uses addictive drugs experiences these effects. In fact, susceptibility to addiction, as with many other disorders, is found in only a minority of people and is presumably due to numerous genetic, social, and environmental factors, such as family history, early drug exposure, developmental immaturity, trauma, and mental illness. Pharmacological and nonpharmacological treatment approaches derived from the brain-disease model of addiction could address any or all of these factors. For example, psychotherapy might be aimed at decreasing the rewarding effect of drugs or increasing the reward intensity of natural stimuli. Other approaches might aim at increasing executive control or at interfering with learned associations between drugs and the environment so as to enhance motivation for non-drug-related activities.

For people trying to recover from addiction and maintain sobriety, a variety of psychological treatments share the concept that achievement of abstinence requires acknowledgment of one's addiction, acceptance of a personal responsibility for the addiction, identification and avoidance of triggers for relapse, and commencement of efforts to change behaviors. Recovery from addiction may also entail a restructuring of one's social world because of the strong influence of relationships with other people on the likelihood of relapse.[5]

A Closer Look at Addiction and the Reward Circuit of the Brain

The preceding discussion of the brain-disease model of addiction makes it clear that dopamine's effects on the brain's reward circuit play a very important role in that model. However, as we will see in this section, other factors also play significant roles, including stress and two other neurotransmitters, GABA and glutamate. In addition, we will discuss how blood levels of brain-derived neurotrophic factor relate to drug use, and we will end the section with a discussion of criticisms of the brain-disease model.

Dopamine and the Initial Pleasurable Response

The core of the reward circuit is one of the brain pathways for dopamine, called the **mesolimbic dopamine pathway** (see Figure 4.1). This pathway begins with a group

[5]Psychological treatment approaches that can aid in recovery from addiction include cognitive-behavioral therapy, relapse prevention therapy, matrix model therapy, motivational therapy, multidimensional family therapy, the 12-step approach, and approaches that help people evaluate whether the individuals in their social circle are supportive of recovery, along with approaches aimed at treating comorbidities such as depression and anxiety.

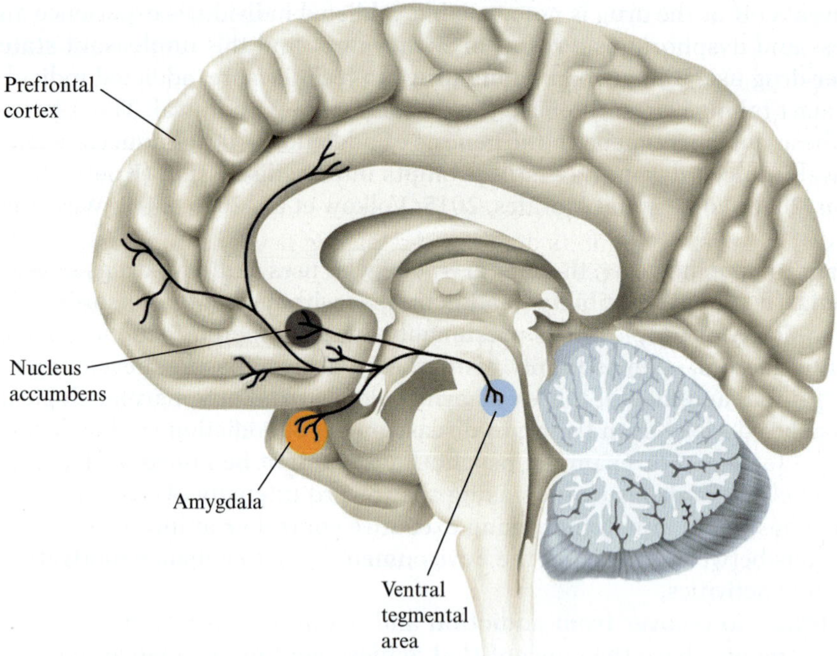

FIGURE 4.1 The Mesolimbic Dopamine Pathway. The pathway starts with dopamine-releasing neurons in the ventral tegmental area. Axons from those neurons release dopamine into the amygdala, hippocampus (not shown), nucleus accumbens, and prefrontal cortex.

of dopamine-releasing neurons in the ventral tegmental area (VTA) in the midbrain. The axons of these neurons extend to several other brain structures—most relevantly, the nucleus accumbens, amygdala, hippocampus, and prefrontal cortex—where they release dopamine when the VTA is activated.

The pathway from the VTA to the nucleus accumbens is critical to addiction: pleasure responses follow from the increase in dopamine-induced neural firing in the nucleus accumbens. This pathway is integrated with the other structures shown in Figure 4.1: the amygdala is involved in mediating the emotions associated with drug use, the hippocampus (not shown in the figure) is crucial to storing memories of drug-related experiences, and regions of the prefrontal cortex are involved in functions that can support or counter drug-related behaviors (e.g., the synthesis and coordination of information, planning, and inhibitory control).

During the last few decades, a converging body of evidence has suggested that regardless of their specific effects, most addictive drugs act similarly with respect to the mesolimbic dopamine pathway, by increasing the amount of dopamine released from the VTA into the nucleus accumbens, amygdala, hippocampus, and prefrontal cortex. But they do not all increase dopamine activity in the same way. In some cases, the dopamine increase is direct; in others, dopamine is increased indirectly; and in still others, dopamine may be increased by more than one mechanism. Nicotine, for example, stimulates dopamine-releasing neurons directly, whereas cocaine indirectly increases the amount of dopamine released into the nucleus accumbens by blocking dopamine reuptake into VTA neurons. Heroin and other opioids can act directly on the nucleus accumbens to produce a reward signal but can also increase dopamine release indirectly, in a different way from cocaine: opioids can bind to receptors on GABA-releasing neurons in the VTA and thereby inhibit GABA release, which increases dopamine release because GABA normally inhibits dopamine-releasing neurons. Similarly, CNS depressants, such as benzodiazepines and alcohol, may also increase dopamine release by inhibiting GABA release, as well as by other mechanisms. Even cannabis and the psychedelic anesthetic ketamine increase the release of dopamine into the nucleus accumbens to some degree (Nutt et al., 2015).

Multiple studies done over the course of more than 30 years support the relationship between the intensity of reward and dopamine increases in the nucleus accumbens and other regions along the mesolimbic dopamine pathway, not only in response to drugs but also in response to natural stimuli such as food, sex, and other enjoyable activities. Consequently, these same regions have also been implicated in nondrug addictions (e.g., compulsive eating, pathological gambling, and sexual addictions) (Nestler, 2005).

The Transition from Pleasure to Addiction

Addiction seems to emerge gradually during chronic exposure to any of several drugs, over a time period that depends on factors such as the genetic characteristics of the person using drugs and the specific drug (e.g., methamphetamine addiction develops more quickly than cannabis addiction) (Volkow and Morales, 2015). During this period of emergence, regions along the mesolimbic dopamine pathway become less responsive to naturally rewarding stimuli, which do not increase the release of dopamine as much as they used to and which are therefore experienced as not being as enjoyable as they once were. This process, which is referred to as *drug-induced neuroplasticity*, is, essentially, the development of tolerance within the pathway (Nestler, 2005). This tolerance and the associated reduction in reward from natural stimuli may contribute to the dysphoria that develops in the periods between drug use or in the period after drug use is stopped. In contrast to natural stimuli, drugs maintain their ability to increase brain levels of dopamine, but the nucleus accumbens becomes less responsive to stimulation by dopamine.

The foregoing description of the process by which addiction emerges raises the question of why only some people using drugs become addicted. Is there something different about their brains? Some evidence suggests that this might be the case. In one study, participants were injected with the stimulant methylphenidate and asked if they found the drug experience pleasant, unpleasant, or neutral. At the same time, they underwent a brain scan that measured the number and activity of their dopamine receptors. Participants who reported that they found methylphenidate to be pleasant had lower levels of D_2 receptor availability than those who reported that the drug was unpleasant. In fact, the participants who enjoyed the drug experience had receptor levels similar to the levels previously reported in people who abuse cocaine, even though these participants were not abusing drugs (Volkow et al., 2004).

Did You Know?

Decreased Dopamine Receptor Availability in Addicted Brains

These brain images indicate that there is less availability of D_2 dopamine receptors in the brain of a person with cocaine addiction than in the brain of a person who does not use drugs. Dopamine-releasing neurons are involved in conditioned learning and in motivation, and the reduced availability of D_2 receptors is presumed to be the basis for the decreased sensitivity to normal rewards that occurs during the development of an addiction (National Institute on Drug Abuse, 2010).

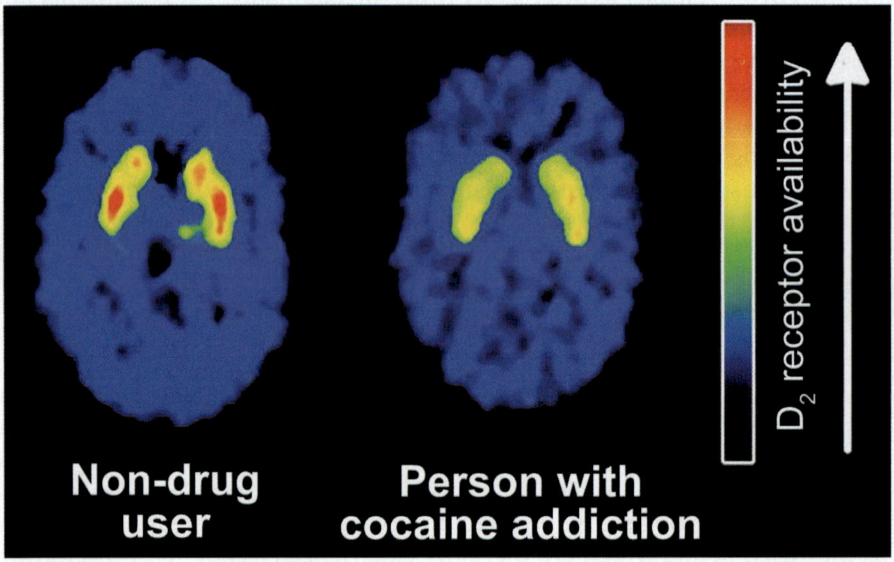

National Institute on Drug Abuse Research Report Series

Does this result mean that people with low levels of D_2 receptors might be biologically vulnerable to addiction? As noted earlier, D_2 receptors are involved in triggering dopamine surges in the reward circuit, so people with a deficiency in those receptors might require a more powerful stimulus (as from a drug) to experience the same intensity of reward that people without a deficiency get from natural stimuli. And for people without a deficiency, the drug stimulus might result in a response that is too strong to be enjoyable.

This interpretation is consistent with studies in which a stimulant (methylphenidate or amphetamine) was given to participants who had never been addicted to drugs and to participants who either were currently addicted or were detoxified after having been addicted. In all these studies, the addicted participants (both current and detoxified) reported a less intense "high" and showed less dopamine increase in their brains than did participants who had never been addicted, suggesting that their brains were less responsive to the drug. Even participants addicted to nonstimulant drugs such as opiates and alcohol had less dopamine increase after stimulant administration (Nutt et al., 2015; Volkow et al., 2011, 2014).

Other experiments have shown differences specific to the frontal lobe between addicted and nonaddicted participants. Like other parts of the reward circuit, the frontal lobe is profoundly altered by chronic drug use, including a reduction in the baseline activity of several regions of the frontal cortex, a phenomenon known as *cortical hypofrontality*. Brain scans have shown that addicted participants not only have fewer dopamine receptors than normal in the nucleus accumbens but also have a lower metabolic rate in wider regions of the frontal lobe, which probably means that their frontal lobe responses to natural stimuli will be "sluggish"; however, the frontal lobes of addicted participants become more activated than normal when they are exposed to stimuli that cause craving, such as drugs or drug-related contextual cues (Volkow et al., 2016). In addition, brain scans have shown that the cortex of regions in the reward circuit, including the prefrontal cortex, is thinner with less volume and surface area in addicted participants than in control subjects, even after months of abstinence, and that those with a thinner cortex are more likely to relapse after one year (Durazzo et al., 2011).

In summary, as a result of chronic drug use, natural stimuli are experienced as less rewarding and cause less release of dopamine. The frontal cortex becomes less active and less responsive to normal stimuli but *overactive* in response to drugs, drug-related cues, and cravings.

Of course, for drug use to continue, with the eventual emergence of addiction, the user has to remember the positive feelings produced by the drug, as well as the contexts in which drug use occurred, including both the internal context (i.e., the user's mental and emotional set) and the external context (i.e., the social and physical settings). Memory of drug use and its contexts is mediated by two other structures associated with the reward circuit, the amygdala and the hippocampus (see Figure 4.2). The importance of contextual memories is shown by the fact that, over time, stimuli associated with the environment in which drugs were used produce a greater response in the reward circuit than the drugs themselves. Conditioned, or learned, responses like these are thought to elicit powerful craving sensations via the frontal cortex—that is, the frontal lobes become sensitized to

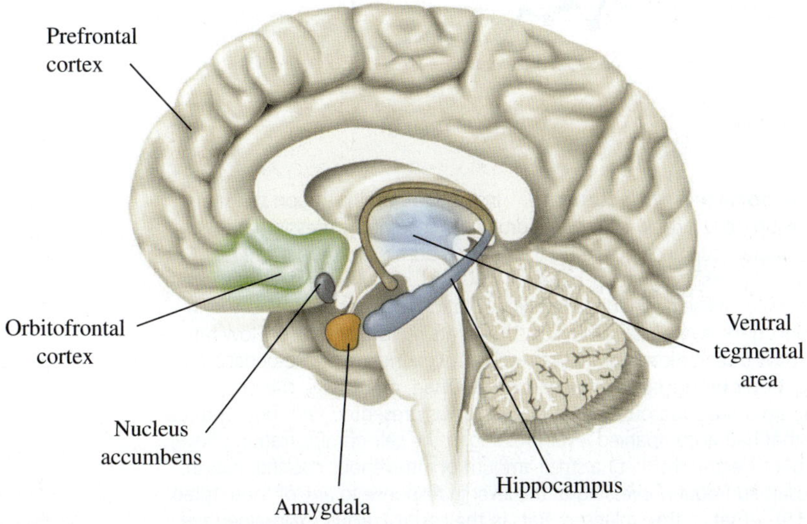

FIGURE 4.2 Brain Structures Involved in Addiction. The drives, emotions, and memories that lead to addiction are coordinated by these key components of the reward circuit: the ventral tegmental area, the nucleus accumbens, the amygdala, the hippocampus, and areas of the prefrontal cortex, including the orbitofrontal cortex.

drug-related stimuli. This can often be seen in the relapse of addicted people after they return to an environment in which they have previously taken drugs, even if they have gone through detoxification and spent time in a rehabilitation program (Chen et al., 2020). Clearly, the ability of drugs to increase dopamine in the nucleus accumbens and other parts of the reward circuit is important, but it cannot account for all the elements of addiction.

Factors That Promote Relapse into Addiction

The brain structures involved in addiction are hypersensitive not only to addictive drugs and drug-associated stimuli, but also to environmental stressors. Studies with animals and with human participants indicate that stress is significantly involved in vulnerability to addiction and to relapse (Haass-Koffler and Bartlett, 2012). In humans, stress may eventually result in a comorbid mood disorder, such as depression, especially during periods of drug withdrawal. In animals, the importance of stress and learned reactions in triggering relapse is shown in Figure 4.3, a composite summary of the

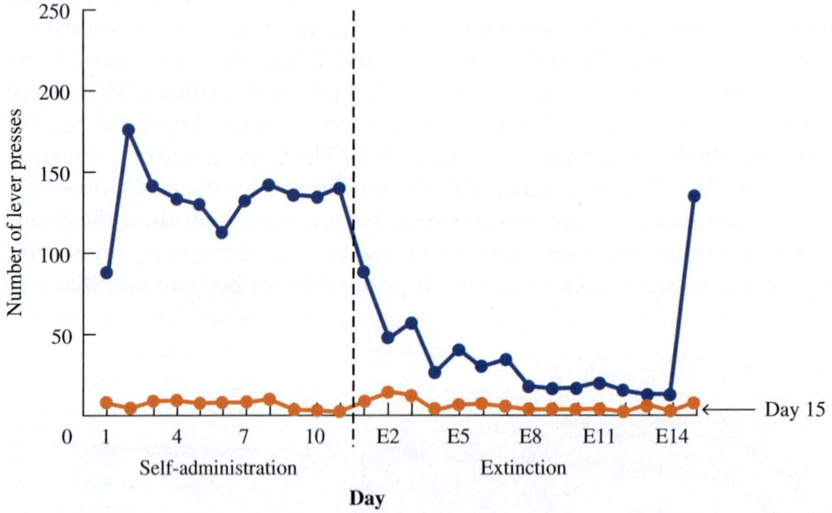

FIGURE 4.3 Factors Associated with Relapse. In the self-administration phase, rats in the experimental group (blue circles) could self-administer cocaine by pressing a lever, which also produced a distinctive cue accompanying the cocaine administration; these rats quickly developed a routine of pressing the lever between 100 and 150 times a day. Rats in the control group (orange circles) could self-administer a saline solution (not cocaine) by pressing the lever, which also produced the same distinctive cue; these rats maintained a very low rate of lever presses. After 12 days (the vertical dashed line), a 14-day extinction phase began, during which lever presses never produced cocaine or the cue. Then, on day 15, the rats in each group were divided into three subgroups, each of which was presented with one of three different stimuli: the cue that had accompanied lever pressing in the self-administration phase, a mild stressor such as a brief electric shock, or a small amount of intravenous cocaine. Rats in the experimental group resumed frequent pressing of the lever in response to any of these three stimuli (blue circle at day 15)—that is, they relapsed. Rats in the control group maintained the same low rate of lever presses as before (orange circle at day 15). [Data from Kalivas et al., 2006.]

results of numerous experiments with rats. In the first phase of these experiments, the experimental group of rats could self-administer cocaine by pressing a lever, and they would quickly begin pressing the lever to get cocaine well over 100 times a day on average. In the second phase (extinction), pressing the lever did not yield cocaine, and the number of lever presses fell dramatically. Then separate groups of rats in the experimental group either were given an injection of cocaine or were presented with a cue that had accompanied self-administration of cocaine in the first phase, or were given a mildly stressful stimulus (e.g., an electric shock). After each of these three treatments (cocaine, cue, or stress), the rats resumed frequent pressing of the lever. Also, a stress-related result of these experiments not shown in Figure 4.3 is that lever pressing resumed at an even higher level after a period of abstinence—that is, after a period during which drug injections were stopped and the lever was not available for pressing. A clear implication of these experiments is that cravings for drugs and relapse into addiction can be triggered by exposure to any of three major factors:

- The drug itself
- Cues associated with the drug
- Stress (including withdrawal symptoms)

The Role of Glutamate in Craving for Drugs

Regardless of how craving sensations are triggered, they are transmitted from neurons in the prefrontal cortex via nerve pathways that feed back into the downstream reward circuit. However, these prefrontal neurons are not primarily dopamine releasing but glutamate releasing, with targets in the nucleus accumbens and the VTA. Evidence from animal experiments and from human brain scans shows that chronic exposure to any of several addictive drugs is associated with complex changes in the prefrontal cortex and in the output of glutamate there. For example, studies with rats showed an increase in the intensity of activation of neurons in the nucleus accumbens that synapse with glutamate-releasing neurons in the prefrontal cortex, even 24 hours after a single exposure to cocaine as well as after exposure to amphetamine, morphine, alcohol, nicotine, and benzodiazepines (Madsen et al., 2012). Other research has demonstrated that activation of glutamate-releasing, but not GABA-releasing, neurons in the prefrontal cortex is associated with both the formation and the retrieval of cocaine-associated memories (Zhang et al., 2020). Figure 4.4 shows the prefrontal cortex and the other major brain structures known to release glutamate into the nucleus accumbens and the VTA.

In summary, the hypersensitivity of the prefrontal cortex to drugs or drug-related cues is the basis of the phenomenon of craving, which is mediated by increased glutamate-related reactivity within the reward circuit. And cravings are believed to be responsible for the profound impulsivity (acting on sudden urges to take a drug) and compulsivity (being driven by irresistible inner forces to take a drug) that characterize addiction (Kalivas, 2009).

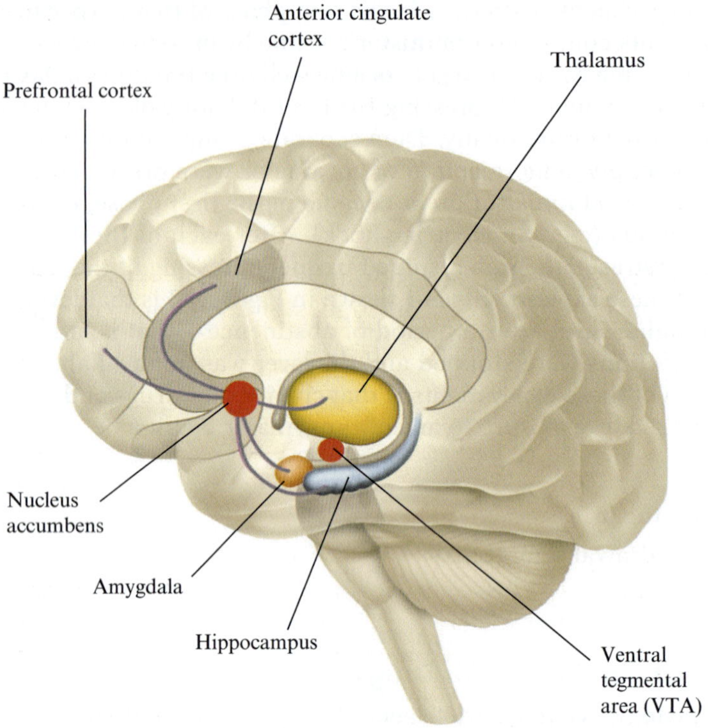

FIGURE 4.4 Glutamate and the Craving for Drugs. The brain structures with glutamate-releasing neurons that interact with the nucleus accumbens and the VTA and mediate the development of drug cravings include the prefrontal cortex, the anterior cingulate cortex, the thalamus, the hippocampus, and the amygdala.

Brain-Derived Neurotrophic Factor and Craving for Drugs

Cravings also seem to be related to blood levels of brain-derived neurotrophic factor (BDNF), a protein in the brain. BDNF levels were found to be significantly increased in opiate-dependent participants, and this increase was significantly associated with craving for heroin (Heberlein et al., 2011). Another study found a similar interaction between BDNF and ethyl alcohol: increases in cortical BDNF signaling were associated with decreases in alcohol consumption in mice, whereas decreases in BDNF signaling were associated with increases in alcohol intake (Logrip et al., 2015).

Criticism of the Brain-Disease Model of Addiction

The brain-disease model of addiction is the predominant model to have emerged from addiction research, but it has not been without its critics. In particular, researchers have questioned both the model's focus on the role of dopamine and the model's depiction of addiction as a compulsion. The main arguments against the focus on dopamine have been as follows (Nutt et al., 2015):

- Evidence for the dopamine hypothesis has been strongest for stimulants (e.g., cocaine and amphetamines), which are the drugs that most directly affect dopamine levels. In contrast, dopamine release has not been as consistently reported in humans in response to alcohol, nicotine, cannabis, or ketamine, even at doses that produce substantial behavioral effects.
- There is no reliable association between the release of dopamine in response to nonstimulant drugs and the experience of reward, particularly in regard to cannabis.
- Blockade of dopamine receptors is not very effective in reducing the rewarding effect of stimulants or in treating human addiction, even addiction to stimulants.
- Neither the administration of opiates nor an expectation of reward from opiate administration affects dopamine levels in the striatum in humans (the striatum is an area in the basal ganglia that includes the nucleus accumbens).
- Lower levels of dopamine receptors in the striatum of people using cocaine than in control groups might be a result of receptor downregulation produced by chronic drug use, rather than a preaddictive condition. Moreover, this phenomenon is not consistently and reliably seen in opiate, cannabis, or nicotine addiction.
- The brain-disease model correctly predicts lower levels of dopamine release in response to a stimulant in opiate- and alcohol-dependent participants, but the model also predicts these lower levels in cannabis-dependent participants, and this has not been seen.
- Research has not established whether changes in dopamine function are present before addiction emerges, or whether such changes mediate vulnerability to addiction, or whether they are a *consequence* of addiction.
- The brain-disease model has not led to any new treatments.

These researchers conclude by noting that the dopamine-focused brain-disease model might be most relevant to stimulant addiction, but that evidence exists for the involvement of other neurotransmitter systems in addiction to other drugs and that these alternative explanations should be further investigated.

Questions about the brain-disease model's depiction of addiction as a compulsion have been based on the following observations (Hall et al., 2015):

- Most people with addiction recover without treatment, and even those who remain addicted can decrease their drug use in response to modest incentives, such as payment for clean urine samples. This argues against a severe compulsive disorder for the majority of users.
- Apparently compulsive self-administration of drugs by nonhuman animals is usually observed in artificial situations that do not parallel the situations in which humans use drugs.
- Vulnerability to addiction has no well-established genetic basis.
- Human neuroimaging studies that find differences in brain structure or function between addicted and nonaddicted participants do not reveal whether these differences are a cause or a result of drug use.

How does the brain-disease model of addiction hold up in light of these critiques? In answering this question, we should begin with the understanding that it is probably unrealistic to expect any single model to explain all the characteristics of addiction to all addictive drugs. That said, it seems likely that the brain-disease model will remain a useful and valid operational model of multiple aspects of addiction to stimulants, including the process by which addiction emerges and the phenomena of withdrawal, cravings, and relapse. It also seems likely that the brain-disease model will need to be modified or supplemented in order to provide an equally useful and valid operational model of addiction to opioids, cannabis, and alcohol.

PHARMACOTHERAPY OF ADDICTIONS

Various therapeutic drugs—including full agonists, partial agonists, and antagonists (all discussed in Chapter 3)—have been used to counter the consequences of drug abuse, such as acute intoxication, cravings, and relapse. Importantly, pharmacological therapies need to be combined with psychological therapies in order to provide the best hope of long-term sobriety, as indicated in a review of the usefulness of cognitive-behavioral therapy (CBT) with or without pharmacotherapy in adults with substance use disorders:

> [B]est practices in addiction treatment should include pharmacotherapy plus CBT or another evidenced-based therapy, rather than usual clinical management or nonspecific counseling services. (Ray et al., 2020)

Full-Agonist Substitution Treatment

Prescribing a full agonist as a substitute for an abused drug is one of the most well-established pharmacological approaches to treating addiction. Full agonists, which bind to and fully activate the same receptors as the abused drug, are carefully chosen not only to provide less reward than the abused drug but also to reduce the discomfort of withdrawal, as well as to improve compliance with the therapeutic procedure and promote healthier behaviors. Two common examples of full-agonist substitution treatments are methadone substituting for heroin and nicotine patches substituting for cigarettes.

The pharmacological advantages of methadone over heroin are that methadone is effective orally, has a slower onset of effect and a longer half-life, so the person needs just one dose each day. Formerly, this meant that everyone taking prescribed methadone had to go to a clinic daily to receive their dose, but in mid-2021 federal rules were changed to include some take-home options: patients deemed sufficiently stable may now be allowed to take home 28 days of doses, while others may be allowed 14 days of doses (Amram et al., in press).

In addition, of course, heroin is obtained illicitly and is usually taken by injection, whereas methadone can be prescribed legally and is taken orally. However, methadone does have serious drawbacks: it is addictive, and it can be fatal in overdose. (See Chapter 10 for a fuller discussion of methadone use and abuse.)

As an example of full-agonist substitution treatment, methadone therapy for heroin addiction contrasts with the use of nicotine patches to break the habit of cigarette smoking. In the former, the full agonist is a different drug (methadone versus heroin), whereas in the latter it is the same drug—that is, compulsive cigarette smoking reflects an addiction to nicotine, and a patch applied to the arm still administers nicotine, only by a different method. However, this different method of administration not only has the well-known and extremely important health advantages of quitting smoking but also has pharmacological advantages: nicotine absorption from a patch is slower, more constant, and much less reinforcing than absorption from cigarette smoking. Patches do, however, maintain a level of nicotine in the blood, thus preventing nicotine withdrawal, and they may not reduce cravings for nicotine. (The advantages and disadvantages of nicotine patches are more fully discussed in Chapter 6.)

Partial-Agonist Substitution Treatment

Unlike a full agonist, a partial agonist is a less potent substitute for the abused drug (it binds to the same receptors but does not fully activate them). The classic partial agonist is buprenorphine, used in treating opioid dependence and addiction (see Chapter 10). Another example is the partial agonist varenicline (Chantix), used to treat nicotine addiction by providing sufficient stimulation to weaken the urge to smoke (varenicline is discussed at length in Chapter 6).

Treatment with Antagonists

The idea behind treating addiction with an antagonist is that an antagonist of an abused drug directly blocks the abused drug's rewarding effect and so might eventually reduce the compulsive use of the drug. In fact, antagonists can be very effective in reducing abuse—but only if they are taken. Antagonists offer no immediate reward, so compliance with treatment is a major problem. The most commonly used antagonist drugs are those used to treat addiction to opioids, including naloxone, naltrexone, and nalbuphine (see Chapter 10). Antagonists of other drugs are available but are not primarily used for treatment of dependence (e.g., flumazenil is used to treat acute benzodiazepine overdose).

CHAPTER REVIEW

1. In DSM-5, what are the three elements required to diagnose an SUD?
2. What is the most commonly observed disorder comorbid with an SUD?
3. In the brain-disease model of addiction, what are three important differences between natural stimuli and addictive drugs in their effects on the reward circuit of the brain?
4. True or false: It is well established that the reward of a drug-induced "high" is much more significant in the genesis of addiction than are the unpleasant feelings associated with withdrawal.

5. Fill in the numbered blanks with the terms in the box (use each term once).

nucleus accumbens	mesolimbic dopamine pathway
VTA	dopamine

Most addictive drugs act similarly with respect to the ___1___, by increasing the amount of ___2___ released from the ___3___ into the ___4___, amygdala, hippocampus, and prefrontal cortex.

6. In the development of addiction, what is drug-induced neuroplasticity?
7. How might low levels of D_2 receptors make a person vulnerable to addiction?
8. Describe three factors in addition to the drug itself that might promote continued use of a drug or relapse into addiction after drug use is stopped.
9. True or false: Increased glutamate-related reactivity within the reward circuit is the basis of the phenomenon of craving.
10. Which two aspects of the brain-disease model of addiction have critics of the model focused on most?
11. Give an example of each of these approaches to treating addiction: full-agonist substitution treatment, partial-agonist substitution treatment, and treatment with an antagonist.

KEY TERMS

addiction
brain-disease model of addiction
comorbid disorder
cravings
mesolimbic dopamine pathway
substance use disorder (SUD)

CHAPTER 5

Ethyl Alcohol and the Inhalants of Abuse

CHAPTER OUTLINE

ETHYL ALCOHOL

Pharmacologically, **ethyl alcohol (ethanol)** is a sedative-hypnotic intoxicant with a history of human use dating from at least Neolithic times—that is, as early as around 10,000 years ago, if not earlier. Because it has a short duration of action, ethanol has no established medical use[1]; furthermore, its excessive use and significant toxicity result in serious negative effects on individuals, families, and society in general. As we will see in this chapter, ethanol is similar in its effects to the sedative-hypnotic compounds that we will discuss in Chapter 13 but differs from those compounds in two important respects: first, ethanol is used primarily for recreational rather than medical purposes; and second, ethanol differs from all other drugs in its pharmacokinetics and in the way it is metabolized.

[1]Unlike ethanol, most other drugs of abuse have some medical use, even if only minimal.

Alcoholism and Alcoholic Beverages: An Overview

The recognition of alcoholism as a multifaceted medical and behavioral disorder is relatively recent. In 1935, Alcoholics Anonymous was founded on a moral model of alcoholism; it offered a spiritual and behavioral framework for understanding, accepting, and recovering from the compulsion to use alcohol. In the late 1950s, the American Medical Association (AMA) recognized alcoholism as an illness and then, in the mid-1970s, redefined it more specifically as a chronic, progressive, and potentially fatal disease. In 1992, the definition was expanded to acknowledge the genetic, psychosocial, and environmental contributions to the condition, as well as the impaired control over drinking despite negative consequences. Currently, the AMA lists the following as the defining behavioral characteristics of alcoholism:

- A prolonged period of frequent, heavy alcohol use
- The inability to control drinking once it has begun
- Physical dependence manifested by withdrawal symptoms when the individual stops using alcohol
- Tolerance, or the need to use more and more alcohol to achieve the same effects
- A variety of social and/or legal problems arising from alcohol use

Terminology

Like the term *addiction* (discussed in Chapter 4), the term *alcoholism* has a long history of formal and informal use. In the first and second editions of the *Diagnostic and Statistical Manual of Mental Disorders* (DSM), the term was used to denote a defined disorder, but it was then dropped in the third and fourth editions in favor of the two terms *alcohol abuse* and *alcohol dependence*. Then, in DSM-5 (2013), these two terms were replaced by the single term **alcohol use disorder (AUD)**, which can be classified as mild, moderate, or severe depending on how many of the 11 diagnostic criteria are met in the individual case.

Despite the DSM's rejection of the term, **alcoholism** finds wide use, both by the AMA—which characterizes alcoholism as a chronic disease with certain well-defined characteristics (which broadly match up with the DSM-5 diagnostic criteria for AUD)—and by the media and the general public as any regular pattern of excessive drinking.

This chapter uses both terms: *alcohol abuse disorder*, or *AUD*, when specifically referring to the disorder defined by the diagnostic criteria in DSM-5, and *alcoholism* to refer somewhat more generally to the chronic disease as viewed by the AMA and to the less strictly defined condition as viewed from the perspective of the media and the general public.

Other terms used to refer to aspects of alcoholism in this chapter include *binge drinking* and *heavy drinking*, which are defined as follows by the National Institute on Alcohol Abuse and Alcoholism (NIAAA):

- **Binge drinking:** drinking that brings **blood alcohol concentration (BAC)** to 0.08 grams%[2] or higher in a span of about 2 hours. (BAC is the weight of alcohol in a

[2]BAC is typically expressed as grams%, which is the weight of alcohol per 100 cc of whole blood. Thus, a BAC of 0.08 grams% means that, on average, there are 0.08 grams of alcohol in each 100 cc of whole blood.

fixed volume of blood, used as a measure of the degree of intoxication; the BAC depends on body weight, the quantity and rate of alcohol ingestion, and the rates of alcohol absorption and metabolism.) For typical adult males, binge drinking means consuming 5 or more drinks in that span; and for typical adult females, it means consuming 4 or more drinks in that span. Binge drinking is among the most important factors in the development of alcoholism, especially if it accompanies drinking initiation at an early age.

- **Heavy drinking:** for typical adult males, consuming more than 4 drinks on any day or more than 14 drinks in a week; and for typical adult females, consuming more than 3 drinks on any day or more than 7 drinks in a week. (In contrast, moderate drinking is no more than 1 drink per day for women and no more than 2 drinks per day for men—i.e., 7 or fewer drinks per week for women and 14 or fewer drinks per week for men.)

Finally, we will often refer in this chapter to **excessive drinking**, which is defined by the Centers for Disease Control as "binge drinking, heavy drinking, and any alcohol use by pregnant women or anyone younger than 21"[3]; and we will discuss **early-onset alcoholism**, defined as alcoholism that develops by age 25 or earlier and is associated with a strong family history of alcoholism and notable antisocial traits.

Alcoholic Beverages and Standard Drinks

Ethanol is a simple organic molecule (see Figure 5.1) that occurs naturally (e.g., in rotting fruit) as a product of the fermentation of sugars by yeast. However, the ethanol in alcoholic beverages is synthesized by fermenting a natural source of sugar with a catalyst, usually yeast. As the source ferments, the starch and sugars in it turn into carbon dioxide and ethanol, which is the basis for different types of alcoholic beverages:

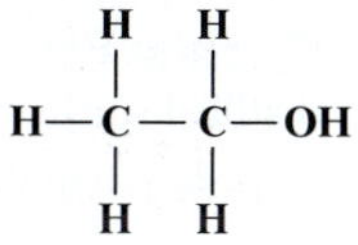

FIGURE 5.1 Structure of Ethyl Alcohol (Ethanol). The ethanol molecule consists of two carbon atoms bound to five hydrogen atoms and a hydroxyl group (OH).

- Beer is made by fermenting grains such as barley and wheat, often flavored with hops and with other ingredients added for color, flavor, and clarity. The alcohol content of beer averages about 5%, but can vary from very low levels to about 12% or even higher in fortified beers when additional ethanol is added.
- Wine is usually made by fermenting grapes, but other fruits or vegetables can also be used. The alcohol content of wine averages about 12–14%.
- Distilled spirits (liquors) are made by first fermenting any of a wide variety of ingredients (e.g., grains for whiskey, sugarcane syrup and molasses for rum, and various other fruits and vegetables for vodka and gin) and then distilling the product to get a concentrated liquid that is usually about 40% alcohol.

Table 5.1 introduces the concept of a **standard drink**, as defined by the NIAAA, and shows the amount of alcohol and number of standard drinks consumed when drinking various quantities of different types of alcoholic beverages.

[3]https://www.cdc.gov/chronicdisease/resources/publications/factsheets/alcohol.htm

TABLE 5.1 How Many Standard Drinks Did You Drink?

Beverage	Alcohol Content*	If You Drink	Total Alcohol Consumed	Standard Drinks
Beer	5%	12 oz	0.6 oz	1.0
		16 oz	0.8 oz	1.3
		22 oz	1.1 oz	1.8
		40 oz	2.0 oz	3.3
Malt liquor	7%	12 oz	0.8 oz	1.4
		16 oz	1.1 oz	1.9
		22 oz	1.5 oz	2.6
		40 oz	2.8 oz	4.7
Wine	12%	A glass (~5 oz)	0.6 oz	1.0
		A bottle (~27 oz)	3.2 oz	5.4
Fortified wine (sherry, port, etc.)	17%	A glass (~3.5 oz)	0.6 oz	1.0
Liqueur, cordial, aperitif	24%	A glass (~2.5 oz)	0.6 oz	1.0
Brandy, cognac	40%	A glass (~1.5 oz)	0.6 oz	1.0
Distilled spirits (gin, vodka, whiskey, tequila, etc.)	40%	A "shot" (~1.5 oz)	0.6 oz	1.0
		A "half pint" (200 ml = 6.8 oz)	2.7 oz	4.5
		A "pint" or "half bottle" (375 ml = 12.7 oz)	5.1 oz	8.5
		A "fifth" (750 ml = 25.4 oz)	10.2 oz	16.9

*The percentages listed here are typical, but the actual alcohol content of beverages in each category can vary widely.

[Source: https://www.rethinkingdrinking.niaaa.nih.gov/How-much-is-too-much/What-counts-as-a-drink/Whats-A-Standard-Drink.aspx.]

Problem Drinking

Despite the well-known negative effects of excessive drinking, efforts to restrict the consumption of ethanol have been failures. In the United States, for example, the Eighteenth Amendment to the Constitution, ratified in 1919, prohibited "the manufacture, sale, or transportation of intoxicating liquors" in the United States, as well as their importation or exportation. The Volstead Act then specified January 17, 1920, as the starting date for the period that became known as Prohibition, which lasted until 1933, when public pressure led to the enactment of the Twenty-first Amendment to repeal the Eighteenth Amendment (the only amendment to the U.S. Constitution ever to have been repealed in its entirety).

Today, excessive drinking remains a significant public health issue, despite being overshadowed in public awareness by the recent surge in abuse of cannabis and various opioids. About 16.6 million Americans older than 18 years are estimated to have an alcohol use disorder. The NIAAA reports that, in 2018, around 26% of U.S. adults over the age of 18 admitted to binge drinking in the past month, with a further 7% admitting they drank heavily (Slater and Alpert, 2021). This staggering statistic is associated with a number of unfortunate social consequences (Esser et al., 2020, 2021; White and Hingson, 2014):

- Binge drinkers are much more likely than nondrinkers to abuse other substances (24% of binge drinkers vs. 6% of nondrinkers).
- More than 10% of children in the United States live in a household where at least one parent abuses alcohol, which is strongly associated with declines in family stability.
- About 25% of college students admit to feeling that alcohol use leads to poorer performance on exams, missing classes, or leaving college altogether.
- About 30% of drinkers continue to drink despite its making them feel depressed or anxious.
- About 22% of drinkers experience withdrawal symptoms when the effects of alcohol are wearing off.
- About 23% of drinkers cut back on important activities or give them up altogether in order to drink.
- About 646,000 college students a year experience alcohol-related assault, with nearly 100,000 of those students experiencing sexual assault.
- An estimated 400,000 students between the ages of 18 and 24 report having had unprotected sex, and nearly 110,000 students between the ages of 18 and 24 report having been too intoxicated to know if they consented to having sex.
- Alcohol use leads to an estimated 95,000 deaths annually in the United States, making alcohol the third leading cause of preventable death in the United States (the first is tobacco and the second is poor diet and physical inactivity). In 2015, alcohol-related driving fatalities accounted for 7,092 deaths (31% of all driving fatalities).

In addition, women, especially younger women, are now ingesting nearly as much ethanol as men, and more women are also drinking "dangerously" and harming themselves as a direct result (Slade et al., 2016). The percentage of people in the United States who drink has not changed much over the years (about 56%), but the percentage who engage in heavy drinking and binge drinking is increasing. And the association between excessive drinking and the simultaneous use of other drugs, such as cannabis, increases the risk of alcohol-related problems. According

Did You Know?

Rejected Male Fruit Flies Turn to Alcohol

Many animals, including mice, rats, and monkeys, are known to drink more alcohol after enduring the stress of isolation for sufficient periods of time. In mice, the stress of enduring aggression or of being bullied also leads to more drinking. To see if stress produces similar effects in fruit flies, researchers allowed one group of males to mate with receptive females, while exposing another group of males to females who had previously mated and were no longer receptive to the males (Carey, 2012). Four days later, both groups of male flies were offered two diets: one was a normal liquid meal of yeast and sugar; the second was the same liquid meal but containing 15% alcohol. On average, the rejected flies consumed the alcohol-spiked diet 70% of the time, while the sexually satisfied flies consumed the alcohol-spiked diet just 50% of the time—a significant difference. Presumably, the sexually deprived flies were using alcohol to make up for their frustration.

to the most recent available data, the 12-month and lifetime prevalence of AUD in the United States are 13.9% and 29.1%, respectively (Grant et al., 2016). Moreover, people who frequently drink to blackout have twice the risk of eventually developing dementia (Kivimaki et al., 2020).[4] (Alcohol-induced blackouts are discussed in detail later in this chapter.)

Comorbidity

Many individuals first begin excessive drinking as a way of relieving psychological distress—that is, as a way of self-medicating—and this is especially true of those who begin drinking at a younger age. If that psychological distress is or becomes a diagnosable disorder and if the self-medicating with alcohol develops into an AUD, the individual then has a comorbidity, or dual diagnosis. For example, an estimated 30–50% of individuals with an AUD meet the diagnostic criteria for major depressive disorder, highlighting just how common this type of comorbidity is. Compared with people who are not depressed, people with a depressive disorder have double the risk of developing an AUD (Pavkovic et al., 2018). A major problem with this comorbidity is that ethanol—the drug being used to relieve depression—is itself a depressant. (See Chapter 12 for discussion of pharmacotherapy for depression.)

Bipolar disorder is also often comorbid with AUD, and this can be a dangerous combination: each can worsen the symptoms and severity of the other, with increased risk of mood swings, depression, violence, and suicide. The reasons for the common association between bipolar disorder and AUD are not clearly understood, but genetics likely plays a role, as do the individual's responses to the symptoms of bipolar disorder

[4]In contrast—and for unknown reasons—low to moderate drinkers, particularly white females, exhibit better cognitive functioning than nondrinkers (Zhang et al., 2020).

(Preuss et al., 2020). Genetic differences appear to affect aspects of brain chemistry linked to bipolar disorder and may also affect the way the brain responds to alcohol and other drugs, increasing the risk of developing an AUD (McIntyre et al., 2020). Drinking to ease depression and anxiety may seem to help, but in the long run it makes those symptoms worse, and this can lead to more drinking—a vicious cycle that is difficult to break. Mania is usually characterized by a euphoric (intensely elated) mood and hyperactivity, as well as by bad judgment and lowered inhibitions, both of which can lead to increased alcohol use. (See Chapter 14 for discussion of pharmacotherapy for bipolar disorder.)

Approximately 33% of people with an AUD have a comorbid anxiety disorder, many have an antisocial personality disorder (Helle et al., 2019), some have schizophrenia (Green et al., 2015), and about 36% have another substance use disorder (SUD) (Serowik et al., 2021). The reasons for the comorbidity of anxiety disorders and AUD are complex, but these factors are probably involved (Kushner et al., 2011, 2012):

- Alcohol temporarily reduces anxiety, which leads to increased drinking.
- Individuals with anxiety disorders transition from regular but unproblematic drinking to excessive drinking more rapidly than do those without anxiety disorders.
- Cessation of drinking leads to anxiety as a withdrawal symptom, and this leads to the resumption of drinking. (See Chapter 13 for discussion of pharmacotherapy for anxiety disorders.)

As many as 38% of people with an AUD have a comorbid impulse-control disorder. Gambling disorder (formerly classified as an impulse-control disorder but reclassified as a behavioral addiction in DSM-5) was associated with a younger age of onset of AUD, a higher number of detoxifications, and a longer duration of AUD (Ooms et al., 2020).

There is a strong association between AUD and personality disorders, especially antisocial, histrionic, and dependent personality disorders (Newton-Howes and Foulds, 2018a, 2018b), an association routinely overlooked within mainstream mental health services. The lifetime prevalence of alcoholism approaches 50% with some personality disorders and is likely similar with others (Helle et al., 2019). (See Chapter 11 for discussion of pharmacotherapy for personality disorders.)

Finally, about 30% of heavy drinkers over the age of 12 years use illicit drugs, indicating that a comorbidity of AUD with another SUD must always be considered.

Pharmacokinetics of Ethanol

As noted at the beginning of this chapter, ethanol has unique pharmacokinetics, including in the way it is metabolized. In this section, we will describe ethanol metabolism in detail (including how it tends to differ between women and men); we will briefly discuss the pros and cons of using biological markers to reveal alcohol use; and we will end with a discussion of concerns related to the use of powdered alcohol products.

Absorption

Ethanol is soluble both in lipids (fats) and in water. Thus, it diffuses easily and rapidly across all biological membranes, which means that, after it is consumed, ethanol is rapidly and completely absorbed both in the stomach and in the upper intestine. This obviously eliminates any need for alternative forms of drug delivery (e.g., by injection). The time from the last drink to maximal concentration in blood ranges from 15 to 60 minutes, largely depending on whether the stomach is empty. With an empty stomach, approximately 20% of a single dose of ethanol is absorbed directly from the stomach and the remaining 80% from the upper intestine, all within 15 minutes or so; food in the stomach increases the time required for complete absorption.

Distribution

After absorption, ethanol is evenly distributed throughout all body fluids and tissues, including the brain (the blood-brain barrier is freely permeable to ethanol). Ethanol is also freely distributed across the placenta and into a developing fetus: fetal blood alcohol levels are essentially the same as those of the pregnant woman (see the section on the teratogenic effects of alcohol later in this chapter, and see Chapter 15 for detailed discussion of alcohol use during pregnancy).

Metabolism and Elimination

The metabolism of ethanol is particularly interesting for two reasons: it involves enzymes that metabolize only ethanol and not other drugs, and unlike the metabolism of almost all other drugs, it occurs at a constant rate regardless of the blood level.

Figure 5.2 shows the normal three-step metabolic process involved in the metabolism of ethanol: First, the enzyme **alcohol dehydrogenase (ADH)**, using the cofactor nicotinamide adenine dinucleotide (NAD^+), converts ethanol to acetaldehyde. Next, the enzyme acetaldehyde dehydrogenase (ALDH), also using NAD^+, converts acetaldehyde to acetic acid. Finally, acetic acid is broken down into carbon dioxide and water. Approximately 95% of the ethanol a person ingests is metabolized by this process. The other 5% is excreted unchanged, mainly through the lungs[5] (very small amounts of ethanol are excreted in the urine). About 85% of the metabolism of ethanol occurs in the liver. Some ethanol metabolism is carried out in the stomach by a gastric ADH enzyme, which can decrease the resulting peak BAC. If the stomach is empty, the time during which ethanol is susceptible to gastric metabolism is reduced, which results in increased blood levels; in contrast, if the stomach is full, ethanol is retained in the stomach for longer, increasing its exposure to gastric ADH and reducing the resulting peak blood levels.

Ethanol's constant rate of metabolism (termed *zero-order metabolism*) means that a constant amount of ethanol is metabolized per unit time (e.g., per hour), regardless

[5]Most of us are familiar with "alcohol breath," the exhalations of a person who has been drinking alcoholic beverages. The Breathalyzer breath analysis test registers the alcohol concentration in these exhalations as a basis for determining whether the person's BAC is above a legal limit (e.g., for driving). The ratio between alcohol in exhaled air and alcohol in venous blood is 1:2300, so the BAC is easily calculated from the alcohol concentration in the exhaled air.

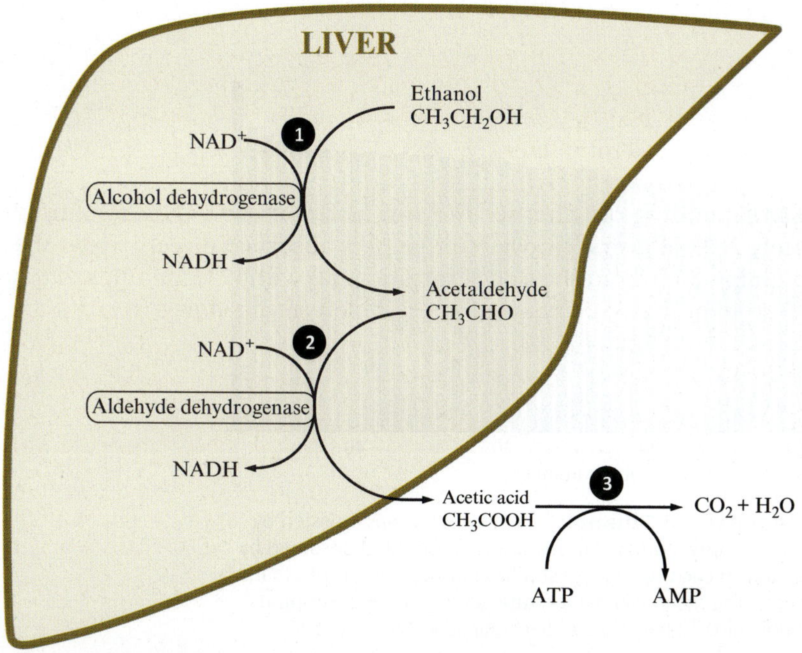

FIGURE 5.2 Metabolism of Ethanol. Ethanol is metabolized in three steps, the first two of which take place within the liver. **(1)** The enzyme alcohol dehydrogenase, using NAD^+ (nicotinamide adenine dinucleotide) as a cofactor, oxidizes ethanol to form acetaldehyde. (The $^+$ in NAD^+ indicates that this is the oxidized form of NAD, which, after the oxidation of ethanol, becomes NADH, the reduced form of NAD, where the H stands for hydrogen.) **(2)** The enzyme aldehyde hydrogenase, again using NAD^+ as a cofactor (which again yields NADH), converts acetaldehyde to acetic acid. **(3)** ATP (adenosine triphosphate) energizes the breakdown of acetic acid into carbon dioxide and water. (AMP = adenosine monophosphate.)

of the BAC.[6] As indicated in Figure 5.3, the average rate is about 0.13 grams of ethanol metabolized per liter of blood per hour (the rate goes up very slightly in persons with very high BAC).

Ethanol metabolism differs between women and men. After consuming comparable amounts of ethanol (i.e., amounts adjusted for differences in body weight), women's BAC tends to be higher than men's, for two main reasons:

- Women have a lower level of gastric ADH, resulting in about 50% less gastric metabolism of ethanol in women than in men and a correspondingly higher BAC (about 7% of ingested ethanol undergoes gastric metabolism in women versus about 15% in men).

[6]Almost all other drugs are metabolized at a rate that depends on the drug's half-life (as discussed in Chapter 1). In this *first-order metabolism*, the BAC decreases by 50% at a constant rate, which means that the absolute amount of drug metabolized per unit time decreases as the BAC decreases.

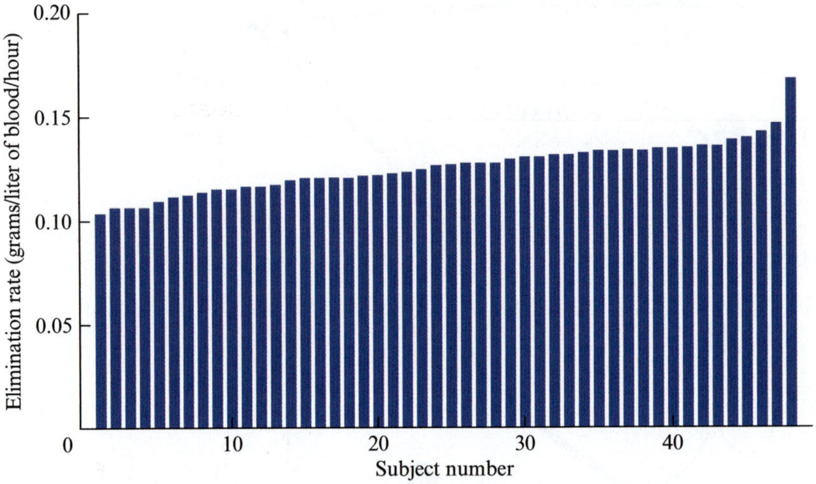

FIGURE 5.3 Elimination Rate of Ethanol. Neat whiskey was ingested by 48 healthy adult males on an empty stomach; the amount of whiskey consumed by each participant was adjusted so each would ingest a total of 0.68 grams of ethanol per kilogram of body weight. The mean elimination rate across the 18 participants was 0.157 grams of ethanol per 0.1 liter of blood per hour. [Data from Jones and Andersson, 2003.]

- Men typically have a greater ratio of muscle to fat than do women, which means that men typically have a larger amount of blood (fat has little blood supply). Therefore, ethanol is somewhat more diluted in men than in women, resulting in a higher BAC in women.

On average, it takes an adult more than an hour to metabolize the amount of alcohol in a standard drink (see Table 5.1). However, drinks poured in bars and restaurants usually contain more alcohol than the amounts shown in Table 5.1—that is, a glass of wine served in a restaurant will usually contain more than 5 oz of wine, and a "neat" (undiluted) glass of 80 proof whiskey (40% alcohol) will usually contain more than 1.5 oz of whiskey, and the same is typically true for home-poured drinks. Interestingly, students tend to overestimate the average number of ounces of liquor in a standard drink by a factor of 3 (White et al., 2005). As a consequence, when they limit themselves to, say, two or three self-poured drinks, they are actually consuming six or nine standard drinks, thus placing themselves at significantly increased risk of alcohol-related adverse events. Clearly, in order to avoid continuously increasing one's BAC and becoming drunk, one needs to be careful about the number of drinks consumed during any single period of time.

Biological Markers

Biological markers that reveal alcohol use up to 96 hours following drinking—that is, even after BAC levels have dropped to zero—are now being widely used to verify abstention in programs where abstinence from alcohol is required. These biomarkers include minor metabolites of alcohol metabolism such as ethyl glucuronide and ethyl sulfate, which can be reliably detected in blood and urine (Shukla et al., 2017). In addition, phosphatidylethanols (a group of phospholipids formed only in the presence of ethanol) have been reported to be the most sensitive biomarkers and to show the best correlation with self-reported alcohol use (Jorgenrud et al., 2021). However, a drawback of testing for biomarkers is that false positives can be obtained in people who have used ethanol-containing products such as mouthwashes and hand sanitizers.

Powdered Alcohol

In 2015, the Alcohol and Tobacco Tax and Trade Bureau of the U.S. Department of the Treasury approved the commercial sale of a powdered alcohol product marketed as Palcohol. Powdered alcohol was defined as any powder or crystalline substance containing alcohol that is produced for direct use or for reconstituted use. Soon after Palcohol was marketed, concern arose that users, especially youth, might mix it with liquid alcohol products rather than with water, which could result in a liquid with extremely high alcohol content, or might use it to "spike" nonalcoholic beverages (Garcia, 2017). In light of these concerns, the majority of state legislatures have banned the sale of this product; however, Internet sales have not been banned.

Effects of Ethanol on Brain, Body, Psychology, and Behavior

Ethanol's lipid solubility enables it to cross biological membranes, and its small molecular size gives it the ability to interact with multiple molecular targets; taken together, these characteristics mean that ethanol's biological effects are numerous and extremely complex, as we will see in the sections that follow.

Brain Effects

Ethanol's effects on the brain include effects on multiple neurotransmitter receptors, as well as effects on memory formation and long-term effects on executive function and cognition. In addition, a recent study suggests that ethanol has deleterious effects on white matter integrity, especially in young drinkers compared with older adolescents (Zhao et al., 2020).

GABA Receptor Effects. Ethanol facilitates the action of inhibitory GABA receptors; more specifically, it acts as an agonist at $GABA_A$ receptors (see Figure 2.18) by binding to a different subunit on the $GABA_A$ receptor than do other GABA agonists and activating an increase in the flow of chloride ions, resulting in increased inhibitory effects. The results of this increased inhibition include sedation, muscle relaxation, and impairment of cognitive and motor skills.

Ethanol's rewarding effects appear to be indirect, in contrast to the direct effects of increased inhibitory $GABA_A$ activity. That is, ethanol appears to promote dopamine release in the mesolimbic dopamine pathway (see Figure 4.1)—the primary neural pathway mediating the rewarding effects of drugs—by indirectly disinhibiting dopamine-releasing neurons and thus increasing the rate of dopamine release into the nucleus accumbens (Loften et al., 2021).

Glutamate Receptor Effects. Ethanol inhibits the responsiveness of the NMDA subtype of glutamate receptors to released glutamate (see Figure 2.17) and thereby potently suppresses the synaptic plasticity mediated by those receptors in certain brain areas, including the hippocampus, amygdala, and striatum (Moykkynen and Korpi, 2012). This inhibition of glutamate receptors generally requires relatively high concentrations and may therefore explain such consequences of severe ethanol intoxication as impairment of motor performance and memory.

With chronic ethanol intake, the persistently inhibited NMDA receptors undergo a compensatory upregulation (see Chapter 3), which means that, if ethanol intake were stopped, the activity of the excess in excitatory receptors resulting from the upregulation would elicit withdrawal symptoms, possibly including seizures and damage to and loss of excitatory neurons (Heinz et al., 2009). (See the discussion later in this chapter of the possible interaction of the drug acamprosate with NMDA receptors as a mechanism for reducing the effects of this upregulation.)

Opioid Receptor Effects. Ethanol's GABA-mediated inhibitory effect appears to activate opioid receptors, and the resulting opioid release triggers dopamine release in the brain's reward circuit (see Figure 2.5), especially in the nucleus accumbens and orbitofrontal cortex (Mitchell et al., 2012). All three types of opioid receptors appear to be involved (mu, delta, and kappa). (See the discussion later in this chapter of the use of opioid receptor antagonists to treat alcohol cravings.)

Serotonin Receptor Effects. Serotonin receptor dysfunction—particularly of the 5-HT2 and 5-HT3 receptors—appears to play a role in the pathogenesis of some types of alcoholism, and antidepressants that inhibit serotonin reuptake, such as sertraline (Zoloft), appear to reduce alcohol consumption in individuals who are considered to be at a lower risk for excessive drinking (Sari et al., 2011). Serotonin receptors also appear to be involved in impulsivity, a core behavior in vulnerability to addiction and relapse (Kirby et al., 2011).

Cannabinoid Receptor Effects. Cannabinoid receptors appear to play an important role in the actions of alcohol. Stimulation of cannabinoid receptors contributes to alcohol's motivational and rewarding effects but also leads to postwithdrawal cravings and then relapse to drinking (Pava and Woodward, 2012). Chronic ingestion of ethanol stimulates the formation of anandamide, a neurotransmitter that activates cannabinoid receptors, eventually leading to the downregulation of these receptors. If the individual then stops drinking, hyperactivity of cannabinoid receptors occurs, which appears to result in a craving for alcohol and a return to drinking. Blockade of cannabinoid receptors by an antagonist results in reduced cravings (see Chapter 9 for discussion of cannabinoid receptors and cannabinoid antagonists).

Memory Effects. Alcohol's effects on memory range from mild deficits to **blackouts**, which can be of two types: fragmentary blackouts (where only bits and pieces of what occurred during the blackout are remembered) and *en bloc* blackouts (where nothing is remembered). Blackouts occasionally occur at BACs of about 0.14 grams% and become more common at BACs of 0.25–0.30 grams% (White et al., 2004). Figure 5.4 shows the results of a study of alcohol-induced blackouts among participants who had been arrested with BACs above the legal limit (Perry et al., 2006). The researchers also found that blackouts at lower BACs correlated with differences in gender, drinking experience,

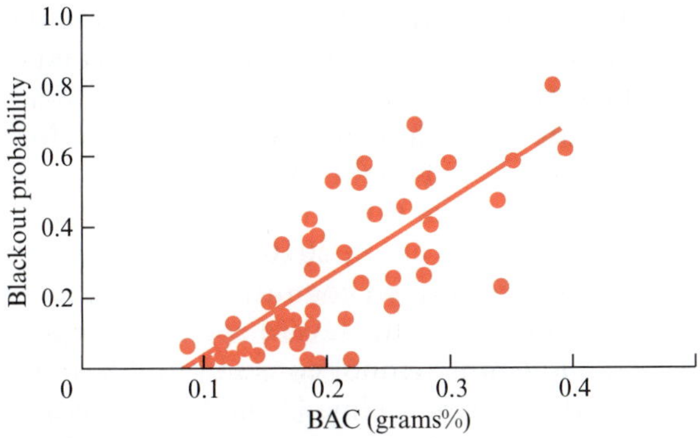

FIGURE 5.4 Probability of Blackouts. Participants who had recently been arrested with a documented BAC above the legal limit were given a questionnaire to determine whether they had experienced a blackout. The graph shows that the probability of experiencing a blackout was 50% or greater in participants with a BAC of 0.310 grams% of blood or greater. [Data from Perry et al., 2006.]

drinking without eating, the rate at which alcohol was ingested, and gulping of alcohol. It is important to understand that, during a blackout, the person is awake and is capable of engaging in complicated and potentially hazardous activities that could lead to adverse legal consequences (e.g.,, driving or engaging in sexual activity), despite later having no memory of what occurred.

The mechanism responsible for a blackout is thought to be a blockade of protein synthesis that is essential for the encoding of long-term memory (Gold, 2008). This state is closely related to organic dementia, which involves severe cognitive dysfunction (Lee et al., 2009). It may also be the case that some persons have an inherent neurobiological vulnerability to alcohol-induced memory impairments (Hermens and Lagopoulos, 2018; Wetherill et al., 2012).

Long-Term Effects on Executive Function and Cognition. It has long been known that chronic alcohol consumption is associated with severe deficits in executive function, even after a protracted period of abstinence. Conversely, persistent executive function deficits could affect the capacity to maintain abstinence if, as is thought, executive functions mediate the suppression of craving and relapse (Le Berre et al., 2017).

A study of 134 adolescents strongly indicated that persistent alcohol use harms the adolescent brain (Squeglia et al., 2015). The investigators compared changes in brain morphology over time in heavy drinkers versus nondrinkers. The participants (72% white, 57% male, and with a mean baseline age of 15 years) were interviewed every three months and underwent magnetic resonance imaging an average of three times over the duration of the study, which averaged 3.8 years across all the participants. During the study, 59 participants were continuous nondrinkers and 75 initiated and maintained heavy drinking. Those who became heavy drinkers had higher baseline rates of depressive symptoms and childhood conduct disorder and, over the course of the study, showed greater reductions than nondrinkers in the volume of frontal and lateral gray matter as well in gray matter in the temporal lobe (in males only). Growth in the volume of white matter in the corpus callosum and pons was seen in both nondrinkers and heavy drinkers but was less in heavy drinkers.

Other research has found that binge drinking by adolescents inhibits the development of new neurons throughout the hippocampus, which might contribute to impaired cognition (Vetreno and Crews, 2015), and in midlife, monthly binge drinking doubles the risk of later, long-term cognitive impairments (Jyri et al., 2010). More generally, problem drinking in midlife is associated with an accelerated cognitive decline and, in people with low baseline cognitive scores, is associated with severe cognitive impairment (Kim et al., 2016). However, long-term *moderate* alcohol consumption in older adults does not appear to exacerbate age-related cognitive decline (Moussa et al., 2015). Finally, it should be noted that excessive, long-term alcohol consumption is associated with increased risk of dementia (Wiegmann et al., 2020). (See below for discussion of other effects of long-term excessive drinking.)

Bodily Effects

The effects of ethanol on the body are mostly negative and often severely negative, although some positive effects have also been reported. In this section, we will describe a range of effects on various bodily systems, effects related to acute and long-term excessive drinking, and teratogenic effects on the developing fetus.

Effects on Various Bodily Systems. In the central nervous system, the primary effect of ethanol is a dose-related, reversible depression of brain functioning, including motor and cognitive abilities. These effects of alcohol are additive with the effects of other sedative-hypnotic compounds, such as the benzodiazepines and marijuana (the sedative-hypnotic drugs most frequently combined with alcohol), potentially resulting in severely deleterious effects on motor and intellectual skills (e.g., driving ability), as well as on alertness. Because ethanol is sedating, people with insomnia may find it effective in inducing sleep, although its short duration of action can lead to counterproductive early morning awakenings.

Alcohol also affects the circulation and the heart. It dilates the blood vessels in the skin, producing a warm flush but a decrease in body temperature, which means that it is pointless and possibly dangerous to drink alcohol to keep warm in cold weather. Long-term use of high doses of alcohol is associated with diseases of the heart muscle, which can result in heart failure. However, daily consumption of low doses of alcohol (up to 2 standard drinks per day for men and 0.5 to 1.0 standard drink per day for women) has been found to reduce the risk of coronary artery disease and peripheral artery disease. This protective effect on blood vessels occurs because of an alcohol-induced increase in high-density lipoprotein ("good" cholesterol) in blood, with a corresponding decrease in low-density lipoprotein ("bad" cholesterol). Unfortunately, the cardioprotective effect of low doses of alcohol is lost on people who also smoke cigarettes or who indulge in binge drinking.

Drinking small amounts of alcohol daily may decrease the likelihood of having a stroke. Consumption of between 1.5 and 2 standard drinks per day is associated with a decreased risk of several types of stroke; however, this apparent protective effect is reversed at doses greater than 2 standard drinks per day (Zhang et al., 2014).

Overall, a sizable amount of evidence indicates that moderate alcohol consumption is associated with decreased rates of cardiovascular disease, but even moderate drinking may produce cardiac damage in older persons. Also, even moderate drinking seems to be associated with increased rates of some cancers, especially breast cancer. In women, the risk of any type of cancer among light to moderate drinkers (less than 30 grams of ethanol per day) was 1.04, compared to 1.30 among heavy drinkers (45 grams or more daily); for alcohol-related cancers (mainly breast cancer), the corresponding risks were 1.13 for light to moderate drinkers versus 1.66 for heavy drinkers. In men, the risk of any type of cancer was elevated significantly among those with daily alcohol intake of more than 30 grams (Cao et al., 2015; Rehm, 2015).

Respiration is transiently stimulated at low doses of ethanol, but as BAC increases, respiration becomes progressively depressed until, at severely toxic doses, respiration ceases, causing death.

Alcohol is high in calories but has little nutritional value, which means that a high-alcohol diet with little else slowly leads to vitamin deficiencies and nutritional diseases. Excessive drinking may be the most common cause of vitamin and trace element deficiencies in adults.

Lastly, patients with chronic widespread pain (a symptom of fibromyalgia but also associated with other conditions) who consume moderate amounts of alcohol have less pain and lower levels of disability (Scott et al., 2018). These researchers reported that moderate levels of alcohol were quite effective at reducing the severity of pain, which may be one reason why so many patients with chronic widespread pain continue to drink despite the adverse consequences.

Bodily Effects of Acute and Long-Term Excessive Drinking. Acute overuse of alcohol (consumption of too much alcohol over too short a period of time) may produce a reversible drug-induced dementia, with disorientation, diminished intellectual capabilities (including impaired insight and judgment), and blackouts.

With more gradual but still excessive consumption during a single period of time, increasing BACs may lead to labile affect, with emotional outbursts precipitated by seemingly innocuous events, and eventually to delusions and hallucinations. In social situations, these alterations often result in unpredictable states of disinhibition (drunkenness), deterioration in driving performance, and uncoordinated motor behavior. Only at very high BACs (perhaps at 0.4 grams% and greater) is consciousness lost, accompanied by a state of "anesthesia" with immobilization. At this point, respiration becomes shallow, and death can result.

Liver damage is a serious long-term consequence of excessive alcohol consumption. Indeed, alcohol-associated liver disease "affects more than 2 million people in the United States and is the leading indication for liver transplant, representing 40% to 50% of all liver transplants in high-income countries" (Singal and Mathurin, 2021). Ethanol produces active oxidants during its metabolism by hepatocytes, which results in oxidative stress on liver cells, leading to **cirrhosis**, a condition characterized by irreversible changes in both the structure and the function of the liver. Not only are 75% of all alcoholism-related deaths caused by cirrhosis of the liver, but cirrhosis is the seventh most common cause of death overall in the United States.

DR. J'S MUSINGS 5.1

Alcohol and Liver Disease

The costs of alcohol-associated liver disease in the United States are enormous, both in terms of lives lost or ravaged and in terms of medical expenses. Who is at risk? Anyone who drinks excessively—for women, on average, that means habitually consuming more than two drinks per day, and for men, more than three drinks per day. And remember, a "drink" is not a full glass of hard liquor, but just 1.5 ounces of 80-proof liquor, or one 12-ounce beer, or one 5-ounce glass of wine. If you are one of the millions of women and men whose regular alcohol consumption exceeds two or three drinks per day, respectively, then you are at risk of liver disease! Truthfully, I myself may be at risk. And of course, the risk of liver disease is in addition to the social and legal risks associated with acute intoxication. Be warned!

Long-term excessive alcohol ingestion may cause an irreversible destruction of nerve cells, producing Korsakoff's syndrome, a permanent type of dementia. Whether or not a diagnosis of Korsakoff's syndrome is made, excessive drinking over the long term can produce more subtle but still persistent cognitive deficits in memory, learning, and other skills, a condition termed *alcohol dementia*. The digestive system may also be affected by long-term excessive drinking, leading to conditions such as pancreatitis (inflammation of the pancreas) and chronic gastritis (inflammation of the stomach lining) with the possible development of peptic ulcers.

As noted in the earlier discussion of the risks of low to moderate drinking versus heavy drinking, chronic excessive alcohol consumption is a major risk factor for cancer. A statement from the American Society of Clinical Oncology notes that 5.5% of all new cancers and 5.8% of all cancer deaths worldwide can be attributed to alcohol ingestion (LoConte et al., 2018), with heavy drinking over the long term carrying the greatest risk. Worldwide, about 3.3 million deaths yearly are attributable to alcohol use. Among the specific types of cancer associated with excessive drinking are oropharyngeal and laryngeal cancer, esophageal cancer, liver cancer, breast cancer, and colon cancer. Even when ethanol use alone may not be strongly carcinogenic, it appears to be a cancer promoter, and those who both drink alcohol and smoke cigarettes are at increased risk of a variety of cancers (Hermans et al., 2021). Worldwide, liver disease accounts for about 2 million deaths per year, with many of those caused by alcohol (Asrani et al., 2019).

Teratogenic Effects. Alcohol is both a physical and a behavioral teratogen—that is, alcohol consumption by a pregnant woman can cause a distinctive pattern of abnormal physical and cognitive-behavioral characteristics in the developing fetus. Children manifesting these abnormal characteristics (or some significant subset of them) are said to have **fetal alcohol syndrome (FAS)**, a devastating developmental disorder that occurs in the offspring of mothers who have high blood levels of alcohol during critical stages of fetal development. FAS affects as many as 30–50% of infants born to women who drink excessively, which may make alcoholism the most common known teratogenic cause of intellectual disability. In fact, it may be that there is no safe level of alcohol intake during pregnancy (i.e., that there is no threshold level of alcohol ingestion that triggers FAS) (Oei, 2020). The defining features of the full form of FAS include the following:

- Central nervous system dysfunction, including microcephaly (reduced cranial circumference), intellectual impairments, and behavioral abnormalities (often presenting as hyperactivity and difficulty with social relationships)
- Retarded body growth rate (fetal growth retardation)
- Facial abnormalities (less-than-normal space between the upper and lower eyelids when the eyes are open, short nose, wide-set eyes, and small cheekbones)
- Other anatomical abnormalities (e.g., congenital heart defects and malformed eyes and ears)

In the United States, an estimated 2.6 million newborns annually have been significantly exposed to alcohol in utero. Many display the full features of FAS, and about 1 newborn out of every 100 live births displays a lesser degree of damage, termed *fetal alcohol spectrum disorder* (*FASD*). The combined rate of FAS and FASD in the United States is estimated to be about 6–9 per 1000 live births (Denny et al., 2020). These statistics mean that excessive alcohol ingestion is the third leading cause of birth defects with associated intellectual disability, and it is the only one that is preventable. The prevention of FAS and FASD obviously involves abstinence from alcohol by pregnant women.

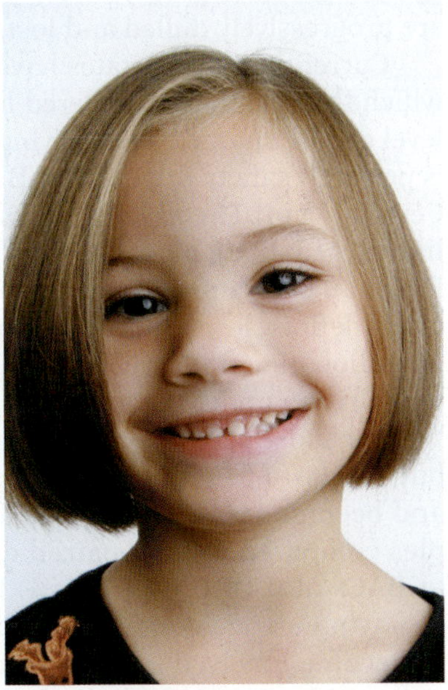

Young girl with symptoms of fetal alcohol spectrum disorder. [Rick's Photography/Shutterstock]

Psychological and Behavioral Effects

The short-term psychological and behavioral effects of ethanol are primarily related to a mixture of the stimulant and depressant effects of low doses in the central nervous system (CNS). The expression of these effects is determined both by the person's mood and expectations (the person's mental set) and by the environment in which drinking occurs (the setting). In one setting, a person may become relaxed and euphoric, and in another, tense and withdrawn or even violent. As BACs increase, mental set and physical setting become progressively less important because the sedative effects of ethanol increase and the person's activity decreases (see Table 5.2).

TABLE 5.2 Effects Associated with Blood Alcohol Concentration Levels

Effect	BAC (Grams%)*
Minimal behavioral change	0–0.04
Intoxication (BAC for legal intoxication is 0.08 grams% in all U.S. states)	0.05–0.10
Gross intoxication	0.12–0.18
Stupor	0.21–0.28
Blackout	0.28–0.34
Sleep	0.35–0.45
Death	0.45–0.50

*The ranges of BAC represent averages across adults.

As doses increase, a person may still function, although with less physical and mental coordination and with markedly impaired perceptual speed, which means that driving and other demanding activities can become dangerous to self and others. At BACs of about 0.05–0.09 grams%, sociability and talkativeness increase, but inhibitions, attention, judgment, and control are decreased; information processing is slowed; and there is an overall loss of efficiency in the performance of tasks. As the BAC increases, the drinker becomes progressively more incapacitated. Memory, concentration, and insight are progressively dulled and lost, even while the person remains awake.

Currently, all U.S. states have set a BAC of 0.08 grams% as the legal threshold above which the person is considered to be intoxicated; that is, a driver with a BAC above this level can be charged with driving under the influence of alcohol. Does this mean that it is perfectly safe to drive with a BAC of 0.07 grams% but not with a BAC of 0.09 grams%? Certainly not! The psychological and behavioral effects of alcohol are not all or none; like all sedatives, alcohol progressively impairs a person's ability to function. Thus, a BAC of 0.08 grams% is only an arbitrary value set to satisfy the requirement for a precisely defined legal limit. A person with alcohol-related impairments detrimental to the operation of a motor vehicle but with a BAC under 0.08 grams/liter can still be charged with driving under the influence.

For most people, driving ability is minimally impaired at a BAC of 0.01 grams%, but at 0.04–0.08 grams%, drivers have increasingly impaired judgment and reactions and become less inhibited. As a result, the risk of their having an accident quadruples compared to unimpaired drivers. The deterioration of driving ability continues at BACs of 0.10–0.14 grams%, leading to a sixfold to sevenfold increase in the risk of having an accident. At 0.15 grams% and higher, drivers are 25 times more likely to become involved in a serious accident. More than 50% of all motor vehicle highway accidents are alcohol related, a number that has changed little in 20 years (Lira et al., 2020). In April 2013, recognizing that over 100 countries on six continents have BAC limits set at 0.05 grams% or lower, the U.S. National Traffic Safety Board recommended that states lower their legal limit to 0.05 grams%. Activities governed by

DR. J'S MUSINGS 5.2

Back-Extrapolation

Since my retirement from the practice of medical anesthesiology about 15 years ago, I have been practicing forensic psychopharmacology, a specialty that functions as a bridge between pharmacology and criminal defense. In that role, I attempt to determine the significance of toxicology results in establishing criminal intent or criminal responsibility. Suppose, for example, that a woman takes an Ambien sleeping pill, putting her into an amnestic state (i.e., awake but unable later to remember anything that occurred while she was in that state). If she then drives recklessly and is arrested, a forensic psychopharmacologist might be asked to provide an opinion, based on the results of toxicology tests done after her arrest, as to whether the woman in her amnestic state could have intended to drive recklessly and whether she should be held responsible for that action, despite having no memory of forming such an intent or of getting in her car and driving.

When alcohol consumption is involved in an event leading to an arrest, a particularly important part of my task as a forensic psychopharmacologist is to determine what the arrested person's blood alcohol concentration was at the time of the arrest in cases where a long period of time elapses (e.g., several hours) between the event and the time when blood was drawn to measure the person's BAC. This process of estimating BAC at the time of an event based on BAC at a time distant from the event is called *back-extrapolation*, and it is the only way of determining whether the person's BAC was above the legal limit. For example, if a person is arrested after being involved in a motor vehicle accident and if a BAC of 0.04 grams% of blood is measured in blood drawn 4 hours after the accident, the question is what the person's BAC probably was at the time of the accident. To answer that question, I might presume an elimination rate of 0.015 grams% per hour, which means that, over a 4-hour period, the BAC would have fallen by 0.06 grams%. Adding this to the measured BAC of 0.04 grams% yields an estimated BAC of 0.10 grams% at the time of the accident, which is above the legal limit of 0.08 grams%.

federal rules already have legal limits under that level: U.S. Department of Transportation regulations prohibit truck drivers from driving at 0.04 grams% or higher, and airline pilots are barred from flying if they have a BAC of 0.02 grams% or higher after 8 hours of abstinence.

Alcohol intoxication plays a major role in a large percentage of violent crimes, including battery, rape, sexual assault, and certain other kinds of deviant behaviors, a fact that is probably related to a dose-related increase in aggressiveness in both males and females (Kuypers et al., 2020). Alcohol is implicated in more than half of all homicides and assaults; about 40% of violent offenders in jail were drinking at the time of the offense for which they were incarcerated. Many drinkers develop a type of "alcohol myopia," defined as shortsightedness in which immediate and only superficially understood aspects of experience have a disproportionate influence on behavior and emotion (Giancola et al., 2011). Cognitive and attentional deficits cause a focus on the present, reduce fear and anxiety, and impair problem-solving ability. Finally, alcohol use increases concerns with power and dominance, which are linked to male violence generally and to violent intimate partner interactions in particular. The effect can be an inappropriate sense of the need for mastery, control, or power.

Finally, it is important to understand that alcohol (like all depressant drugs) is not an aphrodisiac. The behavioral disinhibition induced by low doses of alcohol may involve some loss of restraint, but alcohol depresses bodily functions and thus interferes with sexual performance. As Shakespeare wrote in *Macbeth*: "It provokes the desire, but it takes away the performance."

Ethanol Tolerance, Dependence, and Withdrawal

Tolerance and psychological and physical dependence develop in similar ways with alcohol and other CNS depressants. The extent of tolerance depends on the amount and pattern of alcohol ingestion. People who ingest alcohol only intermittently (even if in large amounts on those occasions) or more regularly but in moderation develop little or no tolerance. People who regularly ingest large amounts of alcohol develop marked tolerance, which takes three different forms:

- *Metabolic tolerance*, involving an increase in the amount of drug-metabolizing enzyme in the liver; metabolic tolerance accounts for at most 25% of the tolerance to alcohol, the remainder being attributable to tissue tolerance.
- *Tissue tolerance* (also called *functional tolerance*), whereby neurons in the brain adapt to the amount of drug present. Drinkers who develop this type of tolerance characteristically have BACs about twice those of nontolerant drinkers showing similar behavioral effects of intoxication; however, *cognitive* impairments are similar at similar BACs in both tolerant and nontolerant drinkers (e.g., at a BAC of 0.15 grams%, both tolerant and nontolerant drinkers display marked deficits in insight, judgment, cognition, and other executive functions); in other words, the tolerant person may just *appear* less intoxicated behaviorally.
- *Associative tolerance* (also called *contingent tolerance* or *homeostatic tolerance*), whereby environmental manipulations are used to counter the effects of ethanol (e.g., drinking black coffee or avoiding activities that would reveal minor impairments).

After physical dependence develops, withdrawal of alcohol results within hours in a period of rebound hyperexcitability that may eventually lead to convulsions, which could be life-threatening in heavy drinkers. Excessive drinking is one of the most common causes of seizures, which occur in about 10% of adults during alcohol withdrawal. The period of seizure activity tends to be relatively short, but the seizures can be very severe (Attilia et al., 2018). Blocking seizure activity during withdrawal is a major goal of detoxification and usually involves two classes of agents: benzodiazepines and anticonvulsants. A "kindling" model of alcohol withdrawal seizures suggests that repeated detoxifications may lead to an increase in the severity of withdrawals and in the likelihood of seizures. In support of this model, a study of detoxification effects found that participants who had experienced two or more detoxifications had higher scores on tests that measure obsessive thoughts about alcohol, drink urges, and drinking behaviors than did participants who had experienced fewer than two detoxifications (Malcolm et al., 2000). The researchers suggested that repeated detoxifications might cause neurological alterations that affect alcohol craving and lead to increased rates of relapse due to a "kindling" of behaviors and thoughts resulting in a compulsion to return to drinking. The researchers added that the kindling effect persists despite treatment with benzodiazepines or other traditional sedative-hypnotic drugs. Other research has supported the use of anticonvulsant "mood stabilizers" (discussed in Chapter 14) for the medical management of alcohol detoxification (Akbar et al., 2018), although "benzodiazepines remain the gold standard, in particular long-acting benzodiazepines administered with a gradual reduction up to cessation" (Attilia et al., 2018).

In addition to seizures, alcohol withdrawal symptoms can include tremulousness with hallucinations, psychomotor agitation, confusion and disorientation, sleep disorders, and a variety of associated discomforts, a syndrome that is sometimes referred to as *delirium tremens* (*DTs*).

Pharmacotherapies for Alcohol Use Disorder or Alcoholism

According to the 2019 National Survey on Drug Use and Health,[7] 5.3% of the U.S. population aged 12 years or older (a total of 14.5 million people) met the DSM-5 criteria for an alcohol use disorder, with the following breakdown by age groups:

- Adolescents aged 12–17 years, 1.7% (414,000 people)
- Young adults aged 18–25 years, 9.3% (3.1 million people)
- Adults aged 26 years or older, 5.1% (11.0 million people)

The same survey found that only 1.6% of the 14.5 million people with AUD (i.e., only 232,000 people) received treatment with medications known to be effective in treating AUD (Han et al., 2021d).

Harm Reduction

Why do so many alcohol-dependent persons fail to seek treatment? Of the survey respondents who recognized they were alcohol dependent and knew they needed treatment for their alcohol problem, almost 50% did not seek treatment because they were simply not ready to completely stop drinking. This is the group that might benefit most

[7]https://www.samhsa.gov/data/sites/default/files/reports/rpt29393/2019NSDUHFFRPDFWHTML/2019NSDUHFFR1PDFW090120.pdf

from a "harm reduction" approach. Support for harm reduction comes from evidence that alcohol-associated mortality risk increases exponentially as daily consumption of alcohol rises above the hazardous drinking threshold, which, in the official U.S. public health definition of hazardous drinking, is 5 drinks per day or 15 drinks per week for men and 4 drinks per day or 8 drinks per week for women. According to one estimate, a decrease in consumption from 100 to 50 grams of alcohol daily would reduce health harms eightfold (Nutt and Rehm, 2014).

Completely eliminating alcohol ingestion is obviously effective in treating alcoholism, but meeting that goal is extremely difficult. This was shown in a remarkable 50-year longitudinal study of two cohorts of men who began abusing alcohol at an early age, one cohort consisting of university undergraduates and the other of nondelinquent inner-city adolescents (Vaillant, 1996). By 60 years of age, 18% of the men in the university cohort had died, 11% were abstinent, 11% were controlled drinkers, and 60% were still drinking excessively. In comparison, among the inner-city cohort, by 60 years of age, 28% had died, 30% were abstinent, 12% were controlled drinkers, and 30% were still drinking excessively. Given the difficulties in achieving complete abstinence, the goals of pharmacotherapy for alcoholism should include the following (along with treatment of any comorbid psychiatric disorders):

- Treatment of the acute pharmacological effects of alcohol (no treatments are yet available that can *reverse* these effects)
- Treatment and prevention of withdrawal symptoms and complications such as neuronal injury during detoxification
- Maintenance of abstinence (or at least a reduction in the number of drinking days) and prevention of relapse into excessive drinking

Treatment of Acute Pharmacological Effects

Currently, there are no pharmacotherapeutic agents that can reverse the acute pharmacological effects of alcohol (Akbar et al., 2017). Treatment of acute effects usually involves supportive care and a quiet environment, both to protect the intoxicated person and to safeguard others against injury. Some drinkers feel that caffeine can counter the effects of alcohol intoxication and increase alertness. In fact, however, caffeine does not reverse alcohol's acute effects but, as a behavioral stimulant, only increases the person's activity without eliminating the motor, cognitive, and other dysfunctions induced by alcohol. This has practical implications in regard to the increasingly widespread consumption of energy drinks (discussed in Chapter 6). In a study limited to youth who had ever drunk alcohol, consumption of energy drinks within the past seven days was associated with a significantly higher likelihood of mixing energy drinks and alcohol (Roemer and Stockwell, 2017). Unfortunately, this combination leads to a greater increase in the person's desire to keep drinking alcohol than does just drinking alcohol alone, without any energy drinks.

Treatment and Prevention of Withdrawal Symptoms

The major goal of managing withdrawal from excessive drinking involves decreasing the activity of glutamate receptors and/or increasing the activity of $GABA_A$ receptors (see Chapter 2 for discussion of these receptor types). Classically, these outcomes have been achieved through use of either benzodiazepines or anticonvulsant medications, both of which can have the desired effects on the target receptors. (Both of these classes of drugs are discussed in detail in Chapter 13.)

Benzodiazepines. When alcohol ingestion is stopped, withdrawal symptoms begin within a few hours. Treatment with long-acting benzodiazepines—the "gold-standard" treatment for alcohol withdrawal syndrome (Minjello et al., 2015)—prevents or suppresses the symptoms, and the medication then can be briefly maintained at a level low enough to allow the person to function or can be withdrawn gradually. Maintenance of even a low level of benzodiazepines, however, should be restricted to only a few days or, at most, a month because of the potential for developing physical dependence on these drugs (unfortunately, current clinical practice is to continue the use of prescribed benzodiazepines indefinitely). The preferred long-acting benzodiazepines for treating the symptoms of alcohol withdrawal are chlordiazepoxide (Librium) and diazepam (Valium). The faster-onset, shorter-acting benzodiazepine lorazepam (Ativan) can be used to control any acute seizure activity associated with alcohol withdrawal. The benzodiazepines, however, have important negative consequences associated with their use in the treatment of alcohol withdrawal: sedation, psychomotor impairments, additive interactions with alcohol, and, as mentioned above, the potential for abuse and dependence.

Anticonvulsant Mood Stabilizers. Seizures are a common acute effect of alcohol withdrawal, so the treatment and prevention of such seizures with an anticonvulsant drug seems intuitively appropriate. The older anticonvulsants (e.g., carbamazepine, phenobarbital, and valproic acid) have historically been shown to be effective but have a significant downside: they can cause liver and pancreatic problems, for example. The newer anticonvulsants—including gabapentin (Neurontin), pregabalin (Lyrica), oxcarbazepine (Trileptal), lamotrigine (Lamictal), and topiramate (Topamax)—are much less liver toxic.

Research on the efficacy of some of these newer drugs includes a review covering a range of older and newer drugs (Maldonado, 2017), two studies of pregabalin (Freynhagen et al., 2016; Mariani et al., 2021), at least eight studies of gabapentin (referenced in Anton, 2020), several studies on oxcarbazepine, a study of topiramate (Manhapra et al., 2019), and a study of cannabidiol (Navarrete et al., 2021). A study of participants with alcoholism and comorbid bipolar disorder showed the usefulness of lamotrigine in improving mood, decreasing alcohol craving, and decreasing alcohol consumption (Naglich et al., 2017).

Ketamine. In a recent report on a clinical trial (Dakwar et al., 2020), treatment of AUD with a 52-minute intravenous administration of ketamine during the second week of a five-week regimen of motivational enhancement therapy was compared to treatment with midazolam during the same period. Results indicated that the ketamine treatment led to significantly better outcomes than the midazolam treatment, including increased likelihood of abstinence, increased time to relapse, and fewer days of heavy drinking. If the results of this study can be verified, ketamine may turn out to be a useful additional treatment for AUD. (The possible use of ketamine in treating AUD and other SUDs is reviewed in Worrell and Gould, 2021; see Chapter 8 for detailed discussion of the pharmacology of ketamine.)

Maintenance of Abstinence and Prevention of Relapse

Three medications have been approved by the FDA specifically to help maintain abstinence and prevent relapse into alcoholism: disulfiram, naltrexone, and acamprosate (Fairbanks et al., 2020; Kranzler and Soyka, 2018; Patel and Balasanova, 2021). However, none of these three is particularly effective when used alone, without intense psychosocial therapy. Alternative agents include the anticonvulsants (discussed later in this section) and three other drugs that have been used off-label to help patients with AUD: nalmefene (an opioid antagonist related to naltrexone), baclofen (a $GABA_B$ agonist), and ondansetron (a serotonin 5-HT3 antagonist). Unfortunately, these three drugs have shown only modest efficacy in well-controlled clinical trials (Minozzi et al., 2018; Palpacuer et al., 2018), but even modest success may be better than the results achieved with the best nonpharmacological clinical approaches.

Disulfiram. In use for over 60 years, **disulfiram** (Antabuse) produces an aversive reaction if the person drinks within several days of taking the drug. Disulfiram inhibits the action of aldehyde dehydrogenase, one of the liver enzymes involved in the metabolism of alcohol. This causes the metabolite acetaldehyde to accumulate (see Figure 5.2), resulting in a syndrome characterized by flushing, throbbing headache, nausea, vomiting, chest pain, unstable blood pressure, and other miserable symptoms. However, controlled trials of disulfiram therapy to maintain reduced alcohol consumption have been disappointing (Skinner et al., 2014).

A common reason that patients give for relapsing while on disulfiram is anxiety, which led investigators to study the coadministration of lorazepam in patients with AUD who were already taking disulfiram (Bogenschutz et al., 2016). Results indicated that lorazepam was safe and effective in treating anxiety but that adherence to taking disulfiram was a problem; only 26 of the original group of 41 patients were available for follow-up at 16 weeks.

Naltrexone and Nalmefene. Opioid antagonists are believed to work in treating AUD by blocking the release of the endogenous opiates that would otherwise create the rewarding effects of drinking alcohol; in other words, opioid antagonists reduce the pleasurable effects of alcohol. Some evidence suggests that treatments with an opioid antagonist work best if the antagonist is taken shortly before the individual expects to drink alcohol (e.g., within an hour). If taken a long time before drinking starts, the blocking effect of the antagonist may not still be strong enough to prevent the rewarding effects of alcohol.

Naltrexone is an opioid antagonist that was initially approved for treating opioid use disorder (specifically, heroin addiction) but then was found effective in treating AUD (Anton, 2008). Naltrexone is marketed as ReVia for once-a-day oral administration and, since 2006, as Vivitrol for administration in a long acting "depot" formulation to be injected once a month. (The cost of the two products is remarkably different: the oral formulation costs pennies per day, while the cost of the injectable formulation averages out to about $40 per day.)

Naltrexone combined with behavioral interventions is an effective antirelapse treatment for alcoholism. Used alone, however, naltrexone's efficacy is poor: not all studies have yielded positive results, and the effect is small. But given that there are many more heavy drinkers who are not dependent than there are dependent drinkers and that nondependent heavy drinkers are not very likely to choose abstinence (instead preferring moderation), it may be that the harm reduction of moving from heavy to moderate drinking is achievable with naltrexone alone.

Some evidence suggests that the efficacy of **nalmefene** (Revex) is similar to that of naltrexone, including when combined with psychosocial interventions (Paille and Martini, 2014). Like naltrexone, nalmefene is an antagonist at the mu and delta opioid receptors, but unlike naltrexone, nalmefene also is a partial agonist at the kappa opioid receptor.

Interestingly, nalmefene was approved in Europe for an unusual "as-needed" use that gives the patient control of the treatment: patients who are concerned that they may drink or who have already begun to drink can immediately take one 18-milligram tablet. Regulators approved this use on the basis of results from three clinical trials in Europe, which demonstrated that this use of nalmefene by heavy drinkers was associated with a more normal amount of alcohol consumption (Lopez-Pelayo et al., 2020).

Acamprosate. Approved by the FDA in 1984 for use in the treatment of alcoholism, **acamprosate** (Campral) was the first pharmacologic agent specifically designed to maintain abstinence in people with alcoholism after detoxification. The drug has been thought to function both as an agonist at GABA receptors and as an antagonist at NMDA glutamate receptors and thereby to restore normal CNS glutamate release altered by chronic alcohol consumption (Kalk and Lingford-Hughes, 2014). Acamprosate has been found to be modestly effective in preventing relapse to drinking in motivated persons. Because the drug is poorly absorbed orally, it is given in relatively high doses (about 2 grams per day). It has a half-life of about 18 hours and is excreted unchanged by the kidneys (i.e., it is not metabolized before excretion). Diarrhea is the most common side effect; nervousness, fatigue, insomnia, and depression have been reported as side effects with high dosages.

In early human studies, acamprosate appeared to be about three times as effective as placebo, with drinking frequency reduced by 30–50%. More recent studies, however, have indicated that its efficacy is comparable to that of naltrexone. Its efficacy is increased when it is combined with established, abstinence-based, cognitive-behavioral rehabilitation programs and when it is combined with naltrexone. Thus, naltrexone and acamprosate, although less than impressively efficacious individually, can be significantly more effective when used together and/or combined with intensive psychotherapy (Avancena et al., 2021; Ray et al., 2020). Coadministration of acamprosate and naltrexone significantly increases the absorption of acamprosate, as indicated by a 33% increase in acamprosate blood level and a 33% reduction in time to peak blood level, compared with absorption of acamprosate administered alone. Also, acamprosate does not affect the pharmacokinetics of naltrexone, which means that, when using the two drugs in combination, the dose of acamprosate can be reduced by 33%, despite the poor oral absorption of acamprosate. According to a review of over 120 studies of medications used for AUDs involving about 23,000 patients (mostly after detoxification or a period of sobriety):

> Both acamprosate and oral naltrexone were associated with reduction in return to drinking. When directly compared with one another, no significant differences were found between acamprosate and naltrexone for controlling alcohol consumption. Factors such as dosing frequency, potential adverse events, and availability of treatments may guide medication choice. (Jonas et al., 2014)

Baclofen. Available since the late 1970s for the treatment of neuromuscular spasticity, **baclofen** (Lioresal) is an agonist at the $GABA_B$ receptor. In AUD, GABA transmission is downregulated, which is why medications under development for AUD often target GABA transmission. Studies during the late 1970s indicated that baclofen has some efficacy in treating alcoholism, but more recent, better-designed studies have indicated that the drug is no better than placebo.

Gabapentin and Other Anticonvulsant Mood Stabilizers. As discussed above, anticonvulsants are useful in ameliorating the severity of alcohol withdrawal. Interestingly, the anticonvulsants also have efficacy in reducing relapse, improving mood and sleep, reducing cravings, and reducing alcohol consumption during longer-term sobriety. With gabapentin, efficacy is further increased when it is combined with naltrexone (Shen, 2018).

Topiramate, another anticonvulsant mood stabilizer used in the treatment of AUD, may reduce symptoms related to relapse, such as anxiety, insomnia, cravings, and anger, and may be superior to placebo at reducing the number of heavy drinking days, reducing the number of drinks per day, alleviating cravings, and increasing the number of abstinent days (Guglielmo et al., 2015). Impaired memory and concentration are among the main side effects of topiramate (Likhitsathian et al., 2012), and lamotrigine may be a viable alternative.

Drugs That Target Serotonin: Combination Treatment with Sertraline and Naltrexone; Treatment with Ondansetron. Serotonin has a complex role in alcoholism (Marcinkiewcz et al., 2016). The combination of **sertraline** (an SSRI) and naltrexone, plus cognitive-behavioral therapy, was studied in a 14-week trial with 170 depressed patients with AUD and was found to be modestly effective in improving abstinence while also reducing depressive symptomatology (Pettinati et al., 2010). Given the high comorbidity of alcoholism and major depression, this may be a reasonable approach to treatment.

Ondansetron (Zofran), typically used as an antinausea medication for patients receiving chemotherapy, is an antagonist at the serotonin 5-HT3 receptor and has shown some positive results in treating AUD, including in reducing alcohol cravings in early-onset alcoholism. In a trial conducted with 271 participants with early-onset alcoholism, researchers found that a twice-daily dose of ondansetron of 4 micrograms per kilogram of body weight (mcg/kg) was better than placebo for reducing cravings, reducing the number of drinks per day, and increasing the number of abstinent days (Johnson et al., 2000). In a second trial, conducted with 321 participants with early-onset alcoholism, a twice-daily dose of 16 mcg/kg was significantly better than placebo for reducing the intensity of symptoms of fatigue, confusion, and general emotional distress, such as depression, anxiety, and hostility (Johnson et al., 2003). Common side effects of ondansetron include constipation or diarrhea, increased liver enzymes, tachycardia, headache, and fatigue.

Cannabidiol. In a study using preclinical (animal) models of alcoholism, cannabidiol (a nonpsychedelic component of marijuana) was found to have protective effects on both the brain and the liver (De Ternay et al., 2019; Navarrete et al., 2021; Turna et al., 2019), and clinical (human) studies are underway to determine whether cannabidiol might represent a new approach to harm reduction in alcoholism while protecting vital organs and perhaps contributing to abstinence.

INHALANTS OF ABUSE

Inhalants—breathable chemical vapors that produce psychoactive effects—are among the most toxic and lethal of abused substances (Cruz and Bowen, 2021). Inhalant abuse (also known as *huffing*, *sniffing*, and *bagging*) is the intentional inhalation of a volatile substance for the purpose of achieving an altered mental state. Although other abused substances can be inhaled (e.g., nicotine, THC, cocaine, and methamphetamine), the term *inhalants* is used only for substances that are rarely, if ever, taken by any route other than inhalation. The extent and consequences of inhalant abuse in the United States were highlighted in this 2021 Senate testimony by Nora Volkow, director of the National Institute on Drug Abuse (NIDA):

> Although many parents are appropriately concerned about illicit drugs such as marijuana, cocaine, and LSD, they often ignore the dangers posed to their children from common household products that contain volatile solvents or aerosols. Products such as glues, nail polish remover, lighter fluid, spray paints, deodorant and hair sprays, whipped cream canisters, and cleaning fluids are widely available yet far from innocuous. Many young people inhale the vapors from these sources in search of quick intoxication without being aware that using inhalants, even once, can have serious health consequences.
>
> National surveys indicate that nearly 21.7 million Americans aged 12 and older have used inhalants at least once in their lives. NIDA's Monitoring the Future (MTF) survey reveals that 13.1% of 8th-graders have used inhalants. Parents and children need to know that even sporadic or single episodes of inhalant abuse can be extremely dangerous. Inhalants can disrupt heart rhythms and cause death from cardiac arrest, or lower oxygen levels enough to cause suffocation. Regular abuse of these substances can result in serious harm to vital organs, including the brain, heart, kidneys, and liver.

As noted in the quotation above, a variety of products common to the home and the workplace contain substances that can be inhaled, and a few inhalants were developed as general anesthetics (e.g., nitrous oxide and halothane). Of course, regardless of their source, none of these agents was meant to be used to achieve a "recreational" intoxicating effect. Table 5.3 lists many of the commonly encountered inhalants of abuse.

The **nitrites** (the "room odorizers" listed in the last row of Table 5.3) are a special class of inhalants. Although other inhalants are used to alter mood, the nitrites are used primarily as sexual enhancers. Formerly, amyl nitrite (or isoamyl nitrite) was often used to relieve chest pain associated with coronary artery disease by dilating veins and thereby reducing the workload on the heart. Today, the drug is infrequently used for this purpose. Isobutyl nitrite and butyl nitrite are sold as video head cleaners, leather cleaners, and so on. These nitrites produce vasodilation, reduced blood pressure, and a "flush" that is claimed to increase sexual satisfaction.

Inhalant abuse disproportionately affects young people. Inhalants are frequently the first mind-altering drugs used by children, occasionally as young as 3 to 4 years of age. Inhalant abuse reaches its peak at some point during the seventh to ninth grades, with eighth graders regularly showing the highest rates of abuse. Inhalants are popular with youth because of peer influence, low cost, availability, and rapid onset of effects

TABLE 5.3 Chemicals Commonly Found in Inhalants

Category	Inhalants	Chemicals
Adhesives	Airplane glue	Toluene, ethyl acetate
	Other glues	Hexane, toluene, methyl chloride, acetone, methyl ethyl ketone, methyl butyl ketone
	Special cements	Trichloroethylene, tetrachloroethylene
Aerosols	Spray paint	Butane, propane (U.S.), fluorocarbons, toluene, hydrocarbons, "Texas shoe shine" (a spray containing toluene)
	Hair spray	Butane, propane (U.S.), chlorofluorocarbons (CFCs)
	Deodorant, air freshener	Butane, propane (U.S.), CFCs
	Analgesic spray	CFCs
	Asthma spray	CFCs
	Fabric spray	Butane, trichloroethane
	PC cleaner	Dimethyl ether, hydrofluorocarbons
Anesthetics	Gas	Nitrous oxide
	Liquid	Halothane, enflurane
	Local	Ethyl chloride
Cleaning agents	Dry cleaning	Tetrachloroethylene, trichloroethane
	Spot remover	Xylene, petroleum distillates, chlorohydrocarbons
	Degreaser	Tetrachloroethylene, trichloroethane, trichloroethylene
Solvents and gases	Nail polish remover	Acetone, ethyl acetate
	Paint remover	Toluene, methyl chloride, methanol acetone, ethyl acetate
	Paint thinner	Petroleum distillates, esters, acetone
	Correction fluid and thinner	Trichloroethylene, trichloroethane
	Fuel gas	Butane, isopropane
	Lighter fluid	Butane, isopropane
	Fire extinguisher	Bromochlorodifluoromethane
Aerosol whipped cream canisters		Nitrous oxide
"Room odorizers" (nitrites)	Locker Room, Rush, poppers	Isoamyl, isobutyl, isopropyl, cyclohexyl, or butyl nitrite (the last is now illegal)

that include euphoria, delirium, intoxication, and alterations in mental state resembling alcohol intoxication or a "light" state of general anesthesia (Nakawaki and Crano, 2015; Tormoehlen et al., 2014). Users are usually not aware of the potentially serious health consequences of abusing inhalants. Especially in children, inhalant abuse is an under-recognized form of substance abuse with significant morbidity and mortality.

Inhalant abuse goes back at least a hundred years, to the introduction of ether, nitrous oxide, and chloroform into medicine as general anesthetics. Concomitant with their discovery as anesthetics was their discovery as intoxicating agents, leading to nitrous oxide and ether parties.

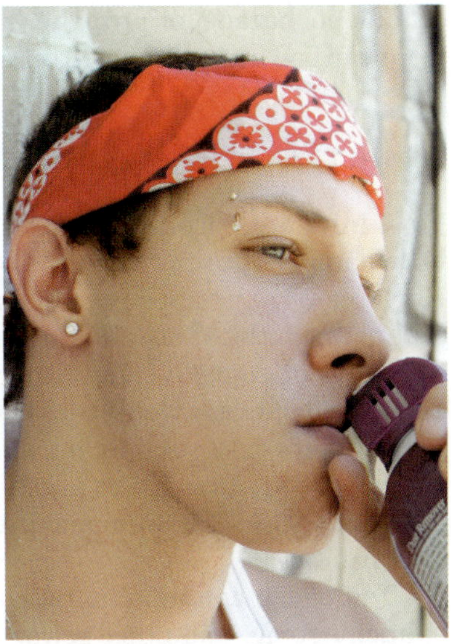

Young man using inhalant to get high.
[AvailableLight/Getty Images]

Acute Consequences of Inhalant Abuse

The acute consequences of inhalant abuse are generally divided into three categories: acute hypoxia, acute intoxication, and medical emergencies. Acute hypoxia follows from the replacement of oxygen in the lungs by gases such as nitrous oxide (found in small metal canisters used in refillable whipped cream containers, or "whippets") and helium (an inert gas often used to fill party balloons), leading to reduced oxygen levels in the lungs and then in the blood and the brain. Hypoxia can cause disorientation, confusion, blackouts, sleep, brain damage, and even death, and these effects are increased by the absorption of nitrous oxide, which leads to an anesthetic state.

Acute intoxication from inhalant abuse is a syndrome similar to alcohol intoxication, consisting of dizziness, incoordination, slurred speech, euphoria, lethargy, slowed reflexes, slowed thinking and movement, tremor, blurred vision, stupor or coma, generalized muscle weakness, and involuntary eye movements, with the associated risks of injury from motor vehicle and other accidents.

Medical emergencies resulting from inhalant abuse include serious cardiac arrhythmias, which can lead to the so-called sudden sniffing death syndrome, even after just the first use (Bowen, 2011). The arrhythmias are produced by the sudden surge of adrenalin that occurs when a person is startled or becomes excited during intoxication (the volatile hydrocarbons in inhalants sensitize the heart and make serious arrhythmias more likely). Arrhythmias can occur during initial experimentation or during any subsequent episode of abuse. Indeed, sudden sniffing death syndrome may account for 50% of fatalities from acute intoxication.

Death is a relatively rare acute consequence of inhalant abuse, but when it does occur, it usually follows from lack of oxygen to the brain (anoxia), cardiac arrhythmias, or trauma. The inhalants most associated with sudden sniffing death syndrome are gasoline (accounting for 46% of such fatalities), butane and propane (due to the production of rapid-onset cardiac arrhythmias), and, increasingly, helium. Inhalation of toluene, butane, or propane (all volatile hydrocarbons) can also lead to sudden death from cardiac arrhythmias (Romolo et al., 2017).

Long-Term Consequences of Chronic Inhalant Abuse

Most inhalants produce intoxication that lasts only a few minutes, usually causing little damage if use is one-time or very sporadic, unless hypoxia or arrhythmias occur. However, *chronic* abuse of inhalants can have serious consequences, including peripheral neuropathies, encephalopathy, liver and/or kidney failure, dementia, disorientation, loss of cognitive and other higher functions due to damage to the cerebellum, gait disturbances, weight loss, loss of coordination, irritability, depression, neurological disorders such as parkinsonism, and loss of muscle strength (Dingwall and Cairney, 2011; Howard et al., 2011). Certainly, when young people engage in chronic inhalant abuse, CNS damage often results in long-term or even permanent intellectual impairment.

Toluene, a common ingredient in abused inhalants, is sought out for the euphoric, hallucinogenic, and other rewarding effects resulting from its activation of the reward circuit of the brain, including the mesolimbic dopamine pathway and the frontal cortex. Over the long-term, toluene inhalation can result in CNS toxicity with cerebellar degeneration, encephalopathy, and dementia, and in peripheral toxicity with kidney and liver dysfunction.

A condition called *fetal solvent syndrome* can result from inhalant abuse during pregnancy, which is associated with significant risks to the developing fetus, both because inhalants readily cross the placental barrier and because maternal hypoxia can damage the fetus (Bowen, 2011).

Many people who abuse inhalants for prolonged periods over many days feel a strong need to continue abusing them. If the person discontinues use after such abuse over the long term, a mild withdrawal syndrome can follow, perhaps similar to the withdrawal syndrome associated with many sedative-hypnotic drugs.

Treatment of Inhalant Abuse

Treatment of acute inhalant intoxication is primarily supportive with the administration of supplemental oxygen. Treatment of chronic inhalant abuse is much more difficult because most people who abuse inhalants have a pessimistic attitude about treatment effectiveness and express little hope of long-term recovery. Education to prevent abuse tends to be ineffective, despite the significant neurological and other damage that can result. Early identification of those who are likely to begin abusing inhalants and rapid interventions are essential in preventing and responding to both short-term and long-term consequences.

Nonpharmacological programs specializing in treatment of inhalant abuse are almost nonexistent, and pharmacological interventions are not indicated, except for the treatment of comorbid disorders. Treatment approaches standardly used for other SUDs are generally ineffective for inhalant abuse because of the need for long-term detoxification and because of the adverse effects that inhalant abuse has on cognitive function. That is, talk therapies are inappropriate for many patients with neurological dysfunction, and the short attention span and poor impulse control of many patients make group therapy a poor choice as well. The best treatment is prevention.

CHAPTER REVIEW

1. Is distillation or fermentation involved in the production of all three main types of alcoholic beverages—beer, wine, and liquor?
2. True or false: Today, excessive drinking is much less of a public health problem than it used to be.
3. True or false: Comorbidity of alcoholism and other psychological disorders is relatively rare.
4. How does the amount of food in the stomach affect the time from the last drink to the time of maximal concentration in blood?
5. Describe the three-step metabolism of alcohol, including the enzymes involved.
6. Where does the metabolism of alcohol mainly occur, in the stomach, in the liver, or in the upper intestine?
7. True or false: Ethanol has a variety of effects on multiple types of neurotransmitter receptors.
8. During a blackout, is the person awake and capable of engaging in complex activities?
9. What are some of the ways in which alcohol use, including binge drinking, harms the adolescent brain?
10. List at least four potential negative effects of low or moderate alcohol use on bodily systems and at least two potential positive effects.
11. Describe four acute or long-term effects of excessive drinking.
12. What are four defining features of fetal alcohol syndrome? Is there a safe level of drinking during pregnancy?
13. Describe some of the psychological and behavioral effects that occur as blood alcohol concentration increases.
14. What are the two main classes of pharmacological agents used to prevent seizures during withdrawal from alcohol?
15. Why might harm reduction be a better approach to treating alcoholism than abstinence?
16. Do medications used to maintain abstinence from alcohol and to prevent relapse tend to work better individually or in combination?
17. What are some of the reasons why inhalant abuse disproportionately affects young people?
18. How does hypoxia result from inhalant abuse and what are some of its effects?
19. Why is inhalant abuse particularly difficult to treat successfully?

KEY TERMS

acamprosate
alcohol dehydrogenase (ADH)
alcohol use disorder (AUD)
alcoholism
baclofen
binge drinking
blackouts
blood alcohol concentration (BAC)
cirrhosis
disulfiram
early-onset alcoholism
ethyl alcohol (ethanol)
excessive drinking
fetal alcohol syndrome (FAS)
heavy drinking
inhalants
nalmefene
Naltrexone
nitrites
Ondansetron
sertraline
standard drink

CHAPTER 6

Caffeine and Nicotine

CHAPTER OUTLINE

CAFFEINE

Caffeine is the most widely consumed psychoactive drug in the world; in the United States, it is consumed daily by 80% or more of the adult population.[1] Pharmacologically, caffeine stimulates the central nervous system (CNS), acts on the kidneys to produce diuresis (increased urination), stimulates cardiac muscle, and relaxes the bronchi.

Caffeine occurs naturally in the coffee bean, the tea leaf, the kola nut, and the cocoa bean. Many tea leaves actually contain more caffeine than coffee beans by dry weight, but because tea is brewed more weakly, there is less caffeine in a standard serving.[2]

---

[1]Caffeine is a member of a family of drugs called xanthines, which includes bronchodilator drugs such as theophylline.

[2]The reason why caffeine is found in so many plants (at least 60) is not known for certain, but because it is toxic to the larvae of several insects, speculation is that it serves as a pesticide (in addition to insects, caffeine is toxic to birds, dogs, and cats). The Dutch began the cultivation of coffee on the island of Java in 1688, which led to the nickname "java" for a cup of coffee.

In addition to occurring in these natural sources, caffeine is often added to soft drinks, bottled water, candies, and medications (see Table 6.1). In particular, since the introduction of the energy drink Red Bull (in Austria in 1987 and in the United States in 1997), many other brands of energy drinks have been marketed, containing on average about 80 milligrams of caffeine per serving, with a range of 50–550 milligrams per can or bottle. However, the caffeine content may not appear on the label; the Food and Drug Administration (FDA) requires added caffeine to be listed in the ingredients panel but does not require the amount of added caffeine to be stated. (Torpy and Livingston, 2013, include a more extensive table than Table 6.1 showing the caffeine content in energy drinks, other beverages, and other consumables; Wickham and Spriet, 2018, discuss the use of other products containing caffeine, such as caffeinated bars and gels, chewing gums, and mouth rinses.)

Caffeine is also available in powdered form in AeroShot Energy, a product that is marketed in a tube containing 100 milligrams of caffeine (about the amount in an

TABLE 6.1 Caffeine Content

Beverage	Caffeine Content
Tea (6 oz)	
Black tea	25–110 mg
Oolong tea	12–55 mg
Green tea	8–16 mg
Coffee (8 oz)	
Brewed	135–150 mg
Instant	60–100 mg
Decaffeinated	1–25 mg
Espresso latte	70 mg
Sodas (12 oz)	
Coke	46 mg
Pepsi	38 mg
Jolt	59 mg
Mountain Dew	52 mg
Surge	52.5 mg
Other	
Chocolate bar (2 oz)	20 mg
Cocoa (5 oz)	2–20 mg
Hot chocolate (7 oz)	4 mg
Vivarin (1 tablet)	200 mg

Did You Know?

The Danger of Consuming Pure Powdered Caffeine

Caffeine is usually thought of as a relatively safe stimulant with little risk of overdose. However, the availability of pure powdered caffeine makes this a dangerous assumption. In May 2014, an 18-year-old Ohio high school senior died after overdosing on caffeine powder that his friend had purchased through Amazon. The official cause of death was "cardiac arrhythmia and seizure, due to acute caffeine toxicity due to excessive caffeine ingestion." (In a subsequent lawsuit, Amazon was found not to be legally liable in the young man's death.) Then, in June 2014, a 24-year-old Georgia man also died after overdosing on pure powdered caffeine. In October 2014, two U.S. senators, Sherrod Brown of Ohio and Richard Blumenthal of Connecticut, wrote to the head of the FDA arguing that the FDA should ban the product. In 2015, Ohio governor John Kasich signed into law a bill banning pure powdered caffeine sales in that state. Also in 2015, the FDA issued warnings to the manufacturers of compounds containing high levels of caffeine, and in 2018 the agency released guidance for consumers on products containing highly concentrated caffeine. However, given that caffeine powder is marketed not as a drug but as a dietary supplement, the FDA has found it difficult to justify an outright ban.

average cup of coffee) and designed to be inhaled into the mouth, deposited onto the mucus membranes of the mouth, and eventually swallowed (however, some of the powder may be inhaled into the lungs). As a dietary supplement intended to be swallowed, AeroShot did not require approval by the FDA, but the FDA issued a warning letter in 2012 about the dangers of inhaling the powder into the lungs, especially for youth.

The caffeine content of one cup of coffee varies widely, of course, depending on many factors. Among popular "gourmet" coffees, for example, one company's coffee averages 200 milligrams of caffeine per 8 fluid ounces, whereas another company's averages 80–90 milligrams, and a third company's averages 100–125 milligrams. People who regularly consume caffeine have an average daily intake of 200–500 milligrams, correlating with two to five cups of coffee daily. The FDA classifies caffeine as "generally recognized as safe" (with consumption of up to 400 milligrams of caffeine per day being considered safe for consumers). However, young-adult-oriented beverages containing caffeine should be avoided, as these also contain large amounts of sugar.

Pharmacokinetics

Taken orally, caffeine is rapidly and completely absorbed. After oral ingestion, significant blood levels of caffeine are reached in 15–20 minutes, and 99% is absorbed within 45 minutes. Caffeine is soluble in both water and lipids; therefore, it is equally distributed throughout the body and the brain and, like all psychoactive drugs, freely crosses the placenta to the fetus.

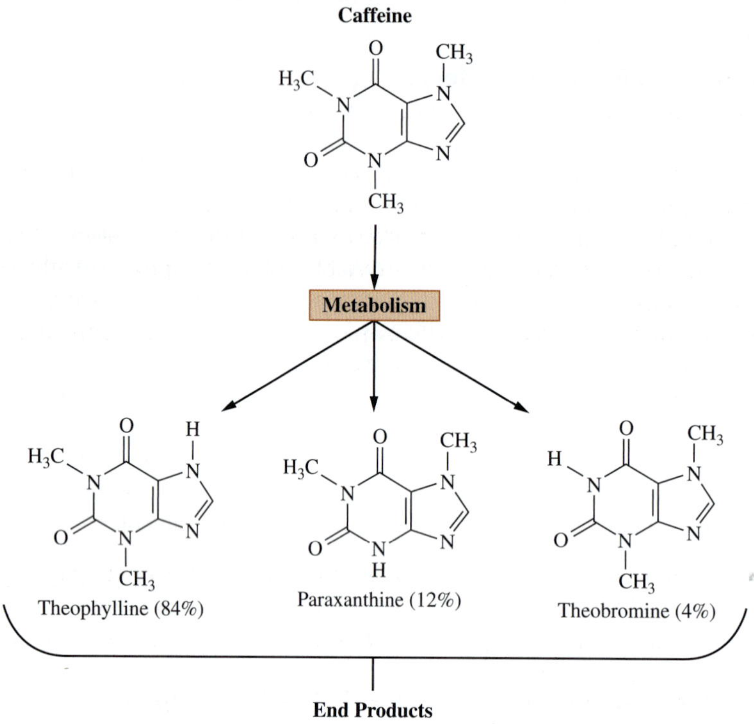

FIGURE 6.1 Structure of Caffeine and Three End Products of Caffeine Metabolism.

Figure 6.1 illustrates the structure of caffeine and its major metabolites. Caffeine is metabolized in the liver by CYP-1A2 enzymes (see Figure 1.8 and the accompanying discussion); the two major metabolites of caffeine, paraxanthine and theophylline, are active, while theobromine (the primary alkaloid in chocolate) is inactive. Caffeine's elimination half-life varies from about 2.5 to 7 hours on average, but the following factors can reduce the rate of metabolism and thereby increase the half-life:

- Asian populations tend to metabolize caffeine more slowly than White populations (Yang et al., 2010).
- Smokers metabolize caffeine 50% faster than nonsmokers. (The fact that caffeine stays in smokers' systems for a shorter period of time explains why smokers tend to consume more coffee than nonsmokers.)
- Alcohol extends the time it takes to metabolize caffeine, which means that caffeine's effects last longer in people who have been drinking.
- Liver disease makes caffeine more difficult to metabolize (the elimination half-life of caffeine in persons with severe liver disease can be as long as 96 hours).

- Oral contraceptives double the time it takes to metabolize caffeine (i.e., the elimination half-life can range from 5 to 10 hours).
- Elderly persons metabolize caffeine more slowly than younger persons (the elimination half-life can be extended by 50–100% in elderly persons).

A reduced rate of metabolism of caffeine can increase plasma caffeine levels and may contribute to caffeine intolerance in some persons, resulting in increased side effects such as anxiety and sleep difficulties. A markedly reduced rate of metabolism of caffeine can result from the use of certain selective serotonin reuptake inhibitor (SSRI) antidepressants, such as fluoxetine and fluvoxamine (discussed in Chapter 12), which are potent inhibitors of CYP-1A2 enzymes; people taking these antidepressants may exhibit increased intolerance to caffeine, which can lead to a condition known as *caffeinism* (discussed below).

Mechanism of Action

Caffeine acts primarily by blocking receptors for the neurotransmitter **adenosine** (see Figure 6.2), a neuromodulator that influences the release of several other neurotransmitters in the CNS (Cappelletti et al., 2015; Ferré et al., 2018). There do not appear to be discrete adenosine-related pathways in the CNS; rather, adenosine-releasing neurons form a diffuse system. Adenosine levels usually increase during the day and exert a sleep-inducing effect in the brain. By blocking adenosine receptors, caffeine weakens this effect and promotes wakefulness; caffeine also increases respiratory and heart rates, constricts blood vessels, and increases the release of the neurotransmitters dopamine, norepinephrine, glutamate, and acetylcholine, with a variety of associated effects (discussed below). In the **striatum**[3] (the largest structure of the basal ganglia), adenosine receptors and dopamine receptors may combine to form a heteromer (a complex formed from multiple types of subunits). When adenosine levels increase during the day, the molecules of adenosine act on this heteromer and reduce the effect of dopamine on dopamine receptors.

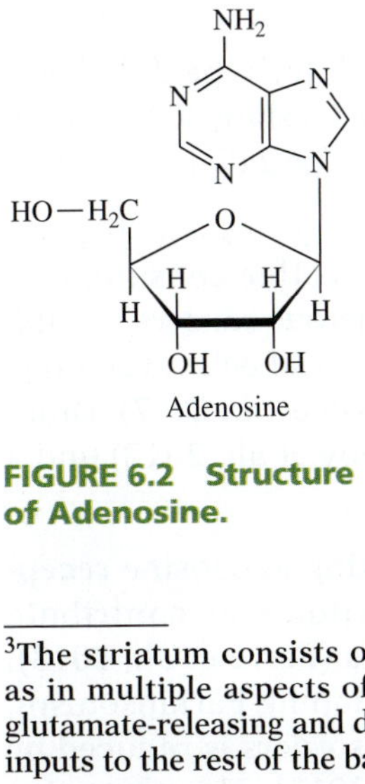

FIGURE 6.2 Structure of Adenosine.

Effects of Caffeine

There is a wide disparity in reactions to caffeine, much of it dose dependent but also with significant dependency on genetics (the gene that specifies caffeine's CYP-1A2 metabolic

[3]The striatum consists of a cluster of neurons critical in the motor and reward systems, as well as in multiple aspects of cognition, decision making, motivation, and reinforcement. It receives glutamate-releasing and dopamine-releasing inputs from various sources and is the primary source of inputs to the rest of the basal ganglia and to the forebrain.

enzyme comes in several varieties; one version of this gene increases the rate at which caffeine is metabolized, while another variant results in a slower rate of metabolism). Most people adjust their intake of caffeine to achieve desired effects and avoid undesired effects.

Beneficial Effects

Not unexpectedly, caffeine has a variety of positive effects, both mental and physical (van Dam et al., 2020; Watson, 2021). In addition to blocking adenosine receptors, caffeine mobilizes intracellular calcium ions, inhibits the enzyme phosphodiesterase, increases postexercise muscle glycogen accumulation, and increases fatty acid oxidation (Cappelletti et al., 2015), and each of these actions may contribute to one or more of the beneficial effects that we discuss next.

Effects on Cardiovascular Function. Caffeine in coffee can transiently raise blood pressure, but the blood pressure elevations are small and typically involve minimal long-term risks. In fact, drinking moderate amounts of coffee is linked to lower rates of pretty much all cardiovascular disease and to overall improvement in cardiovascular health (O'Keefe et al., 2018; Turnbull et al., 2017). The mechanisms underlying these beneficial effects are unclear, although coffee drinkers tend to have lower levels of calcium in their coronary arteries than do nondrinkers, meaning that coffee drinkers are less likely to exhibit subclinical coronary atherosclerosis (Choi et al., 2015). There is also evidence that caffeine dilates coronary arteries, perhaps improving blood flow through them. In contrast, caffeine tends to constrict cerebral blood vessels, decreasing blood flow to the brain but lowering intracranial pressures as a result (Addicott et al., 2009). This action can produce striking relief from headaches, especially migraines, and is the reason why caffeine has historically been an ingredient in many analgesic products.

Gastrointestinal Effects. Regular coffee drinking has been shown to improve glucose metabolism and insulin secretion and to significantly reduce risk for type 2 diabetes (Floegel et al., 2012; Huxley et al., 2009). Research has also revealed a statistical correlation between high consumption of black tea and low prevalence of type 2 diabetes across 50 countries (Beresniak et al., 2012).

Protective Effects Against Cancer and Other Diseases. Moderate coffee consumption (three to six cups a day across studies) can reduce the risk for numerous cancers, including endometrial cancer, prostate cancer, head and neck cancers, basal cell carcinoma, colon cancer, and estrogen receptor-negative breast cancers (Grosso et al., 2017). Other reported benefits include protection against liver diseases (Molloy et al., 2012) and a decreased risk for gout (Park et al., 2016; Zhang et al., 2016).

Neurological and Psychological Effects. Caffeine's action of blocking adenosine receptors and thereby maintaining a higher level of dopamine function may contribute to its beneficial effects in regard to neurodegenerative disorders (Ferré et al., 2018). Numerous epidemiological studies indicate that the risk of developing Parkinsonism, Alzheimer's disease, and a variety of other neurodegenerative disorders is reduced by regular consumption of caffeine (Kolahdouzan and Hamadeh, 2017). The protective effect is thought to be due to the polyphenols in coffee as well as to the caffeine, as both types of compounds are anti-inflammatory and help preserve neurons associated with memory (Vassallo et al., 2014). The development of neurofibrillary tangles and amyloid plaques, which are the main markers of Alzheimer's disease, is also thought to be reduced by caffeine (Laurent et al., 2014).

The increase in acetylcholine release explains caffeine's beneficial effects on learning and memory, in youth as well as in adults (Alhowail, 2019; Cappelletti et al., 2015; Shabir et al., 2018). Elevations of glutamate may contribute to increased attention and alertness in adults, even after a single dose of as low as 60 milligrams (Wilhelmus et al., 2016). Finally, it has been argued that caffeine should be reassessed for the treatment of adult ADHD because of its positive effects on cognition (Cipollone et al., 2020; Liu et al., 2011).

Caffeine consumption might also benefit mental health (Grosso et al., 2016; Tenore et al., 2015). Women who drink two to four cups of coffee per day have a significantly decreased risk for depression compared with those who abstain from caffeine or drink less than one cup per week. This is perhaps not surprising, because caffeine is a psychostimulant and is usually taken because of its positive effects on mood and energy. At low doses, caffeine increases subjective arousal and physical endurance, improves concentration, elevates mood, and enhances cognitive and motor performance. Fatigue is reduced and the need for sleep is delayed.

Other Physical Effects. The elevations in dopamine and norepinephrine explain caffeine's positive effects on physical endurance and on the capacity for exercise. Caffeine also has beneficial effects on physical performance. Specifically, both endurance and muscle power are increased for about 4 hours after ingestion of caffeine. However, high doses of caffeine can be problematic in official athletic competitions—for example, the NCAA considers a urinary caffeine concentration exceeding 15 milligrams per milliliter (which could result from drinking six to eight cups of brewed coffee 2–3 hours before competition) as a positive drug test.

Adverse Effects

Heavy consumption of coffee (12 or more cups per day, or 1.5 or more total daily grams of caffeine) can cause agitation, anxiety, tremors, rapid breathing, and insomnia. The lethal dose of caffeine is about 10 grams, but even ingestion of only 3 grams might be fatal if taken in a short period of time (a blood level of 80 micrograms or more per liter is considered potentially lethal).

Effects Associated with Energy Drinks. There are documented cases of seizures and deaths associated with caffeine consumption in energy drinks. Systolic blood pressure tends to increase by an average of 6.2% within 30 minutes of consuming an energy drink, compared with 3.1% after consuming a placebo drink, and the same holds true for diastolic blood pressure (6.8% increase vs. zero increase after placebo) and serum norepinephrine levels (74% vs. 31%) (Svatikova et al., 2015). And all these potential adverse effects of caffeine in energy drinks may be exacerbated by sleep deprivation (Ishak et al., 2012).

The FDA limits the caffeine content in soft drinks, but energy drinks do not always fit into that classification; depending on the manufacturer, they may be categorized as dietary supplements because they contain so-called natural substances such as ginkgo and vitamins, which are not regulated by the FDA.

Very young children who consume high-caffeine energy drinks (e.g., Red Bull) can suffer seizures, vomiting, chest pain, and erratic heart rhythms. The American Medical Association recommends that high-caffeine energy drinks not be sold to anyone younger than 18 years.

Anxiety Effects. People with anxiety disorders such as panic disorder and social anxiety disorder tend to be sensitive to the anxiogenic properties of caffeine, especially if they usually avoid caffeinated products and do not develop a tolerance to caffeine's effect; however, high doses of caffeine can produce anxiety even in people without such disorders. The wide variability in sensitivity to the anxiogenic effect of caffeine may be due to differences in caffeine metabolism or in the number of adenosine receptors through which caffeine exerts its effects (as discussed earlier in this chapter).

Cardiac Effects. Results of a study of genetic variance (slow metabolizers of caffeine vs. fast metabolizers) among 4000 adults, half of whom had had a prior heart attack, indicated that drinking four or more cups of coffee a day increased the risk of a heart attack by 36% for slow metabolizers but did not increase the risk at all for fast metabolizers (Cornelis et al., 2006). Presumably, the increased risk for slow metabolizers was due to their higher blood concentrations of the drug.

Caffeinism. Habitual consumption of excessive amounts of caffeine can produce a clinical syndrome known as **caffeinism**, with CNS symptoms that can include increases in anxiety, agitation, and insomnia, as well as mood changes, and peripheral symptoms that can include tachycardia, hypertension, cardiac arrhythmias, and gastrointestinal disturbances. The symptoms of caffeinism are usually dose related, with doses higher than about 500–1000 milligrams (equivalent to five to ten cups of coffee) causing the most severe effects. After prolonged consumption of high doses (or after consumption of a single exceptionally high dose), caffeine can produce psychosis in otherwise healthy people, especially during periods of increased stress, and can worsen psychosis in people who are already experiencing it. Fortunately, cessation of caffeine ingestion resolves these symptoms.

Sleep Effects. Perhaps the most concerning adverse effects of caffeine are its effects on sleep (as well as the effects of combining caffeine and alcohol, discussed in the next section). Although caffeine reduces fatigue and improves attention, it disturbs sleep. When taken before bedtime, caffeine tends to impair the duration and quality of sleep and cause repeated awakenings, and these effects may result even from taking caffeine during the day (Burke et al., 2015). Middle-aged adults are typically more sensitive than young adults to the effects of a high dose of caffeine on sleep quantity and quality (Robillard et al., 2015).

Caffeine and Alcohol. Caffeine is often taken along with alcoholic beverages because caffeine can ameliorate some of alcohol's motor impairment, sedation, and intoxication effects; however, caffeine tends to increase the risk of other adverse effects of alcohol, including sexually risky behaviors, fighting, marijuana and other substance abuse, and cigarette smoking (Ishak et al., 2012). The fact that caffeine enhances alcohol tolerance and can counteract some symptoms of a hangover may also contribute to subsequent alcohol dependence (Childs and deWit, 2012). The FDA has characterized drinks containing both caffeine and alcohol as dangerous because caffeine masks some of the cues that people use to tell if they are intoxicated.

Reproductive Effects

Caffeine is consumed by at least 75% of pregnant women, but whether it is safe to ingest during pregnancy is an unresolved issue. As early as 1980, the FDA cautioned pregnant women to minimize their intake of caffeine. More recent studies have explored the connection between caffeine intake and rates of miscarriage, fetal growth restriction, birth weight, and length of gestation. One large epidemiological study found that a caffeine intake of 200–300 milligrams per day was consistently associated with small decreases in birth weight and increased odds of being small for gestational age (Sengpiel et al., 2013). Caffeine itself does not appear to be a human teratogen, nor does it appear to affect the course of normal labor and delivery; however, the current U.S. recommendation is that pregnant women should generally limit their daily intake to about 200 milligrams or less (the World Health Organization recommends an upper limit of 300 milligrams per day).

Tolerance and Dependence

Chronic use of caffeine, even in regular daily doses as low as 100 milligrams, is associated with habituation and a modest degree of tolerance. Discontinuation may produce low-grade withdrawal symptoms. Because tolerance and dependence can occur rapidly, even after low doses, most habitual users are probably physically dependent to some degree. Individuals may become tolerant to several actions of caffeine, including diuresis, elevated blood pressure, and sleep disturbance. Tolerance is more likely with high doses (750–1200 milligrams daily).

With cessation of caffeine use, people who drank a great deal of coffee complain of headache (the most common withdrawal symptom), drowsiness, fatigue, and a generally negative mood. Impaired intellectual and motor performance, difficulty with concentration, and drug craving (for caffeine) are also reported. Withdrawal symptoms typically begin slowly, maximize after one or two days, and cease within a few days. Readministration of caffeine rapidly relieves withdrawal symptoms.

Caffeine use disorder is recognized as a diagnosable condition in DSM-5, with diagnosis being dependent on the presence of the following three criteria (Meredith et al., 2013):

- Chronic craving or an inability to decrease or eliminate caffeine consumption
- Maintained use, even after recognizing that caffeine has caused or worsened some type of mental or physical problem
- Elicitation of withdrawal symptoms or the prevention of withdrawal by continued consumption

DR. J'S MUSINGS 6.1

My Addiction

I love a good cup of coffee! When I worked in anesthesia, I used to drink maybe six to eight cups per day. I seemed to always have a cup in my hands. Now I try and limit my daily intake to three cups of half-caffeinated, half-decaffeinated coffee per day. Am I addicted? I seem unwilling to reduce my intake any further. But even if I am addicted, do the health benefits of caffeine outweigh my dependence? After all, caffeine reduces blood glucose, reduces insulin resistance, and reduces the risk of cardiovascular disease, cancer, and liver disease. And there are psychiatric benefits that include enhanced concentration, improved alertness, and even reduced risk of suicide. Please don't take my caffeine away!

NICOTINE

We will begin our discussion of **nicotine**—a highly addictive alkaloid that is a behavioral simulant and the primary psychoactive component of tobacco—with a review of the epidemiology of nicotine in the United States and the related public policies aimed at reducing its use. After briefly describing nicotine's pharmacokinetics and mechanism of action, we will present a detailed review of nicotine's main effects on brain and body (focusing on the adverse effects of tobacco smoking), describe the development of nicotine tolerance and dependence, discuss the main types of pharmacological treatment of nicotine dependence, and end by summarizing the main conclusions and more detailed information in a 2020 surgeon general's report on cessation of smoking.

Epidemiology and Public Policy

Nicotine is one of the three most widely used psychoactive drugs in the United States, along with caffeine and ethyl alcohol. This and its well-established toxicities give nicotine immense social importance. According to statistics from the Centers for Disease Control:

- In 2019, 13.7% of Americans aged 18 years or older—about 34.2 million people—were current smokers of cigarettes.[4] (But note that current smoking has declined from 20.9% in 2005 and that the proportion of smokers who have quit has increased.)

[4]Current smokers are defined as people who reported smoking at least 100 cigarettes during their lifetime and who, at the time they participated in a survey about this topic, reported smoking either every day or some days.

- Cigarette smoking is the leading cause of preventable disease and death in the United States, accounting for more than 480,000 deaths every year, or about 20% of all deaths. More than 16 million Americans live with a smoking-related disease.
- Nearly 70% of adults who smoke report wanting to quit, and more than 50% reported trying to stop in the year before they were questioned, but only a little over 6% of those who tried were successful despite the dramatic benefits of quitting (see the section on cessation of smoking, later in this chapter).

Electronic Cigarettes and Heated Tobacco Products

Perhaps the most important question associated with the increasing use of **electronic cigarettes (e-cigarettes)**—a question much debated among experts—is whether e-cigarettes can help tobacco smokers stop smoking or whether they are merely a stepping-stone to tobacco cigarette smoking and to use of other tobacco products. In surveys, the main reason cited for regular e-cigarette use is to kick the tobacco habit, and given the lesser toxicity of e-cigarettes compared to tobacco cigarettes, some public health experts support this strategy of harm reduction (e-cigarettes have no tobacco, and laboratory studies suggest that e-cigarettes may be safer than tobacco products because they contain fewer toxic substances and do not produce secondhand smoke). Nevertheless, the main function of both e-cigarettes and heated tobacco products—and the main reason why they were developed—is to deliver nicotine to users, with all the attendant risks of dependence and addiction (along with the health risks associated with nicotine, as discussed later in this chapter).

Users of e-cigarettes add a nicotine-containing liquid to the battery-powered device, which heats the liquid until it emits a nicotine vapor that is inhaled (hence the term *vaping*). Users can adjust the device to increase or decrease the amount of vapor and the amount of nicotine, and they can add ingredients to the liquid such as THC (tetrahydrocannabinol, the main psychoactive component of marijuana) and a range of flavors.

Devices known as *vape pens*, which are larger than typical e-cigarettes, have bigger batteries that can heat the liquid to a higher temperature and consequently increase the nicotine level beyond that of the standard e-cigarette, with a resulting higher blood level of nicotine, closer to the blood level that results from smoking tobacco cigarettes. However, the increased temperature also increases the levels of toxins in the vapor. (Tobacco companies have also introduced cigarettes with higher nicotine levels.)

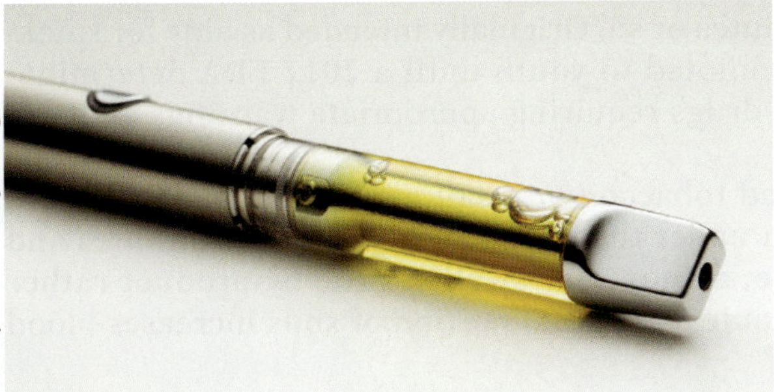

Chimpinski/Getty Images

A vape pen with a refillable tank.

In 2021, the FDA for the first time gave official approval to the sale of an e-cigarette in the United States. The approval, which was given only for tobacco-flavored products, was explained by the director of the FDA's Center for Tobacco Products:

> The manufacturer's data demonstrates its tobacco-flavored products could benefit addicted adult smokers who switch to these products—either completely or with a significant reduction in cigarette consumption—by reducing their exposure to harmful chemicals.

A recent study compared relapse rates among smokers who had switched to e-cigarettes versus former smokers who had begun abstaining completely from nicotine use (Pierce et al., 2021). Discouragingly, results showed that, regardless of the e-cigarette product, smokers who had switched to e-cigarettes were more likely to relapse to cigarette smoking than were former smokers who had tried abstinence. This calls into question the FDA's recent approval of electronic nicotine delivery systems—that is, the relapse rates reported in this study indicate that the FDA's hopes that these products will help reduce cigarette smoking are unfounded.

Heated tobacco products are hybrids between tobacco cigarettes and e-cigarettes. These devices use real tobacco but do not actually burn it; rather, they heat the tobacco to a high enough temperature to produce a tobacco-flavored vapor without smoke or tar, but still with more potentially toxic chemicals than are in the vapor from e-cigarettes. Nevertheless, in 2019, the FDA permitted sale of the IQOS line of heated tobacco products from the Philip Morris International tobacco company (U.S. Food and Drug Administration, 2019a). At the time of this writing, however, the sale and importation of the IQOS product are on hold, pending the outcome of potential patent infringement claims.

Both e-cigarettes and heated tobacco products not only deliver nicotine but also provide the behavioral stimuli associated with the rewards of smoking—the physical act of holding a cigarette and inhaling and exhaling a vapor—and some even produce the typical "throat catch" associated with smoking (i.e., the sensation of smoke in the back of the throat).

Dissolvables, Snus, Hookahs, and Synthetic Nicotine Products

Several other forms of nicotine administration have also become popular, including **dissolvable tobacco products**, snus, hookahs (water pipes), and synthetic nicotine products. Dissolvable products consist of finely powdered tobacco plus a host of other ingredients; they are placed under the tongue, where they dissolve and are swallowed over the course of 15 minutes or so. Originally intended as aids for smoking cessation, they were widely promoted to youth until a 2017 FDA determination that they must be classified as drugs requiring appropriate warnings and sale restrictions.

Snus consists of moist powdered tobacco (with salt and water) in small mesh pouches that are held in the mouth under the upper lip for about 30 minutes and then discarded. To get the nicotine, a snus user swallows the by-product rather than spitting it out (after the 30 minutes, a 2-gram portion of snus increases blood nicotine concentration to around the same level as the level resulting from smoking a tobacco cigarette). In 2019, the FDA granted "modified risk" status to General brand snus products (while smokeless, they still carry a risk of oral cancers, periodontal disease, heart disease, and nicotine addiction) (U.S. Food and Drug Administration, 2019c).

Hookahs pass the smoke from burning tobacco through water, so the smoke is cooled before inhalation. Originating in northern Africa and southwest Asia at least four centuries ago, hookah smoking has long been popular among adult men in Middle Eastern countries and is now spreading worldwide, including with increased adoption by adolescents and young adults in the United States. Apparently, many hookah smokers believe it is less harmful and addictive than cigarette smoking, although studies so far indicate that both the short- and long-term effects of tobacco smoking in hookahs are just as harmful as the effects of cigarette smoking. In addition, exposure to secondhand hookah smoke is an underappreciated health hazard for workers in the increasing number of venues that allow hookah smoking (Zhou et al., 2016).

Synthetic nicotine products (i.e., products containing laboratory-produced nicotine) are available in flavors in disposable vaping products (e.g., products sold under the brand name Puff Bar) and in pouches advertised as "tobacco-free" that are designed to be held in the mouth like snus (e.g., products sold under the brand names NIN, Bidi, and Rush). Because these products are not derived from tobacco, they have not been regulated, despite attempts to regulate them. Certainly, nicotine is nicotine, regardless of whether it is synthetically produced or extracted from tobacco, and addiction to synthetic nicotine is certainly possible; however, it remains to be determined whether synthetic nicotine products will produce the range of toxicities seen with tobacco-extracted nicotine.

Nicotine Use Among Youth

Today, it is well known that drug dependency and addiction begin early in life and that adults with no history of having abused a particular harmful substance will probably not start. Therefore, continuing the intensified efforts aimed at preventing cigarette smoking by youth is vital to smoking reduction overall and to the reduction of smoking-associated disease in adults. The data in Table 6.2, drawn from a large 2020 survey of middle and high school students (Wang et al., 2021), indicate that current prevention efforts are having encouraging results: overall nicotine use declined for middle schoolers from 12.5% in 2019 to 6.7% in 2020 and for high schoolers from 31.2% to 23.6%, with similar across-the-board declines for most of the specific forms of nicotine use covered in the table. Nevertheless, despite these declines, recent reports addressing the consequences of vaping by youth have noted the massive switch from tobacco cigarettes to e-cigarettes in the years following their 2007 introduction into the U.S. market (Chadi et al., 2019) and the difficulties in characterizing the health and addiction risks associated with e-cigarettes (Karey, 2021). Currently, the availability of flavored e-cigarettes remains a strong driver for e-cigarette use among youth (Karey, 2021; Sun et al., 2021).

TABLE 6.2 Nicotine Use Among Middle School and High School Students in 2020*

Nicotine Product	Overall	Girls	Boys
	Middle School Students		
Any product	6.7%	6.8%	6.6%
Electronic cigarettes	4.7%	4.8%	4.5%
Cigarettes	1.6%	2.0%	1.3%
Cigars	1.5%	1.6%	1.4%
Smokeless tobacco	1.2%	1.0%	1.4%
Hookahs	1.3%	1.5%	1.2%
Heated tobacco products	1.3%	1.2%	1.3%
Pipe tobacco	0.4%	—	—
	High School Students		
Any product	23.6%	22.5%	24.7%
Electronic cigarettes	19.6%	18.7%	20.4%
Cigarettes	4.6%	3.9%	5.4%
Cigars	5.0%	4.7%	5.4%
Smokeless tobacco	3.1%	1.4%	4.8%
Hookahs	2.7%	2.9%	2.6%
Heated tobacco products	1.4%	1.5%	1.3%
Pipe tobacco	0.7%	0.4%	1.0%

*Use of any product means use on at least 1 day during the 30 days preceding the survey. All data are from the Centers for Disease Control web page "Youth and Tobacco Use."

Research Needed

Because of their appeal to and use by young persons, the nicotine-delivery products discussed above have generally been unsuccessful as aides in tobacco cessation. The lure of these products and the fact that they are not devoid of toxicity mean that, in the years to come, much effort and research must be directed at finding answers to questions like these:

- Are these products truly safer than tobacco cigarettes?
- Are some of these products safer than others?
- What are the long-term toxicities associated with using these products?
- Is the advertising for these products especially appealing to youth?
- Do these products create new dependency problems in youth?
- Do these products provide a way of avoiding or treating nicotine dependency, or are users more likely to transition to cigarette smoking and continued dependency?
- What works better as part of smoking cessation programs, use of these products or total abstinence?

Pharmacokinetics

Nicotine is the major psychoactive substance in tobacco and is responsible for tobacco dependence. The more than 4000 other compounds released by burning tobacco produce the adverse long-term cardiovascular, pulmonary, and carcinogenic effects of smoking. The psychoactive and dependency-producing effects of nicotine are the reason why nicotine is available in many different formulations and products (all the products listed in Table 6.2 come in many different varieties). Nicotine is readily absorbed from every site on or in the body:

- The lungs absorb the nicotine in cigarette smoke and in vapor from e-cigarettes.
- The mucous membranes of the mouth and nose absorb the nicotine in smokeless tobacco.
- The skin absorbs the nicotine in transdermal patches.

Easy and complete absorption promotes the recreational abuse of smoked or smokeless tobacco, but it also facilitates nicotine's therapeutic use in treating nicotine dependency with chewing gums, nasal sprays, transdermal skin patches, and inhalers (see the section "Pharmacological Treatment of Nicotine Dependence" later in this chapter). Figure 6.3 shows how blood concentrations of nicotine rise and fall with use of four different nicotine products (Benowitz et al., 2009). Note that the fall in blood concentrations is quite rapid after cigarette smoking, whereas blood concentrations are maintained at a high level over a long period with the other products.

The average cigarette contains about 8–10 milligrams of nicotine, but only about 25% of that amount enters the bloodstream; thus, the average smoker will absorb 2.0–2.5 milligrams of nicotine per cigarette, but absorption can range from as little as 0.5 milligrams per cigarette to as much as 3 milligrams per cigarette. This means that a person who smokes 20 cigarettes in a typical day would absorb anywhere from 10 to 60 milligrams of nicotine. Most smokers, consciously or not, regulate the rate of drug intake and consequently the blood level of nicotine by controlling the frequency of breaths, the depth of inhalation, the time that smoke is held in the lungs, and the total number of cigarettes smoked.

Ingesting nicotine can be fatal—the lethal dose is estimated to be between 500 and 1000 milligrams; however, smokers rarely experience acute toxicity because inhalation offers exceptional control of the dose.[5]

Characteristically, smokers wake in the morning in a state of nicotine deficiency, smoke one or more cigarettes fairly rapidly to achieve a blood level of about 15 micrograms per liter, and continue smoking through the day to maintain this level. The elimination half-life of nicotine in a chronic smoker is about 2 hours, necessitating frequent administration of the drug to avoid withdrawal symptoms or drug craving. Use of snus, chewing tobacco, or gum results in blood levels of nicotine that are comparable to the levels achieved by smoking (see Figure 6.3).

The liver metabolizes approximately 80–90% of the absorbed nicotine, primarily by the CYP-2A6 enzyme. People in whom the CYP-2A6 enzyme is deficient have higher

[5]People who harvest or cultivate tobacco may experience green tobacco sickness, a type of nicotine poisoning caused by skin contact with wet tobacco leaves.

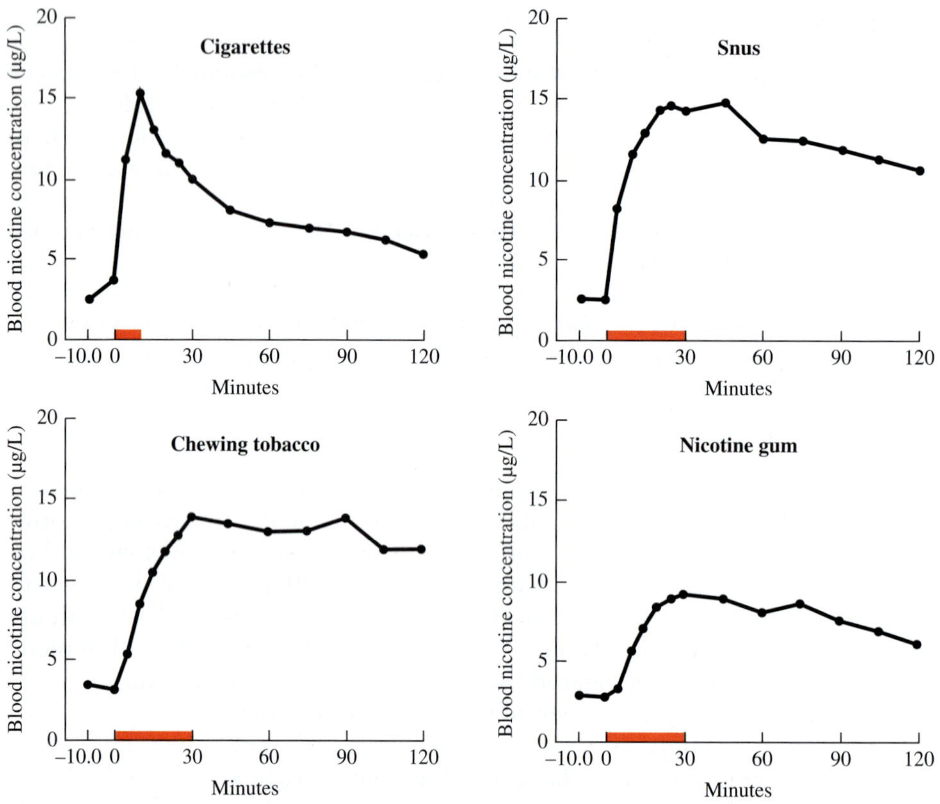

FIGURE 6.3 Blood Nicotine Concentrations During and After Use of Four Different Products. The red bars indicate the time during which participants were using each product: cigarette smoking for 9 minutes, and snus (2.6 grams), chewing tobacco (average of 7.9 grams), and nicotine gum (two 2-milligram pieces) for 30 minutes each. (The concentrations are the average values in micrograms per liter of whole blood for 10 participants.) [Data from Benowitz et al., 2009.]

blood levels of nicotine and lower levels of its metabolite. Interestingly, other constituents of tobacco smoke are capable of stimulating the production of other hepatic drug-metabolizing enzymes (e.g., CYP-1A1 and CYP-1A2), some of which are involved in the metabolism of other drugs, including some antidepressants. As a result, smoking may reduce the blood levels of these medications (by inducing their metabolism in the liver), and smoking cessation may increase their blood levels (because the CYP-2A6 enzyme can now go toward metabolizing these other drugs instead of being used to metabolize nicotine).

Cotinine, the primary metabolite of nicotine, is weakly active and has been used as a biomarker for exposure to tobacco smoke. Interestingly, cotinine was initially developed as an antidepressant and is currently being studied as a treatment not only for depression but also for posttraumatic stress disorder, schizophrenia, Alzheimer's disease, and Parkinson's disease; however, it has never been commercially marketed.

Because cotinine is pharmacologically active, it has been suggested that some of nicotine's effects in the nervous system may be mediated by cotinine and/or by complex interactions of cotinine with nicotine itself (Barreto et al., 2015).

Mechanism of Action

Nicotine exerts virtually all its CNS and peripheral effects by activating specific acetylcholine receptors known as **nicotinic acetylcholine receptors (nAChRs)**—that is, nicotine is an agonist at these receptors, which are divided into two groups, muscle receptors and neuronal receptors:

- Muscle receptors are located on skeletal (voluntary) muscle at the neuromuscular junction, where activation of these receptors by either acetylcholine or nicotine initiates and maintains muscle contraction, which accounts for the muscle fasciculations and tremors that can be induced by cigarette smoking.
- Neuronal receptors are located through the CNS. Activation of these receptors is probably involved in improvements in learning and memory as well as in many other CNS functions.

Effects of Nicotine

Nicotine has a variety of effects on brain and body. Brain effects include nicotine's main rewarding effect and its effects on aspects of cognition; in addition, there are strong associations between cigarette smoking and a number of mental health issues. The main bodily effects are on the cardiovascular and gastrointestinal systems.

Brain Effects

Nicotine's activation of nAChRs results in the release of a variety of neurotransmitters, most importantly the release of dopamine in the ventral tegmental area (VTA) and the nucleus accumbens, as these structures appear to be critical in drug-induced reward; nAChR activation also results in dopamine release in the mesolimbic area and the frontal cortex. Most of this nicotine-mediated release of neurotransmitters occurs via modulation by presynaptic nAChRs functioning as autoreceptors (see the discussion of autoreceptors in Chapter 2), but nicotine may also mediate direct release of neurotransmitters via activation of postsynaptic nAChRs.

Rewarding Effect. Unlike what is seen with caffeine (as discussed earlier in this chapter), nicotine intake from moderate smoking does not alter dopamine synthesis in the striatum (Bloomfield et al., 2014). Instead, nicotine's rewarding effect is believed to be due to the fact that nicotine increases dopamine levels in the limbic system (part of the reward circuit of the brain, discussed in Chapter 4). This increase in dopamine levels may come about in three different ways:

- Activation of nicotinic receptors on neurons in the VTA directly causes dopamine release from these neurons into the nucleus accumbens.

- Activation of nicotinic receptors on neurons in the frontal cortex causes glutamate to be released onto VTA neurons.
- Nicotine desensitizes nicotinic receptors on VTA neurons that release gamma aminobutyric acid (GABA), which by a sequence of steps leads to increased dopamine release in the VTA.[6]

Studies in humans have found that the motivation to smoke (as measured by the smokers' puff rate) predicted the magnitude of dopamine release in the limbic system and that the increased dopamine release correlated with decreased craving to smoke and decreased withdrawal symptoms. Studies also indicate that the motivation to smoke, the anticipation of pleasure from smoking, and the relief of withdrawal symptoms are all related to activity in the limbic striatum (D'Souza, 2016; Le Foll et al., 2014).

Cognitive Effects. Nicotine-induced release of acetylcholine may improve cognitive performance, including memory, and may also be responsible for the arousal effects commonly seen with smoking (Alhowail, 2021). This has raised interest in the development of nicotinic drugs as so-called cognitive enhancers that might be beneficial in treating Alzheimer's disease. In addition, studies suggest that nicotinic receptors may play a protective role in Parkinson's disease; as with caffeine, tobacco smoking is associated with a reduced likelihood of Parkinson's disease (Barreto et al., 2015).

Smoking and Mental Health. More than 25% of U.S. adults are estimated to have a diagnosable mental disorder, and this group is estimated to consume 40–50% of all cigarettes sold (Smith et al., 2015). The association of smoking with substance abuse disorders, attention deficit/hyperactivity disorder, bipolar disorder, and antisocial personality disorder has increased with each of these disorders over the last decades (Talati et al., 2016), and persons with schizophrenia, bipolar disorder, or depression have a significantly increased risk of tobacco-related mortality and of being diagnosed with nicotine withdrawal syndrome. Smoking is also associated with an increased risk of panic attacks, and quitting smoking helps to reduce the risk of such attacks (Bakhshaie et al., 2016). The good news is that smoking cessation treatment can be effective in people with diagnosed mental illness and can improve the psychiatric condition. One study showed that adding smoking cessation treatment to the treatment for illicit stimulant use did not worsen the stimulant use but even enhanced abstinence from the stimulant as well as from nicotine (Winhusen et al., 2014).

Bodily Effects

In the peripheral nervous system, nicotine causes an increase in blood pressure, heart rate, cardiac contractility, and release of epinephrine (adrenaline) from the adrenal glands, as well as an increase in the activity of the gastrointestinal tract.

---

[6]These nicotinic receptors are normally stimulated by acetylcholine to release GABA onto VTA dopamine neurons, and GABA normally inhibits dopamine release. When nicotine desensitizes these receptors, less GABA is released, dopamine-releasing neurons in the VTA are less inhibited, and more dopamine is released.

In normal, nondiseased coronary arteries, nicotine produces vasodilation, which increases blood flow to meet the increased oxygen demand of the heart muscle due to the increased heart rate. Atherosclerotic coronary arteries, however, do not dilate in response to nicotine, which means that the oxygen supply may fail to meet the oxygen demand. This can precipitate angina or a heart attack.

In the early stages of smoking, nicotine may cause nausea and vomiting by stimulating both the vomiting center in the brain stem and sensory receptors in the stomach; however, tolerance to this effect develops rapidly. Nicotine may also reduce weight gain, probably by reducing appetite and altering taste bud sensitivity. Other effects can include stimulation of bowel activity (nicotine is a laxative); stimulation of the hypothalamus to release antidiuretic hormone, which causes fluid retention; and reduction of muscle tone, which may account for the relaxation effects of smoking.

Adverse Effects of Tobacco Smoking

In 1964, a landmark report titled *Smoking and Health: Report of the Advisory Committee to the Surgeon General of the Public Health Service* concluded that cigarette smoking was a cause of lung cancer and laryngeal cancer in men, was a probable cause of lung cancer in women, was the most important cause of chronic bronchitis, and was related to a host of other diseases (U.S. Department of Health and Human Services, 1964). This was the first in a series of 33 surgeon general's reports to expand and update information on smoking-related toxicities with the goal of diminishing the impact of tobacco use on the health of the American people. Over the years, individual citizens, private organizations, public agencies, and elected officials have pursued the 1964 Advisory Committee's call for "appropriate remedial action."

Among the first consequences of the 1964 report was the adoption of the Cigarette Labeling and Advertising Act of 1965, which was followed in 1969 by the Public Health Cigarette Smoking Act. Taken together, these laws required a health warning on cigarette packages, banned cigarette advertising in the broadcasting media, and called for an annual report on the health consequences of smoking.

Reports from the U.S. Department of Health and Human Services since 1964 have focused on such topics as women and smoking (2001), health consequences of smoking (2004), health consequences of environmental exposure to tobacco smoke (2006), smoking among young people (2012), e-cigarettes (2016), and the positive health consequences of quitting smoking (2020).

Since 1964, millions of Americans have given up smoking, and today nearly half of all living U.S. adults who ever smoked have quit (see Figure 6.4). In other words, the antismoking campaign has been a major public health success, despite nicotine's addictive effects and the powerful economic forces promoting its use. However, as noted earlier, more than 34 million American adults still smoke, more than 8 million are living with a serious illness caused by smoking, and about 480,000 Americans die prematurely each year as a result of tobacco use (Centers for Disease Control and Prevention, 2020); further, e-cigarettes and other nicotine delivery devices are contributing to continued nicotine use by youth. In the next few sections, we briefly review some of smoking's disease-producing and other toxic effects.

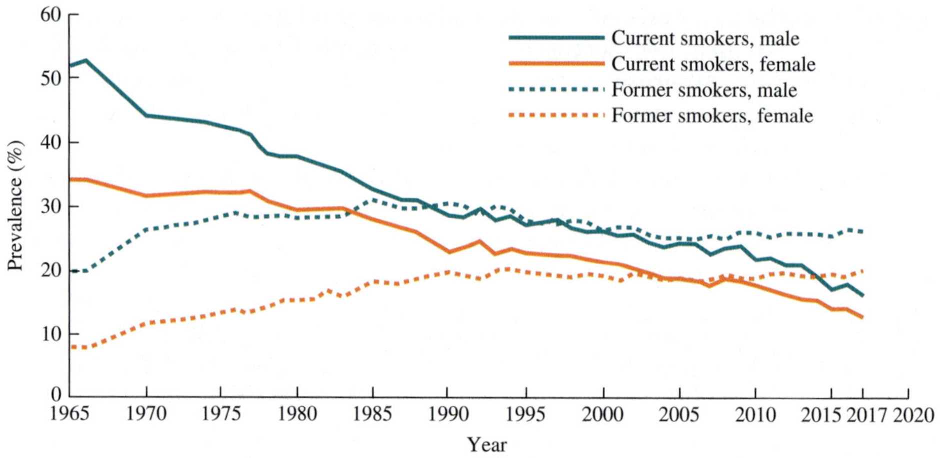

FIGURE 6.4 Current and Former Smokers, 1965–2017. The percent of current smokers among both females and males 18 years of age and older has declined markedly over the past five decades. The percent of former smokers peaked in the 1980s–1990s and has remained fairly constant since. [Data from U.S. Department of Health and Human Services, 2020.]

Cardiovascular Disease

The carbon monoxide in smoke decreases the amount of oxygen delivered to the heart muscle, while nicotine increases the amount of work the heart must do (by increasing the heart rate and blood pressure), and this combination of effects increases the risk of angina or a heart attack. Both carbon monoxide and nicotine promote atherosclerosis (plaque formation) in the coronary arteries. All these effects underlie the dramatic increase in the risk of death from coronary heart disease in smokers compared to nonsmokers.

Smoking also promotes atherosclerosis in other arteries, most notably the aorta (in the abdomen), the carotid arteries (in the neck), and the femoral arteries (in the legs). Cigarette-induced occlusion of these vessels blocks the blood flow to important organs and can result in ischemic damage, strokes, and other disorders.

Lung Disease, Lung Cancer, and Other Cancers

Smokers significantly increase their risk of lung diseases, including chronic obstructive pulmonary disease (COPD), chronic bronchitis, and emphysema. They also significantly increase their risk of lung and other cancers.

Lung cancer is an abnormal growth of cells within the lungs that can result in fatal tumors. It may start in the lining of the bronchi or in other areas of the respiratory system. Smoking, including exposure to secondhand smoke (discussed below), is the leading cause of lung cancer.

Although nicotine itself is not carcinogenic, other components of tobacco smoke are, and the relationship between smoking and cancer is now beyond question. In the United States in 2017, 28.6% of all cancer deaths were attributable to cigarette smoking:

22.9% of cancer deaths in women and 33.7% in men. Regionally, these rates were highest in the South and Appalachia, where as many as 40% of cancer deaths could be attributed to smoking (Islami et al., 2021).

Smoking is also a major cause of cancers of the mouth, voice box (larynx), and throat. Concomitant alcohol ingestion greatly increases the incidence of these problems. In addition, cigarette smoking is a primary cause of bladder and pancreatic cancers, and it doubles the risk of uterine cancer.

Effects of Secondhand Smoke

A 2006 surgeon general's report on the health consequences of exposure to secondhand smoke drew six major conclusions, all of which still stand (U.S. Department of Health and Human Services, 2006):

1. Secondhand smoke causes premature death and disease in children and in adults who do not smoke.
2. Children exposed to secondhand smoke are at an increased risk for sudden infant death syndrome (SIDS), acute respiratory infections, ear problems, and more severe asthma. Smoking by parents causes respiratory symptoms and slows lung growth in their children.
3. Exposure of adults to secondhand smoke has immediate adverse effects on the cardiovascular system and causes coronary heart disease and lung cancer.
4. The scientific evidence indicates that there is no risk-free level of exposure to secondhand smoke.
5. Many millions of Americans, both children and adults, are still exposed to secondhand smoke in their homes and workplaces despite substantial progress in tobacco control.
6. Eliminating smoking in indoor spaces fully protects nonsmokers from exposure to secondhand smoke. Separating smokers from nonsmokers, cleaning the air, and ventilating buildings cannot eliminate exposures of nonsmokers to secondhand smoke.

Effects During Pregnancy

There is no safe level of smoking during pregnancy. Smoking affects the health of the baby before, during, and after childbirth. The nicotine and carbon monoxide in tobacco smoke distribute easily across the placenta, leading to fetal blood levels similar to those in the mother. The effects on the baby of these and other toxins in tobacco smoke can include the following:

- Lower amounts of available oxygen
- Increased heart rate
- Increased risk of miscarriage and stillbirth
- Increased risk of prematurely delivery and/or low birth weight
- Increased risk of respiratory problems

- Increased risk of birth defects
- Increased risk of sudden infant death syndrome

The combination of smoking tobacco and drinking alcohol may be especially dangerous during pregnancy, as shown by a study demonstrating that "combined drinking and smoking after the first trimester of pregnancy, compared with no exposure or quitting before the end of the first trimester, may be associated with significantly increased risk of late stillbirth" (Odendaal et al., 2021).

Tolerance and Dependence

Little tolerance develops to the primary rewarding effects of nicotine, although both physical and psychological dependence do develop in a majority of smokers, as well as in those who absorb nicotine in other ways (e.g., from e-cigarettes or snus). As early as 1988, the surgeon general of the United States concluded that tobacco use is addictive, that nicotine is the substance in tobacco that causes addiction, and that nicotine addiction is pharmacologically as powerful as addiction to other drugs, such as heroin and cocaine (U.S. Department of Health and Human Services, 1988).

A well-defined nicotine withdrawal syndrome has been delineated, which is alleviated by nicotine replacement. Withdrawal symptoms include a severe craving for nicotine, irritability, anxiety, anger, difficulty in concentrating, restlessness, impatience, increased appetite, weight gain, and insomnia. Symptoms usually begin within a few hours after the last dose of nicotine, peak within 24–48 hours, and gradually decline over the next ten days to several weeks. However, mild depression, weight gain, and increased appetite may persist for months. The difficulty of overcoming nicotine dependence is illustrated by the fact that cigarette smokers who seek treatment for other types of drug abuse often find it harder to quit cigarette smoking than to give up the other drugs. Even Sigmund Freud continued his cigar habit (20 per day) until his death, despite many attempts at quitting, persistent heart problems that were probably exacerbated by smoking, and numerous operations for mouth and jaw cancer (his jaw was eventually totally removed).

Unlike withdrawal from other drugs that produce physical dependence, the severity of nicotine withdrawal does not seem to be related to the extent of smoking (or other nicotine use), the duration of the habit, previous attempts at quitting, sex, age, education, or alcohol and caffeine use.

Pharmacological Treatment of Nicotine Dependence

As the reality of nicotine dependence was gradually recognized during the 1990s, a variety of pharmacological products were developed that were aimed at reducing the harm of smoking, presumably with the ultimate goal of promoting cessation.

Among these products are low-nicotine cigarettes. In a six-week trial, participants who smoked low-nicotine cigarettes (with a maximum of 2.4 milligrams of nicotine per gram of tobacco, compared with an average of 15.8 milligrams of nicotine per gram of tobacco in participants' regular cigarettes) decreased the number of cigarettes smoked

DR. J'S MUSINGS 6.2

Doctors Smoking

I grew up in my father's drugstore in the 1950s. We sold cigarettes; but not to youth, and I did not smoke. Cigarettes were widely advertised on the radio, on television, in magazine ads, and in newspapers. In the mid-1960s, concern about the health risks of smoking started to appear, and by the 1970s, cigarette toxicity was well documented. But it was not until one morning in 1981 that I first became shockingly aware of what cigarette addiction really meant.

I was practicing anesthesia at a large hospital in Portland, Oregon. As part of continuing education, I attended a weekly morning seminar at which various anesthesia, surgical, and other medical topics were presented and discussed. On this particular morning, a chest surgeon was lecturing on lung tumors and their removal by surgery, flashing chest X-rays onto a screen, pointing out the tumors—and all the while standing there smoking a cigarette!

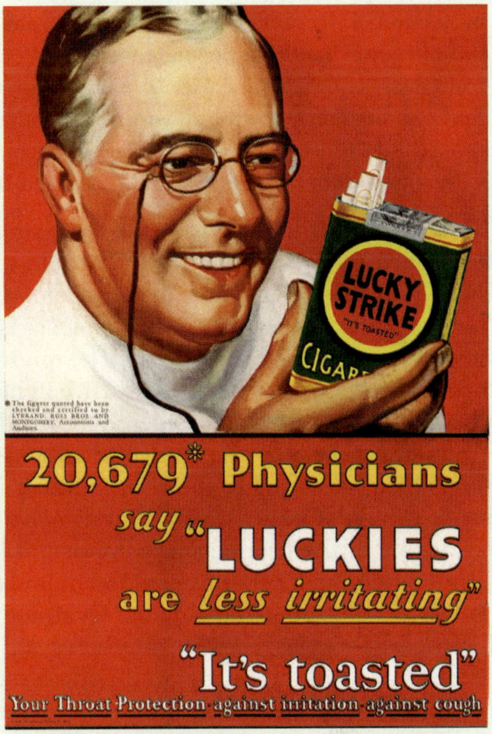

Advertisements like this one, from 1930, were common into the 1950s.

Retro AdArchives / Alamy Stock Photo

I have never forgotten that scene. The memory of it brings to mind the old print ads encouraging smoking, especially the ads placed in the *Journal of the American Medical Association* encouraging doctors to smoke and even implying that cigarettes were beneficial. What a lie! Now we know the truth: they are deadly.

per day compared with participants who smoked their regular brand (Donny et al., 2015). A later study with similar findings reported that switching to very low nicotine cigarettes resulted in reduced tobacco dependence (Shiffman et al., 2019). And another study demonstrated that

> an immediate reduction in nicotine content will result in greater reductions in cigarette satisfaction than a gradual reduction, and this reduction in satisfaction is related to changes in smoking behavior and dependence. (Smith et al., 2019)

In December 2019, the FDA approved the sale of two new low-nicotine products, in line with the study results noted above and other results indicating that switching to very low nicotine cigarettes weakens the motivation to smoke in order to reduce negative affect (Robinson et al., 2020). An FDA news release announcing this approval stated:

> Authorizing these reduced nicotine products for sale in the U.S. is appropriate for the protection of the public health because of, among several key considerations, the potential to reduce nicotine dependence in addicted adult smokers, who may also benefit from decreasing nicotine exposure and cigarette consumption. The agency determined that non-smokers, including youth, are also unlikely to start using the products, and those who experiment are less likely to become addicted than people who experiment with conventional cigarettes. (U.S. Food and Drug Administration, 2019b)

That statement will likely prove to be very controversial. The two low-nicotine cigarettes approved by the FDA have a very low nicotine content (0.2–0.7 milligrams per cigarette vs. 10–14 milligrams in a conventional cigarette), but they are not safer than conventional cigarettes in terms of cancer risks—that is, they are low in nicotine but not lower in tobacco's carcinogens. The question is whether the reduced addictiveness of low-nicotine cigarettes can be effective in helping smokers to quit or at least to switch to other products that are considered to be safer (e.g., e-cigarettes).

Another category of pharmacological treatments consists of the dissolvable tobacco products discussed earlier in this chapter—fine-grained tobacco formed into pellets, strips, or toothpick-size "sticks" that dissolve in the mouth and do not require spitting or discarding of the product. It is important to avoid smoking while using these products, and psychological counseling in conjunction with their use can be helpful.

Other current pharmacological treatments (all discussed below) include nicotine replacement therapies, certain antidepressant drugs, and partial nicotine receptor agonists. Several products associated with these approaches are considered to be first-line options for smoking cessation (Patnode et al., 2015), and both the antidepressant bupropion and the partial nicotine receptor agonist varenicline have received FDA approval for this use.

Nicotine Replacement Therapies

Designed to help smokers quit smoking—that is, eventually abstain completely from cigarettes—**nicotine replacement therapies** supply nicotine in the absence of tobacco and in less harmful ways than cigarettes and other commercial tobacco products—that is, they supply nicotine in controlled amounts and without other chemicals found in tobacco products. Nicotine replacement products—which include nicotine gum, lozenges, inhalers, mouth spray, nasal spray, transdermal nicotine patches, and dissolvable films (Wadgave and Nagesh, 2016)—are generally intended only for short-term use to help manage nicotine cravings and withdrawal. However, the FDA recognizes that some people may need to use these products longer to stay smoke free (U.S. Food and Drug Administration, 2017).

Antidepressants: Bupropion and Nortriptyline

A research review indicated that use of the antidepressants **bupropion** (Wellbutrin, Zyban) and **nortriptyline** (Pamelor) doubles a person's chances of giving up smoking (vs. placebo) and have an acceptable rate of side effects, whereas SSRI antidepressants such as fluoxetine (Prozac) are not effective (Howes et al., 2020; Shoaib and Buhidma, 2018). Of the two, bupropion is the most studied and most widely used, is associated with a longer time until smoking relapse, and results in less weight gain. Interestingly, bupropion and nortriptyline appear to work equally well in both depressed and nondepressed smokers, suggesting that these drugs help smokers quit in some way other than through their action as antidepressants. Perhaps the relevant mechanism of action is revealed by bupropion's inhibition of nicotinic acetylcholine receptors, which indirectly induces dopamine release and thereby reduces the motivation to use nicotine (Shoaib and Buhidma, 2018).

Partial Nicotine Receptor Agonist: Varenicline

In late 2006, FDA approval of the drug **varenicline** (Chantix), based on research showing its greater efficacy than placebo and bupropion in smoking cessation (Jorenby et al., 2006), heralded a new approach to treating nicotine dependence. Pharmacologically classified as a **partial nicotine receptor agonist**, varenicline partially stimulates nAChRs while blocking access of nicotine to those receptors. The effect of this action is that varenicline reduces withdrawal symptoms, makes continued smoking less satisfying, and may thereby help the person to quit and maintain abstinence. Figure 6.5 compares the effect on nAChRs and dopamine release of cigarette smoking, smoking abstinence, and varenicline administration.

A long debate over the safety of varenicline began soon after its 2006 approval, when patients taking varenicline and their doctors started reporting suicidal thoughts, aggression, depression, and agitation. After reviewing the evidence, the FDA gave the drug a black box warning in 2009, which was periodically updated. Then, in 2018, the FDA removed the warning, with this statement:

> Based on an FDA review of a large clinical trial that FDA required the drug companies to conduct, FDA determined the risk of serious side effects on mood, behavior, or thinking with the stop smoking medicines Chantix (varenicline) and Zyban (bupropion) is lower than previously suspected. The risk of these mental health side effects is still present, especially in those currently being treated for mental illnesses such as depression, anxiety disorders, or schizophrenia, or who have been treated for mental illnesses in the past. However, most people who had these side effects did not have serious consequences such as hospitalization. The results of the trial confirm that the benefits of stopping smoking outweigh the risks of these medicines. (U.S. Food and Drug Administration, 2018)

Perhaps the most scientifically interesting study of varenicline revealed that "normal" metabolizers of nicotine were significantly more likely to remain abstinent for up to six months with varenicline than with the nicotine patch. In contrast, varenicline and the nicotine patch were equally effective at helping "slow" metabolizers quit, but users reported more overall side effects with varenicline. The greater effectiveness in normal metabolizers could be due to the fact that varenicline increases dopamine levels, which may reduce the cravings that would otherwise be elicited by the rapid drop in blood nicotine levels. In one such group of normal metabolizers, almost 40% of those taking varenicline were abstinent when the treatment was completed, versus 22% of those on the nicotine patch (Lerman et al., 2015).

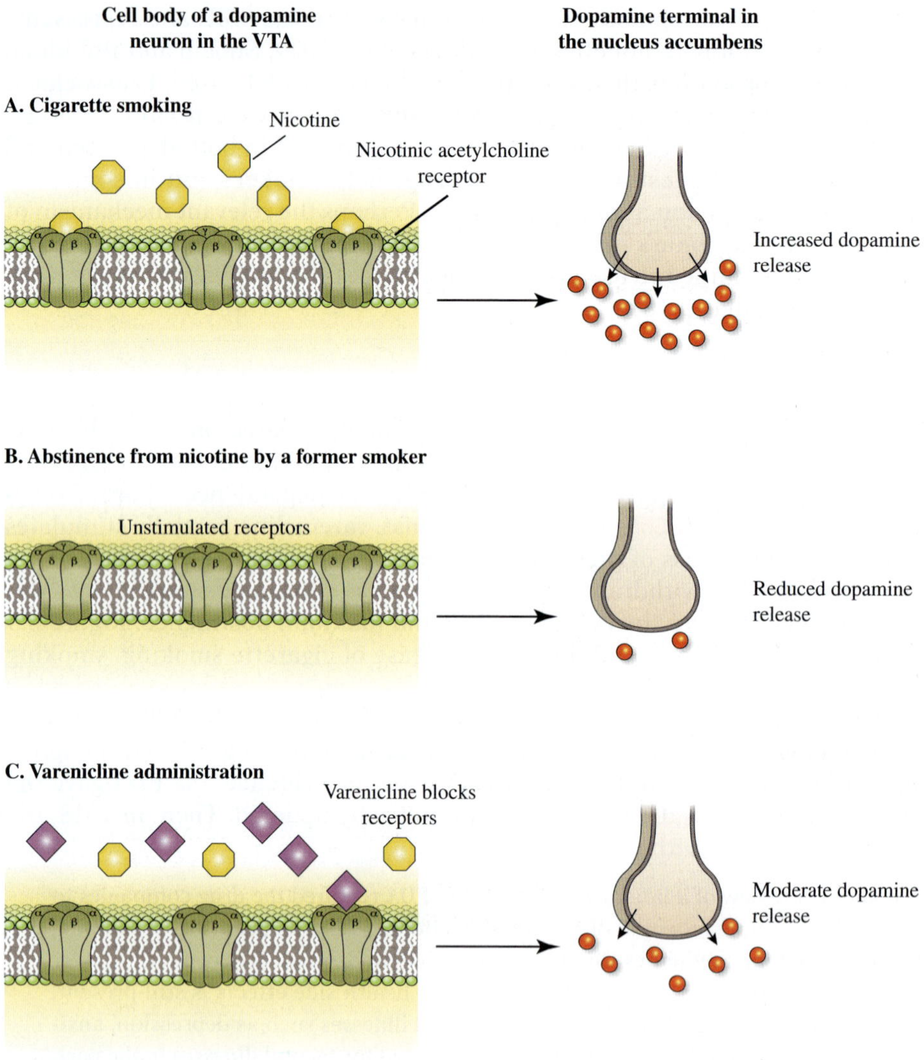

FIGURE 6.5 How Varenicline Works. Nicotinic acetylcholine receptors and dopamine release are affected in different ways by (**A**) nicotine from cigarettes, (**B**) abstinence from nicotine by a former smoker, and (**C**) varenicline administration.

Combination treatment with varenicline and sustained-release bupropion for smokers who were not able to become abstinent with the nicotine patch was more effective than varenicline alone for male smokers and for smokers with a high degree of nicotine dependence. However, varenicline's efficacy as a smoking deterrent was not improved by combining it with a nicotine patch (Baker et al., 2021).

Since 2006, two other partial nicotine receptor agonists have been developed, cytisine (Cahill et al., 2016) and dianicline (Tonstad et al., 2011), though neither has yet received FDA approval as a treatment for smoking cessation (cytisine, a plant-based alkaloid, has been approved as a natural health product by Health Canada). A recent study found that quit rates of persons taking varenicline and those taking cytisine were comparable at about 11–13% of trial participants (Courtney et al., 2021).

Vaccine Therapy

A vaccine would be a novel approach to treating nicotine dependence. Nicotine itself is nonimmunogenic—that is, it does not stimulate an immune response; it must be attached to a carrier protein to induce antibodies that would bind to the nicotine-protein conjugate. The idea is that, once bound in that way, nicotine would not be able to cross the blood-brain barrier, which would reduce its rewarding effect and thereby promote abstinence.

To date, two vaccine products have been tested—NicVAX and NIC002 (or NicQb)—and results have been disappointing: none of the studies detected a statistically significant difference in long-term cessation between participants receiving vaccine and those receiving placebo (Hartmann-Boyce et al., 2012). As noted in a later study, "Current clinically-tested nicotine vaccines have not yet shown enhanced smoking cessation efficacy due to their low immunogenicity" (Zhou et al., 2018). Those researchers go on to suggest that "a hybrid nanoparticle-based nicotine vaccine" might be more effective, as nanoparticles may be better at binding to nicotine molecules and preventing nicotine from crossing the blood-brain barrier. However, no clinical studies have yet been reported.

Cessation of Smoking: Health Benefits and Factors to Consider

A 2020 surgeon general's report on smoking cessation drew ten major conclusions that effectively summarize the health benefits of quitting smoking, as well as some of the main factors to consider in efforts to induce smokers to quit (U.S. Department of Health and Human Services, 2020):

1. Smoking cessation is beneficial at any age. Smoking cessation improves health status and enhances quality of life.
2. Smoking cessation reduces the risk of premature death and can add as much as a decade to life expectancy.
3. Smoking places a substantial financial burden on smokers, healthcare systems, and society. Smoking cessation reduces this burden, including smoking-attributable healthcare expenditures.
4. Smoking cessation reduces risk for many adverse health effects, including reproductive health outcomes, cardiovascular diseases, chronic obstructive pulmonary disease, and cancer. Quitting smoking is also beneficial to those who have been diagnosed with heart disease and chronic obstructive pulmonary disease.
5. More than three out of five U.S. adults who have ever smoked cigarettes have quit. Although a majority of cigarette smokers make a quit attempt each year, less than one-third use cessation medications approved by the U.S. Food and Drug Administration or behavioral counseling to support quit attempts.

6. Considerable disparities exist in the prevalence of smoking across the U.S. population, with higher prevalence in some subgroups. Similarly, the prevalence of key indicators of smoking cessation—quit attempts, receiving advice to quit from a health professional, and using cessation therapies—also varies across the population, with lower prevalence in some subgroups.
7. Smoking cessation medications approved by the U.S. Food and Drug Administration and behavioral counseling are cost-effective cessation strategies. Cessation medications approved by the U.S. Food and Drug Administration and behavioral counseling increase the likelihood of successfully quitting smoking, particularly when used in combination. Using combinations of nicotine replacement therapies can further increase the likelihood of quitting.
8. Insurance coverage for smoking cessation treatment that is comprehensive, barrier-free, and widely promoted increases the use of these treatment services, leads to higher rates of successful quitting, and is cost-effective.[7]
9. E-cigarettes, a continually changing and heterogeneous group of products, are used in a variety of ways. Consequently, it is difficult to generalize about efficacy for cessation based on clinical trials involving a particular e-cigarette, and there is presently inadequate evidence to conclude that e-cigarettes, in general, increase smoking cessation.
10. Smoking cessation can be increased by raising the price of cigarettes, adopting comprehensive smoke free policies, implementing mass media campaigns, requiring pictorial health warnings,[8] and maintaining comprehensive statewide tobacco control programs.

The 2020 report also notes a variety of more specific benefits and significant factors associated with some of these major conclusions, the most important of which are as follows:

- Smoking cessation reduces the risk of stroke and of many cancers, including cancers of the lung, larynx, oral cavity and pharynx, esophagus, pancreas, bladder, stomach, colon and rectum, liver, cervix, and kidney, as well as acute myeloid leukemia; it also benefits the health of pregnant women, their fetuses, and their newborns.
- Progress has been made in inducing smokers to quit or at least to try quitting, but success depends on a wide variety of factors. Consider:
  - Among adult cigarette smokers over the past two decades, quit attempts and actual cessation have increased; health professionals have increasingly given

[7]All insurers under the Affordable Care Act must cover screening for tobacco use and pay for at least two tobacco cessation attempts per year. That coverage would include four counseling sessions of at least 10 minutes each (including telephone, group, and individual counseling) as well as all FDA-approved tobacco cessation medications (whether prescription or over the counter) with a 90-day supply as prescribed. That coverage is to be without prior authorization or cost sharing for the patient.

[8]Unfortunately, graphic warning labels on cigarettes, on their own, are not a strong enough tobacco control measure to reduce cigarette consumption among smokers not ready to quit (Strong et al., 2021).

advice to quit (however, almost half the smokers who saw a health professional during the past year did not receive advice to quit); and use of evidence-based cessation counseling and/or medications has increased (however, more than two-thirds of smokers who tried to quit during the past year did not use evidence-based treatments).

- Attempts to quit and success in quitting vary widely across groups defined by differences in race/ethnicity, age, education, income, health insurance status, and where they live.

- Strategies and tactics that have been effective in helping smokers try to quit include quit-line counseling (either alone or in combination with cessation medications); short text message services about quitting (particularly if they are interactive or tailored to individual text responses); Internet-based interventions (especially when they include behavior change techniques and interactive components); and combining short- and long-acting forms of nicotine replacement therapy.
- Life events such as hospitalization, surgery, and lung cancer screening can lead to quit attempts and to actual cessation (including through smoking cessation treatments).
- The rate at which clinicians deliver smoking cessation treatments can be increased by the dissemination of evidence-based clinical practice guidelines and by payments to clinicians, clinics, or health systems linked to their success in helping patients quit smoking.

CHAPTER REVIEW

1. What are the main sources of caffeine?
2. How is caffeine metabolized? Describe at least four factors that affect the rate of caffeine metabolism.
3. Describe the mechanism of action of caffeine.
4. What are the main beneficial effects of caffeine? What are the main adverse effects?
5. How would you know whether you have caffeine dependency or even caffeine use disorder?
6. What types of statistics reveal the serious problems associated with nicotine use in the United States?
7. Describe the differences among these nicotine delivery devices: e-cigarettes, heated tobacco products, dissolvable tobacco products, snus, and hookahs.
8. Describe nicotine metabolism and how nicotine use can affect the metabolism of other drugs.
9. What are nicotinic acetylcholine receptors? How are they involved in some of the brain effects of nicotine?

10. Summarize the history since 1964 of the recognition of the adverse effects of tobacco smoking. What are the main adverse effects related to cardiovascular disease, cancer, secondhand smoke, and pregnancy?
11. Describe nicotine withdrawal syndrome and how withdrawal from nicotine differs from withdrawal from other drugs.
12. What are the main types of pharmacological treatment of nicotine dependence? Describe at least one example of each type.
13. According to the 2020 surgeon general's report on smoking cessation, what are some of the main challenges faced by efforts to get smokers to quit, and what are some of the main ways of increasing the success of such efforts?

KEY TERMS

adenosine
bupropion
caffeine
caffeinism
cotinine
dissolvable tobacco products
electronic cigarettes (e-cigarettes)
heated tobacco products
hookahs
nicotine
nicotine replacement therapies
nicotinic acetylcholine receptors (nAChRs)
nortriptyline
partial nicotine receptor agonist
snus
striatum
synthetic nicotine products
varenicline

CHAPTER 7

Psychostimulants: Cocaine, Amphetamines, and Nonamphetamines

CHAPTER OUTLINE

Psychostimulants are drugs that exert their primary behavioral effects by augmenting the action of the neurotransmitters norepinephrine, epinephrine, and dopamine, the most important of which is dopamine. Sometimes psychostimulants are referred to as *sympathomimetics* because their effects mimic the effects of those neurotransmitters in stimulating the sympathetic nervous system, which results in feelings of arousal and reward. In particular, by activating the sympathetic nervous system, the psychostimulants produce the characteristic "fright-flight-fight" physiological response characterized by an increased heart rate, increased blood pressure, vasodilation, and bronchodilation, as well as by a rise in body temperature, dilation of the pupils, an increase in blood glucose levels, and increased blood flow to the muscles.

DR. J'S MUSINGS 7.1

How Do Psychostimulants Differ?

The drugs discussed in this chapter resemble one another in being psychostimulants, but how do they differ? In a nutshell, they differ primarily in their metabolic half-lives: cocaine's being only a few minutes and the amphetamine's being several hours. This guides their potential for clinical use, methods of administration, and even intensity of action.

In addition to cocaine and amphetamines (including methamphetamine), psychostimulants include naturally occurring plant products such as ephedrine and cathinone, as well as synthetic drugs such as methylphenidate and modafinil. Although some synthetic psychostimulants have approved medical uses, this chapter primarily covers their recreational use as drugs of abuse. Most recently, recreational use of synthetic cathinones (psychostimulants known as "bath salts") has become a public health concern.

COCAINE

Cocaine is an alkaloid derived from the leaves of any of the four varieties of the coca plant (genus *Erythroxylum*, also called *Erythroxylon*) that grow naturally and are cultivated in the high altitudes of the Colombian, Peruvian, and Bolivian Andes of South America.[1] Cocaine may have evolved in the coca plant because it is toxic to insects that eat the plant's leaves, protecting them from damage.

History of Use

The Indigenous peoples of the regions where the coca plant grows discovered the plant's psychoactive properties at least 5000 years ago, including its ability to reduce fatigue, thirst, and hunger and help alleviate the adverse effects of high-altitude sickness.[2] In fact, the practice of chewing the leaves or brewing a tea from the leaves persists even today in those regions of the Andes and among people who have emigrated from those regions (Bauer, 2019[3]). When the Incas conquered parts of those Andean

[1]Methodology has been developed to identify which of the 19 known coca-growing regions in Colombia, Peru, and Bolivia is the source of any given sample of cocaine (Mallete et al., 2016).

[2]Bauer (2019) notes that current high-altitude medicine recommends chewing coca leaves along with acetazolamide (Diamox) to alleviate altitude sickness and increase endurance.

[3]Bauer makes a careful distinction between cocaine (as a pure drug) and coca leaves, which are usually chewed: "The clinical effects of *coca* and cocaine must be kept distinct, e.g., a cocaine user would consume 60% pure cocaine alkaloid nasally or intravenously immediately vs. a *coca* chewer obtaining 0.5% cocaine in gradual release over 1 hour."

regions in about the tenth century, they treated the plant as sacred and restricted its use to priests and nobility for special ceremonies. After the Spanish conquered the Incas in the sixteenth century, they initially banned coca use, but they then realized how useful it was as a form of money and as a way of increasing the productivity of Indigenous workers.

The Spanish sent samples of the plant to Europe, where the Swedish scientist Carl Linnaeus later classified it in its own family (*Erythroxylaceae*) (the most important species was named *Erythroxylon coca* by the French scientist Jean-Baptiste Lamarck). Europeans, however, remained unaware of the psychoactive properties of the plant until the second half of the nineteenth century, perhaps because its potency deteriorated during the long trip from South America to Europe. It was not until 1857 that the psychoactive compound was isolated and named *cocaine* by the German chemist Albert Niemann, who noted its bitter taste and its anesthetic effect on his tongue.

Cocaine soon became very popular as an additive to drinks and elixirs, most famously when added to wine by the French Corsican chemist Angelo Mariani in 1863. This product, Vin Mariani, was extremely successful and was endorsed by a long list of celebrities.

In 1884, Sigmund Freud published a booklet titled *Über Coca*, praising cocaine and advocating its use to treat depression and to alleviate chronic fatigue. He described cocaine as a marvelous drug with the ability to cure opioid addiction. While using cocaine to relieve his own depression, Freud described the drug as inducing exhilaration and a lasting euphoria that was no different from the normal euphoria of the healthy person. Unfortunately, Freud did not immediately recognize the drug's side effects—tolerance, dependence, a state of psychosis, and withdrawal depression—and became addicted. After he recovered, Freud called cocaine the "third scourge" of humanity, after alcohol and heroin.

DR. J'S MUSINGS 7.2

How I Used Cocaine

A young man came out the loser in a bar fight, with a severely fractured jaw requiring lengthy surgery with general anesthesia. To protect his airways during the surgery, I had to pass a breathing tube through his nose and into his throat before inducing anesthesia—that is, with the young man awake. So I obtained from the pharmacy a vial of powdered cocaine hydrochloride that I dissolved in a teaspoonful of water. I then soaked several cotton swabs in the solution and placed them in his nostrils. After a few minutes, the nasal mucosa shrank, opening the airway, and the mucosa also became quite numb. I then removed the swabs and was able to pass the breathing tube through his nose and into the back of his throat without causing him pain. At that point, I induced anesthesia and passed the breathing tube into his trachea. Following surgery, I woke the patient, and when he could breathe on his own, I pulled the breathing tube back out of his throat and nose.

In the United States, in 1886, a Georgia pharmacist, John Pemberton, developed a product similar to Vin Mariani. But when the city of Atlanta prohibited the sale of alcohol, he changed the formulation, removing alcohol, adding soda water, and combining the coca (about 60 milligrams in 8 ounces of liquid) with syrup of the kola nut, containing 2% caffeine. This drink, which Pemberton named Coca-Cola, was promoted as a health drink, which is a reason why soda fountains in the United States were often found in drugstores. Around the same time, the introduction of the syringe and hypodermic needle prompted many attempts to use cocaine as a local anesthetic for surgery,[4] while also facilitating the use of cocaine (and morphine) as drugs of abuse.

In the late 1800s, concern about cocaine's toxicities increased, with several hundred reports of cocaine intoxication and several reported deaths. At that time, however, there were no restrictions on the sale or consumption of cocaine, which became popular with writers and other artists. Robert Louis Stevenson is said to have conceived of the fictional characters Dr. Jekyll and Mr. Hyde with cocaine in mind, and some of the behavioral effects of the drug were exhibited by Sir Arthur Conan Doyle's fictional character Sherlock Holmes, who used the drug under the supervision of his companion, Dr. Watson. In the United States, President Howard Taft (served 1909–1913) proclaimed cocaine "public enemy number one," and in 1914, the Harrison Narcotics Tax Act banned the incorporation of cocaine into patent medicines and beverages. With the enforcement of the Narcotics Act, cocaine use decreased during the 1930s, largely replaced by use of the newly available amphetamines, which were cheaper and produced longer-lasting yet similar effects. Cocaine all but disappeared until the late 1960s, when tight federal restrictions on the distribution of amphetamines raised their cost, once again making cocaine attractive.

In the 1980s, a new epidemic of cocaine use began with the widespread availability of crack cocaine, intended for use by inhalation (smoking) rather than injection. This stimulant epidemic continues today, although the relatively inexpensive and widely available methamphetamine is currently more commonly encountered. With the increased availability of lower-cost methamphetamine, the number of cocaine users stabilized for a time, but then once again began increasing. Indeed, as of 2018, cocaine was the second leading cause of illicit drug overdose deaths in the United States (Bentzley et al., 2021).

Forms of Cocaine

Coca leaves contain about 0.5–1.0% cocaine. Soaking and mashing the leaves yields coca paste, which is 40–85% cocaine. Coca paste, which is produced during the cocaine-extraction process, is smokable and is consumed mainly in South America.

[4]Today, cocaine's vasoconstrictive and local anesthetic effects give it limited use in head, face, and oropharyngeal surgeries.

It has high potential for abuse, and chronic consumption induces severe complications and dependency (Schwarzkopf et al., 2018).

Treating coca paste with hydrochloric acid yields **cocaine hydrochloride**, the less potent form in which cocaine is usually exported. Powdered cocaine hydrochloride (known as *crystal* or *snow*) can be either "snorted" (sniffed into the nose, where it is absorbed directly from the nasal mucosa) or dissolved in water and injected intravenously (the powder is very water soluble).

However, cocaine hydrochloride cannot be smoked (inhaled) because it is destroyed by heating. In contrast, **cocaine base**, crystals of which are produced by treating cocaine hydrochloride with an alkaline solution and adding a solvent,[5] can be heated until the crystals convert to a stable vapor that can be inhaled, allowing the drug to reach the brain within seconds. But the process of producing cocaine base can be dangerous, with a considerable risk of explosion. Consequently, given the large profits to be made from selling a smokable form of cocaine, illicit factories sprang up for the safe production of cocaine base crystals (also known as *freebase*, *crack cocaine*, or just *crack*, the crystals are somewhat less pure than cocaine base itself; the term *crack* is derived from the sound of the crystals popping when heated for smoking).

Pharmacokinetics

When snorted as a line of drug, cocaine hydrochloride provides a dose of about 25–50 milligrams; thus, sniffing two lines of drug at a time would provide a dose of about 50–100 milligrams. In contrast, smoking crack cocaine provides a dose in the range of 250–1000 milligrams (1 gram). Table 7.1 shows average doses and other pharmacokinetic data for various common methods of administration.

Absorption

Cocaine is absorbed from all sites of application, including mucous membranes, the stomach, and the lungs, but different modes of administration yield differences in the percentage of the drug that is absorbed (see Table 7.1). Cocaine hydrochloride crosses mucosal membranes poorly because the drug is a potent vasoconstrictor, which limits absorption of the cocaine in the snorted drug into blood to only about 20–30%; in addition, 70–80% of the amount absorbed may be metabolized in the liver before it reaches the brain.

In contrast, intravenous injection of cocaine hydrochloride bypasses all the barriers to absorption, placing the total dose of drug immediately into the bloodstream (the 30- to 45-second delay in the onset of action simply reflects the time it takes the drug to travel from the site of injection through the pulmonary circulation and into the brain). Similarly, absorption after smoking cocaine base is rapid and quite complete; effects begin within seconds and peak at around 5 minutes.

[5]Similarly, the Incas mixed coca leaves with lime for chewing, which made saliva more basic (alkaline), thereby enhancing absorption.

TABLE 7.1 Pharmacokinetics of Cocaine

Mode	Average Acute Dose (mg)	Purity (% Cocaine)	Bioavailability (% Absorbed)	Onset of Action (sec)	Duration of "High" (min)	Peak Plasma Levels (mg/l)
Chewing coca leaf	20–50	0.5–1	25	300–600	45–90	150
Snorting cocaine HCl	25–50	20–80	20–30	120–180	30–45	150
Injecting cocaine HCl	25–50	10–100	100	30–45	10–20	300–400
Smoking						
Coca paste	60–250	40–85	6–32	8–10	5–10	300–800
Cocaine base	250–1000	90–100	6–32	8–10	5–10	800–900
Crack	250–1000	50–95	6–32	8–10	5–10	?

Information from M. S. Gold, "Cocaine (and Crack): Clinical Aspects," in J. H. Lowinson, P. Ruiz, R. B. Millman, and J. G. Langrod, eds., Substance Abuse: A Comprehensive Textbook, 3rd ed. (Baltimore: Williams & Wilkins, 1997), p. 185.

Distribution

Cocaine penetrates the brain rapidly, which accounts for the "rush" experienced by users; initial brain concentrations far exceed the concentrations in plasma. After it penetrates the brain, cocaine is rapidly redistributed to other tissues. It freely crosses the placental barrier, achieving blood levels in the fetus equal to those in the mother. (The effects on fetuses and newborns of cocaine or methamphetamine use by pregnant females are discussed in the section "Psychostimulant Use During Pregnancy," at the end of this chapter.)

Metabolism and Elimination

Cocaine has a biological half-life in plasma of only about 50 minutes, as it is rapidly and almost completely metabolized by enzymes located both in plasma and in the liver. Butyrylcholinesterase, which is made in the liver but found mainly in plasma, is the major enzyme for metabolizing cocaine in humans. Cocaine is rapidly removed from plasma but removed more slowly from the brain, where it can be detected for 8 or more hours after initial use. Urine can test positive for cocaine for up to 12 hours. The major metabolite of cocaine is the inactive compound benzoylecgonine, which can be detected in urine for about 48 hours (and for as long as one to two weeks in chronic users) and in hair for several months (hair closest to the scalp takes three to four months to become negative). Detection of benzoylecgonine is the primary basis of urine testing for cocaine use.

There is an important metabolic interaction between cocaine and ethanol in people who use the two drugs concurrently. As shown in Figure 7.1, the liver enzymes that

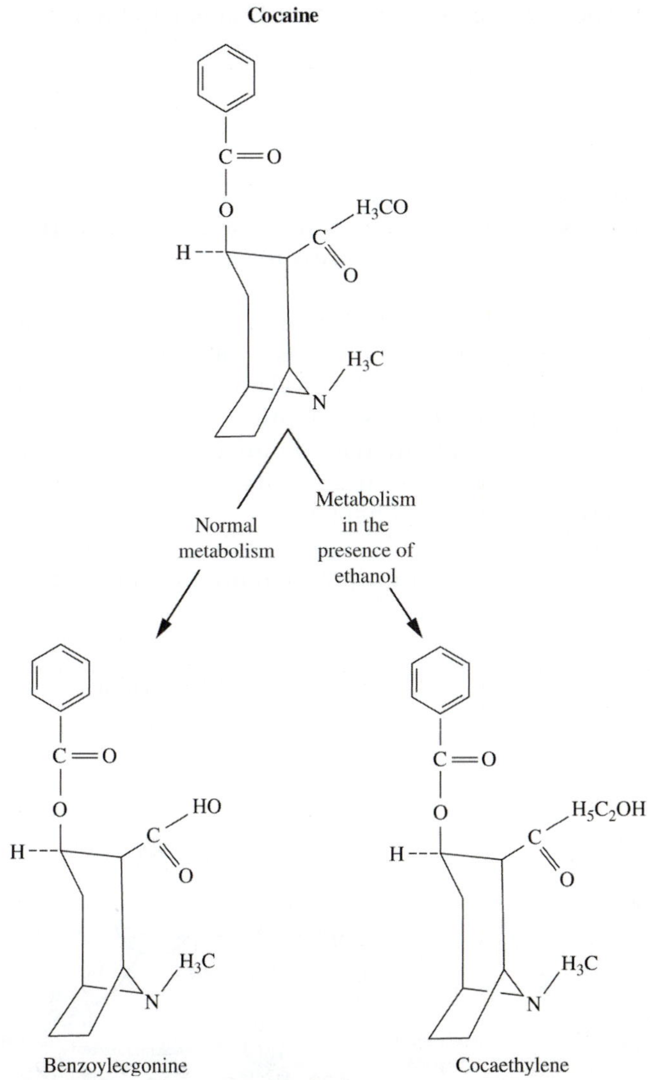

FIGURE 7.1 Cocaine Metabolism. Benzoylecgonine is the primary end product of the normal metabolism of cocaine. In the presence of ethanol (when cocaine and ethanol are used concurrently), the pharmacologically active metabolite cocaethylene is formed.

metabolize the two drugs produce a metabolite called **cocaethylene** (an ethyl ester of benzoylecgonine) that is as pharmacologically active as cocaine; it potentiates the euphoric effect of cocaine, increases the risk of a dual dependency, and increases the severity of withdrawal symptoms. With chronic use of cocaine and ethanol together, cocaethylene's toxic effects on the heart and liver are more severe than the effects of cocaine used alone (Jones, 2019). The half-life of cocaethylene is about 150 minutes, more than twice that of cocaine.

Mechanism of Action

Cocaine has three main pharmacological actions that account for virtually all its physiological and psychological effects: it is a potent local anesthetic; it is a vasoconstrictor, strongly constricting blood vessels and raising blood pressure; and it is a powerful psychostimulant.

Cocaine blocks the presynaptic reuptake of epinephrine, norepinephrine, and dopamine. However, most of cocaine's psychostimulant effects appear to result from the blockade of dopamine reuptake, which increases the levels of dopamine within the synaptic cleft and prolongs the activation of postsynaptic G-protein-coupled receptors (GPCRs) (see Figure 7.2). The resulting increased dopamine levels in the nucleus accumbens and other components of the brain's reward circuit seem to be responsible for the euphoric effects of the drug (see Chapter 4 for a discussion of the reward circuit). Brain imaging studies have historically suggested that at least 47% of the presynaptic dopamine transporters in the brain's reward circuit must be blocked

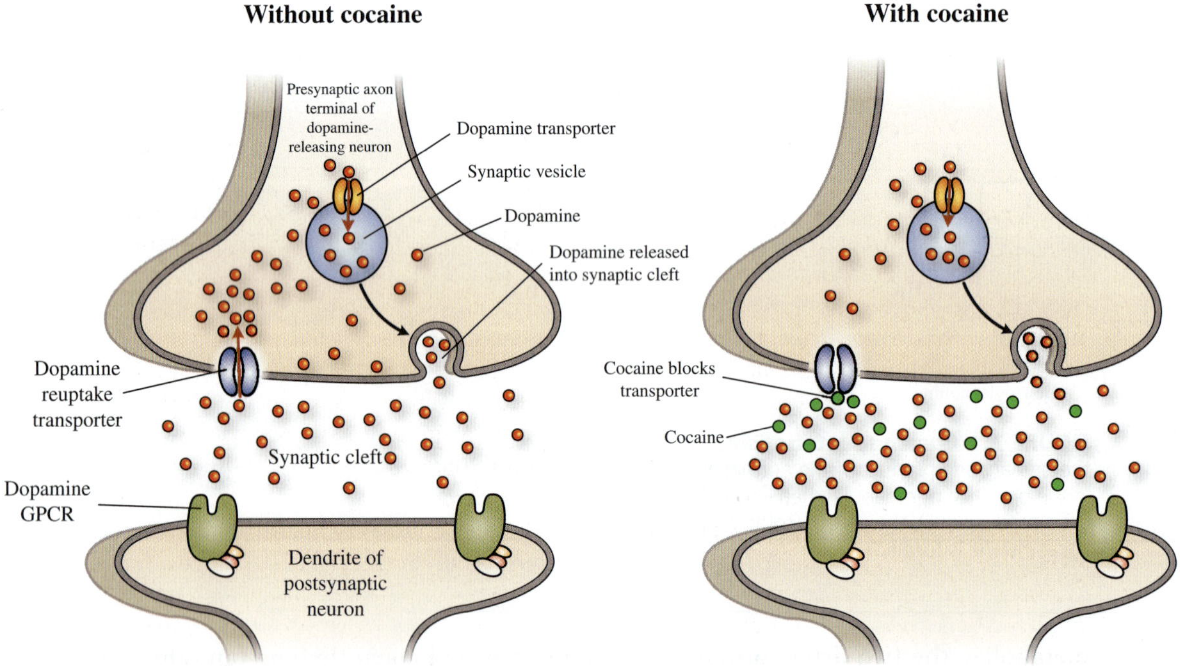

FIGURE 7.2 Dopamine Reuptake and Cocaine. Without cocaine, dopamine reuptake transporters bring dopamine back into the presynaptic axon terminal from the synaptic cleft, to be recycled into synaptic vesicles for future release. With cocaine, the drug blocks the dopamine reuptake transporters, resulting in prolonged activation of dopamine GPCRs in the postsynaptic neuron.

for cocaine to produce its "high" (Volkow et al., 1997); however, more recent studies indicate that the "high" might be produced through blockade of as few as 2% of the transporters (Brodnik et al., 2017). The difference in these results suggests that the relationship between dopamine reuptake inhibition and the cocaine "high" may need reexamination.

Pharmacological Effects

In addition to the "fright-flight-fight" physiological effects described at the beginning of this chapter, cocaine even at low doses (25–75 milligrams) produces feelings of increased energy and alertness, decreased fatigue, increased libido, and a general sense of euphoria or elevation of mood, as well as a reduction in appetite, increased physical activity, and prevention of sleep. If cocaine is snorted, there may first be a numbing sensation known as the "freeze"; if injected, the euphoric effect is so rapid, it is called a "rush." The typical duration of the positive feelings may be 10–20 minutes, followed by a mild depression, called a "letdown" or "comedown." An acutely toxic dose of cocaine has been estimated to be about 2 milligrams per kilogram of body weight; thus, 150 milligrams of cocaine would be a toxic one-time dose for a 150-pound (70-kilogram) person.

Tolerance to the euphoric effects of cocaine develops rapidly, and this can result in continuous cycles of cocaine use lasting for hours (known as "coke runs"). Tolerance may also result in a switch from the intranasal route to injection or to smoking crack cocaine, routes that provide a more intense and more euphoric rush.

As the dose of cocaine or its duration of use increases, all the effects are intensified. Higher blood levels of cocaine may elicit agitation, impulsiveness, anxiety, suspiciousness, paranoia, or even a toxic paranoid psychosis (also known as *substance-induced paranoid psychosis*), which is indistinguishable from true paranoid schizophrenia. A not uncommon and very disturbing symptom of such a cocaine-induced psychosis is formication (from the Latin *formica*, meaning "ant"), the sensation of bugs crawling around under the skin. This may be accompanied by a stereotyped, compulsive, repetitive pattern of behavior in which the person becomes absorbed in taking apart and putting together an object such as a bike or a computer or becomes absorbed in an otherwise aversive activity such as housecleaning (but note that this behavioral phenomenon is more common with formication induced by amphetamine use than by cocaine use). During this behavior, the person might not eat or drink or even use the bathroom and may become annoyed if the behavior is interrupted.

Other possible adverse effects of cocaine use include cardiac arrhythmias, convulsions, strokes, and irreversible cardiac damage or even lethal cardiorespiratory arrest—indeed, cardiac side effects are the single greatest cause of premature deaths due to the use of cocaine. Research indicates that chronic cocaine users have increased aortic stiffening, higher systolic blood pressure, and greater thickness of the heart's left ventricle, effects that led one researcher to call cocaine "the perfect heart attack drug" (Kozor et al., 2014).

When the acute effects of cocaine wear off, depression, dysphoria, anxiety, somnolence, and drug craving typically follow. Cocaine may seem to heighten sexual interest, and high doses (injected or smoked) are sometimes described as orgasmic, but cocaine is not an aphrodisiac. In fact, sexual dysfunction is common in heavy users because they lose interest in sexual and other interpersonal interactions.

Dependence on cocaine can produce changes in the brain, as shown by a brain-scanning study with 120 participants, half of whom were cocaine dependent (Ersche et al., 2011). Not only was there widespread loss of gray matter (neurons) in the brains of the cocaine-dependent participants, but the amount of the decrease was related to the duration of the cocaine abuse—that is, the longer they had been abusing the drug, the greater the loss of gray matter; also, the greater the loss of gray matter, the greater was the craving for cocaine. Another study showed that, although cocaine-dependent participants performed normally on a computer-based spatial learning task, they had abnormal neural responses in cortical areas that mediated reward (Tau et al., 2014), and other studies have shown a deficiency in D_2 receptors in the brains of cocaine-dependent participants (Payer et al., 2014). Over time, as cocaine use continues, cognitive function deteriorates, including negative effects on memory; however, this effect appears to be reversible with cessation of drug use (Vonmoos et al., 2014). Finally, cocaine use appears to be associated with an increased risk of physical injury: according to one study, 24% of the chief complaints among cocaine-positive emergency room patients were related to violent trauma, and the most common cause of death among cocaine-positive patients (37%) was violent injury (Walton et al., 2009).

Comorbidity

People dependent on cocaine are typically young (12–39 years of age), male, and also dependent on at least two other drugs. In addition, they tend to have coexisting psychopathology: 30% have an anxiety disorder, 67% have clinical depression, and 25% exhibit paranoia. Other comorbidities include bipolar disorder, antisocial personality disorder, posttraumatic stress disorder, and attention deficit/hyperactivity disorder (ADHD) (Juteau et al., 2018). Intravenous drug users often take cocaine and heroin together in a mixture known as a "speedball" (the heroin reduces the jitteriness and hypervigilance caused by the cocaine, while the cocaine reduces the sleepiness caused by the heroin).

Treatment of Cocaine Dependence

Psychotherapy is the primary method of treating cocaine dependence, with the best results being achieved by contingency management programs (which use motivational incentives and tangible rewards) (Bentzley et al., 2021). However, given the limited success of even this most successful psychotherapeutic approach, various attempts have been made to augment such therapies with medications.

In a 12-week trial with 81 cocaine-dependent adult participants, a combination of mixed amphetamine salts (Adderall), topiramate (Topamax), and supportive behavioral interventions led to three consecutive weeks of abstinence in 33% of participants receiving the combination treatment versus 17% in participants receiving placebo

(Mariani et al., 2012). Eight years later, a replication trial with 127 participants led to three consecutive weeks of abstinence in 14% with treatment versus 0% in controls. Other studies with topiramate alone (Prince and Bowling, 2018), with other anticonvulsants (Minozzi et al., 2015a), with a variety of dopamine agonists[6] (Minozzi et al., 2015b), with antidepressants (Pani et al., 2011), and with antipsychotics (Indave et al., 2016) reported modest or no efficacy. However, another study found some benefit in the use of dopamine agonists:

> The most promising pharmacological strategies for cocaine use disorder treatment thus far include the use of dopamine agonists, such as long-acting amphetamine and modafinil or glutaminergic and GABAergic agents such as topiramate. Combination drugs may be especially promising. (Kampman, 2019)

Finally, some evidence suggests that cannabidiol may have efficacy in reducing withdrawal symptoms, craving, impulsivity, and paranoia (Calipe-Lopez et al., 2019).

Obviously, more research is needed.

AMPHETAMINES

The **amphetamines** comprise a variety of compounds in the class of phenylethylamines (sometimes called *phenethylamines*), including amphetamine itself, methamphetamine, and MDMA,[7] among others. Figure 7.3 shows the structure of phenylethylamine and how that structure is included in the structures of amphetamine and methamphetamine, as well as in the neurotransmitters dopamine, norepinephrine, and epinephrine. The amphetamine molecule has two isomers. The more pharmacologically potent isomer is **dextroamphetamine** (or *d-amphetamine*), marketed under the trade names Dexedrine and DextroStat; the less potent isomer is levoamphetamine (or l-amphetamine). The two isomers are combined in the medication Adderall, approved for treatment of ADHD (see Chapter 16). **Methamphetamine** is a modified version of dextroamphetamine formed by substituting a methyl group (CH_3) for the hydrogen atom at one end (see Figure 7.3), which allows the drug to cross the blood-brain barrier much faster than amphetamine does. (Methamphetamine is separately discussed in detail below.)

History

Amphetamine was first synthesized in 1887, by the Romanian chemist Lazar Edeleanu, who called it *phenylisopropylamine*. But the actions of amphetamine were not studied until much later, because there were no known therapeutic uses for it at that time. The structure of amphetamine is similar to that of **ephedrine**, which occurs naturally in the herb *Ephedra sinica* and which had been isolated at around

[6]Amantadine, bromocriptine, L-dopa/Carbidopa, pergolide, cabergoline hydergine, and pramipexole.

[7]Due to its psychedelic effects, MDMA is covered in detail in Chapter 8.

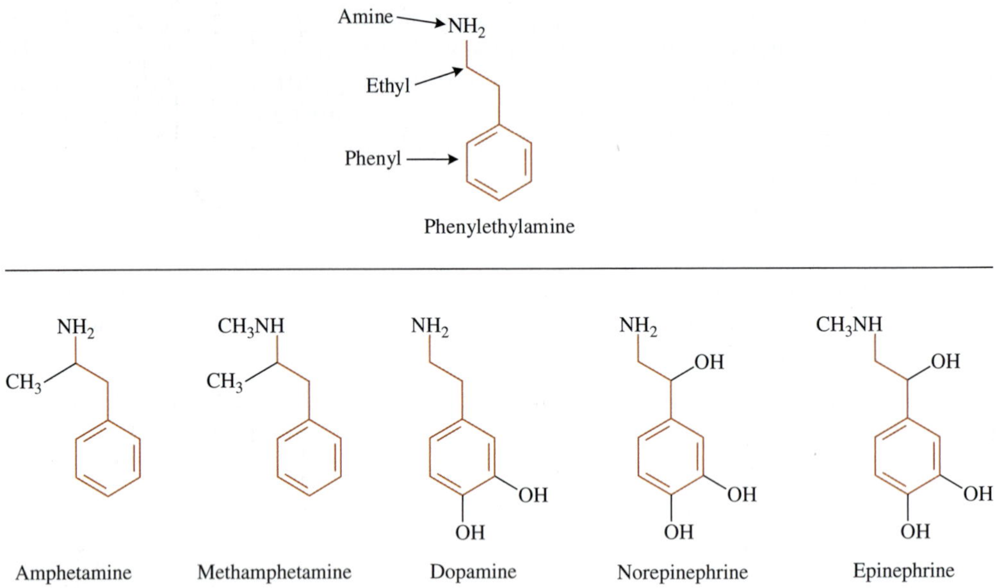

FIGURE 7.3 Phenylethylamine: The Basic Sympathomimetic Amine Nucleus. The structure of phenylethylamine is central to the structures of amphetamine and methamphetamine and the neurotransmitters dopamine, norepinephrine, and epinephrine.

the same time.[8] (Ephedrine is discussed in more detail later in this chapter, in the section on nonamphetamines.)

Ephedrine was found to have an effect similar to that of the neurotransmitter epinephrine, which was already being used as a nasal decongestant to treat asthma. But epinephrine's decongestant effect was short-lived and it had to be injected; ephedrine was better because it could be taken orally and was longer-lasting. However, there were concerns that supplies of ephedrine might be limited because it was a natural plant product, so intense efforts were made to find an alternative.

Amphetamine is an effective nasal decongestant and, in the early 1930s, began to be sold over-the-counter (without a prescription) in inhalers under the brand name Benzedrine. This lack of regulation on the sale of amphetamine set up a potential for abuse, but it was not until 1965 that these inhalers were made available only by prescription.[9]

During World War II, various amphetamines were given to soldiers as a treatment for battle fatigue and to enhance their performance in battle. Between 1935 and 1946, 39 conditions were identified for which amphetamines could be used in treatment,

---

[8]The medicinal preparation ephedra (also known as *ma-huang*) is obtained from the same herb (as noted later in this chapter, ephedra has been banned by the FDA). In 1919, Akira Ogata used ephedrine derived from that same herb to synthesize methamphetamine in a crystalized form soluble in water, a process that continues to be used today.

[9]I remember selling these inhalers in the 1950s in my father's pharmacy in Seattle.

including schizophrenia, morphine addiction, tobacco smoking, head injury, radiation sickness, hypotension, seasickness, severe hiccups, and caffeine dependence. In 1935, racemic amphetamine (i.e., a mixture of d- and l-amphetamine) was found to be effective in promoting wakefulness, leading to its use for the treatment of the neurological disorder narcolepsy, and in 1937 it was reported to have a calming effect on hyperactive children. Large-scale abuse (usually by oral ingestion of amphetamine tablets) began in the 1940s, beginning with students and truck drivers who used it to maintain wakefulness, temporarily increase alertness, and delay sleep. Advertising directed toward women promoted use of methamphetamine to reduce appetite and relieve depression. However, users soon developed tolerance to its anorexic and antidepressant actions, although this was poorly recognized at the time. Today, the legitimate use of the various amphetamines is largely restricted to the clinical treatment of ADHD, occasionally in the treatment of narcolepsy, and rarely (off-label) in the treatment of resistant depression.

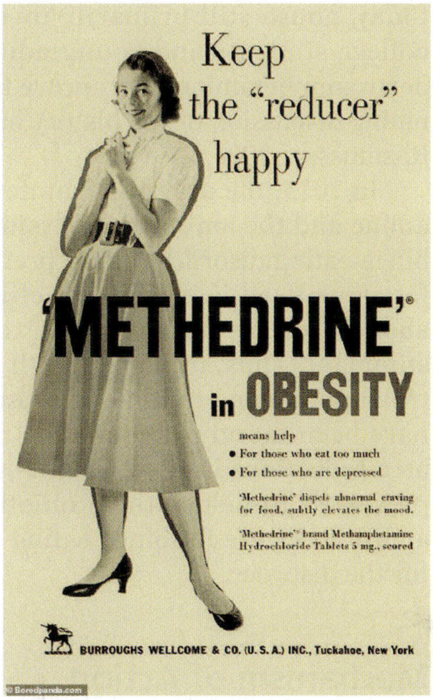

Methamphetamine was once thought to be safe enough to promote in ads like this (under the brand name Methedrine, from the early 1950s) and safe enough to be sold without a prescription. The small print claims that the drug means help "for those who eat too much" and "for those who are depressed" and that it "dispels abnormal craving for food" and "subtly elevates the mood."

In the late 1960s, the abuse pattern changed with the advent of injectable forms of the amphetamines. During the next decades, there was an epidemic of abuse that saw the appearance of the "speed freak"—users who took intravenous doses continuously for days.

In 1965, after decades of reported abuse, the FDA restricted the amphetamines (especially dextroamphetamine) to prescription use, but nonmedical abuse remained widespread. In 1971, under the Controlled Substances Act, amphetamines became Schedule II drugs, and eventually the epidemic slowed, for several reasons:

- First, users became aware of the dangers of compulsive use (as expressed in the phrase "speed kills").
- Second, at the same time, the government exerted pressure on drug companies to decrease their legal production of amphetamines; medical use was discouraged, and physicians who prescribed amphetamines unethically were prosecuted.
- Third, alternative and more effective treatments for depression were discovered.
- And fourth, during the 1970s and 1980s, cocaine abuse reemerged (at that time, more people could afford cocaine).

Then, in the mid-1990s, amphetamine abuse resurfaced, becoming even more of a scourge when the smokable form of methamphetamine ("ice") was developed;

today, abuse still primarily involves methamphetamine, not uncommonly among college students and young adults who also used other amphetamines (especially dextroamphetamine) to improve their performance in school or on the job. (For a fascinating discussion of the history of amphetamine abuse during the years 1929–1971, see Rasmussen, 2008.)

In 2015, the drug lisdexamfetamine (Vyvanse)—a combination of dextroamphetamine and the amino acid l-lysine—became the first drug approved for treatment of binge-eating disorder (it had previously been approved for treating ADHD). Lisdexamfetamine itself is initially inactive, but after it is swallowed, the amino acid is metabolically separated from dextroamphetamine in the gut, which releases the active stimulant. Thus, treatment with lisdexamfetamine is a barely disguised form of dextroamphetamine treatment. Doses of 50–70 milligrams of lisdexamfetamine per day have been found to reduce the number of binge-eating days per week, with associated reductions in body weight of 5.2–6.25% (Ward and Citrome, 2018). The FDA had previously forbidden the promotion of lisdexamfetamine for treatment of obesity but approved its use for binge eating because there was no other approved drug treatment for the disorder.

Mechanism of Action

Like cocaine, amphetamines amplify the actions of norepinephrine, epinephrine, and dopamine in the brain, most importantly dopamine. But amphetamines do this in several different ways:

- At low doses, amphetamines bind to the presynaptic membrane of the axon terminals of dopamine-releasing neurons, which induces increased release of dopamine from the terminal into the synaptic cleft. Also at low doses, amphetamines block the presynaptic dopamine reuptake transporters on the axon terminals, similar to the blocking action of cocaine illustrated in Figure 7.2; however, the effects of this reuptake block differ from the effects with cocaine. As illustrated in Figure 7.4, the blocked reuptake transporters begin to transport the amphetamine into the axon terminal, and the amphetamine there begins interfering with the transporter that normally conveys dopamine into synaptic vesicles for release. This leads to increased dopamine levels in the cytoplasm of the terminal, which induces the reuptake transporter to reverse direction and begin transporting dopamine out of the terminal, thereby increasing the amount of dopamine available in the synaptic cleft for activation of postsynaptic dopamine receptors.
- At high doses, amphetamines taken into the axon terminal interact directly with dopamine-containing synaptic vesicles, causing the vesicles to release dopamine into the cytoplasm of the terminal, which, as described above, induces presynaptic reuptake transporters to reverse direction and transport dopamine out of the terminal. Also at high doses, amphetamines taken into the axon terminal bind to the enzyme monoamine oxidase (MAO), preventing the degradation of dopamine there, which results in increased release of dopamine into the synaptic cleft and thus increased stimulation of postsynaptic dopamine receptors.

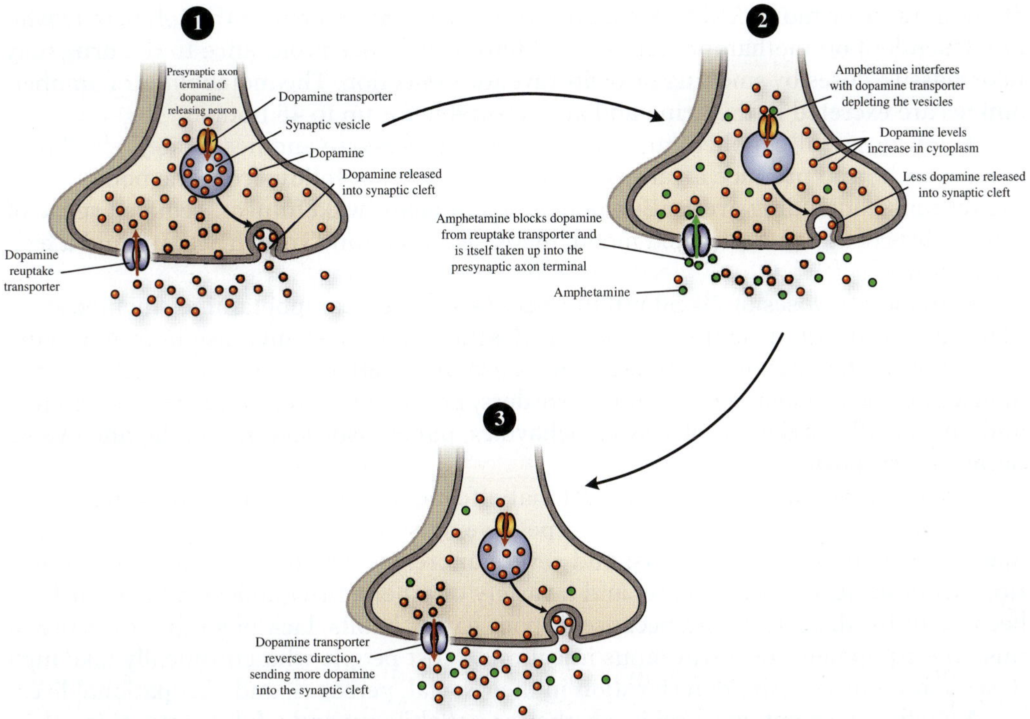

FIGURE 7.4 Dopamine Reuptake and Amphetamines. **(1)** Normally, without the presence of amphetamines, dopamine reuptake transporters convey dopamine back into the axon terminal for rerelease into the synaptic cleft. **(2)** Amphetamine blocks the dopamine reuptake transporter, preventing the reuptake of dopamine, but allowing the transport of amphetamine into the terminal, where it interferes with the transport of dopamine into synaptic vesicles, thereby increasing dopamine levels in the cytoplasm of the terminal. **(3)** As a result, the direction of the dopamine reuptake transporters reverses, which increases the amount of dopamine released into the synaptic cleft.

These actions all serve to amplify the action of dopamine and thus account for the psychostimulant and rewarding effects of the amphetamines. Given that the amphetamines and cocaine have the net effect of increasing the amount of available dopamine (although through different mechanisms), it is not surprising that people who abuse cocaine have difficulty distinguishing between the subjective effects of equivalent intravenous doses of cocaine and dextroamphetamine.

Pharmacological Effects

Pharmacological responses to amphetamines vary with the specific drug, the dose, and the route of administration. For example, with racemic amphetamine, effects may be categorized as those produced by low to moderate doses (5–50 milligrams, usually administered orally) and those observed at high doses (approximately 100 milligrams or more, often administered intravenously). But dextroamphetamine alone is more potent: low to moderate doses range from 2.5 to 20 milligrams, while high doses are

50 milligrams or more. Methamphetamine is even more potent, although people who are dependent on methamphetamine and have developed a tolerance to the drug may take massive doses by smoking or by intravenous injection. The metabolites of amphetamines are excreted in the urine and are detectable for up to 48 hours.

At low doses, all amphetamines increase blood pressure and heart rate, relax bronchial muscle, and produce a variety of other actions that follow from the body's alerting response, including arousal, euphoria, excitement, wakefulness, reduced sense of fatigue, loss of appetite, elevated mood, increased motor and speech activity, and a feeling of power.

At moderate doses of 20–50 milligrams, the effects of amphetamines include stimulation of respiration, slight tremors, restlessness, a greater increase in motor activity, insomnia, and agitation. As doses increase, these effects are accompanied by the appearance or worsening of anxiety disorders, possibly progressing from restlessness and nonspecific anxiety to obsessive behaviors, panic disorders, paranoia, and even a paranoid psychosis.

Chronic high doses produce additional effects, including stereotypical behaviors such as continual, purposeless, and repetitive acts; sudden outbursts of aggression and violence; paranoid delusions; and severe anorexia. Weight loss, skin sores, infections from neglected health care, and a variety of other consequences may occur both because of the drug itself and because of poor eating habits, lack of sleep, or the use of unsterile equipment for intravenous injections. Most people who chronically take high doses show a progressive deterioration in their social, personal, and occupational lives.

A vitally important question is whether or not children and adolescents taking therapeutic doses of prescribed amphetamine (e.g., Adderall) may be at risk of developing neurotoxicity with subsequent long-term cognitive and other mental impairments. In a study of the effects of amphetamine in adult nonhuman primates, with doses and plasma concentrations of amphetamine calculated to resemble those seen in children and adolescents receiving amphetamine for ADHD treatment, the primates had damage to the axon terminals of dopamine-releasing neurons in the striatum (Ricaurte et al., 2005). Other research on the effects of amphetamine in adolescents suggests neurotoxic effects, although less profound than in adult animals (Teixeira-Gomes et al., 2015). However, all the evidence still leaves unanswered the question of whether or not youth treated with amphetamine for ADHD will suffer any long-term neurotoxicity in the form of memory or behavioral impairments.

Interestingly, some subjective effects of amphetamines, such as arousal and euphoria, seem to be related to personality traits, such as impulsivity. For example, research indicates that people who gamble pathologically have different blood pressure and cortisol responses to amphetamines than do healthy controls, suggesting that norepinephrine-related disturbances in the gamblers may account for this difference in response to the drug (Zack et al., 2015). During short-duration, high-intensity activity, such as an athletic competition, amphetamines may enhance performance despite any impairment of dexterity and fine motor skills. Importantly, all amphetamine products used by athletes with ADHD are very tightly controlled by antidoping agencies (Nazeer et al., 2014; White et al., 2013).

The toxic dose of amphetamine varies widely among people. Severe reactions can occur even from doses as low as 20–30 milligrams, whereas people who have developed tolerance have survived doses of 400–500 milligrams. (The slogan "speed kills" refers not only to a fatal effect of single doses of amphetamine but also to the deteriorating mental and physical condition of the addicted person.)

Amphetamines are prone to compulsive abuse, and physical dependence is readily induced (the treatment of amphetamine use disorder is discussed later in this chapter). Once drug use is stopped, a person experiences a withdrawal syndrome with symptoms that may include increased appetite, weight gain, decreased energy, and increased need for sleep. Suddenly discontinuing amphetamine use may result in severe depression and suicidal behavior. The paranoia mentioned above as a possible symptom of chronic use may persist after withdrawal, but it generally does not develop as a result of withdrawal.

Methamphetamine

Most methamphetamine in the United States is smuggled from Mexico, where the drug is readily available and inexpensive (Mullen et al., 2021). The rest comes mainly from clandestine U.S. laboratories (the drug is easily synthesized from readily obtainable chemicals, including pseudoephedrine). Methamphetamine is FDA approved for the treatment of ADHD and narcolepsy but is rarely used for those legitimate clinical treatments because of its well-established neurotoxicity (discussed below).

Like cocaine hydrochloride, methamphetamine hydrochloride (the form in which it is usually produced) breaks down at high temperatures and so cannot be smoked. But when converted to its crystalline form (variously known as *ice*, *speed*, *crystal*, *crank*, and *go*), methamphetamine can be effectively vaporized and inhaled, like crack cocaine.

Pharmacokinetics

Smoking crystalline methamphetamine results in its near-immediate absorption into plasma, with additional absorption continuing over the next 4 hours. The blood level then progressively declines. However, methamphetamine has a much longer half-life than cocaine (more than 11 hours), resulting in an intense, persistent drug action, or "high." After distribution to the brain, about 60% of the drug is slowly metabolized in the liver, and the end products of metabolism (including small amounts of the pharmacologically active metabolite, amphetamine) are eliminated in urine, along with the unmetabolized methamphetamine (about 40% is eliminated unchanged).

Toxicity, Including Neurotoxicity

Methamphetamine produces acute psychotic symptoms, including delusions and hallucinations. In a study with nearly 300 participants who met the DSM criteria for methamphetamine dependence, psychotic symptoms were just over five times more likely to occur during periods of methamphetamine use than during periods of no use (McKetin et al., 2013). The risk of psychotic symptoms was dose dependent and doubled if the participant also used marijuana or alcohol. The most common psychotic symptoms are persecutory delusions and auditory hallucinations (Mullen et al., 2021). Recovery can take more than a month. Treatment begins with antipsychotics, with electroconvulsive therapy added for patients with psychoses lasting more than a month (Zarrabi et al., 2016). Research suggests that methamphetamine-induced psychosis may result from an overflow of dopamine in the cortex, leading to excessive cortical glutamate release, ultimately damaging cortical interneurons, with this damage manifesting itself as psychotic symptoms (Hsieh et al., 2014).

Neurotoxicity is a long-term consequence of methamphetamine toxicity and includes damage to the axon terminals of serotonin- and dopamine-releasing neurons, neuronal death, and replacement of dead neurons with astroglial and microglial cells in the brain (Halpin et al., 2014; Shaerzadeh et al., 2018; Yu et al., 2015). Dopamine-related neurotoxicity has been associated with slower motor function and memory deficits, perhaps with a predisposition to future development of neurodegenerative disorders such as Parkinson's disease (Callaghan et al., 2012). To what extent these neurodegenerative changes are reversible over time is unclear; some effects may be irreversible. Reductions in gray matter, increases in white matter scar tissue, and increases in the size of ventricles are all consistent with irreversible loss of brain matter; also, neuronal loss in the hippocampus, the brain's center for making new memories, is comparable to the loss seen in early Alzheimer's disease, and recovered methamphetamine users perform significantly worse on average on memory tests than healthy people of the same age (Thompson et al., 2004). In a study with mice consuming doses of methamphetamine mixed with sweetened oatmeal, significant memory problems and hippocampal neurotoxicity were found after 28 days of drug administration (Avila et al., 2018).

In sum, the evidence is mixed as to whether or not methamphetamine abuse causes cognitive decline in humans; most of the data indicate intellectual decline for an indefinite duration in some users (Mizoguchi and Yamada, 2019).

Tolerance and Dependence

Tolerance to methamphetamine-induced euphoria rapidly develops, which can lead people to taking higher and higher doses and can start a cycle of drug use, dependence, and withdrawal. The increases in feelings of well-being in nonusers given doses of 5 or 10 milligrams of methamphetamine twice daily continue only for the first couple of days and are followed by increases in negative feelings (dizziness, nausea, depression, and so on) (Panenka et al., 2013). Chronic methamphetamine users who become abstinent have low brain levels of stored dopamine, which then recover to normal levels in some abstinent users, raising the question of whether users who cannot maintain abstinence have a more persistent dopamine depletion (Boileau et al., 2016).

Treatment of Amphetamine Use Disorder, Including Methamphetamine Use Disorder

Methamphetamine use disorder is skyrocketing, at least as measured by overdose deaths. From 2015 to 2019, methamphetamine overdose deaths increased by 180%, methamphetamine use increased by 43%, frequent methamphetamine use increased by 66%, and the number of people with diagnosable methamphetamine use disorder increased by 105% (Han et al., 2021). In absolute numbers, there were 15,489 methamphetamine overdose deaths in 2019. The reasons for the large increase in number of overdose deaths are unclear, but contamination of methamphetamine with illicit fentanyl and increased use of methamphetamine in combination with heroin (a combination known as a "goofball") or with fentanyl are possibilities.

A recent review of the treatment of amphetamine use disorder (including methamphetamine use disorder) not only noted the relative effectiveness of brief cognitive-behavioral therapy versus no therapy but also reached the following conclusions about pharmacological treatments (Khoramizadeh et al., 2019):

> Risperidone reduced positive psychotic symptoms while aripiprazole reduced negative psychotic symptoms. Methylphenidate reduced craving and depression compared with placebo. Topiramate reduced addiction severity and craving for methamphetamine. . . . Buprenorphine reduced methamphetamine craving more than methadone. Haloperidol [also] reduced psychosis. Riluzole[10] reduced craving, withdrawal and depression. . . .

In other research, one study highlighted the significance of dopamine-related dysfunctions in amphetamine use disorder and the potential use of that knowledge in the development of new therapies (Ashok et al., 2017b), while the authors of another study had this to say about the possible use of cannabidiol (CBD) in the treatment of stimulant use disorders: "Observational studies suggest that CBD may reduce problems . . . such as withdrawal symptoms, craving, impulsivity and paranoia" (Calipe-Lopez et al., 2019).

The rise specifically in methamphetamine use in the 1990s spurred research into potential treatments of methamphetamine abuse, dependence, and addiction (i.e., methamphetamine use disorder). By the early 2000s, however, researchers had become well aware of the difficulty in finding effective ways of treating this disorder: "Treatment of methamphetamine intoxication is primarily supportive. Treatment of methamphetamine abuse is behavioral. . . . Pharmacological treatments are under investigation" (Winslow et al., 2007).

Behavioral treatments of methamphetamine use disorder that have shown some efficacy include cognitive-behavioral therapy, behavioral activation, and contingency management (Paulus et al., 2020; Winslow et al., 2007). Pharmacological approaches that have been tried include drugs that block euphoria; drugs that reduce withdrawal symptoms, including negative mood symptoms (e.g., depression); and drugs that ameliorate craving by inhibiting the release of glutamate in the prefrontal cortex (as discussed in Chapter 4). To date, however, as with cocaine use disorder, no specific pharmacotherapies have been developed that show significant improvement in abstinence rates in the treatment of methamphetamine use disorder (Hartel-Petri et al., 2017; Morley et al., 2017; Paulus et al., 2020).

Nevertheless, some pharmacological treatments do seem to have some effectiveness in the treatment of specific symptoms of methamphetamine use disorder. For example, a review of studies on the treatment of methamphetamine-induced psychosis suggests the use of pharmacological agents that target psychotic symptoms, along with agents that target any comorbid psychiatric disorders such as depression and anxiety, plus behavioral treatments to prevent relapse because "[p]revention of methamphetamine relapse is the most direct means of preventing recurrence of psychotic symptoms and syndromes" (Glasner-Edwards and Mooney, 2014). Certainly, comorbid

---

[10]A drug used to treat amyotrophic lateral sclerosis (Lou Gehrig's disease).

depression can be treated with an appropriate antidepressant drug (see Chapter 12); antipsychotic drugs can be used to treat paranoid or psychotic reactions or behaviors, as well as personality disorders (see Chapter 11); and appropriate drugs can be used to treat bipolar disorder (see Chapter 14). In terms of particular drugs, as noted above, risperidone, aripiprazole, and haloperidol may have some effectiveness in treating methamphetamine-induced psychosis (Khoramizadeh et al., 2019). And other researchers discuss possible pharmacological approaches to ameliorating neurocognitive and memory disorders associated with methamphetamine abuse (Calipe-Lopez et al., 2019).

A review of pharmacological treatments for methamphetamine addiction stated that "clinical trials examining the potential pharmacotherapies for methamphetamine use disorders have largely been negative" (Ballester et al., 2017). In fact, however, four medications that have been tested in clinical trials (methylphenidate, bupropion, modafinil, and naltrexone) have shown some limited efficacy; although none of these was clearly effective, any of them could be tried, depending on the clinical situation.

In sum, research indicates that these are the most promising pharmacological approaches to treating methamphetamine use disorder, especially if combined with behavioral therapies (all these types of medications will be discussed at length in subsequent chapters):

- A dopamine agonist (e.g., long-acting methylphenidate) may help prevent craving.
- An antipsychotic agent may assist with treatment of psychotic symptoms.
- An anticonvulsant (e.g., topiramate) may assist with withdrawal symptoms and craving.
- An opioid partial agonist (e.g., buprenorphine) may also assist with craving.
- Antidepressants may help with treatment of comorbid or residual depression and anxiety.
- Cannabidiol may help in treating multiple aspects of postwithdrawal syndromes.

NONAMPHETAMINES

In this section, we will discuss a variety of nonamphetamine stimulants that have been subject to abuse, including ephedrine and pseudoephedrine; the herbal substance khat; synthetic cathinones ("bath salts," including flakka); DMAA; and four prescription-only drugs (methylphenidate, pemoline, modafinil, and armodafinil).

Ephedrine and Pseudoephedrine

In anesthesiology, ephedrine is sometimes administered intravenously to temporarily elevate blood pressure and heart rate when such action is needed. Most nonmedical use of ephedrine has been as an ingredient in dietary supplements to help with energy increase and weight loss. However, ephedrine can cause a toxic (even fatal) reaction when combined with caffeine or other stimulants, and in 2004 the FDA banned its use in dietary supplements.

The structurally similar drug pseudoephedrine is used in cough and cold medicines to relieve nasal congestion, but as mentioned earlier, it is also used in the illicit manufacture of methamphetamine, leading the FDA to restrict it to prescription-only use.

Khat

The leaves and fresh shoots of *Catha edulis*, a flowering shrub native to East Africa commonly known as **khat**, can be chewed (like loose tobacco) or brewed as a tea, at a daily dose of up to several hundred grams. Khat has effects similar to, but less powerful than, amphetamine and cocaine, including excitement, loss of appetite, and euphoria, and it is being increasingly encountered as a substance of abuse in the United States and elsewhere. The active components of khat are cathinone and cathine, which are closely related in structure but differ in the strength of their pharmacological effects. Cathinone, the pharmacologically more active substance, deteriorates within about 48 hours after khat is harvested, which means that khat must be used fresh. Cathine appears to be a mild psychostimulant, comparable to caffeine in potency.

Synthetic Cathinones

By far, the most concerning development in stimulant abuse in the past few years has been the increased abuse of **synthetic cathinones** (i.e., synthesized derivatives of cathinone), in particular those derivatives known as "bath salts," a name that apparently comes from their being sold in packages labeled as such to avoid detection as drugs.

Synthesis of cathinone derivatives has been reported since the late 1920s—for example, methcathinone was synthesized in 1928 and mephedrone in 1929—and by 1933, some concern about detrimental effects had arisen, but it was not until the 1990s that outbreaks of abuse were seen in various places, eventually reaching the United States around 2009. In early 2011, emergency rooms began to see an increase in admissions from ingestion of these drugs, and in September of that year the Drug Enforcement Administration (DEA) gave notice that it intended to temporarily "schedule" the three drugs that were the main synthetic cathinones being abused at that time: **mephedrone**, **methylone**, and **MDPV** (methylenedioxypyrovalerone), all of which were officially classified as Schedule I drugs in 2013. A fourth frequently abused synthetic cathinone, **flakka** (α-PVP), was classified as a Schedule I drug in 2014 ("la flaca" is Spanish slang referring to a slender woman or a beautiful woman). Figure 7.5 shows the chemical structure of cathinone and the four drugs mentioned above, along with a number of other synthetic cathinones.

Typical clinical effects of synthetic cathinones include agitation and anxiety, paranoia, impaired concentration and memory, headache, rapid heart rate, hypertension, vertigo, abdominal pain, muscle damage, and convulsions, which can be lethal (Karila et al., 2015). In addition, besides the acute side effects generally associated with psychostimulants, use of synthetic cathinones is associated with a high incidence of psychosis, including hallucinations and delusions, as well as with problems with concentration,

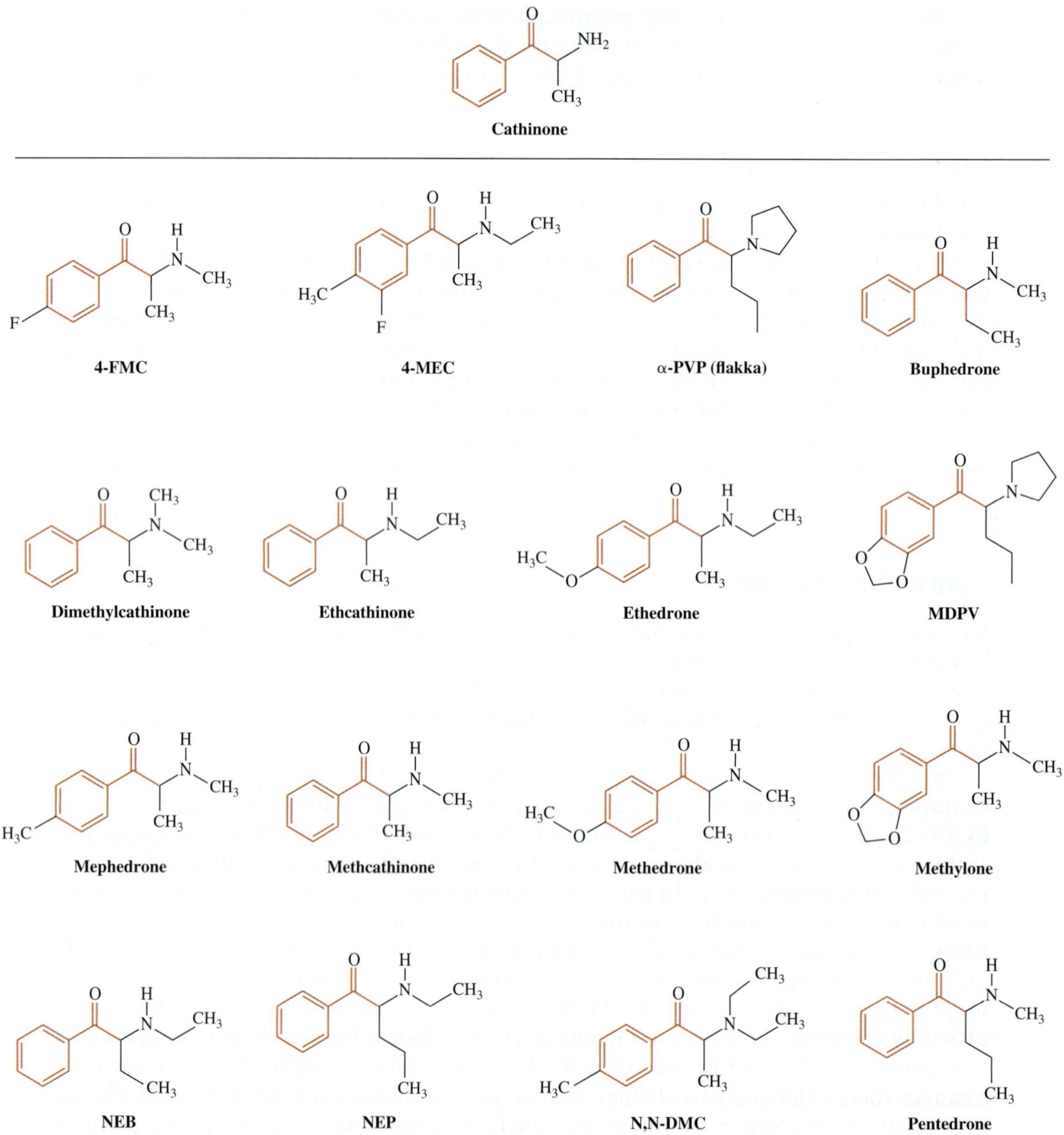

FIGURE 7.5 Structures of Some Synthetic Cathinones. The highlighted part of the cathinone molecule (top) is part of the structure of each of the synthetic cathinones below.

memory, and problem solving. Repeated use of high doses of synthetic cathinones leads to tolerance, dependence, and craving (Ross et al., 2011), and sudden termination of chronic use may elicit symptoms of withdrawal, with treatment being symptomatic (Miliano et al., 2016).

Mephedrone, Methylone, MDPV, and Second-Generation Synthetic Cathinones

According to users, doses of mephedrone and methylone are 100–200 milligrams orally, with effects beginning about 30–45 minutes after ingestion and lasting about 2–5 hours. MDPV appears to be more potent, with effects beginning 15–30 minutes after a typical oral dose of 10–15 milligrams and lasting 2–7 hours. Routes of administration other than oral are also effective, including nasal inhalation and intravenous and intramuscular injection.

All three of these drugs produce subjective effects similar to the effects of amphetamine and cocaine, due to dopamine release in the reward circuit of the brain, including a sense of euphoria and well-being but also including mild changes in perceptions accompanied by paranoia. They also produce peripheral nervous system effects due to the release of serotonin, including pupillary dilation and increases in pulse rate, blood pressure, and glucose utilization. Toxic reactions produced by high doses of these drugs include hyperthermia and hallucinations, which may be associated with aggressive behaviors and violence (John et al., 2017).

In experimental animals, doses of mephedrone and methylone lead to increased release of dopamine, norepinephrine, and serotonin, whereas MDPV acts as a cocaine-like dopamine reuptake inhibitor (Kolanos et al., 2013).

It is important to note that MDPV is 50 times more potent than cocaine as a blocker of the dopamine transporter (see Figure 7.2), that it is anywhere from three to ten times more potent than mephedrone and methylone in potentiating motor activity, and that it is detected in either urine or blood in most cases of fatal overdoses of bath salts in the United States (Baumann et al., 2014). Among patients admitted to emergency rooms, those who tested positive for MDPV in urine or blood showed a tenfold increase in overall dopamine levels compared with those who had used cocaine (Islam et al., 2015).

After mephedrone was classified as a Schedule I drug, several so-called second-generation synthetic cathinones came into use, including 4-MEC (shown in Figure 7.5), which causes serotonin release and blocks dopamine reuptake, and 4-MePPP, which can block both dopamine and serotonin reuptake, although it is more potent at the dopamine transporter. Both of these agents have been available since about 2010 and, in 2017, were listed as Schedule I controlled substances (Drug Enforcement Division, 2017).

Flakka

After mephedrone, methylone, and MDPV were banned in 2011, reports of MDPV use dropped precipitously, but DEA monthly surveillance reports of flakka use increased from about 20 to more than 3000. Originally synthesized in the 1960s, flakka is an inexpensive drug that comes in the form of crystals of different colors (this gives it another nickname, "gravel," because of its similar appearance to whitish pink aquarium gravel). It can be taken orally (the crystals dissolve in the mouth), dissolved in water and injected, powdered and then snorted, or heated and vaporized for inhalation (Marusich et al., 2016). Overdoses are more likely as a result of injection or inhalation because these forms of administration increase the rate at which blood levels of the drug rise. Flakka is more potent than cocaine or amphetamine because of its greater effectiveness in blocking reuptake of dopamine and norepinephrine. Heart rate and blood pressure might be dangerously elevated by the rapid increase in norepinephrine, while sudden increases in dopamine may elicit euphoria, along with delusions, hallucinations, and agitation. Other behavioral effects of flakka are comparable to those of other psychostimulants, such as increased alertness and energy, but with flakka these may progress to bizarre effects including delirium accompanied by paranoia and possibly delusions of great power and strength (Olson, 2015).

Intoxication due to flakka is treated with supportive care to reverse the effects and prevent further problems. Therapy includes intravenous benzodiazepines to sedate the patient and mitigate seizures until the effects of the drug wear off. Intravenous fluids are also administered, especially if rhabdomyolysis is evident. It is difficult to identify flakka intoxication with a laboratory assay because special testing of blood or urine is required. (For a review of the pharmacology and health risks of flakka, see Patocka et al., 2020.)

DMAA

DMAA (1,4-dimethylamylamine), a stimulant that has some structural similarity to ephedrine and amphetamine, was first patented in 1944 and marketed as a nasal decongestant (like Benzedrine). It was withdrawn from the market in 1970 but was remarketed in 2004 after the FDA banned the sale of the stimulant ephedra in dietary supplements. Supplement manufacturers used DMAA as a substitute for ephedra and claimed it was a natural component of the geranium plant.

The FDA has received dozens of adverse event reports on products containing DMAA; the drug raises blood pressure and constricts blood vessels, which may contribute to heart attacks. Although the FDA's current position is that DMAA cannot be sold as a "dietary ingredient," it remains as an ingredient of multiple dietary energy products. DMAA has been added to the group of banned substances by the World Anti-Doping Agency.

Prescription-Only Nonamphetamines

The last group of psychostimulants that we will discuss in this chapter consists of three prescription-only nonamphetamines: methylphenidate, modafinil, and armodafinil. The structures of these three drugs are shown in Figure 7.6.

Methylphenidate

The primary medical use of **methylphenidate** (Ritalin) is in the treatment of ADHD (discussed in Chapter 15). Like cocaine, methylphenidate increases the synaptic concentration of dopamine by blocking presynaptic dopamine reuptake transporters and perhaps also by slightly increasing the release of dopamine (an amphetaminelike or ephedrinelike action). Experienced cocaine users who inject methylphenidate intravenously report a cocainelike or amphetaminelike rush, an effect not usually experienced when methylphenidate is taken orally. At clinically relevant doses, methylphenidate blocks more than 50% of the dopamine transporters 60 minutes after oral administration, with a relatively low level of rewarding effects due to the slow uptake of methylphenidate into the brain. The half-life of the regular-release formulation of methylphenidate is 2–4 hours, which contrasts markedly with the approximately

12-hour half-life of the three other prescription-only nonamphetamine stimulants that we discuss next—pemoline, modafinil, and armodafinil.

Modafinil and Armodafinil

As shown in Figure 7.6, **modafinil** (Provigil) is a racemic mixture, and only the R-isomer, **armodafinil** (Nuvigil), is pharmacologically active. As noted in Chapter 3 in the case of citalopram and escitalopram, when a patent expires on a racemic medication and cheaper generic versions become available, a manufacturer can market the active isomer of the drug under a new patent and sell it at a higher price under a new name, which seems to be the situation with armodafinil. (Of course, armodafinil is twice as potent as modafinil because it is not diluted by the inactive isomer, so the recommended dosages of armodafinil are half those of modafinil.)

Modafinil and armodafinil have the same FDA indications and have primarily been used for "wakefulness promotion," including for treatment of sleepiness due to jet lag. The drug also has FDA approval for the treatment of three disorders: narcolepsy, shift-work sleep disorder, and obstructive sleep apnea with residual excessive sleepiness despite the use of a continuous positive airway pressure device. It has also been used in the treatment of ADHD, although the FDA has not approved it for this use, and one study did not find it effective for ADHD in adults (Arnold et al., 2014).

The mechanism of action behind the drug's "wakefulness" effect is not well established. Like cocaine, modafinil blocks dopamine transporters in the human brain, but perhaps less potently than cocaine (Loland et al., 2012). Nevertheless, as with most drugs with abuse potential, modafinil's blockade of dopamine transporters increases

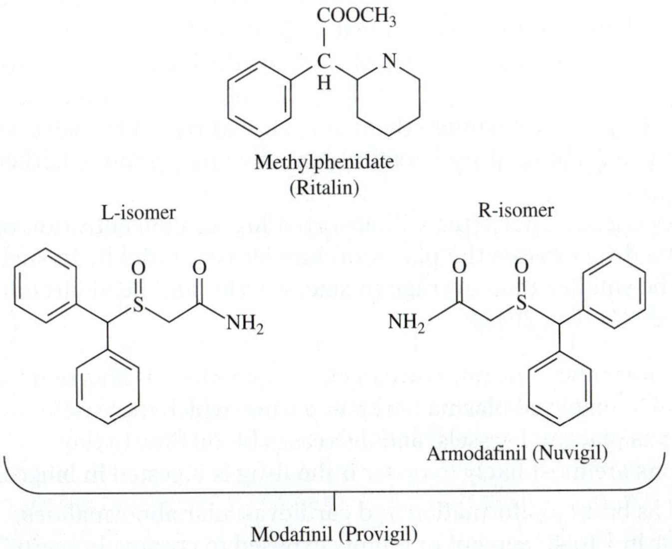

FIGURE 7.6 Structures of Methylphenidate, Modafinil, and Armodafinil. Note that modafinil is a racemic mixture of left (L) and right (R) optical isomers; only the R-isomer (armodafinil) is pharmacologically active. (See Chapter 3 for discussion of racemic mixtures.)

dopamine levels in the nucleus accumbens to levels similar to those induced by other psychostimulants (Wuo-Silva et al., 2016).

Laboratory investigations of putative cognitive enhancement from modafinil in healthy volunteers have shown consistent but relatively modest benefit, perhaps due to an effect of increased "motivation" in that participants described feeling more pleasure in performing the experimental tasks (Müller et al., 2013). In a review of modafinil's actions in non-sleep-deprived persons, the researchers argue that the cognitive effects of this drug may depend on the type of assessment used, given that benefits are not consistent or very impressive when "basic" assessments are used, whereas "complex" assessments show enhancement of attention, executive function, and learning (Battleday and Brem, 2015). This study did not find any substantial evidence for side effects or mood changes, but other researchers observed that this is not consistent with reports of headache, dizziness, tachycardia, nervousness, insomnia, and gastrointestinal complaints, as well as other serious adverse effects (but almost half of such effects occurred when the drug was used for nonindicated reasons) (Nicholson et al., 2015). A review of an extensive literature on the use of modafinil and armodafinil in humans concludes that there is no serious risk of seizure, even in patients with ADHD, head injury, brain tumors, or seizure disorders, but notes that the drug may affect the levels of some anticonvulsant drugs by pharmacokinetic interactions and that this possibility needs to be considered in individual situations (Andrade, 2016). Overall, use of the drug is limited by the risk of a potentially fatal skin eruption (Stevens-Johnson syndrome).

PSYCHOSTIMULANT USE DURING PREGNANCY

A wide-ranging review of the use of psychostimulants by pregnant women in the United States notes that "stimulants are the second most widely used and abused substances during pregnancy and pregnant women using stimulants during pregnancy are at increased risk of adverse perinatal, neonatal, and childhood outcomes" (Smid et al., 2019); in addition, of course, the pregnant women themselves are at risk of the adverse effects associated with the use and abuse of psychostimulants by any person, whether pregnant or not (see Table 7.2).

If a pregnant woman uses cocaine, her fetus will absorb a higher concentration of the drug than she does, as the drug crosses the placental barrier very quickly. In such cases, the newborns tend to be smaller than average in size, weight, and head circumference. According to one study (Malek, 2012):

- During the early months of pregnancy, cocaine use can cause spontaneous abortion, "probably due to an increase in maternal plasma norepinephrine, which increases uterine contractility, constricts placental vessels, and decreases blood flow to the fetus." Spontaneous abortions are most likely to occur if the drug is ingested in binges.
- Congenital anomalies, such as brain malformation and cardiovascular abnormalities, "have been reported to occur in 7 to 40 percent of infants exposed to cocaine in utero."
- Withdrawal symptoms may occur in about one-third of babies born to cocaine-using mothers. These include seizures, lethargy, hyperactive reflexes, vomiting, diarrhea, high-pitched crying, and restlessness. Such babies have a harder time feeding and are more likely to be sick in their first year of life.

TABLE 7.2 Maternal, Perinatal, Fetal, and Childhood Outcomes Associated with Use of Psychostimulants During Pregnancy

Cocaine	
Maternal effects Cardiovascular complications • Hypertension • Myocardial ischemia and infarction • Cardiotoxicity Infectious disease (HIV, hepatitis B and C) Renal failure Hepatic rupture Thrombocytopenia Cerebral ischemia and infarction Maternal death **Perinatal effects** Preterm birth Low or reduced birth weight Small for gestational age infant Shorter gestational age at delivery Perinatal infection (HIV, hepatitis, syphilis) Placental abruption	**Structural fetal anomalies** Genitourinary defects Limb reduction Intestinal atresia **Childhood neurodevelopmental effects** Some evidence of adverse behavioral, growth, cognition and learning outcomes, which may be attributable to other social and other perinatal factors
Amphetamine/Methamphetamine (Illicit)	
Maternal effects Cardiovascular complications • Hypertension • Myocardial ischemia and infarction • Cardiomyopathy Infectious disease (HIV, hepatitis B and C) Dental disease Adolescent pregnancy **Perinatal effects** Intrauterine growth restriction Preterm birth Fetal death Earlier gestational age Lower birthweight Smaller head circumference	**Structural fetal anomaly** Cleft palate **Childhood neurodevelopmental effects** Increased anxiety and depression and attention problems at 3 and 5 years old Poorer cognitive outcomes at 7.5 years old Frontal and striatal brain changes at age 7–15 years old with differential effects by sex

(Continued)

TABLE 7.2 *Continued*

MDMA (Ecstasy)**	
Maternal effects* Work and social problems **Perinatal effects***	**Structural fetal anomalies** Cardiovascular anomalies Musculoskeletal anomaly (clubbed foot) Gastroschisis **Childhood neurodevelopmental effects** Poor motor quality and lower milestone attainment at 4 and 12 months of age Fine and gross motor delays at 24 months of age
Ephedra	
Maternal effects* (based on data from nonpregnant populations) Cardiovascular complications Death Among those with coexisting psychiatric conditions: psychosis, severe depression, mania, suicidal ideation	Other effects*
Synthetic Cathinones ("Bath Salts")*	

*Limited or no information available.
**See Chapter 8 for detailed coverage.
SOURCE: Smid et al., 2019.

Prenatal cocaine exposure may impair attentiveness and emotional expressivity in childhood, producing a condition that resembles ADHD. Although one study found that cocaine exposure in utero was not a strong predictor of adolescent delinquent behaviors (Gerteis et al., 2011), another group of researchers reported that adolescents between the ages of 14 and 17 exposed to cocaine in utero had lower gray matter volume in brain regions involved in emotion, reward, memory, and executive function compared with nonexposed adolescents (Rando et al., 2013).

Other effects associated with cocaine use by pregnant women include a greater likelihood of poor prenatal care, greater prevalence of tobacco and alcohol use, and greater likelihood of infant abuse and neglect. In addition, cocaine decreases appetite, which means that both the mother and the fetus are at risk of malnutrition. Clearly, many indirect negative effects of cocaine use are due to psychiatric problems experienced by the pregnant women and to social and environmental risk factors such as domestic abuse and the absence of a significant other. As these types of issues increase, a substance-abusing pregnant woman or new mother may be overwhelmed and have little time for careful prenatal care or for effective parenting. Overall, the effects of cocaine use by pregnant women are typically a combination of direct effects of drug exposure and the effects of multiple psychiatric, social, and environmental factors.

Methamphetamine use and abuse during pregnancy tends to produce adverse maternal and perinatal effects similar to those associated with cocaine (see Table 7.2). In addition, fetal brain structures known to be sites of neurotoxicity in adult methamphetamine abusers are more vulnerable to methamphetamine exposure than to alcohol exposure, and the more severe the damage to those structures, the more severe tend to be later cognitive deficits (Sowell et al., 2010).

Other adverse effects associated with methamphetamine use during pregnancy include a much higher incidence of preterm births (50% vs. 17% among nonusers), fewer prenatal care visits, a higher incidence of infant death soon after birth (4% vs. 1%), and a higher incidence of poor response on measures of newborn health (6% vs. 1%) (Good et al., 2010). On the positive side, although methamphetamine levels in breast milk tend be about 14% of maternal blood levels, no adverse consequences have been reported on breast-feeding babies.

CHAPTER REVIEW

1. Why are psychostimulants sometimes referred to as *sympathomimetics*?
2. True or false: Powdered cocaine hydrochloride can be sniffed into the nose, dissolved in water and injected intravenously, or vaporized and smoked.
3. True or false: The effects of injecting cocaine hydrochloride or of smoking cocaine base occur much more rapidly and completely than the effects of snorting cocaine hydrochloride.
4. What is cocaethylene?
5. Describe how cocaine causes an increase in dopamine levels in the brain's reward circuit.
6. Describe some of the "positive" effects of cocaine and at least three adverse effects, including formication.
7. How do cocaine and amphetamine differ in their mechanism of action?
8. Describe some of the pharmacological effects of amphetamines, including differences in the effects of low doses, high doses, and chronic high doses, and describe the risks to children and adolescents of taking prescribed amphetamines for treatment of ADHD.
9. Why does methamphetamine use result in a more persistent "high" than cocaine use?
10. What are some common psychotic symptoms associated with methamphetamine toxicity, and what are the neurotoxic effects associated with long-term methamphetamine toxicity?
11. True or false: Various pharmacological approaches have shown some effectiveness in the treatment of methamphetamine use disorder, especially if combined with behavioral therapies.

12. What is khat?
13. True or false: The synthetic cathinones MDPV and flakka are significantly more potent than cocaine as blockers of dopamine reuptake.
14. Describe the structural difference between modafinil and armodafinil.
15. Describe the adverse effects of stimulant use during pregnancy, including effects on the pregnant woman, the fetus, and the child. Distinguish between direct effects of the drugs and indirect effects associated with drug use.

KEY TERMS

amphetamines
armodafinil
cocaethylene
cocaine
cocaine base
cocaine hydrochloride
dextroamphetamine
DMAA
ephedrine
flakka
khat
MDPV
mephedrone
methamphetamine
methylone
methylphenidate
modafinil
psychostimulants
synthetic cathinones

CHAPTER 8

Psychedelic Drugs

CHAPTER OUTLINE

Psychedelic drugs (or *psychedelics*) act on various neurotransmitter pathways in the brain to produce hallucinatory perceptual experiences, which may be accompanied by marked changes in cognition and mood. In contrast to other drugs of abuse, which are mainly taken for their direct rewarding effects, many psychedelics are taken specifically to alter subjective states of consciousness (the term *psychonaut* refers to a person who uses psychedelics to explore such experiences). In fact, it is not uncommon for these substances to produce dysphoric, rather than euphoric, effects. Moreover, nonhuman animals are less likely to self-administer these drugs than they are to self-administer classically rewarding drugs such as amphetamines or opioids.

Primarily for this reason, psychedelics have long been considered to have little or no therapeutic potential. This situation, however, is beginning to change; some psychedelics are being investigated for use in treating pain and such psychiatric disorders as anxiety, depression, and posttraumatic stress disorder (PTSD) (with one drug having already received FDA approval for treatment of depression), and these therapeutic uses are leading to reevaluations of drug classifications, of the kinds of treatments that could be considered medical use, and of DEA drug scheduling. The use of psychedelic drugs as medicines—referred to as **psychedelic medicine** (Tupper et al., 2015; Yaden et al., 2021)—is explored at length at the end of this chapter.

The best overall term for describing these drugs has been debated for years. The term *hallucinogen* reflects the drugs' ability, in high enough doses, to induce hallucinations, defined as "perceptions in the absence of the appropriate sensations." However, that definition is problematic because it also describes perceptual illusions and distortions, which are more common than are true hallucinations. The term *psychotomimetic* reflects these drugs' alleged ability to produce effects that mimic psychoses or to actually induce psychotic states. However, research has shown that people who used any of three classic drugs—lysergic acid diethylamide (LSD), psilocybin, and mescaline—were in fact at *reduced* risk of developing symptoms of mental health problems (Hendricks et al., 2015). For those reasons, we will use the term *psychedelic* (meaning "mind manifesting") because it groups the drugs' disparate array of effects under a recognizable descriptive umbrella. Many psychedelics occur in nature; others are synthetically produced. Regardless of their origin, most psychedelic drugs appear to act on one of the known neurotransmitter systems. Based on similarities in chemical structure, mechanism of action, and pharmacological effects, psychedelics have been categorized as shown in Table 8.1.

TABLE 8.1 Classification of Psychedelic Drugs

Categories	Drugs
Catecholaminelike and amphetaminelike compounds	Naturally occurring compounds, including mescaline, myristicin, and elemicin Synthetic compounds, including MDMA, MDA, DOM, TMA, DMA, MDE, MDAI, BZP, and TFMPP
Serotoninlike compounds	LSD, ayahuasca (DMT and harmine), psilocybin and psilocin, bufotenine, ololiuqui (with lysergic acid amide), 2C-B, mCPP, and the psychoactive tryptamines 5-MeO-MiPT and AMT
Acetylcholine muscarinic receptor antagonist	Scopolamine
Glutamate NMDA receptor antagonists	Phencyclidine, ketamine, and esketamine
Opioid receptor agonists	Salvinorin A, kratom, and tianeptine

As indicated by the names of the categories in Table 8.1, the psychedelic drugs discussed in this chapter share neurochemical similarities with the major types of neurotransmitters: the catecholamines (dopamine and norepinephrine), serotonin, acetylcholine, glutamate, and the opioid peptides. The actions of the psychedelics range from amphetaminelike (more stimulatory, less hallucinogenic) to LSD-like (more hallucinogenic, less stimulatory).

CATECHOLAMINELIKE AND AMPHETAMINELIKE PSYCHEDELICS

Figure 8.1 shows the structural similarities and differences among the catecholamine neurotransmitters dopamine and norepinephrine, the psychostimulant amphetamine, and ten of the psychedelic drugs discussed in this section. As you can see, the psychedelics in this figure are structurally similar both to the catecholamine neurotransmitters and to amphetamine, but with this crucial difference: the psychedelics are all oxygenated—that is, they all contain one or more oxygen atoms attached to the basic ring structure, either as one or more methoxy (–OCH_3) groups or as two oxygen atoms connected by a single carbon atom (of the drugs in the figure, only myristicin has both these features). These structural differences are what give these compounds their psychedelic properties.

Naturally Occurring Compounds

The naturally occurring catecholaminelike and amphetaminelike psychedelics that we will discuss in this section include mescaline (from the peyote cactus) and myristicin and elemicin (found in the spices nutmeg and mace). Of these, mescaline is the more widely known and used.

Mescaline

Mescaline is a psychedelic component of the **peyote** plant (*Lophophora williamsii*), a spineless cactus that is common in the southwestern United States and in Mexico. The plant has a small crown, or "button," and a long root. When the plant is used for its psychedelic effects, the crown is cut off and dried into a hard brown disk (frequently referred to as a "mescal button") that is then softened in the mouth and swallowed.

Historical Background. The use of peyote as a psychedelic extends back perhaps 5000 years or more in North America; the cactus was used in the religious rites of the Aztec and other Indigenous peoples of North America in present-day Mexico and the United States (el-Seedi et al., 2005). The name "mescaline" derives from the Mescalero Apache people, who adopted ceremonial use of peyote in the eighteenth century, having learned of it from Indigenous peoples of present-day Mexico, who had been using peyote for thousands of years. Currently, use of peyote is legal in the religious practice of the Native American Church of North America, which was chartered in 1918. Such use of peyote for religious purposes is not considered abuse, and peyote is, in fact, seldom abused by the members of the Native American Church (Fickenscher et al., 2006).

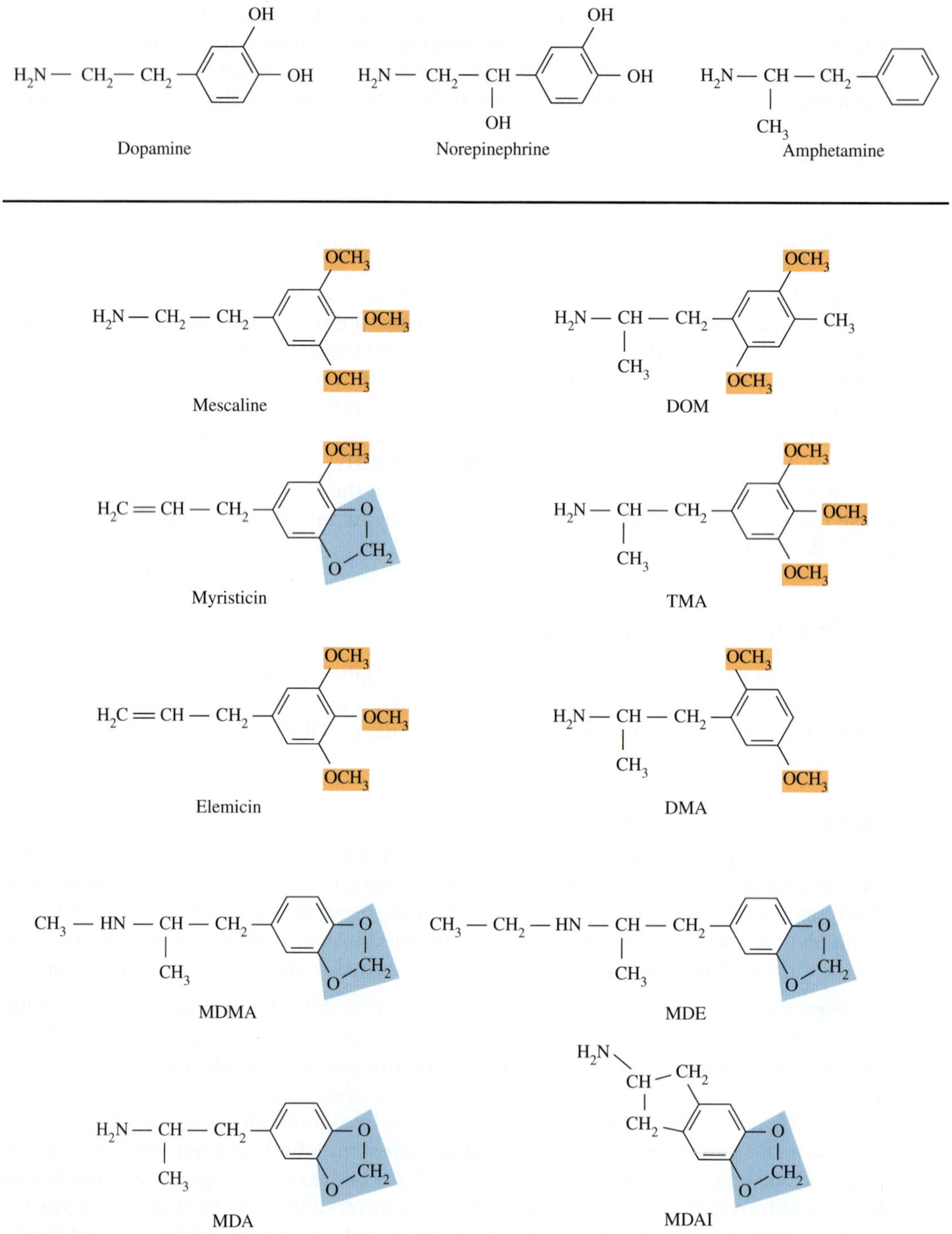

FIGURE 8.1 Structures of Dopamine, Norepinephrine, Amphetamine, and Ten Structurally Related Psychedelic Drugs. In contrast to the catecholamine neurotransmitters (dopamine and norepinephrine) and to amphetamine, the psychedelics all contain one or more –OCH_3 groups (orange shading) or two oxygen atoms connected by a single carbon atom (blue shading). Only myristicin has both features.

Pharmacological Effects. Early research on the peyote cactus led, in 1896, to the identification of mescaline as its pharmacologically active compound. After the chemical structure of mescaline was elucidated in 1918, the compound was produced synthetically, and a wide variety of mescaline derivatives have now been synthesized, all with methoxy groups or similar additions on their benzene ring.

When taken orally, mescaline is rapidly and completely absorbed, with significant concentrations appearing in the brain within 1–2 hours. Between 3.5 and 4 hours after drug intake, mescaline produces an acute psychotomimetic state, with prominent effects on the visual system. The effects of a single dose of mescaline persist for approximately 10 hours and are thought to involve interaction with 5-HT$2_{A\text{–}C}$ receptors (Dinis-Oliveira et al., 2019).

The usual oral dose of 5 milligrams per kilogram body weight typically causes anxiety, sympathomimetic effects, hyperreflexia of the limbs, tremors, and visual hallucinations that consist of brightly colored lights, geometric designs, animals, and occasionally people; color and space perception is often concomitantly impaired, but otherwise the sensorium is normal and self-awareness is retained.

Myristicin and Elemicin

Nutmeg and mace are common household spices sometimes abused for their psychedelic effects, which are due to the presence of **myristicin** and **elemicin**. Ingestion of large amounts of either compound (1–2 teaspoons—i.e., 5–15 grams—usually obtained by brewing the spices to make a tea) may, after 2–5 hours, induce feelings of unreality, confusion, disorientation, impending doom, depersonalization, euphoria, visual hallucinations, and acute psychotic reactions. Considering the close structural resemblance of myristicin and elemicin to mescaline (see Figure 8.1), these psychedelic actions are not surprising. Ingestion of large quantities of nutmeg in particular, however, produces many physically unpleasant side effects.

Synthetic Compounds

The psychedelics discussed in this section (sometimes referred to as "designer psychedelics") all produce effects similar to the effects produced by mescaline and amphetamine due to their structural similarity to those compounds (see Figure 8.1). At low doses, they have moderate behavioral stimulant effects, and at higher doses, psychedelic effects dominate, with increased self-reports of "mystical" types of hallucinogenic effects, including visual alterations. However, these drugs are considerably more potent and more toxic than mescaline, with side effects that can include nausea, anxiety, panic attacks, and paranoid ideation.

MDMA

MDMA (methylenedioxymethamphetamine, with the street name "ecstasy") was developed in about 1914 as an appetite suppressant, but this use was not pursued (Freudenmann et al., 2006). By the 1970s, there was interest in it as a therapeutic aid for patients undergoing psychological treatment, but in the 1980s, college students started abusing the drug, and its potential therapeutic uses were put aside (Sessa et al., 2019). Since the 1990s, it has been associated with the social phenomenon of the rave.

MDMA resembles MDA (discussed next) in structure but may be less hallucinogenic. It is a releaser and/or reuptake inhibitor of serotonin, dopamine, and norepinephrine. As with other psychedelic compounds, the psychological experience resulting from MDMA use is not always predictable but is most commonly described in terms of "empathy," "insight," "enhanced communication," and "transcendent religious experiences" (Papaseit et al., 2018b). The most frequent adverse reactions include increases in blood pressure and heart rate, muscle tension, fatigue, insomnia, sweating, blurred vision, loss of motor coordination, and anxiety. However, when MDMA is used during periods of intense activity (e.g., at raves), severe symptoms such as high fever, cardiac arrhythmias, and even death may occur.

More disturbing and more controversial are questions about the potential toxicities associated with chronic use of MDMA:

- Will psychedelics that are structurally similar to methamphetamine, such as MDMA, turn out to be similarly neurotoxic, including with MDMA-induced dysfunction of dopamine pathways in the CNS (Costa et al., 2020)? (The neurotoxicity of methamphetamine was discussed in Chapter 7.)
- Will serotonin reuptake transporters be reversibly damaged, with resulting display of deficits in executive functioning (Roberts et al., 2016)?

MDA

MDA (3,4-methylenedioxyamphetamine) is not well studied, and its pharmacokinetics in humans are unknown (Baggott et al., 2019). Like MDMA, MDA increases blood pressure and heart rate and produces vivid and hallucinogenic effects. Its duration of action appears to be modestly longer than MDMA's (8 hours vs. 6 hours). MDA is also a metabolite of MDMA, and much of MDMA's effects may actually be due to the presence of MDA. MDA is sometimes passed off as MDMA, with potentially dangerous consequences because MDA is more lethal than MDMA in lower doses, and its effects are longer lasting. The side effects and toxicities (including fatalities) associated with MDA use are similar to those associated with MDMA.

DOM

DOM (2,5-dimethoxy-4-methylamphetamine, with the street name STP, standing for "serenity, tranquility, and peace") is a partial agonist at 5-HT2_A receptors. This property mediates its psychedelic effects, which are similar to those of mescaline; however, DOM is 100 times more potent than mescaline (though much less potent than LSD). Doses of 1–6 milligrams produce euphoria, which is followed by a 6- to 8-hour period of hallucinations. The use of DOM is not widespread because it is associated with a high incidence of overdose (due to its potency and the fact that street doses are poorly controlled), and acute toxic reactions are common, typically consisting of tremors that may eventually lead to convulsive movements, prostration, and even death.

TMA

TMA (trimethoxyamphetamine) is structurally similar to several of the other synthetic psychedelics discussed in this section, as well as to mescaline (see Figure 8.1). People who have used TMA report that it elicits a range of emotions, from sadness to empathy and euphoria, similar to that seen with MDMA (Kolaczynska et al., 2019).

DMA

DMA (dimethoxyamphetamine) refers to any of a series of six psychedelic drugs that differ from each other structurally in the attachment points of the two $-OCH_3$ groups (the structure shown in Figure 8.1 is that of 2,5-dimethoxyamphetamine). Little is known about the effects, risks, or toxicities associated with use of DMA in any of its structural variations (Passie and Benzenhofer, 2018).

MDE

MDE (3,4-methylenedioxy-N-ethylamphetamine, also called *MDEA*, with the street name "eve") is somewhat less potent than MDMA but otherwise has very similar effects. In smaller doses, MDE's physical and tactile effects are generally perceived as being less intense than MDMA's. The emotional opening and empathic effects for which MDMA is famous, although present with MDE, also do not seem to be as pronounced. Because of this more subtle effect, MDE has a possible advantage as a recreational substance over MDMA when used in public (e.g., at raves). That is, people using MDE are less likely to embarrass themselves in public through inappropriate touching and emotional bonding while still being able to enjoy a heightened sense of connection with others (in addition, MDE's duration of action is only about 2–4 hours). At large doses, MDE's effects may somewhat resemble MDA's, but with less intense psychedelic effects; however, some people report a "stoning" effect that MDA lacks, and MDE can make walking or dancing difficult.

MDAI

MDAI (5,6-methylenedioxy-2-aminoindane) is a reuptake inhibitor of serotonin, dopamine, and norepinephrine, especially of serotonin (Murnane, 2019). It does not appear to be as neurotoxic as methamphetamine or MDMA. Some people who have used MDAI report spiritual experiences (a phenomenon quite common to this class of drugs) and other effects similar to those of MDMA, including euphoria, empathy, and intensified sensory experiences. However, use of MDAI is also associated with reports of serious adverse effects on the kidneys, liver, and lungs (Palenicek et al., 2016; Richter et al., 2019).

BZP and TFMPP

While structurally unrelated to the psychedelics discussed above and shown in Figure 8.1, some drugs in the class known as *piperazines* have similar stimulant and psychedelic effects. The best known of these psychedelic compounds are **BZP** (benzylpiperazine) and **TFMPP** (trifluoromethylphenylpiperazine), whose psychedelic properties are attributable to their unique side chains (see Figure 8.2). BZP and TFMPP

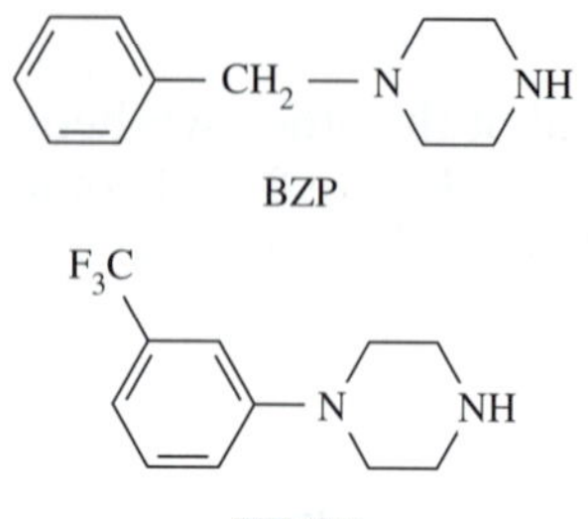

FIGURE 8.2 Structures of BZP and TFMPP. The psychedelic actions of these drugs are due to the unique side chains attached to their benzene ring.

are sometimes taken together as a combination "party pill" (Cohen and Butler, 2011). Both drugs facilitate the release of dopamine, TFMPP facilitates serotonin release directly, and BZP raises serotonin levels by blocking its reuptake. The limited pharmacokinetics information about these drugs indicates that BZP doses are typically 75–150 milligrams and that the effects last about 6–8 hours. Onset of effect may take up to 2 hours, with peak plasma concentrations reached 60–90 minutes after oral administration; this delay sometimes leads users to take multiple doses before experiencing onset, which can be dangerous. Elimination is essentially complete in 44 hours for BZP (which is eliminated unchanged) and 24 hours for TFMPP (which undergoes metabolic breakdown). When taken recreationally, low doses of either drug cause stimulant effects, while hallucinogenic actions predominate at higher doses. Side effects are many and sometimes serious (Lin et al., 2011).

SEROTONINLIKE PSYCHEDELICS

Figure 8.3 shows the structures of serotonin and ten of the structurally related serotoninlike psychedelics discussed in this section. Because of their structural resemblances to one another and to serotonin, it has long been presumed that these agents exert their effects through interactions at serotonin receptors, but only in recent years has it become generally accepted that the hallucinogenic effects of these drugs are mediated by an agonistic or partial agonistic action at postsynaptic 5-HT2_A receptors. This is consistent with the observation that the drugs' affinity for these receptors is highly correlated with their hallucinogenic potency (Kim et al., 2020). Also, it is well established that many other psychedelic drugs exert their hallucinogenic effects by acting as agonists at 5-HT2_A receptors.

Serotonin 5-HT2_A receptors are widely distributed in the CNS, especially in brain regions essential for learning and cognition (Zhang and Stackman, 2015). Various research studies have shown that antagonists of these receptors have antipsychotic and antidepressant effects, whereas agonists have cognition-enhancing and hallucinogenic effects. The fact that 5-HT2_A receptors are part of a stress response system and have been implicated in the genesis of PTSD (Murnane, 2019) implies that they could be a target for psychedelic medications in the treatment of this disorder (treatment of PTSD with psychedelic agents is discussed in the section on psychedelic medicine at the end of this chapter). Additional evidence of a relationship between 5-HT2_A receptors and psychiatric disorders is provided by research showing that abnormalities in the structure or function of these receptors are associated with a number of disorders, including schizophrenia, depression, anxiety, and drug addiction (dos Santos and Hallak, 2020).[1]

[1]As we will see in Chapter 11, many of the newer "atypical antipsychotic" drugs exert a major part of their antipsychotic effect by acting as antagonists at 5-HT2_A receptors.

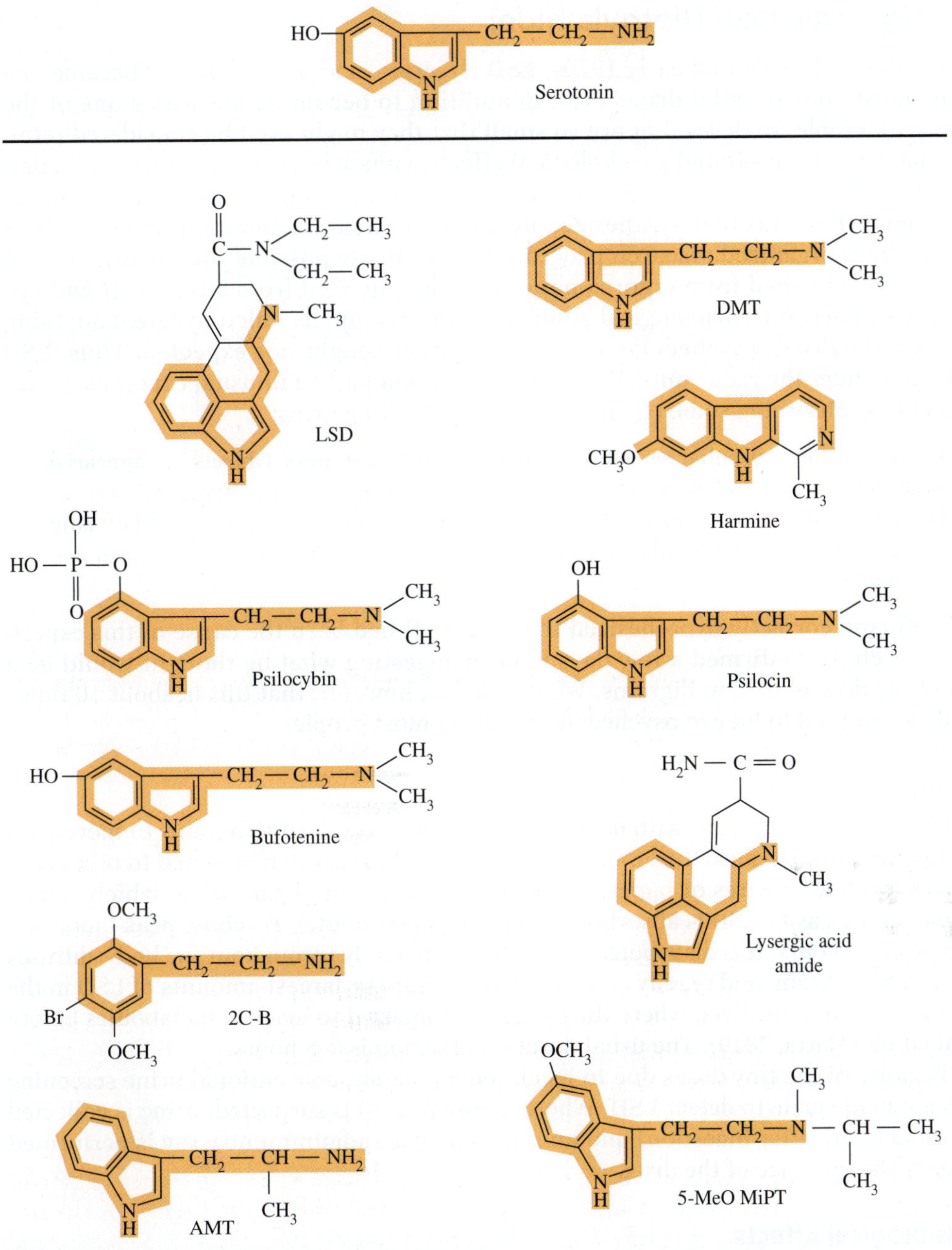

FIGURE 8.3 Structures of Serotonin and Ten Serotoninlike Psychedelic Drugs. The psychedelic effects of these drugs are thought to result from their agonistic actions at 5-HT2_A receptors in the brain.

LSD (Lysergic Acid Diethylamide)

During the mid-1960s and early 1970s, **LSD (lysergic acid diethylamide)** became one of the most controversial drugs ever, in addition to becoming known as one of the most remarkable. In doses that are so small that they might even be considered infinitesimal, LSD has profound psychological effects, enhancing self-awareness and altering internal reality, while causing relatively few alterations in the general physiology of the body. LSD was first synthesized by the Swiss chemist Albert Hofmann in 1938 as part of an organized research program to investigate possible therapeutic uses of compounds obtained from ergot, a natural product derived from a fungus (*Claviceps purpurea*). Early pharmacological studies of LSD in animals failed to reveal anything unusual; the drug's psychedelic action was neither sought nor expected. Thus, LSD remained under the radar until 1943, when Hofmann had an unusual experience after accidentally absorbing some of the drug through his fingertips:

> I was seized by a peculiar sensation of vertigo and restlessness. Objects . . . appeared to undergo optical changes. . . . In a dream-like state I left for home, where . . . I . . . immediately fell into a peculiar state similar to drunkenness. . . . [F]antastic pictures of extraordinary plasticity and intensive color seemed to surge toward me. (Hofmann, 1994)

Hofmann correctly hypothesized that that LSD had been the cause of this experience, which he confirmed a few days later by ingesting what he thought would be a minuscule dose of 0.25 milligrams. We now know, however, that this is about 10 times the dose required to induce psychedelic effects in most people.

Pharmacokinetics

LSD is usually taken orally, with doses ranging from about 25 micrograms to more than 200 micrograms. Because the amounts are so small, LSD is often attached to other substances, such as squares of paper, the backs of stamps, or sugar cubes, which can be handled more easily. LSD is absorbed within about 60 minutes, reaching peak blood levels in about 3 hours. It is distributed rapidly and efficiently throughout the body, diffuses easily into the brain, and readily crosses the placenta. The largest amounts of LSD in the body are found in the liver, where the drug is metabolized to inactive metabolites before elimination (Marta, 2019). The usual duration of action is 6–8 hours.

Because of the tiny doses due to its extreme potency, conventional urine screening tests are inadequate to detect LSD. When the use of LSD is suspected, urine is collected (up to 30 hours after ingestion) and an ultrasensitive radioimmunoassay is performed to verify the presence of the drug.

Physiological Effects

Although the LSD experience is characterized by hallucinogenic effects, subtle physiological changes also occur. People who use the drug may experience a slight increase in body temperature, dilation of the pupils, slightly increased heart rate and blood pressure, and increased levels of glucose in the blood, as well as dizziness, drowsiness, nausea, and other effects that, although noticeable, seldom interfere with the psychedelic experience.

LSD has a low level of toxicity, with an effective dose of about 50 micrograms and a lethal dose of about 14,000 micrograms. These figures provide a therapeutic index of 280, making the drug a remarkably nonlethal compound (most deaths attributed to LSD result from accidents, homicides, or suicides). The use of LSD during pregnancy is certainly unwise, although a distinct fetal LSD syndrome has not been described.

Psychological Effects, Including Adverse Reactions

The psychological effects of LSD are intense. Doses of 25–50 micrograms produce alterations in perception, thinking, emotion, arousal, and self-image.

Sensory Phase and Psychic Phase. The sensory phase (or perceptual phase) is characterized by sensory distortions and hallucinations, which usually are the effects desired by the person using the drug. Time seems slowed or distorted. Sensory input is intensified, especially visual input, with alterations that typically include colored lights, distorted perception of actual or imagined objects, and vivid and fascinating images and shapes. Synesthetic effects can include hearing colors and seeing sounds. In addition, during this phase, the person has a decreased level of vigilance and a decreased capacity for logical thought.

The onset of the psychic phase signals a maximum drug effect, with changes in mood, disruption of thought processes, altered perception of time, depersonalization, true hallucinations, and psychotic episodes. A loss of boundaries and fear of fragmentation may create a need for a structuring or supportive environment, including experienced companions. During the "trip," distressing thoughts and memories can emerge, and mood may be labile, shifting from depression to gaiety, from elation to fear. Tension and anxiety may mount and may even reach panic proportions: such an experience is considered a "bad trip."

Neurobiological Effects. A study investigating the neurobiological effects of LSD in 20 healthy volunteers found that the drug increased activity in the visual areas of the brain, which was associated with perceived hallucinations even though the participants closed their eyes, and that many other brain areas were also activated (Carhart-Harris et al., 2016a). In effect, the drug appeared to enhance the visual aspect of imagined experiences (i.e., hallucinations) by increasing the connectivity between the visual cortex and other brain regions. Similarly, listening to music after taking LSD results in intensified auditory neural responses as well as associated visual imagery (Kaelen et al., 2016).

Adverse Reactions. Unpleasant experiences with LSD may involve an uncontrollable drift into confusion or into dissociative, psychotic, or acute panic reactions, perhaps triggered by a reliving of earlier traumatic experiences. Uniquely with LSD and related substances, some of the acute effects (mainly, the visual effects) may return long after the drug has been completely eliminated. These recurring effects are described either as **flashbacks** or as **hallucinogen persisting perception disorder (HPPD)** (Martinotti et al., 2018), two terms that are used fairly synonymously but typically with this difference:

> Flashback is a usually short-term, non-distressing, spontaneous, recurrent, reversible, and benign condition accompanied by a pleasant affect. In contrast, HPPD is a generally long-term, distressing, spontaneous, recurrent, pervasive, either slowly reversible or irreversible, non-benign condition accompanied by an unpleasant dysphoric affect. (Johnson et al., 2008)

These phenomena can occur without warning but are most likely to appear just before sleep or when a person enters a dark environment.

Treatment of flashbacks and HPPD has been symptomatic. Case reports note the success of benzodiazepines as well as other drugs, but there is no consensus on appropriate therapy and no specific treatment. Most commonly, an atypical antipsychotic drug is used to treat both acute LSD toxicity and HPPD (see Chapter 11 for discussion of atypical antipsychotic drugs).

Tolerance and Dependence

Tolerance of both the psychological and physiological effects of LSD readily and rapidly develops, and cross-tolerance occurs between LSD and other psychedelics. Tolerance is lost within several days after the person stops taking the drug.

Physical dependence on LSD does not develop, even when the drug is used repeatedly for a prolonged period of time. In fact, most heavy users of the drug say that they ceased using LSD because they tired of it, had no further need for it, or simply had had enough. Even when the drug is discontinued because of concern about bad trips or about physical or mental harm, few withdrawal signs are exhibited. Laboratory animals do not self-administer LSD.

Other Serotoninlike Compounds

As we will see in this section, the serotoninlike psychedelics other than LSD include both naturally occurring and synthetic compounds, all with a range of effects based mainly on their action as agonists at 5-HT2_A receptors.

Ayahuasca (with DMT and Harmine)

Ayahuasca (meaning "vine of the soul" in the Quechuan languages of South America) is a hallucinogenic tea brewed from parts of two plants: the vine *Banisteriopsis caapi* and the shrub *Psychotria viridis*, both of which are native to the Amazon basin in South America. Indigenous peoples of that region use the tea in religious, spiritual, and medicinal contexts (Barker, 2018; Cameron and Olson, 2018; Hamill et al., 2019; Heise and Brooks, 2017). The psychedelic effects of ayahuasca result from two of the tea's constituent compounds, **DMT** (dimethyltryptamine) and **harmine**, a monoamine oxidase inhibitor that seems to potentiate the effects of DMT. Like LSD, DMT is an agonist at 5-HT2_A receptors, and its psychedelic effects are like those of LSD, including rapidly moving, brightly colored visual displays (auditory effects are less common). "Loss of control" associated with a brief but overwhelming "rush" may lead to a dissociated state in which euphoria alternates or coexists with anxiety. Physiological effects include nausea; vomiting; elevated blood pressure, heart rate, and body temperature; dilated pupils; and increased levels of endorphins and hormones. Effects have an onset of about 30–60 minutes, peak at 1–2 hours, and persist for about 3–4 hours. In most cases, effects are well tolerated, but disorientation, paranoia, and anxiety may occur. Ayahuasca has been reported to be useful in treating alcohol- and cocaine-use disorders (Brierley and Davidson, 2012; Mertens and Preller, 2021).

Psilocybin and Psilocin

The compounds **psilocybin** (4-phosphoryl-DMT) and **psilocin** (4-hydroxy-DMT) are found in many species of mushrooms of the genera *Psilocybe*, *Panaeolus*, *Copelandia*, and *Conocybe*. As Figure 8.3 shows, the only difference between psilocybin and psilocin is that psilocybin contains a molecule of phosphoric acid. After the mushroom has been ingested, the phosphoric acid is enzymatically removed, thus producing psilocin, which is the active psychedelic agent. Psilocybin-containing mushrooms grow throughout much of the world, including the northwestern United States; the mushrooms are eaten raw to obtain their psychedelic effects.

Psilocin is an agonist at serotonin 5-HT2_A and 5-HT1_A receptors, with effects becoming noticeable at a dose of about 0.25 milligrams per kilogram of body weight when ingested. Psilocin and psilocybin are approximately 0.05% as potent as LSD; effects peak after about 2 hours and last about 6–10 hours (both compounds are absorbed effectively when taken orally).

There is great variation in the concentration of psilocybin and psilocin among the different species of mushrooms, as well as significant differences among individual mushrooms of the same species. For example, the usual oral dose of *Psilocybe semilanceata* (liberty caps) may range from 10 to 40 mushrooms, while the dose for *Psilocybe cyanescens* may be only two to five mushrooms.[2]

The psychedelic effects of *Psilocybe mexicana* are part of the folklore of Indigenous peoples in Central America and Mexico, but the mushroom's psychedelic effects were not more formally described until 1955, by Gordon Wasson, a New York banker who traveled through Mexico, mingled with Indigenous groups, and was allowed to participate in a *Psilocybe* ceremony, during which he consumed the mushrooms and had hallucinatory experiences.

Today, there is a resurgence of interest in psilocybin (along with other psychedelics) as a medical treatment for drug-resistant anxiety and depression (see the discussion in the section on psychedelic medicine at the end of this chapter).

Bufotenine

Bufotenine (5-hydroxy DMT, or dimethylserotonin), like LSD and DMT, is a potent serotonin agonist psychedelic with an affinity for several types of serotonin receptors, especially the 5-HT2_A receptor, and with a half-life of about 2 hours in rats after subcutaneous injection. The name *bufotenine* comes from the name for a toad of the genus *Bufo*, whose skin and glandular secretions supposedly produce hallucinogenic effects when ingested.

Bufotenine is not normally found in the human body; however, it can be an end product of an unusual pathway for the metabolic breakdown of serotonin. Indeed, some have attempted to correlate the presence of bufotenine in urine with various psychiatric disorders, although this theory is not generally accepted (Emanuele et al., 2010).

[2]Be aware! Some extremely toxic species of mushrooms bear a superficial resemblance to mushrooms that contain psilocybin and psilocin. Also, because the effects of psilocybin closely resemble those of LSD, illicitly sold drugs advertised as psilocybin may actually be LSD, and ordinary mushrooms laced with LSD may be sold as psilocybin-containing "magic mushrooms."

Ololiuqui (with Lysergic Acid Amide)

Ololiuqui is the Nahuatl name for the plant *Rivea corymbosa*, a species of morning glory native to an area extending from Mexico to Peru. It is a climber vine that grows rapidly and is often kept as an ornamental plant due to its beautiful white flowers. The seeds, when ingested, produce hallucinations and intoxication, characteristically including a hypnotic, euphoric, dreamlike state with visions. These are similar to the effects induced by ingesting psilocybin-containing mushrooms or peyote buttons but with slow onset and fairly long duration. Ololiuqui was used in pre-Columbian times by the Aztec and neighboring peoples in religious ceremonies and magical healing practices, a use that continues among some groups, in rituals to enable communication with the gods and to predict the future using the visions that ololiuqui induces.

The ritual use of ololiuqui seeds was first described by the sixteenth-century Spanish explorer Francisco Hernández de Córdoba, who is said to have reported, "When the priests wanted to commune with their Gods, they ate ololiuqui seeds and a thousand visions and satanic hallucinations appeared to them" (Brecher and Editors of Consumer Reports Magazine, 1972). The seeds were analyzed by Albert Hofmann, the discoverer of LSD, who identified the active ingredient as **lysergic acid amide** (see Figure 8.3), which has approximately one-tenth the potency of LSD as a psychoactive agent.

Side effects of ololiuqui can include extreme nausea, vomiting, headache, increased blood pressure, dilated pupils, and sleepiness. As these side effects dissipate, they are replaced by distorted perceptions, hallucinations, and confusion, with continued sleepiness (Carod-Artal, 2015). Flashbacks have been reported but not frequently.

2C-B

With effects similar to those of MDMA, **2C-B** (4-bromo-2,5-dimethoxyphenethylamine) has been appearing more frequently at raves and club venues. Like MDMA, it is a partial agonist at 5-$HT2_A$ receptors; also, like MDMA (and unlike methamphetamine), it is a norepinephrine and serotonin reuptake inhibitor more than a dopamine reuptake inhibitor; and like classic amphetamines, it releases monoamines from presynaptic vesicles. Oral doses of about 20 milligrams are reported to produce psychedelic perceptual effects (Papaseit et al., 2018a). A report from the Netherlands notes an increase in social media posts about the drug (Blankers et al., 2021).

5-MeO-MiPT and AMT

A number of compounds belonging to a group described as *novel psychoactive tryptamines* have psychedelic effects based on their partial or full agonist actions at 5-$HT2_A$ receptors (Rickli et al., 2016). In this section, we will discuss two of these compounds: 5-MeO-MiPT (5-methoxy-*N*-methyl-*N*-isopropyltryptamine, with the street name "moxy") and AMT (alpha-methyltryptamine).

Little is known about the pharmacological properties of **5-MeO-MiPT**. Anecdotal reports describe its effects as more stimulating than psychedelic, without typical psychedelic visual distortions. Many users report strong physical and tactile effects that enhance pleasure. Side effects include uncomfortable muscle tension and nausea. The psychedelic effects are believed to come from a partial agonist action at 5-$HT2_A$ receptors. In addition, 5-MeO-MiPT is moderately potent as a serotonin and norepinephrine reuptake inhibitor, which may help account for anecdotal reports of antidepressant and anxiolytic effects from relatively low doses (Rickli et al., 2016).

5-MeO-MiPT can be ingested orally or smoked, with reportedly more prominent visual and sensory effects after oral ingestion. The effects occur in two stages: first, stimulating and empathic effects, and then effects more similar to those of psychedelics like psilocybin mushrooms and LSD. When the drug is smoked, the physically and cognitively stimulating effects become emphasized.

AMT was originally developed as an antidepressant but was never marketed for this use, except briefly in Russia. It is structurally closely related to serotonin (see Figure 8.3) and is a reuptake inhibitor of serotonin, norepinephrine, and dopamine. It is also an agonist at serotonin receptors.

Administered orally, AMT is of slow onset (3–4 hours) and prolonged duration (12–24 hours). Psychedelic and other effects reported by people who used the drug recreationally include hallucinations, an altered state of mind, mood elevation, nervousness, anxiety, insomnia, muscle tension, jaw tightness, pupil dilation, tachycardia, headaches, nausea, and vomiting (Araujo et al., 2015).

mCPP

A metabolite of the antidepressant drug trazodone and a difficult psychedelic to classify, **mCPP** (meta-chlorophenylpiperazine) is structurally a piperazine similar to the catecholaminelike psychedelic piperazines BZP and TFMPP discussed above. However, its psychedelic effects result from its agonistic action at almost all 5-HT receptors and possibly from an action in blocking serotonin reuptake and release. As a psychedelic agent, mCPP produces effects that are generally considered to be undesirable. Also, it reduces appetite, an effect that has prompted a clinical trial of other, selective 5-HT2_C receptor agonists for the treatment of obesity (Higgins et al., 2013; Thomas et al., 2018).

ACETYLCHOLINE MUSCARINIC RECEPTOR ANTAGONIST: SCOPOLAMINE

In contrast to the psychedelic compounds discussed previously in this chapter, which act as agonists at dopamine, norepinephrine, and/or serotonin receptors, **scopolamine** is an antagonist at acetylcholine muscarinic receptors, which primarily occur in the CNS (see the discussion of acetylcholine receptors in Chapter 2; Figure 8.4 shows the structures of acetylcholine and scopolamine). Scopolamine is one of the two most common naturally occurring acetylcholine muscarinic antagonists, the other being atropine, which cannot have psychedelic effects as it does not cross the blood-brain barrier and does not enter the CNS (a third, less common naturally occurring compound is L-hyoscyamine, a common ingredient in many gastrointestinal medications). Medically, scopolamine has long been used to treat motion sickness, including in motion-sickness–prevention patches.[3]

[3]Certain other medicines also have anticholinergic properties and can have similar effects—for example, antihistamines such as diphenhydramine, as well as Benadryl and medicines such as Cogentin, used in the treatment of Parkinsonism.

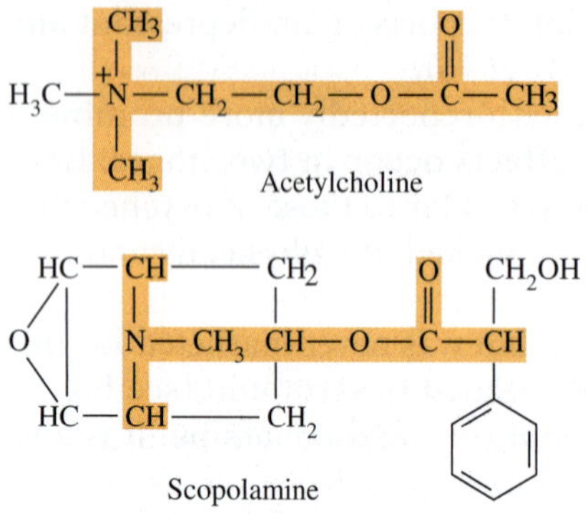

FIGURE 8.4 Structures of Acetylcholine and Scopolamine. Scopolamine is an antagonist at acetylcholine muscarinic receptors. The orange shading highlights the two compounds' structural similarities.

Historical Background

The history of scopolamine is long and colorful (Holzman, 1998). The drug is distributed widely in nature and is found in especially high concentrations in the plants *Atropa belladonna* (deadly nightshade), *Datura stramonium* (variously referred to as "Jamestown weed," "jimsonweed," "stinkweed," "thorn apple," and "devil's apple"), *Mandragora officinarum* (mandrake), and *Datura inoxia* (moonflower), species that have been known as sources of poison since ancient times.[4] In addition, scopolamine-containing plants have been used and misused for centuries for their psychedelic and other effects, including delirium and intoxication. For example, the delirium caused by scopolamine may have persuaded some people that they could fly, a phenomenon associated with Halloween images of flying witches. At one time, marijuana and opium preparations from eastern Asia were fortified with material from *Datura stramonium*. Today, cigarettes made from the leaves of *Datura stramonium* and *Atropa belladonna* are smoked occasionally to induce delirium and intoxication, and throughout the world, the leaves of plants that contain scopolamine are used to prepare intoxicating beverages.

Pharmacological Effects

Scopolamine acts on the peripheral nervous system to produce a syndrome characterized by dry mouth, reduced sweating, dry skin, increased body temperature, dilated pupils, blurred vision, tachycardia, and hypertension (the phrase "red as a beet, hot as a hare, dry as a bone, blind as a bat, and mad as a hatter" has been used to describe a person with this syndrome). Low doses reaching the CNS produce drowsiness, mild euphoria, profound amnesia, fatigue, mental confusion, dreamless sleep, and loss of attention (Renner et al., 2005). Thus, rather than expanding consciousness, awareness, and insight (effects associated with certain other psychedelics, such as LSD), scopolamine clouds consciousness and inhibits memory. As doses increase, psychiatric symptoms include restlessness, excitement, hallucinations, euphoria, and disorientation. Delirium (i.e., mental confusion) may progress to stupor and even coma and may be

---

[4]Deadly nightshade's genus name, *Atropa*, is derived from Atropos, one of the three Fates, who was believed to cut the thread of life; the species name *belladonna* means "beautiful woman," which refers to the drug's ability to dilate the pupils when it is applied topically to the eyes and which reflects the idea that widely dilated pupils are a mark of beauty. Accidental ingestion of berries from *Datura inoxia* has been associated with the incapacitation of whole armies (e.g., the defeat of Marc Antony's army in 36 BCE), and tea made from this plant is said to have contributed to the defeat of British soldiers by American settlers in the conflict known as Bacon's Rebellion near Jamestown, Virginia, in 1676–1677 (hence the name "Jamestown weed").

followed by respiratory depression. While scopolamine intoxication can convey a sense of excitement and loss of inhibitions, the clouding of consciousness and the loss of memory of the episode (amnesia) render scopolamine rather unattractive as a psychedelic drug. Although historically used as poisons, the margin of safety for these drugs is large, and death is usually a result of accidents (wandering into traffic or falling) or of inadvertent ingestion (e.g., eating of the berries by children). Typically, the sensory and psychosislike effects clear within 36–48 hours. If necessary, the antidote to scopolamine poisoning is the drug physostigmine, which blocks the enzyme acetylcholinesterase and thereby increases the concentration of acetylcholine.

Tolerance to scopolamine is generally modest, and psychological dependence is uncommon. However, physical dependence can develop, particularly in conjunction with long-term use of medications that have anticholinergic actions or side effects. Withdrawal symptoms include vomiting, excessive sweating and salivation, and general malaise.

GLUTAMATE NMDA RECEPTOR ANTAGONISTS: PHENCYCLIDINE, KETAMINE, AND ESKETAMINE

Phencyclidine (phenylcyclohexyl piperidine, or PCP, with the street name "angel dust"), **ketamine** (a racemic mixture, with the street name "Special K"), and ketamine's more active isomer, **esketamine**, are structurally unrelated to other psychedelic drugs (see Figure 8.5).

Phencyclidine was developed in 1956 as a "safer" surgical anesthetic that produced less respiratory depression than did other anesthetics of the time (Mion, 2017); also, unlike other anesthetics, the lethal dose of phencyclidine is ten times the anesthetic dose, and at appropriate doses it reduces pain reactions while maintaining stable blood pressure and heart rate (Castellanos et al., 2020). However, its use as an anesthetic in humans was brief because it was soon found to have psychedelic properties and to produce a high incidence of psychiatric reactions (but it is still used as a veterinary

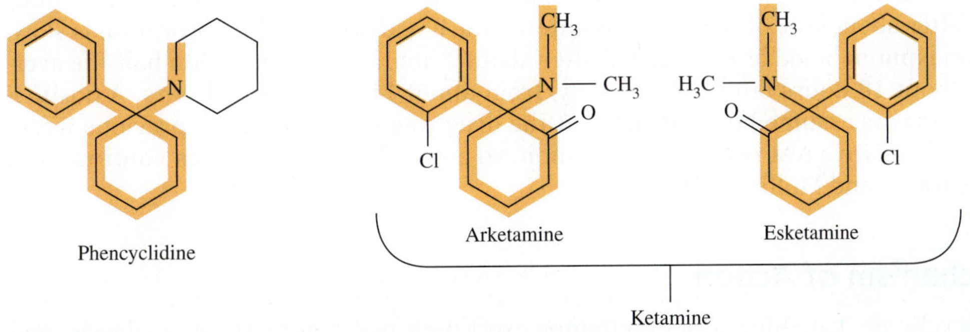

FIGURE 8.5 Structures of Phencyclidine and Ketamine. Ketamine is a racemic mixture in which esketamine is a much more pharmacologically active isomer than arketamine. The orange shading highlights the compounds' structural similarities.

anesthetic). Racemic ketamine (Ketalar) is a mixture of two isomers (arketamine and esketamine); it was developed as a replacement for phencyclidine shortly after the prominent psychedelic properties of phencyclidine were identified. Introduced in 1960, ketamine induces a phencyclidinelike anesthetic state in low doses, with similar but less severe psychiatric side effects. Ketamine is still used as an anesthetic in special situations, such as in pediatric anesthesia, in cases of trauma requiring emergency surgery, and in very "brittle" or highly compromised patients. Esketamine (Spravato) has been separately (and more expensively) marketed as an antidepressant (see the discussion of these uses for both ketamine and esketamine in the section on psychedelic medicine later in this chapter). Pharmacologically, phencyclidine, ketamine, and esketamine exhibit a unique combination of four actions:

- They are powerful analgesics.
- They are powerful amnestics.
- They induce psychedelic and dissociative experiences, including hallucinations and out-of-body experiences.
- They have antidepressant effects.

In toxic doses, all three compounds produce effects that resemble both the positive and negative symptoms of schizophrenia, and they exacerbate psychosis in people with schizophrenia (these effects have led to a glutamate-related model of schizophrenia, as discussed in Chapter 11). However, people who use these drugs infrequently do not actually develop schizophrenia.

Abuse of phencyclidine and ketamine began in the mid-1960s but did not become common until the 1990s, when ketamine began showing up as an adulterant in MDMA tablets. The two drugs are essentially interchangeable in recreational use, with a typical street dose of about 5 milligrams. Popular at times as club drugs, they are most often smoked, including sprinkled on tobacco or marijuana.

Pharmacokinetics

When phencyclidine and ketamine are smoked, peak effects occur in about 15 minutes, after about 40% of the dose has entered the bloodstream. Oral absorption is slow, with maximum blood levels reached after about 2 hours. The elimination half-life averages about 18 hours but ranges widely, from about 11 to about 51 hours. A positive urine assay is assumed to indicate that the drug was used within the previous week, but false-positive test results are common, so a positive assay requires confirmation (Rengarajan and Mullins, 2013).

Mechanism of Action

Phencyclidine, ketamine, and esketamine exert their psychotomimetic, analgesic, and amnestic actions primarily as a result of binding as noncompetitive antagonists at glutamate NMDA receptors (Ingram et al., 2018). In addition, these drugs may, to a far lesser extent, block acetylcholine and dopamine receptors (Morgan and Curran, 2011). The drugs inhibit NMDA receptors by two mechanisms:

- Blockade of the open channel by occupying a site within the channel in the receptor protein
- Reduction in the frequency of NMDA channel opening by binding to a second attachment site on the outside of the receptor protein

Similarly, the drugs seem to exert their powerful analgesic action by two mechanisms:

- Blockade of glutamate NMDA receptors in the spinal cord
- Activation of descending analgesic pathways that appear to involve norepinephrine and dopamine

Psychological and Physical Effects

Phencyclidine and ketamine are both known as *dissociative anesthetics*, meaning that their analgesic, amnestic, and sensory effects occur without loss of consciousness. That is, they produce an unresponsive state with intense analgesia and amnesia, although the person's eyes remain open (with a blank stare) and the person may even appear to be awake. In low doses (1–5 milligrams), phencyclidine may have any of a range of effects, including mild agitation, euphoria, disinhibition, and excitement; the person will appear to be grossly drunk and exhibit a blank stare and may be communicative but will not respond to pain. Ketamine at low doses produces similar effects, including distortions of time and space, hallucinations, and mild dissociation (Hashimoto, 2020; Mihaljevic et al., 2020). People who have used the drugs have described the effects as "melting into the surroundings," "visual hallucinations," and "out-of-body experiences."

High doses of phencyclidine induce a state of coma or stupor, during which even surgery can be performed without subsequent memory of it. The patient may recover physically within 2–4 hours, but a state of confusion and reduced cognition may last for as long as 8–24 hours. The disruption of sensory input causes unpredictable, exaggerated, distorted, and even violent reactions to environmental stimuli, which may be augmented by phencyclidine-induced analgesia and amnesia. Massive oral overdoses of up to 1 gram of street-purchased phencyclidine result in prolonged periods of stupor or coma, followed by a prolonged recovery phase marked by confusion and delusions lasting as long as two weeks. (Of course, people who use the drug recreationally tend to titrate their dose to maximize the intoxicant effect while attempting to avoid unconsciousness.)

Ketamine at large doses induces a more severe dissociation in which the detachment experienced by users is so intense that their perceptions appear completely divorced from their previous reality (Morgan and Curran, 2011). The person may become withdrawn, negativistic, and unable to maintain a cognitive set and may give overly concrete, impoverished, idiosyncratic, and bizarre responses to questions.

Tolerance to phencyclidine and ketamine does develop, but gradually. People who abuse these drugs may escalate their abused doses as a way of compensating for the drugs' disruptive effects, rather than for a direct physiological cause. The incidence of dependence is not known, and no specific withdrawal syndrome has been described (cravings seem to be the most common symptom).

Phencyclidine and ketamine have wide margins of safety. The highest mortality risk comes from accidents while intoxicated. Symptoms of toxicity include agitation, violent behaviors, altered states of consciousness, hallucinations, and a catatonic trance in which the person does not talk, move, or react (even to pain).

In cases of acute intoxication, ketamine is associated with increases in transient psychopathology with both positive and negative schizophrenialike symptoms (Beck et al., 2020). Therapy for such symptoms is aimed at keeping the patient calm and sedated and preventing the patient from doing harm to self or others. There are no specific antidotes. To minimize disturbing sensory inputs, the intoxicated person can be placed in a quiet environment, with physical restraints if necessary. Agitation can be reduced by administering either a benzodiazepine (discussed in Chapter 13) or an atypical antipsychotic (discussed in Chapter 11). Hyperthermia, hypertension, convulsions, renal failure, and other potential medical consequences should be treated as necessary.

OPIOID KAPPA RECEPTOR AGONIST: SALVINORIN A

Salvinorin A is a psychedelic compound found in the leaves of the perennial herb *Salvia divinorum* (known under various names, including "magic mint," "diviner's sage," and "Sally-D"). A member of the mint family, *Salvia divinorum* is native to cloud forest in the mountains of Oaxaca, Mexico, and has been used for centuries for curing and divination in traditional spiritual practices by the Mazatec peoples of Oaxaca. Among the various species of *Salvia*, only *divinorum* is known to contain salvinorin A. Generally, the leaves of the plant are chewed or brewed in a tea, but the dried leaves can also be smoked in the manner of marijuana or cocaine freebase. Compared with other naturally occurring and synthetic psychedelics, salvinorin A differs structurally (see Figure 8.6), in its mechanism of action, and perhaps in its clinical effects (Butelman et al., 2010; Doss et al., 2020).

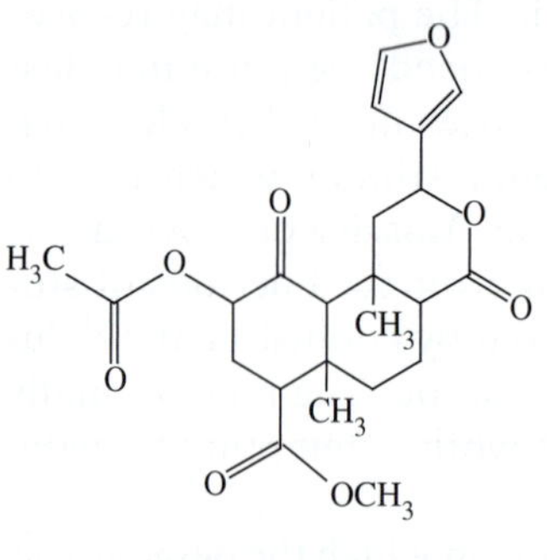

FIGURE 8.6 Structure of Salvinorin A. The structure of this psychedelic compound is unlike that of the other psychedelics discussed in this chapter.

Mechanism of Action

Unlike classical hallucinogens, salvinorin A has no action at $5\text{-HT}2_A$ receptors; rather it is an agonist at opioid kappa receptors and is the first naturally occurring compound known to exhibit such an action (Roth et al., 2002). Laboratory studies in nonhuman animals confirm that salvinorin A's effects differ from the effects of $5\text{-HT}2_A$ agonists, LSD, psilocybin, THC (tetrahydrocannabinol), glutamate NMDA receptor antagonists, and opioid delta or mu receptor agonists, but are similar to the effects of other kappa receptor agonists and are blocked by kappa receptor antagonists (Addy, 2012). This is unusual because the drug is not structurally like other kappa agonists and because its effects are also similar to those of 5-HT2_A agonists (Cunningham et al., 2011; Johnson et al., 2011).

Psychological and Physical Effects

When smoked in doses of 200–500 micrograms, the leaves of *Salvia divinorum* have a short-acting hallucinogenic action, lasting about 30 minutes, with effects that have been described in many different ways: laughter, visions, peace, understanding, experiencing multiple realities, traveling to other places or times, contacting other entities or spirits, entering the realm of the dead, feeling of being underground, flying, floating, twisting, losing one's individuality, and connecting to a larger whole. Smoking also rapidly elicits intense sensory effects, loss of normal awareness of self and surroundings, and, in some cases, delusional experiences. Adverse effects include intense anxiety, dysphoria, confusion, and a hangover with headache and drowsiness lasting several hours. There are no characteristic physical signs except for some tachycardia and hypertension. But because the drug is often taken with other substances, specific reactions are difficult to determine. The risks of dependence and addiction are unknown, and there is no recognized antidote for intoxication.

PSYCHEDELIC MEDICINE: THERAPEUTIC APPLICATIONS OF PSYCHEDELIC DRUGS

The naturally occurring psychedelic compounds covered in this chapter have long been used by Indigenous peoples, including medicinally in healing practices, as well as in other ritual and social practices. We have briefly discussed some of these practices in the cases of mescaline (from the peyote cactus), DMT and harmine (from the plants *Banisteriopsis caapi* and *Psychotria viridis*, parts of which are brewed into ayahuasca), psilocybin and psilocin (from various species of mushrooms), lysergic acid amide (from ololiuqui, the seeds of the plant *Rivea corymbosa*), scopolamine (from the plants *Atropa belladonna*, *Datura stramonium*, *Mandragora officinarum*, and *Datura inoxia*, among others), and salvinorin A (from the plant *Salvia divinorum*). Now, in this section, we will discuss recent scientific research into pharmaceutical uses of some of these naturally occurring psychedelics as well as into such uses of a variety of synthetic psychedelic compounds.

Scientific interest in the use of psychedelic drugs for psychiatric treatment of nonpsychotic disorders began in the 1950s. In 1970, in the context of widespread recreational use of psychedelics and their association with the counterculture, most of the psychedelics in use were classified under Schedule I of the United Nations convention on drugs, meaning that they had no known medical use and were considered potentially very harmful (Chi and Gold, 2020). Although this classification made possession or sale of these drugs illegal and essentially ended research into their possible therapeutic uses, it had little practical impact on their recreational use (Nutt, 2019).

Over the years since, however, the situation has changed. The relative ineffectiveness of currently approved medications for difficult-to-treat psychiatric disorders has been widely recognized, scientific interest in potential therapeutic uses of psychedelic compounds has undergone a resurgence, and the new field of psychedelic medicine has emerged (Andersen et al., 2021; Carhart-Harris, 2019; De Gregorio et al., 2021; Inserra et al., 2021; Nutt and Carhart-Harris, 2020; Reiff et al., 2020; Tupper et al., 2015). This field encompasses research into psychedelic treatments for a wide range of psychiatric disorders, including treatment-resistant depression (Benko and Vrankova, 2020; Bouso et al., 2021; Reiff et al., 2020), persistent anxiety, treatment-resistant OCD, treatment-resistant PTSD, substance-related disorders (including alcohol abuse and cigarette dependence), end-of-life depression and anxiety, and anxiety associated with advanced cancer diagnoses (Chi and Gold, 2020; dos Santos and Hallak, 2020; Muttoni et al., 2019; Nutt, 2019).

Despite this range of research, only one of the psychedelics discussed here has received FDA approval, while two others have been given breakthrough therapy designation by the FDA[5] (all three for treatment of depression, as discussed below)—a lack of widespread approval that is probably due to the following factors affecting studies of psychedelic medicine:

- Most studies have been small, with few subjects, and may not be applicable to wider populations.
- Studies are typically case reports, usually retrospective, noncontrolled, and not blinded.
- Research funding is poor, with few or no research grants available, because most of the drugs being investigated are classified as Schedule I compounds by the DEA.[6]
- The drugs available for study vary in quality (e.g., in purity), which can make dosages difficult to control.

At this point, the most that can be said is that studies indicate only potential application to poorly treatable mental disorders. Larger, better controlled studies are needed to determine the true impact and clinical utility for each disorder (Daniel and Haberman, 2017; Phelps et al., 2022). Here is an even more general assessment of the current status of psychedelic psychiatry:

> Psychedelics are neither a cure for mental disorders nor a quick fix for an unfulfilled life and should not be portrayed as a panacea. Ominously, propsychedelic subcultures are increasingly fostering utopian visions for society based on research findings that, while intriguing, still must be considered preliminary. (Yaden et al., 2021)

---

[5]According to the FDA, breakthrough therapy designation is meant to "expedite the development and review of drugs that are intended to treat a serious condition [where] preliminary clinical evidence indicates that the drug may demonstrate substantial improvement over available therapy" (https://www.fda.gov/patients/fast-track-breakthrough-therapy-accelerated-approval-priority-review/breakthrough-therapy).

[6]Of the scheduled psychedelics discussed in this chapter, mescaline, MDMA, MDA, DOM, TMA, DMA, MDE, MDAI, BZP, LSD, DMT, bufotenine, psilocybin, psilocin, 5-MeO-MiPT, AMT, and 2C-B are classified as Schedule I, phencyclidine as Schedule II, and ketamine as Schedule III.

DR. J'S MUSINGS 8.1

Psychedelic Psychiatry: A New Era

I began my study of psychopharmacology in the late 1960s, just as research into the use of psychedelics to treat psychiatric disorders was being shut down by the FDA. As a result, when I began teaching about these drugs, I focused on their intense immediate effects, including hallucinations, dissociative behaviors, and alterations in the perception of reality; largely overlooked was the use of psychedelics by Indigenous peoples in religious and healing practices stretching back hundreds or even thousands of years (Guimaraes dos Santos et al., 2021; Pollan, 2021). Of the psychedelic drugs that were banned at that time (and that are still classified as Schedule I compounds by the DEA), psilocybin has attracted the greatest current interest, for its potential as a treatment for resistant depression and anxiety. As the legal status of psilocybin and other psychedelics changes and as research into their potential pharmacological benefits expands, other uses will surely emerge—for instance, in treating addictions, PTSD, and chronic pain. Judging by the research done to date, these future uses will involve drugs such as mescaline, DMT, and perhaps even LSD. However, investigators must keep this important point in mind: carefully crafted research and not emotions must guide assessments of clinical usefulness (Harris, 2021).

As this area of psychopharmacology develops further and more drugs are approved, new medical infrastructure will be required to handle these powerful psychoactive substances while simultaneously providing appropriate psychotherapeutic support (Heifets and Malenka, 2019), including through the development and evaluation of therapist training programs for psychedelic-assisted psychotherapy (Harris, 2021; Tai et al., 2021). Clinicians will have to deal with safety issues (including patient selection), substance abuse potential, and emergent psychiatric and medical crises. Clearly, many challenges lie ahead, but the need is so great that the required efforts are well justified—for example, as noted in a study of the need for a reexamination of psychedelic drugs (specifically 5-HT2_A agonists) in the treatment of chronic pain:

> Given the current state of the opioid epidemic and limited efficacy of non-opioid analgesics, it is time to consider further research on psychedelics as analgesics in order to improve the lives of patients with chronic pain conditions. (Castellanos et al., 2020)

Similarly, a review of clinical studies of several serotoninlike psychedelics (including LSD, ayahuasca, and psilocybin) in treating patients suffering from anxiety, depression, OCD, and tobacco and alcohol use disorders came to this conclusion:

> The resurgence of clinical psychedelic research provides early evidence for treatment efficacy and safety for a range of psychiatric conditions and constitutes an exciting new treatment avenue in a health area with major unmet needs. (Andersen et al., 2021)

Psilocybin

In a handful of studies from a few years ago, psilocybin showed efficacy in the treatment of a variety of mental health conditions (Daniel and Haberman, 2017), including end-of-life distress secondary to cancer (i.e., cancer-related psychiatric distress); substance use disorders (i.e., addictions), especially nicotine dependence and alcoholism; treatment-resistant depression and anxiety; and OCD (Johnson and Griffiths, 2017).

Later studies have shown that the actions of psilocybin (and other psychedelics) are of rapid onset (Witkin et al., 2019), with minimal side effects and prolonged duration (Goldberg et al., 2020; Muttoni et al., 2019), and have suggested a significant role for psilocybin in the treatment of depression. For example:

- Research indicates that the combination of psilocybin therapy and mindfulness training in the treatment of depression could be efficacious (Heuschkel and Kuypers, 2020; Smigielski et al., 2019).
- A randomized clinical trial using the GRID Hamilton Depression Rating Scale "found that psilocybin-assisted therapy was efficacious in producing large, rapid, and sustained antidepressant effects in patients with major depressive disorder" (Davis et al., 2021).
- In a comparative study of patients with long-standing moderate to severe treatment-resistant depression, psilocybin exhibited an efficacy similar to that of escitalopram (Carhart-Harris et al., 2021). (See Chapter 12 for detailed discussion of escitalopram.)
- A study demonstrated that psilocybin altered the functioning of the amygdala in a way that indicated that the drug was having positive effects on treatment-resistant depression (Mertens et al., 2020).
- In open trials, psilocybin had positive effects on both depression (as measured by the Beck Depression Inventory) and anxiety (as measured by the State-Trait Anxiety Inventory) (Vargas et al., 2020). Other research suggests that such effects might be especially beneficial in patients with advanced states of cancer (Agin-Liebes et al., 2020).

As acceptance and use of psilocybin therapy have gained momentum, industry has attempted to produce and market psilocybin for profit on the model of traditional pharmaceuticals (Phelps et al., 2022). For example, in a development that is both exciting and challenging for the medical community, the British company Compass Pathways is poised to become the first legal provider of psilocybin, having received breakthrough therapy designation from the FDA in 2018 on the basis of a clinical study testing the drug as a treatment for depression. Similarly, in 2019, the FDA also granted the nonprofit Usona Institute breakthrough therapy designation for psilocybin for the treatment of major depressive disorder, implicitly acknowledging that effective treatment of that disorder is an unmet critical medical need and that psilocybin therapy might offer substantial clinical improvement over existing therapies. This possibility is strengthened by the results of a study finding that 71% of patients given psilocybin-assisted therapy (i.e., along with psychotherapy) experienced a "clinically significant response" (an improvement that lasted at least four weeks after treatment) and that 54% met the criteria for total "remission of depression" (Davis et al., 2021). Finally (and encouragingly), an earlier study found that psilocybin had relatively low abuse potential and would be appropriately classified as safe for medical use (Johnson et al., 2018), and a more recent study describes the synthesis of psilocybin, a critical need if psilocybin is to find wider use in therapeutics (Sherwood et al., 2020).

Interestingly, by 2021, six cities in the United States (Santa Cruz and Oakland, California; Denver, Colorado; Somerville and Cambridge, Massachusetts; and Washington, DC) had passed ordinances to decriminalize psilocybin and other natural psychedelics (including peyote and ayahuasca) for medical use, and Oregon voters passed a ballot measure to decriminalize psilocybin statewide for therapeutic use (Smith and Appelbaum, 2021). Synthetic psychedelics such as LSD and MDMA have been excluded from these measures, but of course that could change, as it has with marijuana legalization efforts. Certainly, controversy will continue.

LSD

Studies of LSD in the 1950s and 1960s (before it was classified as a Schedule I drug) were consistent with the notion that LSD might have psychiatric uses but also suggested that it might cause or exacerbate psychiatric problems. The latter notion has been essentially refuted by subsequent studies, and the drug's safety has been confirmed.

LSD has been shown to be beneficial in the treatment of alcoholism, initially in the case of the founder of Alcoholics Anonymous, who used LSD to provide insights that helped him overcome his disorder (Nutt, 2019). Other studies have suggested LSD's potential benefits as an adjunct to psychotherapy for treatment-resistant depression, anxiety and depression associated with life-threatening diseases, and tobacco and alcohol dependence (Das et al., 2016; dos Santos et al., 2016).

Ayahuasca

As discussed earlier in this chapter, ayahuasca is a tea brewed from Amazonian plants, with psychedelic properties due to the presence of DMT and harmine. Originally used by Indigenous peoples for the purposes of spirit communication, magical experiences, healing, and religious rituals, ayahuasca has been incorporated into folk medicine and spiritual healing practices. More recently, it is being used recreationally in Europe and North America, while also being considered for use in psychedelic medicine on the basis of studies indicating that it may be helpful in treating various psychiatric disorders—including addictions, pain, depression, and anxiety—and that its side effects appear to be relatively mild (Hamill et al., 2019; Orsolini et al., 2020). For example, one study reported on the efficacy of ayahuasca in the treatment of eating disorders (Renelli et al., 2020), and an earlier study found that people who used ayahuasca reported less problematic drinking and greater well-being than did people who used classical psychedelics (i.e., LSD and "magic mushrooms" containing psilocybin) (Lawn et al., 2017).

Mescaline and MDMA

Of the catecholaminelike psychedelics covered earlier in this chapter, currently only mescaline and especially MDMA merit some discussion as possible agents in psychedelic medicine. Regarding mescaline, the Canadian company XPhyto added industrial production of medical-grade mescaline to its psychedelic medicine program in 2021, claiming that mescaline holds promise for the treatment of addiction, PTSD, and depression.

MDMA, in contrast, has already received FDA breakthrough therapy designation for treatment-resistant depression and for PTSD, and it seems likely to be fully licensed by the FDA for treatment of PTSD in the not-too-distant future—that is, "MDMA would become a medicine," with an action that has been described like this:

> MDMA produces a more gentle and easily tolerated state compared to LSD. It is shorter acting, which makes it more clinically manageable, [and] it enhances feelings of empathy and bonding and allows users to access and process memories of emotional trauma. (Sessa et al., 2019)

Several recent articles have pointed to the efficacy and safety of MDMA for treatment-resistant PTSD as an adjunct to psychotherapy (Bahji et al., 2020a; Gorman et al., 2020; Jerome et al., 2020; Krediet et al., 2020). In particular, studies indicate that MDMA-assisted psychotherapy for PTSD seems to reduce the severity of symptoms for at least 12 months posttreatment (Jerome et al., 2020) and that the mechanisms underlying MDMA's effects on PTSD may be memory reconsolidation and fear extinction (Feduccia and Mithoefer, 2018). In addition, a Phase 3 clinical study of 90 adults with severe PTSD in which MDMA was used together with three preparatory and nine integrative therapy sessions found that those receiving MDMA experienced much better results than did controls, leading the authors to conclude that "MDMA-assisted therapy represented a potential breakthrough treatment that merits expedited clinical evaluation" (Mitchell et al., 2021).

Moreover, according to one team of researchers, future clinical trials studying the effects of MDMA in nonpsychedelic doses may validate the idea that "MDMA and MDMA-like molecules have a role in the management of the social impairments in autism" (Chaliha et al., 2021).

However, in a recent review, the researchers found only "moderate" evidence for the effectiveness of MDMA in combination with psychotherapy in treating PTSD (Varker et al., 2021), and other studies raise the question of whether the potential toxicities associated with chronic use of MDMA (as discussed earlier in this chapter) may limit its therapeutic use (Bahji et al., 2020; Feduccia et al., 2019).

Salvinorin A

Research suggests that the naturally occurring compound salvinorin A (a component of the leaves of the plant *Salvia divinorum*, as discussed earlier in this chapter) has therapeutic potential as a treatment for chronic pain, anxiety, depression, opioid withdrawal and maintenance of abstinence, cocaine withdrawal and craving, and personality disorders (Cunningham et al., 2011; Gonçalves et al., 2021; Siegel, 2021). For example, a case study describes a patient with severe depression unrelieved by traditional antidepressant medications and cognitive-behavioral therapy who claimed total remission of depressive symptoms based on a regimen of chewing two or three *Salvia divinorum* leaves at a time three times per week (Hanes, 2001). Given that doses of about 200–300 milligrams of salvinorin A can cause hallucinations, potentially therapeutic doses should be below that level. *Salvia divinorum* is not scheduled by the DEA and is therefore legal to use, so further research into its possible therapeutic benefits should not be difficult.

Ketamine and Esketamine

According to a recent study, ketamine and its pharmacologically more active isomer, esketamine, have multiple potential therapeutic uses, including treatment of depression, relief of chronic pain, and treatment of substance use disorders (especially cocaine dependence) (Gautam et al., 2020). The molecular mechanisms underlying these antidepressant and analgesic effects appear to involve an interaction between the drug and central cannabinoid receptors (Hashimoto, 2020). For example, coadministration of cannabidiol and ketamine results in stronger antidepressant effects (Sartim et al., 2021), while the central analgesic effects of ketamine appear to be exerted through activation of cannabinoid receptors (Pacheco et al., 2019). More research on this interaction should be forthcoming.

Esketamine as an Antidepressant

Research indicates that ketamine (and especially its isomer esketamine), in low, non-psychedelic doses, might be useful in treatment-resistant depression (Molero et al., 2018; Shouan and Grover, 2018). This would extend the pharmacological uses of ketamine beyond its applications as an anesthetic and an amnestic and of course beyond its use (or abuse) for its psychedelic effects (as discussed earlier). Indeed, injections of subanesthetic doses of ketamine produce a very rapid onset of antidepressant effects, faster than any relief afforded by conventional antidepressants (Katz et al., 2022).

Intranasal administration of esketamine also appears to be rapidly effective in treatment-resistant depression, improving mood and reducing suicidal ideation (Canuso et al., 2018). This was confirmed in 2019 when the FDA formally approved the esketamine nasal spray Spravato for use as an antidepressant in treatment-resistant patients (Kim et al., 2019) and in 2020 when Spravato was approved for the treatment of adults with major depression who are experiencing suicidal ideation (Fu et al., 2020). In addition, a Phase 3 study of 705 patients with treatment-resistant depression found that, among participants who achieved stable remission, those who received esketamine nasal spray plus an oral antidepressant were 51% less likely to relapse than those who received a placebo plus an oral antidepressant (Daly et al., 2019).

However, the use of esketamine to treat depression is not without limitations and not without critics, for the following reasons:

- Several doses of the drug are required (the current requirement is six to eight doses).
- The drug must be administered in specialized clinics, which makes the treatment costly: a full course of treatment currently costs several thousand dollars. (Dozens of these clinics are already operating in the United States.)

DR. J'S MUSINGS 8.2

"Doc, What Was That Stuff?!"

I had on-call duty for anesthesia services. It was around midnight when I received a call about a serious emergency: a middle-aged male had come to the emergency room with very low blood pressure, severe pain, and a ruptured aneurism in the abdominal aorta. He was brought directly to an operating room, where I rapidly explained to him that because of his condition, I didn't know how much anesthesia he could handle and the drug I was going to give him might cause some bizarre mental effects. However, use of this drug was necessary to give him a chance at survival. When all was ready, I injected a dose of ketamine followed by additional doses every 30 minutes. (Ketamine was the only anesthetic that would also provide amnesia and help maintain blood pressure.) After several hours of surgery, which involved several total body blood transfusions, the repair was made, and the patient survived. The next day I saw him awake in the ICU, and I introduced myself. He glared at me and said, "Doc, I know who you are! What was that stuff? I knew I was dead. I was floating on the ceiling looking down at my dead body!" My answer was simple: "I'm so very happy that you are here to tell me about it." We talked several times during the following weeks, and I explained what ketamine was and why I had to use it in his situation, which usually results in death. To this day, similar use of ketamine is relied upon in battlefield situations.

- No long-term effectiveness studies have yet been reported. Advertising from for-profit ketamine clinics claims a 70–80% success rate in formerly treatment-resistant patients, but evidence of this has been called "flimsy" at best (Simons, 2019).

The controversy over this drug and its use will likely continue, which probably means that financial interests will determine its future.

Ketamine as an Analgesic

With the ongoing opioid crisis, when people with complaints of severe pain come to emergency rooms, physicians are often unwilling to prescribe opioids for relief. An alternative emergency-room treatment consists of injection, infusion, or sublingual administration of low ("subdissociative") doses of ketamine (Motov et al., 2016; Orhurhu et al., 2019; Pourmand et al., 2017), which is about as effective an analgesic as morphine.

Guidelines for the use of ketamine as an analgesic, especially in emergency situations where opioid use needs to be avoided, have facilitated the emergence of ketamine as a leading option for rapid pain relief and possibly long-term analgesia (Schwenk et al., 2018). Before the publication of these guidelines, there had been few recommendations on how to use ketamine for pain relief.

Ketamine for Cocaine Dependence

A trial in 55 cocaine-dependent persons compared the effects of a single 40-minute infusion of a subdissociative dose of ketamine plus mindfulness-based relapse prevention therapy to the effects of a placebo drug (midazolam) plus the same mindfulness-based therapy (Dakwar et al., 2019). The results were that 48.2% of the participants in the ketamine group maintained abstinence from cocaine use over the last two weeks of the trial, compared with 10.7% in the midazolam group. The ketamine group was 53% less likely than the midazolam group to relapse (i.e., drop out of the trial or use cocaine) and had craving scores that were 58.1% lower. The authors concluded that a "single ketamine infusion improved a range of important treatment outcomes in cocaine-dependent adults. . . . Further research is needed to replicate these promising results in a larger sample."

Methoxetamine

Structurally similar to ketamine, **methoxetamine** (MXE) also acts like ketamine pharmacologically, as a noncompetitive antagonist at NMDA receptors, with psychedelic effects that include euphoria and perceptual hallucinations like those that are typical of ketamine (Botanas et al., 2021; Marti et al., 2021). Recent research shows a variety of other actions, including potent reuptake inhibition of the neurotransmitters dopamine, norepinephrine, and serotonin (Hondebrink et al., 2017). In human studies, MXE showed robust antidepressant effects within 30 minutes of administration, which lasted for at least 24 hours (Botanas et al., 2021; Sayson et al., 2019). Not surprisingly, MXE also seems to have analgesic properties (Botanas et al., 2019). The drug's

DR. J'S MUSINGS 8.3

Who Would Have Thought?

As a graduate student in the 1960s, I knew the scientists who developed ketamine (and PCP) as novel analgesic drugs. Ketamine was introduced clinically as an anesthetic drug in 1970, but its use was frequently accompanied by psychiatric reactions, which eventually relegated it to specific types of uses, such as battlefield anesthesia (Mion, 2017). During the 1980s, ketamine became an abused drug, causing it to be classified as a Schedule III drug under the Controlled Substances Act. In the 1980s, I used ketamine as a surgical anesthetic on very ill patients only and wrote (in earlier editions of this text) of it as a psychedelic drug that dissociates the user from reality. Now, some 40 years later, ketamine has been recast as a therapeutic drug for resistant depression, PTSD, and chronic pain syndromes (so-called ketamine psychedelic therapy). Infusions of ketamine to treat these conditions occur "off-label" at specialized ketamine infusion clinics, and FDA approval was recently granted for use in a nasal spray for treatment-resistant depression. Ketamine is the first (and so far the only) psychedelic agent with an FDA-approved therapeutic use.

analgesic and anesthetic properties seem to be weaker than those of ketamine but with a longer duration of action.

Dextromethorphan

Dextromethorphan (DXM; also known as "poor man's PCP") is a common ingredient in more than 140 varieties of over-the-counter cough suppressants. Recreational ingestion is referred to as "roboing," "dexing," "robo-tripping," or "robo-copping" (the "robo" nomenclature comes from the cough suppressant Robitussin DM, which contains DXM). In a recent study in human volunteers, high doses (over 1500 milligrams per day) produced a mental state similar to that produced by PCP (phencyclidine), with hallucinations, delusions, and paranoia (Martinak et al., 2017; Schifano et al., 2021). Like ketamine and PCP, DXM is an antagonist at NMDA receptors, and as such it has antidepressant and analgesic effects, although those have been poorly elucidated (Boas et al., 2019; Kreutzwiser and Tawfic, 2019; Marti et al., 2021). In a study of DXM's effects at maximal doses, participants displayed unresponsiveness to questions, anxiety or fearfulness, and confusion or disorientation, while also endorsing the drug's positive effects in regard to "mysticism" (Reissig et al., 2012). Acute psychotic reactions have occasionally been reported (Martinak et al., 2017), and a recent study describes DXM toxicity and its treatment (Journey et al., 2020).

Kratom

Kratom is the common name for the plant *Mitragyna speciosa* (also known as "thang," "kakuam," "thom," "ketum," and "biak"), which is native to Southeast Asia. Kratom leaves have been used medicinally by Indigenous peoples of the region for thousands of years, by chewing, smoking, brewing in a tea, and oral ingestion. In low doses, kratom has a stimulant action, but high doses produce sedation and opioidlike effects. More than 40 alkaloids have been isolated from kratom, but most research has been conducted on the predominant alkaloid, **mitragynine**, which was first isolated in 1921. The alkaloid 7-hydroxymitragynine is also present as another active ingredient (Figura et al., 2020).

Mitragynine is believed to be a partial agonist at the mu opioid receptor and an antagonist at the delta opioid receptor. A study in mice found that mitragynine pseudoindoxyl (a semisynthetic opioid obtained from the mitragynine in kratom) was a more effective pain reliever than morphine; produced less tolerance, addiction, and dependence than are usually associated with opioids; and did not suppress respiration and did not seem to produce constipation (as most potent opioids do) (Váradi et al., 2016). A review of the pharmacology of kratom and its potential clinical uses noted that a recent rise in kratom use was a cause for concern but that

> The problem must be understood within the greater context of the current epidemic of opioid abuse, as the desire to alleviate opioid withdrawal symptoms is a crucial factor accounting for patients who seek out and abuse kratom. (Eastlack et al., 2020)

Similarly, a survey of 2800 people taking kratom orally found that 91% used it for pain, 67% for anxiety, and 65% for depression, with high ratings of efficacy, and that

DR. J'S MUSINGS 8.4

So Where Do We Go from Here?

Naturally occurring psychedelic compounds such as mescaline, psilocybin, and salvinorin A have been used for millennia by Indigenous peoples for healing and other purposes but were largely unknown in Western society until the 1960s. At that time, following the synthesis of LSD and its wide abuse, other psychedelic drugs (both natural and synthetic) found wide use as intoxicants. In 1967, the FDA banned most psychedelics by classifying them as Schedule I compounds, but as we have seen in this chapter, the recent resurgence of investigation into therapeutic uses of subintoxicating doses of these agents has already led to FDA approval of one such agent, esketamine, for treatment-resistant depression.

Many mental health disorders remain unresponsive to medication, even when supplemented by psychotherapy. Evidence suggests that trials of psychedelic drugs should be considered for treatment of depression, chronic pain (as opioid substitutes), cocaine and opioid addiction, PTSD, severe anxiety, and other disorders. Perhaps it is time to recognize the legitimacy of psychedelic medicine, develop guidelines, and encourage research, controlled experimentation, and publication of results, which may also require reconsideration of government scheduling of these agents. Dependency can result from use of psychedelics (as it can with alcohol, nicotine, benzodiazepines, and opioids), but their therapeutic potential for treatment of currently treatment-resistant mental health disorders may outweigh that risk (Nutt, 2019; Rucker et al., 2018; Tupper et al., 2015).

41% used it to reduce or end their use of illicit or prescription opioids (Garcia-Romeu et al., 2020). Adverse effects were mild, and only 2% of the respondents met the criteria for kratom use disorder.

The FDA recognizes kratom as a concern, but it has not been added to federal scheduling, and it remains classified as a dietary supplement. In 2016, when the DEA attempted to temporarily ban the substance, more than 22,000 people responded, mostly telling stories about how they relied on the plant for easing their anxiety, PTSD, chronic pain, or struggles with opioid withdrawal, and how restricting access to it would have serious adverse effects on their lives. In 2017, the FDA released a public health advisory related to potential risks associated with the use of kratom or its active ingredient mitragynine, but at the time of this writing, kratom remains legal in the United States (with the exception of a few states). For the foreseeable future, concern over kratom's abuse potential and its toxicity, as well as study of its therapeutic potential, will continue (Fluyau and Revadigar, 2017; Kruegel and Grundmann, 2018; White, 2018).

Finally, a note of warning: kratom is sometimes found in combination with another mu agonist, O-desmethyltramadol, the active metabolite of the opioid analgesic tramadol (discussed in Chapter 10). This combination (with the street name "Krypton") is potentially fatal (Kronstrand et al., 2011).

Tianeptine

Tianeptine (Stablon) is an atypical antidepressant of the class of tricyclic antidepressants (discussed in Chapter 12). Tianeptine works by increasing serotonin reuptake in the brain, modulating the system of glutamate NMDA receptors, and functioning as an indirect partial opioid agonist, leading to a range of positive effects experienced by users but possibly also to "our next kratom problem" due to its opioidlike risks (Bettinger and Cleary, 2020). As with many of the psychedelic drugs presented in this chapter, Tianeptine's potential for abuse has to be weighed against its potential clinical benefits, including enhanced cognitive functioning and relief from anxiety (panic disorder), depression, and PTSD, as well as pain relief.

CHAPTER REVIEW

1. What are some of the ways in which psychedelic drugs differ from other drugs of abuse?
2. Match the letter for each psychedelic drug with the number of the category to which it belongs:
   A. ketamine; **B.** psilocybin; **C.** MDMA; **D.** LSD; **E.** salvinorin A; **F.** mescaline; **G.** scopolamine.
   1. naturally occurring catecholaminelike compound; **2.** synthetic catecholamine-like compound; **3.** naturally occurring serotoninlike compound; **4.** synthetic serotoninlike compound; **5.** acetylcholine muscarinic receptor antagonist; **6.** glutamate NMDA receptor antagonist; **7.** opioid receptor agonist.
3. What structural features differentiate the catecholaminelike and amphetaminelike psychedelics from the catecholamine neurotransmitters and amphetamine?
4. What are the natural sources of mescaline and of myristicin and elemicin?
5. What are some of the positive and negative effects associated with MDMA?
6. True or false: MDA, MDE, and MDAI have effects similar to those of MDMA.
7. Which of the following compounds are piperazines: BZP, DMA, DOM, TFMPP, TMA?
8. Choose the correct term in the parentheses: The serotoninlike psychedelics exert their effects mainly through an (agonistic/antagonistic) action at 5-$HT2_A$ receptors.
9. Describe the discovery of LSD, its potency, and its psychological effects, including adverse reactions.
10. Compare and contrast the three naturally occurring serotoninlike psychedelics ayahuasca, psilocybin, and ololiuqui in terms of their sources and their effects.
11. Which of the following are classified as novel psychoactive tryptamines: AMT, 2C-B, bufotenine, 5-MeO-MiPT, mCPP?
12. Describe scopolamine's history of use and its pharmacological effects.

13. Compare and contrast the history of use and psychological and physical effects of phencyclidine and ketamine/esketamine.
14. What is the natural source of salvinorin A, and how does its mechanism of action set it apart from other psychedelics?
15. Summarize the history of psychedelic medicine, including recent developments and the current status of the field.
16. If you were diagnosed with depression and had poor results from treatment with FDA-approved nonpsychedelic medications and psychotherapy, which psychedelic medications would you consider trying, if any? Answer the same question with regard to treatment for PTSD and for chronic pain. Explain your answers.

KEY TERMS

AMT
ayahuasca
bufotenine
BZP
dextromethorphan
DMA
DMT
DOM
elemicin
esketamine
5-MeO-MiPT
flashbacks
hallucinogen persisting perception disorder (HPPD)
harmine
ketamine
kratom
LSD (lysergic acid diethylamide)
lysergic acid amide
mCPP
MDA
MDAI
MDE
MDMA
mescaline
methoxetamine
mitragynine
myristicin
ololiuqui
peyote
phencyclidine
psilocin
psilocybin
psychedelic drugs
psychedelic medicine
salvinorin A
scopolamine
TFMPP
tianeptine
TMA
2C-B

CHAPTER 9

Cannabis

CHAPTER OUTLINE

Cannabis is both another name for the drug **marijuana** and the genus name of the plant species from which the drug is derived. The genus *Cannabis* includes three accepted species: *Cannabis sativa*, *Cannabis indica*, and *Cannabis ruderalis*, of which *Cannabis sativa* is the most widely known and cultivated.[1] Plants of that genus contain a large variety of **cannabinoids** (compounds found in *Cannabis*), the most important of which for the purposes of this chapter are the pharmacologically active compounds **tetrahydrocannabinol (THC)** and **cannabidiol (CBD).**

---

[1]Varieties of *Cannabis sativa* that are grown specifically for industrial uses are known as *hemp* (which has also become a street name for the drug). *Cannabis sativa* is a fast-growing plant that can be used in manufacturing a variety of commercial items. Hemp has negligible levels of psychoactive compounds, which limits its use as a drug.

The chapter begins with a discussion of the general characteristics of cannabis and cannabinoids. This is followed by a history of cannabis use (including economic, medicinal, religious, and recreational uses) and then by a discussion of current cannabis-related issues, including legal and epidemiological issues as well as issues arising from the abuse of synthetic cannabinoids. We then describe the neurobiology of cannabis, the pharmacokinetics of both THC and CBD, and the pharmacological effects of THC. The chapter continues with an extensive discussion of therapeutic applications of cannabinoids and ends with a discussion of cannabis tolerance, withdrawal, dependence, and addiction.

WHAT IS CANNABIS?

Cannabis sativa grows throughout the world and flourishes in most temperate and tropical regions. At least 140 cannabinoids have been identified in the plant, including THC and CBD, but note that neither THC nor CBD are found in the "raw" plant. Rather, the cannabinoids tetrahydrocannabinolic acid (THCa) and cannabidiolic acid (CBDa), which are not pharmacologically active, are converted into THC and CBD in a reaction called *decarboxylation* when the plant is burned or heated (as in a cigarette or in cooking). The process of drying cannabis leaves also slowly converts THCa to THC by decarboxylation (heat simply expedites the conversion). Interestingly, the same process of decarboxylation that converts THCa to THC converts THC into its inactive metabolite, **carboxy-THC**, which is slowly excreted in urine and is the basis for urine testing to detect cannabis use.

THC is a partial agonist at **cannabinoid receptors** in the brain, for which **anandamide** is the natural neurotransmitter (cannabinoid receptors and anandamide are discussed in more detail later in this chapter). CBD, in contrast, is a competitive antagonist at those receptors, despite the structural similarity of THC and CBD and the dissimilarity of anandamide (see Figure 9.1). Unlike THC, CBD does not produce any psychedelic effect, but it may have a variety of therapeutic uses.

Although cannabis has an ancient history of medical and recreational use, we have only recently begun to understand how it acts in the brain to produce its effects.

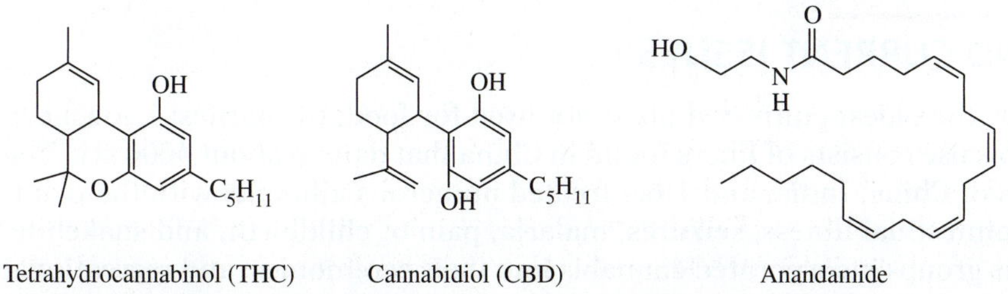

FIGURE 9.1 Structures of THC, CBD, and Anandamide. THC is an agonist at cannabinoid receptors where anandamide is the natural neurotransmitter, which means that THC and anandamide produce similar effects, despite their dissimilar structures. CBD is an antagonist at cannabinoid receptors, which means that its effects are very different from the effects of THC, despite their very similar structures.

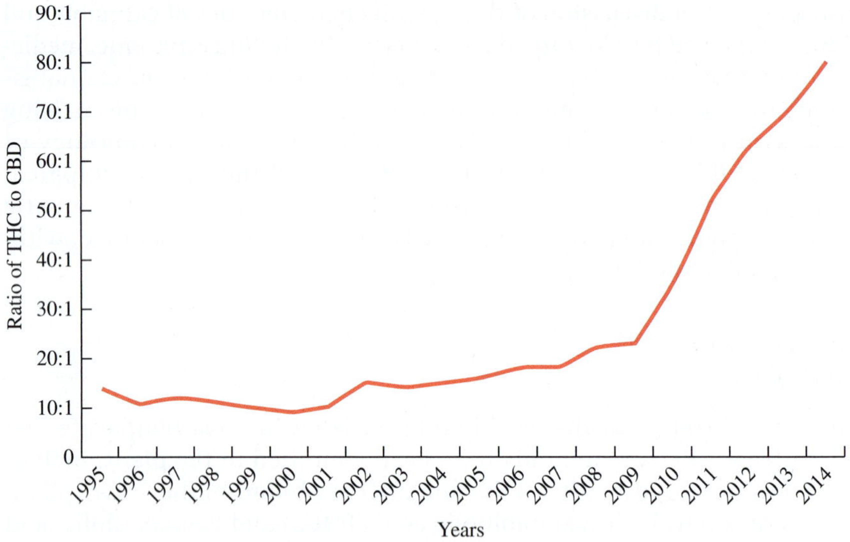

FIGURE 9.2 Increasing Ratio of THC to CBD. During the period from 1995 to 2014, strains of cannabis were bred with increased levels of THC and decreased levels of CBD. [Data from ElSohly et al., 2016.]

Its main psychoactive ingredient, THC, is unique because it has stimulatory, sedating, analgesic, and psychedelic effects without being chemically related to the classical psychostimulants, sedative/hypnotics, analgesics, or psychedelics.

In recent years, as shown in Figure 9.2, strains of cannabis have been bred with increasing levels of THC and decreasing levels of CBD. Strains have also been bred in which the reverse is true, with increasing levels of CBD and decreasing levels of THC. Thus, certain strains (high in THC) are more potent as psychedelics, while other strains (high in CBD) have little psychedelic action but perhaps more therapeutic potential (Leas et al., 2020).

HISTORY AND CURRENT ISSUES

Cannabis may be the oldest cultivated plant not used for food; the earliest known evidence of cannabis use consists of fibers found in China that date to about 4000 BCE. The ancient cultures of China, India, and Tibet treated numerous ailments with the plant, including gastrointestinal illness, seizures, malaria, pain of childbirth, and snakebite. Various religious groups incorporated cannabis into their ceremonies, and recreational use was widespread. Gradually, cannabis use spread elsewhere in Asia and into the Middle East. Everywhere, the plant's primary behavioral effects were well known.

In 1545, Spaniards brought cannabis to America, where hemp was cultivated to manufacture rope for naval use—crucial for overseas empires dependent on sailing

DR. J'S MUSINGS 9.1

Marijuana Potency and Changing Pharmacodynamics

Cheech and Chong's stoner comedies in the 1970s introduced marijuana into mainstream American culture. At that time, THC concentrations in marijuana tended to be about 1.5–2.0%, and the drug's psychoactive effects were modest. Over the next 50 years, improvements in farming have increased THC concentrations close to tenfold, with many strains having 15% or more THC content. Furthermore, chemical refinement techniques have yielded concentrations of 75% and higher. This drastic increase in THC concentration (and consequently in the potency of the drug) has necessitated drastic revisions in our ideas about THC's classic dose-response measurements and its therapeutic effects (including analgesia, anxiolysis, and sedation) and toxicities (including psychotic reactions), all of which vary among patients, at least partly based on patient expectations. Until recently, I never used products containing THC, but now I have found THC "cookies" very useful for relief from very painful ischemic lesions on my feet. Pain relief from these cookies seems better than that from NSAIDs (nonsteroidal anti-inflammatory drugs) and gabapentin, but not as great as what can be achieved with opioids. I find that the combined use of an NSAID, gabapentin, and THC/CBD cookies has largely eliminated my need for opioid medication.

ships. For this reason, and since cannabis did not grow well in England, in 1611 Sir Walter Raleigh was ordered to cultivate hemp in Virginia alongside another important cash crop, tobacco. From that time onward, hemp became a staple crop of the American colonists for making rope, clothes, and paper. George Washington grew hemp on his plantation.

After Napoleon's army brought cannabis back to Europe from Egypt in the early nineteenth century, its use for both medical and recreational purposes began to spread in the West. In the United States, drug companies marketed cannabis tinctures for medicinal use until the Pure Food and Drug Act of 1906 and the Harrison Narcotic Act of 1914 began to impose constraints. The use of recreational cannabis, not specifically outlawed, increased in the United States after 1920, when the Eighteenth Amendment went into effect, prohibiting alcohol consumption. In 1930, Harry Anslinger, the first commissioner of the Federal Narcotics Bureau, began trying to eradicate recreational use of cannabis. In the wake of the repeal of the Eighteenth Amendment in 1933, Anslinger devised dramatic media attacks on marijuana use, which led to the enactment of the Marijuana Tax Act of 1937. This law did not directly outlaw cannabis but imposed a tax on the sale of marijuana. The Marijuana Tax Act was repealed in 1969 and replaced in 1970 by the Controlled Substances Act, under which marijuana was classified as a Schedule I drug (the legal status of marijuana is discussed in more detail below).

During the past few years, cannabis-related social changes have led to a variety of social challenges, as discussed in the sections that follow:

- Advances in cultivation have produced much more varied and potent strains of the plant than were available in the past, and even more potent manufactured products have been developed. Not only has this led to more frequent and more serious adverse effects, but it has also made the older literature less relevant to the effects of current use.
- At the national level, cannabis is still placed in the most restrictive legal category, making scientific study very difficult. At the same time, changes in legal status at the state level have had a range of other effects.
- The epidemiology of cannabis use is changing, due to changes in social attitudes and legal status, which have exposed a greater number of people to cannabis than ever before, especially young people.
- Synthetic cannabinoid use has become much more common and dangerous because of dozens of new formulations, collectively known as **spice**.

Cultivation and Manufacture

Modern cultivation techniques have produced strains of both *Cannabis sativa* and *Cannabis indica* (as well as hybrid strains) with THC concentrations of 20–30%, an order of magnitude higher than the 2–3% concentrations that formerly prevailed (the increasing ratio of THC to CBD shown in Figure 9.2 reflects this development).[2] These high-THC strains are claimed to make users feel happy and uplifted and to have many other beneficial effects, including increased energy, pain relief, reduced stress, and relief from anxiety and depression. In addition, very high THC "concentrates" are being manufactured with THC levels ranging from 60% to 90%, for vaping or for adding to edibles. Use of products with such high concentrations of THC can result in significant cognitive and psychomotor impairments and has led to rising numbers of calls to poison control center calls and visits to emergency rooms (Dilley et al., 2021). (Also see the discussion of vaping-related lung issues in the section on the pharmacological effects of THC later in this chapter.)

Research has not yet caught up with these high-THC strains and concentrates, but it is known that side effects can include increased heart rate (tachycardia), slow reaction times, driving problems, panic reactions, memory loss, and hallucinations and that neuropsychiatric side effects appear to be dose related, especially in the elderly (Velayudhan et al., 2021). Clearly, clinical studies of marijuana's effects should, whenever possible, include information about the THC concentrations in the cannabis products involved and the THC blood concentrations found in the people who used those products (Englund, 2017).

---

[2]Currently, high-THC strains of *sativa* are being marketed under names such as Laughing Buddha, Hawaiian, Thai, Silver Haze, and Memory Loss; high-THC strains of *indica* include Kosher Kush and Triangle Kush; and hybrid strains include Death Star, Ghost OG, White Tahoe Cookies, Banana OG, and The White.

Legal Issues

In the United States, at the federal level, marijuana in all its forms except for hemp[3] remains a Schedule I drug. This classification implies that marijuana has great potential to cause harm and that it has no known medical uses. These implications, especially the latter, are clearly no longer true, despite the fact that "[t]he FDA has not recognized or approved the marijuana plant as medicine" (National Institute on Drug Abuse, 2019). The federal government's unchanged position on marijuana has led individual states to pass laws easing regulation of medical and/or recreational uses of marijuana and its derivatives:

- In November 1996, California passed into law Proposition 215, the Compassionate Use Act, which allows patients with a valid physician's prescription to possess and cultivate marijuana in the state for medical use in the treatment of severe conditions, including cancer, AIDS, chronic pain, and spasticity.
- As of February 2022, 37 states and the District of Columbia had legalized medicinal uses of marijuana, and 18 states had legalized recreational use by adults.

The outcomes of these state-level changes remain to be assessed, including their effects on driving behavior (Fink et al., 2020) and, more broadly, on youth (Cerdá et al., 2020; Dilley et al., 2019). One study provides a thoughtful analysis of the public health and legal consequences that need to be considered as a result of cannabis legalization (Kilmer, 2019), and another study reports on an association between state-level policy liberalization and past-year cannabis use and the prevalence of **cannabis use disorder**, finding that "liberal" states had modestly higher rates of cannabis use than "conservative" states but lower rates of cannabis use disorder (Philbin et al., 2019).

Epidemiology

Information about the prevalence and nature of drug use comes from a variety of sources and from different points in time. Large-scale surveys provide the best available evidence, but they are based primarily on self-reports in questionnaires. A national survey covering the years 2016–2017 found that 8.3% of adults said they had used marijuana at least once in the previous month, while 3.6% considered themselves to be daily smokers. Of adults with one or more medical conditions, 8.8% reported using marijuana at least once in the previous month, while 3.9% reported daily use. The difference between those with and those without medical conditions seems slight but is statistically significant (Dai and Richter, 2019). Another national study found significant differences in cannabis use associated with differences in gender, race, age, marital status, education, and socioeconomic status (Jeffers et al., 2021).

Increasing numbers of middle and high school youth report vaping marijuana (Dai, 2020; Dai and Siahpush, 2020), and there is increasing concern about the long-term

[3]The 2018 federal Farm Bill removed hemp (defined as *Cannabis* with a THC concentration of less than 0.3%) from the list of Schedule I controlled substances, thereby making hemp an ordinary, unscheduled agricultural commodity.

effects of vaping on cognitive development, attentional and inhibitory control, depression, anxiety, and future suicidality, especially when vaping involves high-THC marijuana or other concentrated cannabis products (Gobbi et al., 2019; Paige and Colder, 2020). In addition, polysubstance vaping (e.g., vaping a combination of nicotine and cannabis) is becoming more common (Lanza et al., 2020), which raises additional concerns over both acute and long-term effects. (See, for example, the discussion below of outbreaks of vaping toxicities in 2019, in the section on the pharmacological effects of THC.)

Synthetic Cannabinoids

After 1964, when THC was identified as the main psychoactive ingredient in cannabis, efforts were made to develop synthetic cannabinoids for possible therapeutic applications. By 1985, this had been accomplished, with FDA approval of two synthetic THC drugs, dronabinol (Marinol) and nabilone (Cesamet) as antiemetic drugs for the treatment of nausea and vomiting associated with cancer chemotherapy. (Other potential therapeutic uses of synthetic cannabinoids are noted in the section on therapeutic applications later in this chapter.) Other synthetic cannabinoids include drugs that can be classified as follows (Potts et al., 2020):

- Cyclohexylphenols such as CP-50,556-1 and CP-47,497, both of which are 30 times more potent than THC, and the more recently developed NE-CHMIMO[4] (Angerer et al., 2016).
- Aminoalkylindoles such as pravadoline, WIN-55212–2, JWH-018 JWH-073, and JWH-015.
- Benzoylindoles such as AM-694 and RCS-4 (Rosenbaum et al., 2012).

More important than the difficult nomenclature of these compounds is the fact that they are all full agonists at cannabinoid receptors, exerting much more powerful effects at those receptors than the partial agonist THC (Kelly and Nappe, 2021), which accounts for the toxicity of synthetic cannabinoid products (Kourouni et al., 2020) and for the many reports of serious toxicity following their recreational use (Alexandre et al., 2020), including psychotic effects such as extreme anxiety, confusion, paranoia, and hallucinations. In the words of one group of researchers:

> [T]he available evidence suggests that synthetic cannabinoids can trigger the onset of acute psychosis in vulnerable individuals and the exacerbation of psychotic episodes in those with a previous psychiatric history. (Papanti et al., 2013)

A study of synthetic cannabinoid users who had been admitted to a psychiatric hospital found that they were generally younger males who had greater severity of

[4]NE-CHMIMO has been found along with the synthetic cannabinoid 5F-ADB (also known as 5F-MDMB-PINACA) in a so-called herbal mixture marketed as Jamaican Gold Extreme.

Did You Know?

Mass Intoxication from a Synthetic Cannabinoid

In July 2016, 33 people in a New York City neighborhood consumed a drug containing a synthetic cannabinoid that produced intoxicated behavior likened to a "zombie" outbreak. Of the 33 people who used the drug, 18 were admitted to local hospitals. The drug was a so-called herbal incense product labeled AK-47/24 Karat Gold, which, when tested, was found to contain the synthetic cannabinoid AMB-FUBINACA at a concentration of about 16 milligrams per gram (Adams et al., 2017). AMB-FUBINACA is known to be a powerful depressant, which accounts for the "zombie" behavior.

psychotic symptoms at admission, were more likely to be admitted by criminal court order, and required longer hospitalization periods than did cannabis users (Shalit et al., 2016).

Nonpsychotic clinical symptoms of synthetic cannabinoid toxicity include excited delirium, acute injury to the kidneys, seizures, cardiotoxic effects, coma, and even death (Trecki et al., 2015).

Synthetic cannabinoids either are sprayed on dried, shredded *Cannabis* plant material so they can be smoked or are made into liquids so they can be vaporized and inhaled in e-cigarettes and other devices (such products are also known as herbal or liquid incense, respectively). Despite efforts to limit their availability, synthetic cannabinoids have become increasingly common drugs of abuse, marketed under various street names (e.g., K2, Spice, and Black Mamba). In the early 2000s, several generically labeled synthetic cannabinoids became widely available in "head shops" and convenience stores, as well as through Internet vendors. According to 2019 data from the National Institute on Drug Abuse, use of these synthetic cannabinoids by middle and high school students has remained steady over recent years, with about 2.5–3.5% of students reporting use in the past year. A study of adult patients in residential facilities for treatment of substance use disorders found that the most frequently cited motives for synthetic cannabinoid use included curiosity or experimentation (91% of participants), a desire to feel good or get high (89%), a desire to relax (71%), and a desire to get high without risking a positive drug test (71%) (Bonar et al., 2014).

Several factors make treatment of synthetic cannabinoid toxicity difficult. First, there is as yet no antidote, which means that no matter how intense or unexpected the symptoms, the only available remedy is medical support. In addition, there are no quick urine assays to confirm the presence of synthetic cannabinoids (complicated analyses of blood in specialized laboratories are required), and this makes it hard to be sure that symptoms are the result of synthetic cannabinoid intoxication.

Despite the dangers inherent in the use of synthetic cannabinoids, they have gained worldwide popularity because they produce intense psychoactive effects, are easily available, are inexpensive, and are difficult to detect. In the United States, synthetic cannabinoids have been classified as Schedule I compounds and are now banned in all states.

CANNABINOID RECEPTORS AND THE ACTIONS OF THC, CBD, AND THE NEUROTRANSMITTER ANANDAMIDE

In 1988, the first type of cannabinoid receptor, designated CB1, was discovered, followed by the 1993 discovery of a second type of receptor, designated CB2. Both types of cannabinoid receptors are G-protein-coupled receptors (GPCRs, discussed in detail in Chapter 3). CB1 receptors are located throughout the body but are found in their highest concentration in the central nervous system (CNS); in fact, CB1 receptors are the most common of the GPCRs in the CNS, with concentrations similar to those of GABA and glutamate receptors. In the CNS, CB1 receptors are most abundant in the hippocampus, basal ganglia, cerebellum, and frontal cortex; they are also found in the amygdala, ventral striatum, hypothalamus, brain stem, and spinal cord, which is consistent with the well-known involvement of CB1 receptors in the functions of those brain structures (see Figure 9.3). CB1 receptors are even found in the retina of the eyes, where they may function as part of a neuroprotective mechanism (as discussed later in this chapter). CB2 receptors are mostly (but not completely) found outside the CNS, primarily in tissues of the immune system, such as the tonsils and thymus.

As noted earlier, THC and CBD differ in their actions at cannabinoid receptors: THC is a partial agonist at both CB1 and CB2 receptors, whereas CBD does not stimulate

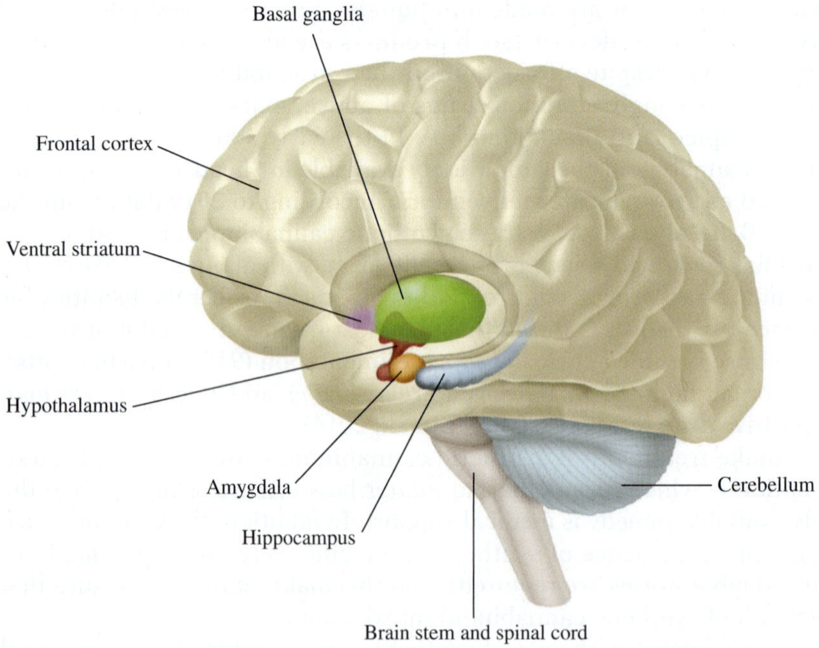

FIGURE 9.3 Cannabinoids in the Brain. Cannabinoids produce their psychoactive effects by binding to CB1 receptors concentrated in brain structures that regulate functions such as attention and judgment (frontal cortex), learning and memory (hippocampus), fear and anxiety (amygdala), movement (basal ganglia and cerebellum), ingestion (hypothalamus), drug "high" (ventral striatum), and pain and the vomiting reflex (brain stem and spinal cord).

either receptor but acts as an antagonist at CB1 receptors, which means that CBD can antagonize many of the effects of THC. For example, THC can precipitate psychotic reactions, whereas CBD may block this action and may therefore be useful in treating THC-induced psychosis (this and other therapeutic applications of CBD are discussed later in this chapter). The range of CBD's actions has been summarized like this:

> CBD has broad actions on multiple systems, such as modulating opioid, serotonin, and adenosine neurotransmission. CBD's modulatory actions on these diverse biological systems would be expected to affect multiple functions including anxiety, cognition, inflammation, mood, and nociception (pain). (Hurd, 2020)

The discovery of the receptors through which THC produces its effects was significant: "[R]eceptors are not present in the body because there is a plant outside there. They are present in the body in order to be activated by something the body produces when and where needed" (Mechoulam, 2010). This implication led to the 1992 identification of the neurotransmitter anandamide, which, like THC, is a partial agonist at both CB1 and CB2 receptors (Seely et al., 2011). Since the discovery of anandamide, several other endogenous compounds have been postulated to act on cannabinoid receptors (Pertwee, 2015), but to date none have been sufficiently confirmed to include in this discussion. However, studies have suggested that these anandamidelike compounds may be involved in functions such as feeding behaviors, sexual behaviors, pleasure and other emotional states, and cravings and may turn out to be useful in cannabinoid-based therapeutics (Bettinger et al., 2019; Cristino et al., 2020; Pacher et al., 2020).

PHARMACOKINETICS OF THC

In this section, we will discuss how the absorption of THC into the bloodstream depends on the mode of administration, how storage of THC in body fat increases the effects of subsequent doses of the drug, and how THC is metabolized and eliminated in urine, with implications for drug testing.

Absorption

THC is usually administered by inhalation of the smoke created by burning dried, shredded marijuana in a pipe (including in a water pipe) or in a hand-rolled "joint" (a marijuana cigarette). In general, about one-fourth to one-half of the THC in the plant material is available in the smoke. In practice, the amount absorbed into the bloodstream depends not just on the amount of THC in the smoke but also on how deeply the smoker inhales and how long the smoke is kept in the lungs. Estimates of the amount of the available THC absorbed into the body range from 5% to 60%. Whatever the amount, absorption of THC from smoking is rapid and complete. Once absorbed, THC is distributed to the various organs of the body, especially those that have significant concentrations of fatty material, such as the brain. The behavioral effects occur almost immediately after smoking begins and correspond with the rapid attainment of peak concentrations in plasma.

Note that smoking marijuana in a water pipe tends to increase the amount of THC absorbed in a given time, as the cooling effect of the water pipe enables deeper, lengthier inhalations (the use of water pipes in smoking tobacco is discussed in Chapter 6). The authors of a study of marijuana smoking with water pipes proposed, consistent with earlier research, that rapid absorption of THC might mimic the effects of other illicit drugs and might thereby put smokers at greater risk by predisposing them to initiate use of such other drugs, even after as long as 5.5 years (Tsai et al., 2021). Thus, efforts to limit the use of this and other methods of rapidly absorbing THC might help lower the risk of using more addictive drugs with more dangerous effects.

Other methods of rapidly inhaling high levels of THC include **dabbing** and vaping. Dabbing involves preparing highly concentrated THC by passing butane through a tube packed with dried cannabis (a process called "blasting"). Once the butane evaporates, the remaining product, butane hash oil, has THC concentrations of up to 80% or more. This hash oil is then vaporized by heating it (e.g., with a blow torch), and the vapor is inhaled ("dabbed") through a water pipe. Not only have fires and burns been attributed to this process, but also little is known about the long-term risks of dabbing.

Vaping involves putting hash oil or marijuana in an e-cigarette or other vaping device (vaping of nicotine products is discussed in Chapter 6). Some vaping devices use regular marijuana, heated to a temperature sufficient to release the THC as an aerosol, while preventing actual combustion. Others use concentrates such as hash oil. For people who have not smoked marijuana before, absorbing high concentrations of THC from vaping hash oil requires caution (Giroud et al., 2015).

Marijuana can also be taken orally (i.e., ingested), which delays onset of the "high" as it takes more time for the drug to get through the liver. In addition, acidic degradation of THC, enzyme action, and first-pass metabolism (discussed in Chapter 1) may reduce the potency of the drug by two-thirds. However, once the THC is absorbed, oral administration results in a more intense and longer lasting "high," with no associated effects on the lungs and no odor. Despite these "positives," the negative consequences of ingesting marijuana have come more to the fore as the use of edible marijuana has increased.

Did You Know?

Maureen Dowd's Experience with Edible Marijuana

In 2014, the *New York Times* columnist Maureen Dowd described her experience with edible marijuana in the form of a caramel and chocolate flavored candy bar, illustrating how easy it is to eat too much of a THC-infused food product and suffer the consequences. She relates how she began by just nibbling the end of the bar and then, when nothing happened, eating some more. For an hour or so, she says, she felt no effects, but then . . .

> I felt a scary shudder go through my body and brain. . . . I was panting and paranoid. . . . I strained to remember where I was or even what I was wearing. . . . I became convinced that I had died and no one was telling me.

The next day, she found out novices were supposed to consume candy bars like that in small pieces; unfortunately for her, there was nothing to that effect on the label.

Distribution

Much of the THC taken into the body is stored in body fat, from which it is only slowly released over a period that can last from several days to about two weeks or even longer in people who smoke marijuana chronically or are obese (Huestis, 2005). Such a delay tends to prolong and intensify the activity of subsequently smoked marijuana, forming a type of "reverse tolerance" to THC, where the persistent low levels are increased by subsequent uses. The delayed release also means that very low, clinically insignificant amounts of THC may be present in blood for a considerable time after drug use ceases.

Metabolism and Elimination

Because of its rapid and almost complete metabolism, only minor amounts of nonmetabolized THC are ultimately eliminated and can be identified in urine. The initial metabolite, 11-hydroxy-THC, is psychoactive in the same way as THC itself, only somewhat less potent, and is quickly broken down into the inactive metabolite carboxy-THC (11-nor-9-carboxy-THC).

Urine testing for THC use focuses on identification of carboxy-THC, which is only slowly excreted. The half-life of carboxy-THC in urine varies: people who use THC infrequently (less than twice per week) will generally test positive for 1–3 days after using the drug, whereas people who use it regularly (i.e., at least several times per week) can test positive for 7–21 days (daily use for prolonged periods of time can yield positive results for 30 days or longer after use stops). Thus, a positive urine test does not necessarily mean that a person was under the influence of THC at the time the urine specimen was collected—that is, there is little or no correlation between the presence of carboxy-THC in urine and the presence of a pharmacologically significant amount of THC in the blood. This can become quite important in certain legal situations, such as when a person is charged with driving while under the influence of marijuana (see the discussion of driving under the influence in the section on psychomotor effects of THC later in this chapter).[5] Exposure to secondhand smoke will usually not result in a positive result for carboxy-THC in urine.

PHARMACOKINETICS OF CBD

CBD, the most abundant nonpsychoactive ingredient in marijuana, attracted a surge of interest when a high-CBD, low-THC strain of marijuana appeared to help reduce convulsions in a case of epilepsy (see the discussion in the section on therapeutic applications later in this chapter). The pharmacokinetic effects of CBD have not been well elucidated, but a technique developed for the detection of CBD in urine revealed that CBD could be detected for 24 hours after dosing (Wertlake and Henson, 2016)

[5]Use of a product high in CBD and low in THC (i.e., less than 0.3% THC) does not ensure that urine will test negative for carboxy-THC (Dahlgren et al., 2021).

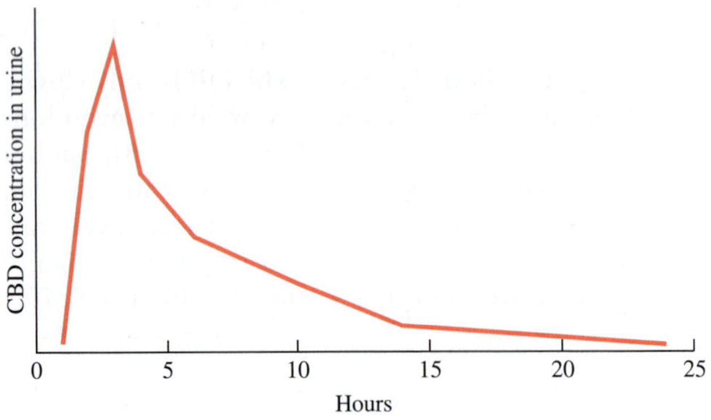

FIGURE 9.4 CBD Concentration in Urine over Time. In a 24-hour time study of a single individual following a single dose of CBD oil capsules, the peak urinary level occurred after about 3 hours, and urine continued to test positive after 24 hours. [Data from Wertlake and Henson, 2016.]

(see Figure 9.4). However, forensic testing currently does not routinely look for CBD in urine because CBD is not psychoactive.

It is known that following oral intake, CBD undergoes first-pass metabolism, leading to a number of metabolites, most notably 7-hydroxy-CBD; the half-life appears to be 8–33 hours following intravenous administration (not routinely done), 27–35 hours following smoking, and 2–5 days following oral administration (Zhornitsky and Potvin, 2012). In addition, CBD is known to be a potent inhibitor of multiple cytochrome enzymes, and this inhibitory action may result in elevated blood concentrations of other drugs (Geffrey et al., 2015).

PHARMACOLOGICAL EFFECTS OF THC

Our understanding of cannabis pharmacology has become more complicated as a result of three main factors: the realization of the opposing actions of CBD and THC, the variability of the CBD-to-THC ratio among diverse cannabis plant products, and the cultivation and development of high-THC cannabis products with greatly increased potency. In addition, there is growing concern about understanding how cannabis interacts with standard medications (Melton, 2017). The following sections summarize the major pharmacological effects of THC (but also see the discussions of cannabis pharmacology in the sections below on therapeutic applications of cannabinoids).

Physiological Effects

As we will see in this section, THC has significant effects on a variety of important physiological systems and functions.

Cardiovascular Effects

Perhaps the most well-known cardiovascular effects of smoking marijuana are bloodshot eyes (due to dilation of the corneal blood vessels) and pupillary dilation. Smoking marijuana also elicits an initial dose-dependent increase in heart rate. Blood pressure changes are generally slight and variable.

Effects on Respiration

Marijuana smoking involves repetitive, deep inhalation of unfiltered material, which is usually smoked as completely as possible in order not to waste any of the drug. So it is no surprise that smoking a single marijuana cigarette may be more harmful than smoking a single tobacco cigarette, both in causing changes in lung tissues and in causing bronchial irritation and inflammation (Turcotte et al., 2016). After controlling for tobacco use, however, there is no definitive evidence that marijuana smokers are at increased risk for lung cancer.[6]

Of more concern in recent years has been the dangers of vaping marijuana. Beginning in mid-2019, multiple cases of vaping-associated lung injuries and death were being reported (Bonner et al., 2021; Friedman, 2021). By the end of 2019, more than 2700 such cases had been reported in young persons, including more than 60 deaths. At first, the etiology of these cases was unclear, but by mid-2020 it had been determined that more than 85% involved vaping of marijuana products rather than nicotine, that more than 65% of the people involved were male, and that their median age was 27 years (Heinzerling et al., 2020). In more than 75% of the cases, the marijuana product was reportedly received from informal sources (e.g., friends, acquaintances, and unlicensed retailers), and in more than 85% of the cases, the product used was found to contain the oils of vitamin E or vitamin E acetate (Blount et al., 2020; Christiani, 2020). In most cases, the drug was contained in counterfeit street cartridges produced by using volatile oil cutting agents, with vitamin E acetate as the key agent (Cherian et al., 2021; Hartnett et al., 2020), although other agents could not be excluded (Muthumalage et al., 2020). Vaping of contaminated marijuana is considered to be dangerous to lungs and life.

Effects on Sleep

Several types of sleep disturbances have been linked to chronic cannabis use. In adults, chronic daily marijuana use is significantly associated with trouble falling asleep, trouble maintaining sleep, and feeling groggy the next day (Conroy et al., 2016). However, persons experiencing poor sleep quality due to chronic pain find that marijuana use improves sleep quality, likely due to reduced stress and anxiety, as well as to marijuana's analgesic effects (Cranford et al., 2017; Volkow et al., 2017). (See also the discussion of pain relief in the section on therapeutic applications later in this chapter.)

---

[6]This conclusion may be premature, however, because, in general, fewer marijuana cigarettes are smoked than tobacco cigarettes, and the cohort of people who habitually smoke marijuana cigarettes may only now be reaching the age when lung cancer typically appears.

Effects on the Immune System

Given that CB2 receptors are found primarily in the immune system, it should not be surprising that long-term marijuana use is associated with some degree of immunosuppression. Although cannabinoid-induced immunosuppression is not currently known to be involved in any diseases, the potential for such involvement is certainly there.

Effects on Appetite, Nausea, and the Gastrointestinal System

One of the classic effects attributed to marijuana use is appetite stimulation, especially for sweet and fattening foods. THC and other CB1 receptor agonists stimulate appetite in test animals, even when the animals are sated (Seely et al., 2011). A study of the relationship between marijuana use and body weight drew the following tentative conclusions (Sansone and Sansone, 2014):

- In wasting disorders, such as AIDS or cancer, cannabis may increase appetite and weight gain, but not more than the amount produced by other medications.
- Cannabis may actually regulate body weight, having no effect when weight is normal or excessive, but increasing it in those who are underweight.
- Alternatively, the effect of the drug on body weight may be associated with long-term versus short-term use, the presence of other drugs, or the competition between cannabis and food for brain sites that mediate reward.

Use of cannabinoids to treat gastrointestinal conditions is discussed in the section on therapeutic applications later in this chapter.

Effects on the Reproductive System and Pregnancy

Chronic use of marijuana by males can reduce levels of the hormone testosterone and reduce sperm count and viability (DuPlessis et al., 2015). However, there is no reported evidence of male infertility or reduced sexual potency or of pregnancy complications in the female as a result of male marijuana use. Still, the risk to a pregnant female and her fetus of being exposed to environmental smoke is ever present.

In females, the levels of follicle-stimulating hormone and luteinizing hormone are reduced by the use of marijuana. Menstrual cycles can be affected, including the occurrence of cycles without ovulation. All these actions reverse when drug use is discontinued.

Marijuana is currently the most widely used illicit drug during pregnancy, and its use is increasing, from about 3.4% in 2002 to 7% or more in 2020 during the COVID-19 pandemic (Young-Wolff et al., 2021). Much use is for the relief of stress and anxiety, made worse by the pandemic (Meinhofer et al., 2022). Other uses include the inappropriate treatment of pregnancy-induced nausea and vomiting, a use that should be avoided (Volkow et al., 2016). A recent survey found that 9.8% of women who had recently given birth reported using marijuana before pregnancy, 4.2% during pregnancy, and 5.5% after pregnancy (Ko et al., 2020).

THC freely crosses the placenta and achieves the same blood concentration in the fetus as it does in the mother. THC is also found in breast milk and is readily passed to a breast-feeding infant. A developing brain exposed to the effects of cannabis both during gestation and afterward would be expected to exhibit some neurodevelopmental consequences. In addition, some researchers conclude that cannabis increases the likelihood of preterm birth and small size for gestational age (Nguyen and Harley, 2022); others, however, report only a small, clinically unimportant drop in birth weight and no effect on preterm births or neurodevelopmental outcomes for at least the first three years (Zhang et al., 2017). Although cannabis use does not appear to increase the incidence of birth defects, one report concluded that newborns of women who smoked marijuana when pregnant may display mild, transient withdrawal signs, such as hyperactivity, reduced cognitive functioning, and changes in the functioning of the dopamine system (Metz and Stickrath, 2015). Another report, however, contained a more negative assessment:

> Recent reviews found an association between marijuana use and adverse perinatal outcomes, especially with heavy marijuana use. . . . [L]ongitudinal cohort studies demonstrate a possible effect of prenatal marijuana exposure on long-term neurobehavioral outcomes. Marijuana use may be associated with growth restriction, stillbirth, spontaneous preterm birth and neonatal [ICU] admission. (Metz and Borgelt, 2018)

A recent study reported that prenatal cannabis exposure was associated with greater risk for psychopathology during middle childhood (Paul et al., 2021), and another recent study noted that "there are remarkably consistent effects of prenatal cannabis exposure on externalizing behaviors, such as delinquency and substance use, which persist into adulthood" (DeGenna et al., 2022). In contrast, an earlier study reported that prenatal cannabis exposure was *not* associated with clinically significant negative cognitive effects in persons aged 0 to 22 years (Torres et al., 2020).

Psychological and Psychomotor Effects

The psychological effects of THC vary with the dose, the route of administration, how experienced the person is with using the drug, the person's vulnerability to psychoactive effects, and the setting in which the drug is administered.

Psychomotor effects of THC can include impairments in perception, attention, coordination, and reaction time that may persist for several hours beyond the person's perception of the "high," depending on the dose and the blood concentration. These effects have obvious implications for driving a motor vehicle (discussed in more detail below), as well as for performance in the workplace or at school. (In this context, it is worth noting that, unlike THC, CBD does not seem to impair driving performance [Arkell et al., 2020].)

Subjective Effects

The subjective effects of THC reported by people who smoke marijuana include an increased sense of well-being, mild euphoria, relaxation, and relief from anxiety, as well as sensory intensification and alterations in the perception of time. Events may seem especially funny, and laughter is easily elicited. Mundane ideas can seem profound, and an inflated sense of creativity may be experienced due to the loosening of associations and to thought intrusions. Infrequently, the person might experience illusions and hallucinations, perhaps following high doses or when blood concentrations peak.

The rewarding effects of THC are likely due to indirect activation of the dopamine reward system in the brain (Volkow et al., 2017). In people who formerly used marijuana but have been abstaining, cues related to marijuana use also activate reward circuitry (Filbey and Dewitt, 2012). Dopamine release is increased by short-term THC use, while chronic use may reduce such release—research into the detailed effects of long-term use has not yet produced clear results (Bloomfield et al., 2016). Although it seems clear that dopamine release is responsible for many of the positive subjective effects of THC, the relationship between the brain's cannabinoid and dopamine systems is complicated, and studies of that relationship in humans and animals have produced conflicting results.

Effects on Driving

Driving under the influence of marijuana doubles or triples the risk of a crash (Li et al., 2020). Drivers tend to compensate by driving slower, but when the task intensity of driving increases, drivers become more impaired: lane weaving increases, performance of critical tracking tasks declines, reaction time increases, and attention becomes divided between driving and other focuses. People who use marijuana regularly do poorly at evaluating their own impairment (but impairment is usually resolved within 4.5 hours after usage stops) (Marcotte et al., 2022). Police who suspect drivers of being under the influence of marijuana often subject them to standardized field sobriety testing to ascertain their blood THC concentrations. In general, concentration levels of 2–5 nanograms per milliliter are associated with moderate impairments in driving performance (Brubacher et al., 2022), with much greater impairments seen at levels of 5–10 nanograms per milliliter (Doroudgar et al., 2018). State laws vary with respect to allowable THC levels while driving, with some states permitting levels below 5 nanograms per milliliter. The risk of driving under the influence of THC is greatly increased when the driver is also under the influence of alcohol, but guidelines for such concomitant use have not been legislated.

Cognitive Effects

THC produces a range of acute effects on several neurocognitive systems, including executive control, emotional reward, and memory processing. These effects occur via THC's direct actions on cannabinoid receptors and indirect actions on the body's glutamine, GABA, and dopamine systems (Bloomfield et al., 2019). Heavy cannabis use, especially during adolescence, has particularly disadvantageous adverse effects, including anxiety, paranoia, impaired psychomotor performance, and cognitive dysfunction. However, adverse effects on cognitive functioning may lessen during abstinence (Scott et al., 2018).

Perhaps the best-known adverse cognitive effect of marijuana use is memory impairment (Bloomfield et al., 2019; Borgan et al., 2019). THC impairs all three stages of memory processing: encoding, consolidation, and retrieval. These effects appear to be mediated by CB1 receptors in the hippocampus, as indicated by the results of a large study of nearly a thousand participants who used marijuana, which found that marijuana use was associated with abnormally low blood flow in virtually every area of the brain, but especially in the hippocampus (Amen et al., 2017).

Other adverse cognitive effects of THC include disruption of the ability to focus attention and filter out irrelevant information, fragmentation of speech and presumably the underlying thought patterns because of the distracting intrusions of other ideas, and difficulty remembering what has been recently said. This difficulty in concentration impairs performance on many cognitive tasks. Furthermore, THC may also reduce the motivation to perform well.

Cognitive deficits may persist for a month or more following discontinuation of heavy use, but it is generally believed that only minimal effects are likely to persist over the longer term. One study, however, found that heavy cannabis users with a certain form of the CB1 gene have smaller hippocampi and amygdalae than control subjects (Schacht et al., 2012). Given the importance of these two structures for cognition, such long-term changes are troubling, especially considering that the mean age of the men and women in the study was between 27 and 28. Also troubling are the results of a longitudinal study that found that participants who were persistently diagnosed with cannabis abuse when they were teenagers had significant decreases in IQ over the years between age 7 and age 38, whereas participants who were non-cannabis abusers tended to have some increase in IQ over those years.

THERAPEUTIC APPLICATIONS OF CANNABINOIDS

The therapeutic uses of cannabinoids, including THC and CBD, as well as synthetic cannabinoids, are many and varied, with such use constituting one of the greatest stimulants to cannabinoid use overall (Hurd, 2020). People who use cannabis therapeutically on their own, generally without medical supervision, most frequently report using it for back pain, sleeping disorders, stress, depression, pain resulting from injury or accidents, and multiple sclerosis (Lake et al., 2019). More broadly, recognition of the inability of current prescription medications to effectively treat these and other conditions has prompted research into the question of whether use of cannabis products can increase the effectiveness of those medications. (See the section on legal issues earlier in this chapter for discussion of the differences between federal and state views on the therapeutic potential of THC, which remains illegal at the federal level.)

When discussing therapeutic uses of cannabinoids, the effects of THC (a cannabinoid receptor agonist) must be distinguished from those of CBD (a cannabinoid receptor antagonist), either alone or in combination, with varying routes of administration and at varying concentrations in different products. Use of CBD alone (without THC) has been suggested for treatment of a wide range of conditions, including anxiety disorders, depression, schizophrenia, psychosis, cancer pain, autism, insomnia, epilepsy, cannabis use disorder, Crohn's disease, Parkinsonism, and more, including other substance abuse disorders (Navarrete et al., 2021). Thus, according to one researcher, "the major question now being asked is whether CBD is hype or if there is true medical potential" (Hurd, 2020).

Daily cannabis use is associated with significantly lower daily use of illicit opioids (Lake et al., 2020) and with lower rates of addiction and overdose than occur with opioids (Fitzcharles et al., 2019). Note, however, that use of cannabis to treat opioid dependence has not been medically substantiated and that cannabis is not an approved drug for this disorder (Shover et al., 2020).

Many people are able to decrease their use of prescription medications for pain, anxiety, migraine headaches, and insomnia after starting medical cannabis use (Piper et al., 2017). This is extremely important both because of the current opioid crisis (discussed in Chapter 10) and because of the overuse of addictive benzodiazepine anxiolytics (discussed in Chapter 13).

A large-scale review of research on the therapeutic uses of cannabis products rated treatments for a variety of medical disorders as beneficial, probably beneficial, harmful, probably harmful, no effect, or unclear (Montero-Oleas et al., 2020). The disorders studied included multiple sclerosis, movement disorders, psychiatric disorders, Alzheimer's disease, epilepsy, acute and chronic pain, neuropathic pain, symptoms associated with cancer and chemotherapy, rheumatic disorders, HIV-related symptoms, glaucoma, and COPD (chronic obstructive pulmonary disease). Overall, treatment with cannabis products was considered most beneficial for multiple sclerosis, pain, and cancer-related symptoms. A more recent study of primary care patients using medical cannabis found that 44% had conditions for which cannabis might confer benefits and 54% had conditions for which cannabis might confer risks, suggesting that primary care physicians should be prepared to discuss the potential risks and benefits of cannabis use with patients (Matson et al., 2021). Studies like these, which attempt to bring science to bear on the discussion of whether and how to use cannabis products as medical treatments, should help both clinicians and the people contemplating such use. Of course, the decision will also depend on the person's willingness to experience the psychoactive effects of cannabis and on any former experiences with the drug.

Cannabinoids for Nonpsychiatric Disorders

As we will see in this section, research suggests that cannabinoids could be beneficial in treating a wide range of nonpsychiatric disorders.

Pain and Spasticity

Studies of the pain-relieving effects of cannabinoids have yielded a range of results, some similar and some conflicting. For example:

- Both THC and CBD were found to have analgesic effects in both humans and animals, especially against pain resulting from persistent inflammation and neuropathic pain, an effect that distinguishes these cannabinoids from opioids such as morphine (Boychuk et al., 2015).
- One study found that patients using medical marijuana to control chronic pain reported a 64% reduction in their use of opioid prescription pain medication (Boehnke et al., 2016), whereas other studies have concluded that smoking marijuana is *not* efficacious for managing chronic noncancer pain (Johal et al., 2020; Wong et al., 2020).

- A recent study noted sex differences in the results of using THC to treat chronic pain (Blanton et al., 2021).
- An analysis of results from 2800 patients with cancer-related pain concluded that adding cannabinoid therapy to opioids did not reduce cancer pain and had undesirable side effects (primarily sedation and dizziness) (Boland et al., 2020); in contrast, another study concluded that cannabinoids are effective in treating pain in patients with advanced cancer who were already taking maximum doses of opioids (Meng et al., 2020).
- Compelling evidence exists that CBD can reduce sensations of painful burning, pins and needles, numbness, neuropathic pain, and other painful conditions (Jensen et al., 2015). (See Fine and Rosenfeld, 2013, for a review of the analgesic effects of cannabinoids, focusing on CBD.)

Smoking marijuana may specifically reduce spasticity-related pain in people diagnosed with multiple sclerosis (MS). The oral medication nabiximols (Sativex), which contains THC and CBD in a 1:1 mixture and is delivered in a mouth spray, has been approved in Canada, New Zealand, and eight European countries for the relief of muscle spasms and poor sleep quality associated with MS, as well as for pain associated with end-stage cancer. A review of the efficacy of nabiximols found that 60% of patients reported some pain relief, 26% discontinued the drug for lack of effectiveness, and 18% discontinued the drug due to side effects (Patti et al., 2016). These results suggest that any analgesic effect of the drug may be due to muscle relaxation from its antispastic action rather than a direct analgesic action.

Epilepsy

The use of medical marijuana as a treatment for epilepsy has been reported numerous times in the popular press. Many of these reports are anecdotal accounts of children with refractory epilepsies, such as Dravet syndrome and Lennox-Gastaut syndrome. Interest in the use of medical marijuana to treat these conditions surged after 2013, with widespread reporting of the case of Charlotte Figi (2006–2020), who had Dravet syndrome and experienced remarkable improvement (a massive reduction in seizures) after her mother started treating her with a laboratory-tested oil (given under the tongue in a measured amount) derived from an unusual strain of cannabis now known as **Charlotte's Web**. This strain of medical marijuana has very little THC, with a CBD-to-THC ratio of 30:1 or greater (Kolikonda et al., 2016).

In 2016, GW Pharmaceuticals announced positive results of the first randomized, double-blind trial of its investigational medicine Epidiolex (CBD in a liquid solution, taken by mouth) for the treatment of Lennox-Gastaut syndrome. In this trial, Epidiolex, when added to patients' current treatment, significantly reduced the monthly frequency of drop seizures over the entire 14-week treatment period, compared with placebo. In 2018, Epidiolex was approved for medical use in the United States for treatment of Lennox-Gastaut and Dravet syndromes. Currently, Epidiolex is classified as a Schedule V controlled drug, meaning that it has a low potential for abuse. However, use of Epidiolex is complicated by the expense of the product.

Finally, it is important to note that synthetic cannabinoids may eventually be developed to treat epilepsy (Smolyakova et al., 2020).

Neuroprotection

Research suggests that CBD combined with THC can have neuroprotective effects following brain injury or damage associated with various neurodegenerative disorders (Fernandez-Ruiz et al., 2012; Li et al., 2022).

Interestingly, CB1 receptors are widely distributed in all layers of the retina of the eyes, where they are thought to be involved in visual processing and neuroplasticity, and where they may also function as part of a neuroprotective mechanism to prevent or delay neuronal death and maintain cellular integrity in vision loss due to glaucoma or retinal neurodegenerative disease (Rapino et al., 2018). How cannabis products affect these receptors and protect retinal functioning is under study (Schwitzer et al., 2016; Zantut et al., 2020).

Cancers

Studies of the efficacy of THC and CBD in treating the severe pain associated with advanced cancers have produced conflicting evidence (Glogauer and Blay, 2022). Marijuana has been used to treat side effects of cancer chemotherapy (nausea and vomiting, anorexia, and pain), and this has prompted studies of possible antitumor effects of cannabis and in particular CBD, which may have potential beneficial effects on many types of cancer, including glioblastoma and cancers of the breast, lung, prostate, and colon (Huang et al., 2015; McAllister et al., 2015). (For an extensive review of the potential role of cannabinoids in treating cancers, emphasizing actions that are not mediated by CB receptors, see Soderstrom et al., 2017.)

In September 2021, the state of Texas expanded its medical marijuana program to include the treatment of all forms of cancer (previously, only terminal cancer was an approved condition), as well as posttraumatic stress disorder (PTSD). Unfortunately, the state mandates that the medical marijuana products dispensed can have a maximum THC concentration of 1%, which means that the products are unlikely to be of much benefit. Furthermore, only edible products are allowed, not products that can be smoked.

Gastrointestinal Conditions

Cannabinoids have been used for appetite stimulation to clinical advantage in treating a variety of conditions. The synthetic cannabinoid nabilone has been FDA approved to treat nausea and vomiting associated with cancer chemotherapy, and dronabinol has been approved as an antiemetic for similar situations. In 1992, approval was extended for dronabinol to be used to stimulate appetite in wasting conditions, such as AIDS; then, in August 2017, an easy-to-swallow dronabinol solution (Syndros) was approved for oral use, allowing better control of the dosage.

Anecdotal evidence suggests that cannabinoids may affect gastric emptying and colonic motility, and strong evidence exists of an intestinal anti-inflammatory effect (Izzo et al., 2015). This may mean that CBD has the potential to treat gastrointestinal tract disorders such as irritable bowel syndrome and inflammatory bowel disease, in addition to its possible role in inhibiting colon cancers (Romano et al., 2014).

Glaucoma

In the section on neuroprotection, we discussed the possible neuroprotective role of CB1 receptors in mitigating vision loss in glaucoma and other eye conditions. In 2014, however, the American Academy of Ophthalmology reiterated that it does not recommend the use of medical marijuana or other cannabis products to treat glaucoma, particularly when standard therapies are available and effective. This statement was based on an analysis by the National Eye Institute and the Institute of Medicine indicating that reductions in intraocular pressure following medical marijuana use were short-lived. Nevertheless, the controversy continues, as later research disputes this interpretation (Turner and Agrawal, 2020).

Cannabinoids for Psychiatric Disorders

Research indicates that cannabinoids could be of benefit in the treatment of at least three types of psychiatric disorders: Alzheimer's disease, anxiety disorders (particularly PTSD), and psychoses, including schizophrenia.

Alzheimer's Disease

There is conflicting evidence regarding the use of cannabinoids to treat symptoms of Alzheimer's disease. One study found that, in patients already diagnosed with Alzheimer's disease, up to 4.5 milligrams daily of oral THC was well tolerated but did not reduce symptoms such as aggression and agitation (Van den Elsen et al., 2015); in contrast, later studies found that cannabinoids had beneficial effects on certain symptoms, especially night-time agitation, disturbed eating behavior, and aggression (Ruthirakuhan et al., 2019; Talarico et al., 2019).

Other research suggests that CBD and other cannabinoids may facilitate the elimination of amyloid beta from brain cells and thus reduce the neuroinflammation induced by amyloid beta, which means that cannabinoids may hold promise for reducing the neuronal loss seen in Alzheimer's disease (Abate et al., 2021).

Anxiety Disorders

PTSD is difficult to treat because most patients do not respond to current medications. In addition, many people with PTSD also have a substance use disorder, which significantly complicates treatment. Recent data suggest that cannabis may help patients cope with PTSD and may reduce their use of opioids and other risky drugs (J. Cohen et al., 2020). Moreover, according to the authors of another study:

> Present data show that cannabis and synthetic cannabinoids, both acting on the endocannabinoids system, may have a potential therapeutic use for improving PTSD symptoms, e.g., reducing anxiety, modulating memory-related processes, and improving sleep. (Orsolini et al., 2019)

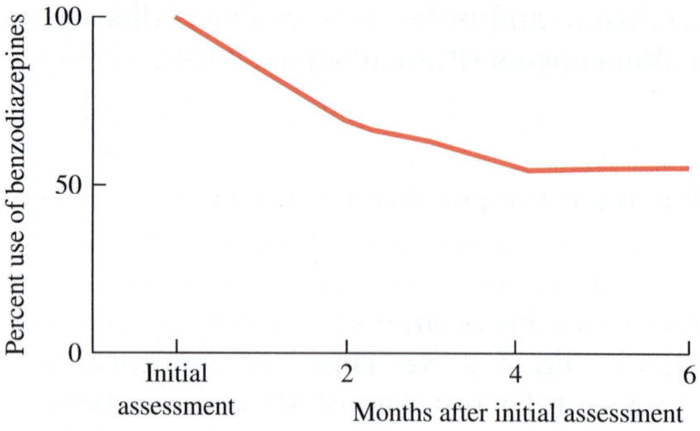

FIGURE 9.5 Benzodiazepines Use Declines with Cannabis Use. At their initial assessment, all the patients in this study (100%) were using benzodiazepines to treat their psychiatric disorder. They all then began using medical cannabis as well. After two months, only about 70% of the patients were still using their benzodiazepines (i.e., 30% had stopped benzodiazepines and were just using cannabis), and after six months, only about 55% were still using benzodiazepines (i.e., 45% had stopped). [Data from Purcell et al., 2019.]

Some states already allow the use of medical marijuana to treat PTSD. At the federal level, in 2016 the U.S. Drug Enforcement Administration approved the first U.S. clinical trial using marijuana to treat PTSD, with the aim of developing the *Cannabis* plant into a prescription medicine. Sponsored by the nonprofit Multidisciplinary Association for Psychedelic Studies, the trial, currently in Phase 2, will study the effects of smoking marijuana on 360 patients (all war veterans) with chronic, treatment-resistant PTSD.

Early evidence strongly supports CBD as a treatment for a variety of sleep and anxiety disorders (Shannon et al., 2019), including generalized anxiety disorder (Sarris et al., 2013), panic disorder (Soares and Campos, 2017), and social anxiety disorders (Blessing et al., 2015). Given that benzodiazepines are a mainstay in the current treatment of anxiety disorders and that long-term benzodiazepine use is known to have adverse consequences (as discussed in Chapter 13), studies comparing long-term dosing with CBD versus benzodiazepines could be useful. One such study in Canada of 146 patients using benzodiazepines who had then been prescribed medical marijuana found that 30% had voluntarily stopped using benzodiazepines after two months and that 45% had stopped after six months (see Figure 9.5), a number that then remained stable over several more months (Purcell et al., 2019). Not all the patients in this study had an anxiety disorder, but the results do suggest that cannabis might help patients with anxiety disorders reduce their use of benzodiazepines.

Despite these results, other researchers emphasize the limitations of clinical research to date and remain wary about using cannabinoids to treat mood and anxiety disorders (Botsford et al., 2020). The authors of a review of eight studies of the use of cannabinoids for anxiety disorders, including PTSD, reached the following conclusion:

> Medical cannabis should not be recommended for treating patients with these disorders [affective disorders, anxiety disorders, or PTSD]. Further research should investigate the safety and efficacy of managing psychiatric disorders with cannabinoids. (Stanciu et al., 2021)

Schizophrenia and Other Psychotic Conditions

Of all the areas of potential therapeutic uses of cannabinoids, nowhere is the distinction between THC and CBD more important than in the treatment of schizophrenia and other psychoses.

THC and Psychosis. There is extensive evidence that smoking marijuana is a risk factor for precipitation of psychotic episodes in susceptible persons, with young people being at greatest risk. As early as 1958, a study described psychotic-like behavior in healthy volunteers after a single instance of smoking marijuana (Ames, 1958; Bartolucci et al., 1969). In 1987, a comprehensive review covering more than 45,000 Swedish military conscripts found that those who had used cannabis more than 50 times by the age of 18 years were 6 times more likely to have schizophrenia than nonusers. In 2002, this result was replicated in a study showing that the risk of schizophrenia had increased to 6.7 times in heavy users of cannabis.

These and many other longitudinal studies indicate a relationship between chronic, high-dose cannabis use and psychotic behaviors (Bidwell et al., 2020; Hines et al., 2020). One study found that subclinical psychotic symptoms related to weekly cannabis use persist in adolescents for as long as one year after stopping the drug (Bechtold et al., 2016). A factor in such effects of long-term use is the increased potency of cannabis (DiForti et al., 2015). During the last 20 to 30 years, the THC content in all parts of the *Cannabis* plant has increased, with some reports finding 25% THC or more, compared to "classic" levels of 3%. Many cannabis users do not modify their smoking behavior if the potency increases (e.g., by smoking less or changing the way they inhale). Some users with more experience may alter their intake, depending on how strong they think the material is, but they are not capable of making accurate adjustments when potency varies or of overcoming the negative emotional effects of the drug (Stuyt, 2018). Also, research indicates that long-term use of cannabis is associated with long-term neurocognitive disorders; however, stopping cannabis use can lead to recovery of neurocognitive functioning to the level seen in people who have never used cannabis (Setien-Suero et al., 2019).

It is now clear that use of THC-containing cannabis products is associated with increased risk of psychosis, including schizophrenia (Hindley et al., 2020). Probably, the higher the concentration of THC in the product being used (and thus the higher the blood levels of THC likely being reached), the greater the risk of psychotic reactions. Other research discusses the possibility of genetic contributions to this association (Gillespie and Kendler, 2021) and the possibility that the increasing use of more potent cannabis products is contributing to the rising incidence of major depressive disorder and the alarming increase in suicides over the past decade, which may reflect psychotic

DR. J'S MUSINGS 9.2

CBD for Pain Relief and Timely Sedation

As I age, I suffer from some chronic medical problems, among them diabetes and peripheral neuropathies. I reviewed the literature on using cannabinoids to treat neuropathies and decided they were worth a try. I had never smoked either cigarettes or marijuana and so am not used to inhaling smoke. This left oral CBD as an option to supplement the ibuprofen and gabapentin I was already taking. I started on 25 milligrams twice daily, but I found the sedation undesirable. I am now successfully taking 50 milligrams (two gummy bears) at bedtime. So far, I consider this to be an optimal therapy that has allowed me to avoid use of opioids.

thinking (Han et al., 2021). However, the authors of the latter study were careful not to draw causal inferences from these reported associations.

CBD and Psychosis. In contrast to THC, CBD appears to exert beneficial effects as an adjunct to the treatment of schizophrenia. An early study reported that CBD reduced psychotic symptoms in patients with acute schizophrenia (Leweke et al., 2012). The next year, a study reported that CBD inhibited psychotic and paranoid symptoms produced by smoking THC-containing marijuana and even improved the memory impairment produced by marijuana (Englund et al., 2013). In contrast, a later review of four studies relevant to this effect found that only one of the studies had identified a CBD-induced reduction in adverse THC-induced symptoms (Hindley et al., 2020). These kinds of mixed results have led researchers to make conflicting statements such as the following:

- "Isolated positive studies have . . . revealed tentative support for cannabinoids (namely cannabidiol, CBD) for reducing social anxiety, with mixed (mainly positive) evidence for adjunctive use in schizophrenia" (Sarris et al., 2020).
- "There is a lack of evidence that cannabinoids improve depressive disorders and symptoms, anxiety disorders, . . . or psychosis" (Black et al., 2019).

A review of CBD trials for various disorders included coverage of four trials studying cognitive impairment and psychotic symptoms in patients with schizophrenia (Larsen and Shahinas, 2020). CBD was administered orally in capsules with doses ranging from 600 to 1000 milligrams per day (much higher than the usual daily doses of 50–100 milligrams). In one of the four studies reviewed, there was improvement in positive symptoms and in clinicians' impressions of cognitive function and overall level of functioning; however, the other studies reviewed showed no improvement. Another review came to a similar conclusion of no or limited efficacy (Ghabrash et al., 2020), in contrast to a study that found limited, but likely real, efficacy in the use of CBD as an adjunct to existing medications (Schoevers et al., 2020). Clearly, the controversy continues over the efficacy or lack thereof of THC and/or CBD in the treatment of mental illnesses (Sarris et al., 2020).

CANNABIS TOLERANCE, WITHDRAWAL, DEPENDENCE, AND ADDICTION

In this section, we first discuss the question of whether tolerance develops to cannabis (despite some controversy, we will see that tolerance does indeed develop). Then we describe the nature and varying severity of cannabis withdrawal symptoms, followed by a discussion of cannabis dependence and addiction and concluding with a description of treatments for cannabis use disorder.

Tolerance

People who use marijuana often report that they become more rather than less sensitive to its psychoactive effects with continued use—in other words, that they become sensitized (i.e., they get "high" more quickly) rather than tolerant. Laboratory studies, however, routinely find that tolerance to cannabis develops. This difference between anecdotal reports from the "real world" and experimental results is believed to be due to several factors. First, people smoking marijuana in the real world have to learn how to get enough of the smoke into the lungs to provide a THC dose sufficient to produce a "high"—that is, apparent sensitization with continued use may just be an effect of learning to take in more drug. Second, people also have to learn to recognize the subjective effects of the drug and to be aware of experiencing them. Third, because the drug accumulates in fat tissue, people who use the drug regularly will always have some residual amount of THC in their bodies, which increases the apparent effect of each new dose by producing a quicker "high." These factors explain any apparent sensitization to cannabis and leave little doubt that tolerance to cannabis does develop.

In what was probably the first study to correlate the development of tolerance with plasma concentrations of THC, results demonstrated that tolerance rapidly developed (over four days) to oral THC at a dose of 260 milligrams and that plasma concentrations remained steady as tolerance developed to THC's subjective effects (Gorelick et al., 2013). This shows that tolerance was not metabolic (i.e., that it was not due to increased breakdown of THC), but that it was the result of either cellular adaptation or behavioral conditioning.

Tolerance to the beneficial effects of cannabis (such as pain relief in cancer patients) can increase the amount of drug needed and thus the cost of the drug. To control this, some have recommended **cannabinoid cycling**, a process of periodically switching from high-THC, low-CBD strains of *Cannabis* to high-CBD, low-THC strains. What the cycling period should be is unclear but is probably a period of one to four weeks. It is important to note, however, that no formal medical research has been done on the effectiveness of cannabinoid cycling as a way of reducing tolerance.

Withdrawal

Symptoms of cannabis withdrawal commonly occur after the person stops heavy and long-term cannabis use (Bahji et al., 2020). These symptoms often include irritability, anxiety, marijuana craving, disrupted sleep with strange dreams, anger and aggression, depressed mood, restlessness, decreased appetite, and weight loss. Less common symptoms include chills, headache, physical tension, sweating, stomach pain, and general physical discomfort. Symptoms tend to begin within 48 hours after drug use stops and last at least two days, usually seven to ten days, and sometimes longer; and electroencephalographic changes associated with withdrawal persist for at least 28 days. The intensity of cannabis withdrawal symptoms has been compared to the intensity of symptoms of recovering from the flu or of nicotine withdrawal, but as with other drugs of abuse, the intensity of withdrawal symptoms depends on the severity of the dependence. That is, the greater the dependence, the more intense the withdrawal syndrome, and the more likely that relapse will occur (Allsop et al., 2015). As would be expected, reinstituting cannabis use relieves the discomfort of withdrawal symptoms.[7]

Dependence and Addiction: Cannabis Use Disorder

Cannabis dependence used to be thought of as a relatively benign and infrequent condition. In fact, however, cannabis dependence occurs in about one of every ten persons who start smoking the drug, yet it is an uncommon reason for admission to drug treatment programs. In 2015, about 4 million people in the United States met the diagnostic criteria for cannabis use disorder (CUD), but only 138,000 voluntarily sought treatment for it (National Institute on Drug Abuse, 2020b). A study of the demographics of people with CUD and the treatments they did or did not receive found that, overall, only 7.8% received cannabis-specific treatment; that Asian Americans, women, and college-educated adults tended to underutilize treatment; that the odds of developing CUD varied by racial or ethnic groups; and that young adults, men, and less-educated adults were at greater risk for developing CUD (Wu et al., 2017). These findings support the idea that medical personnel should monitor the treatment needs of people with CUD.

When people using cannabis were asked to rate the effects of their own use as positive, neutral, or negative, they gave overwhelmingly negative ratings of the effects that cannabis had on their social life (70%), their physical health (81%), their cognition (91%), their memory (91%), and their career (79%) (Elkashef et al., 2008).

According to one team of researchers, there are four general areas of concern related to cannabis dependence and addiction (MacDonald and Pappas, 2016):

- A predicted increase in the number of people driving under the influence of cannabis and of cannabis plus alcohol
- Evidence of profound negative effects related to cannabis addiction in a range of important spheres, including education, employment, income, interpersonal relationships, and overall life satisfaction; these effects being especially noticeable in people who began cannabis use in adolescence
- The cannabis–psychosis link, as well as the negative effect of cannabis use on other mental disorders
- Evidence that cannabis produces neuropsychological impairments found with other abused substances, including blunted dopamine function

[7]There is as yet no evidence of a withdrawal syndrome following abrupt discontinuation of CBD (Taylor et al., 2020).

Treatment of Cannabis Use Disorder

A study conducted a few years ago noted the adverse effects associated with heavy cannabis use and the lack of effective treatments for CUD, while also noting an increase in clinical trials of pharmacological agents as adjuncts to psychosocial treatments (Sherman and McRae-Clark, 2016). A later study again noted that no pharmacotherapies have been approved for the treatment of CUD and that therapies with antidepressants, anticonvulsants, and mood stabilizers were probably ineffective (Nielsen et al., 2019). One team of researchers offered this overall assessment: "[C]annabis use disorder is a clinical diagnosis with high prevalence . . . and . . . often has its genesis in adolescence and in vulnerable individuals associated with psychiatric comorbidity, genetic and environmental factors" (Ferland and Hurd, 2020).

One of the studies cited above classified potential pharmacotherapies as follows (Nielsen et al., 2019):

- Therapies that attenuate withdrawal symptoms
- Therapies that reduce the subjective reinforcing effects of THC
- Therapies that may help reduce the risk of relapse

The drugs evaluated in that study included antidepressants (e.g., bupropion), mood stabilizers (e.g., divalproex), and synthetic THC compounds (e.g., dronabinol and nabilone). Of these, dronabinol and nabilone were most effective, with dronabinol (at a dose of 10 milligrams taken five-times per day) reducing ratings of cannabis craving, anxiety, misery, chills, sleep disturbances, and weight loss associated with cannabis withdrawal. This might be termed *agonist substitution therapy*, similar to the use of varenicline to treat nicotine dependence and of methadone or buprenorphine to treat opioid dependence.

Important newer studies have noted that antipsychotic medications may be useful in treating CUD (Lees et al., 2021) and that the antipsychotic quetiapine specifically has been found to reduce heavy use of marijuana but not light use (Mariani et al., 2021). Also, a report on eight patients receiving motivational enhancement therapy plus ketamine infusions during a six-week study noted that "combining ketamine with behavioral therapy is feasible, tolerable, and potentially helpful in treating cannabis-dependent individuals" (Azhari et al., 2021).

Another study found that the fatty acid amide hydrolase inhibitor PF-04457845, which inhibits the enzyme that degrades anandamide, reduced withdrawal symptoms and cannabis use in 46 men with CUD, with no serious adverse events during the study (D'Souza et al., 2019). The results of studies of other compounds being evaluated for use in treating CUD, including nicotine patches (Gilbert et al., 2020), will be interesting and important because of the great need for effective therapies.

CBD has also been proposed as a potential treatment for CUD (Chye et al., 2019), and the efficacy of CBD in this use has been demonstrated in a Phase 2a study in which CBD at doses of 400 or 800 milligrams appeared effective and was well tolerated with no severe adverse events and in which 94% of the participants completed the CBD treatment (Freeman et al., 2020). There is no evidence that CBD induces psychotic symptoms or that it exacerbates other undesired effects of THC. Finally, a recent report indicates that N-acetyl cysteine might be useful in the treatment of CUD (Sharma et al., 2022).

N-acetyl cysteine is FDA approved for the treatment of acetaminophen (Tylenol) poisoning; other uses are more poorly documented.

Clearly, more study is needed in this important area of investigation.

CHAPTER REVIEW

1. What is the process by which the cannabinoids tetrahydrocannabinolic acid and cannabidiolic acid are converted into THC and CBD?
2. How do THC and CBD differ in their action at cannabinoid receptors?
3. True or false: Both THC and CBD have psychedelic effects.
4. Discuss the social challenges related to the cultivation of increasingly potent strains of *Cannabis*.
5. Summarize the current situation regarding cannabis legalization in the United States, at both federal and state levels.
6. Discuss some of the current concerns related to vaping of cannabis products by youth.
7. Summarize the risks associated with the use of synthetic cannabinoids.
8. True or false: CB1 receptors are most highly concentrated in the CNS, whereas CB2 receptors are mostly found outside the CNS.
9. True or false: Anandamide is structurally dissimilar to both THC and CBD.
10. Describe dabbing and vaping as methods for rapidly absorbing THC.
11. True or false: There is significant correlation between the presence of carboxy-THC in urine and the presence of a pharmacologically significant amount of THC in the blood.
12. Why is vaping of cannabis products associated with a high risk of lung injuries?
13. True or false: THC freely crosses the placenta and achieves the same blood concentration in the fetus as it does in the mother.
14. Describe the dopamine-related subjective effects of THC.
15. What are the adverse effects of cannabis use on driving performance?
16. Describe the cognitive effects of THC.
17. What conditions do people most frequently attempt to treat with cannabinoids?
18. Discuss the results of research studying the use of cannabinoids for pain relief.
19. Why is a particular strain of cannabis known as "Charlotte's Web"?
20. Name two synthetic cannabinoids that have been used as treatments for gastrointestinal disorders and proposed as treatments for cannabis use disorder.
21. How might cannabinoids help in the treatment of Alzheimer's disease?
22. True or false: Use of THC may cause or exacerbate psychotic symptoms, whereas use of CBD may ameliorate such symptoms.

23. What is cannabinoid cycling?
24. Discuss the prevalence and seriousness of cannabis use disorder and the research aimed at finding effective treatments.

KEY TERMS

anandamide
cannabidiol (CBD)
cannabinoid cycling
cannabinoid receptors
cannabinoids
cannabis
cannabis use disorder
carboxy-THC
Charlotte's Web
dabbing
marijuana
spice
tetrahydrocannabinol (THC)

CHAPTER 10

Opioids

CHAPTER OUTLINE

An **opioid** is any drug that binds to and activates the functioning of any of the various types of **opioid receptors**, producing analgesia and other pharmacological effects.[1] The natural neurotransmitters at opioid receptors are the opioid peptides (discussed in Chapter 2 and later in this chapter).

Opioid drugs can be categorized in different ways: by their agonistic action (full or partial), by their origin (natural, semisynthetic, or synthetic), and by the opioid receptors at which they act (mu, kappa, or delta). Table 10.1 shows how the opioid medications discussed in this chapter are so classified (the table also shows how three medically important opioid antagonists are classified). The source of the natural opioids is the **opium poppy (*Papaver somniferum*)** (see Figure 10.1). Over 82% of opium poppies are grown in Afghanistan.[2] In addition to the two natural opioids listed in Table 10.1—morphine and codeine—the natural opioids papaverine and thebaine can also be isolated from the poppy plant. These four natural opioids have been chemically modified to produce both semisynthetic opioids (such as heroin) and totally synthetic opioids (such as fentanyl).

The agonistic and antagonistic actions of opioids and opioid antagonists can be described as follows (each of the "prototypical" drugs mentioned in this list is discussed in its own section in this chapter; see Chapter 3 for general discussion of the concepts of agonism and antagonism):

- *Full agonists.* Full opioid agonists activate their opioid receptors to the same extent as the natural neurotransmitters at those receptors. Morphine is a prototypical full opioid agonist, but there are many others.
- *Partial agonists.* Partial opioid agonists activate their receptors to a lesser extent than full agonists. That is, they have lower efficacy than full agonists, with an analgesic **ceiling effect** less than that of morphine (a ceiling effect is the maximum effect of a drug regardless of dosage). Buprenorphine is a prototypical partial opioid agonist.
- *Mixed agonist–antagonists.* Mixed opioid agonist–antagonists have an agonistic effect at one opioid receptor and an antagonistic effect at another. Like partial agonists, mixed agonist–antagonists usually display a ceiling effect for analgesia, with less efficacy than morphine. Pentazocine (Talwin) is a prototypical mixed agonist–antagonist. Today, mixed agonist–antagonist opioids are infrequently used clinically.
- *Antagonists.* Opioid antagonists have affinity for opioid receptors but do not activate their receptors; that is, after binding to an opioid receptor, they elicit no change in cellular functioning. However, by competing with agonists for the receptors, they can precipitate withdrawal in opioid-dependent people. Naloxone is a prototypical opioid antagonist.

---

[1]Opioid drugs may sometimes be referred to as *narcotics* (from the Greek word *narke,* meaning "numbness," "sleep," or "stupor"). Originally used to refer to any drug that induced sleep, the term *narcotic* later began to be used to refer to opioids such as morphine and pheroin and, in legal contexts, to non-opioids such as cocaine and marijuana. The term is not useful in a pharmacological context.

[2]A different variety of poppy, the "Norman poppy," is high in an opioid called thebaine, which is a precursor to oxycodone production and is legally grown in Tasmania.

TABLE 10.1 Opioid Medications

Medication	Origin	Opioid Receptor Action
Full Opioid Agonists		
Morphine	Natural	μ
Codeine	Natural	μ
Hydrocodone	Semisynthetic	μ
Oxycodone	Semisynthetic	μ
Hydromorphone	Semisynthetic	μ
Oxymorphone	Semisynthetic	μ
Propoxyphene	Synthetic	μ
Meperidine	Semisynthetic	μ
Fentanyl	Synthetic	μ
Methadone	Synthetic	μ
Oliceridine	Synthetic	μ
Levo-alpha acetylmethadol (LAAM)	Synthetic	μ agonist
Partial Opioid Agonists		
Tramadol	Semisynthetic	μ
Tapentadol	Synthetic	μ
Buprenorphine	Semisynthetic	μ
Cebranopadol	Synthetic	*
Mixed Opioid Agonist–Antagonists		
Pentazocine	Synthetic	κ agonist μ antagonist
Butorphanol	Synthetic	κ agonist μ antagonist
Nalbuphine	Semisynthetic	κ agonist μ antagonist
Targiniq-ER**	Semisynthetic	μ agonist/antagonist
Troxyca***	Semisynthetic	μ agonist/antagonist
Pure Opioid Antagonists		
Naloxone	Semisynthetic	μ
Naltrexone	Semisynthetic	μ
Nalmefene	Semisynthetic	μ

* Agonist at multiple opioid receptors including the nociceptin/orphanin peptide receptor (NOP), kappa opioid receptor, and mu, delta, and kappa receptors.
** Combination of oxycodone and naloxone.
*** Combination of oxycodone and low-dose naltrexone.

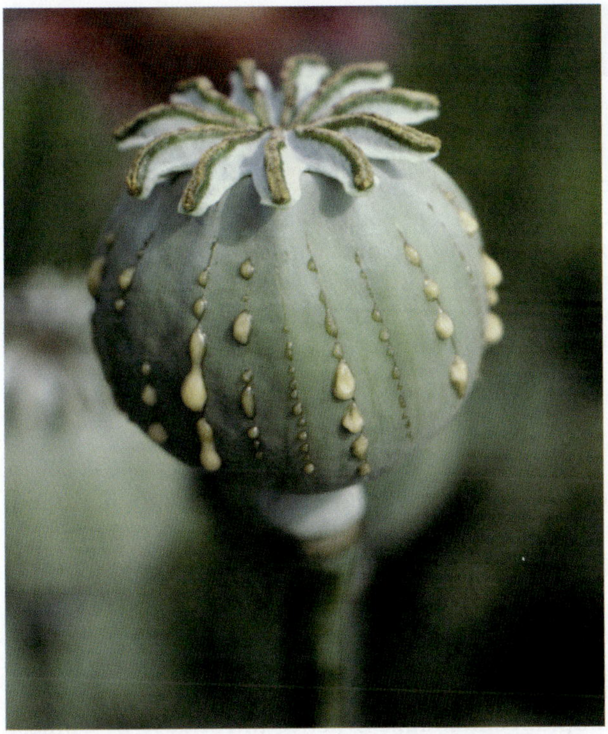

FIGURE 10.1 Opium Poppy. This immature seedpod of the opium poppy (*Papaver somniferum*) has been scored to release a milky resin, which is dried to produce opium. [Dr. Jeremy Burgess/ Science Source.]

HISTORY OF OPIOID USE

Opium, a resinous exudate from the seed pods of the opium poppy (see Figure 10.1), is an ancient drug that contains morphine and codeine as active opioids (the word *opium* is derived from the Greek *opion*, which means "poppy juice"). There is evidence that the opium poppy was cultivated 10,000 years ago, although the earliest definite evidence of its use as an analgesic dates to about 3500 to 3000 years ago. Besides its use as an analgesic, opium has also been used for thousands of years to produce euphoria, sleep, and relief from diarrhea and cough. In ancient times, opium was used primarily for its constipating effect, then for its sleep-inducing properties (noted by writers such as Homer, Hippocrates, Virgil, and Ovid). During the Middle Ages, opium was used to treat practically every known disease, and its beneficial effects earned it the name "stone of immortality." Often, it was combined with alcohol, a mixture that the sixteenth-century Swiss physician Paracelsus called *laudanum,* meaning "something to be praised." Although it was also used recreationally, not much is known about such use before the eighteenth century.

Morphine, isolated from opium in 1806 and its chemical formula determined in 1847, is considered the model opioid analgesic against which all others are compared.

DR. J'S MUSINGS 10.1

Paregoric

I vividly remember my father, a pharmacist, bringing home a bottle of **paregoric** (a tincture containing powdered opium) whenever I had childhood diarrhea. A dose of 1 teaspoonful by mouth corresponds to a dose of about 16 mg of opium, or 1.6 mg of morphine. Paregoric was available without a prescription until about 1970, when it was classified as a Schedule III drug, making it a controlled substance. Despite its effectiveness, this treatment for diarrhea is little used today.

After the invention of the hypodermic needle in 1853, its use in medicine increased, with its especially liberal use on the battlefield and in military hospitals often resulting in morphine addiction. (During and after the Civil War, morphine addiction was referred to as "soldier's disease.")

During the second half of the nineteenth century, both clinical and recreational use of morphine and opium expanded. Morphine, being unregulated, was added to patent medicines and elixirs as an unidentified ingredient, which resulted in addiction among the civilian population. Recreational opium smoking, a practice introduced by Chinese immigrant workers in the United States, also increased.[3] By the year 1900, more than 4% of the U.S. population was addicted to opium or another opioid. A survey of 35 Boston drugstores in 1888 found that 78% of the prescriptions that had been refilled three or more times contained opium (Levinthal, 2013).

By the turn of the century, physicians had become increasingly concerned about the extent of opioid addiction, especially about addiction resulting from the overprescription of opioid drugs and the widespread use of opioids in patient medicine. That concern—and the almost epidemiclike abuse of opioids in the United States—led to the passage of the Pure Food and Drug Act of 1906, which required that manufacturers list their products' ingredients on the labels. When people saw that their medicines contained questionable compounds, the unregulated use of opioids began to decline.

The Harrison Narcotic Act of 1914 had an even greater impact on the use of morphine and opium by mandating that only licensed physicians and dentists could

[3]Opium smoking took hold in China early in the nineteenth century as a result of trade with the West, especially Britain. Needing to balance their large purchases of tea from China, Britain traded Indian-grown opium for Chinese tea. The Chinese government saw what opium addiction did to its people and outlawed the drug, but after the First Opium War of 1839–1842 and the Second Opium War of 1856–1860, won by Britain and its allies because of British naval superiority, China was forced to accept the opium trade. Not only did the trade resume, but China was also forced to cede Hong Kong to Britain as a treaty port.

prescribe opioids (and cocaine). The law also required medical professionals to register with the Internal Revenue Service to write such prescriptions. Over time, court decisions interpreted this law to mean that opioids could be prescribed and taken for medically approved purposes only and not for nonmedical reasons; that is, it became illegal for people addicted to opioids to get these drugs just to maintain a drug habit.

Since the early twentieth century, periodic cycles of opioid abuse have been followed by efforts to reduce the recreational use of opioids—but without much success. An important part of such efforts has been an ongoing search for drugs that would alleviate pain without the potential for addiction. This search has produced an expanding formulary of natural, semisynthetic, and synthetic opioid analgesics but has failed to achieve the goal of finding opioids with analgesic properties and without euphoric-addictive properties. Nevertheless, the ongoing epidemic of abuse of prescription opioids, with an epicenter in the United States, is prompting further development of opioid formulations that are pharmacologically designed to prevent recreational misuse (Coplan et al., 2016).

THE OPIOID EPIDEMIC

It appears that we are now experiencing the so-called third wave of the opioid epidemic (Volkow and Blanco, 2021). The first wave began in the 1990s with massive increases in the prescription of strong opioids such as oxycodone, and the second wave resulted from an explosion in heroin use (discussed later in this section).

Currently, an average of about 190 people in the United States die each day after overdosing on opioids, either with prescription drugs such as oxycodone or with illicit opioids such as heroin (frequently mixed with fentanyl), and that number is still increasing. In the year ending in April 2021, there were more than 100,000 drug overdose deaths in the United States, an increase of almost 16% over the year ending in April 2020[4] (Centers for Disease Control and Prevention, 2021). Of these deaths, 80,800 resulted from opioids in 2021, up from about 70,029 deaths from opioids the year before. Approximately 64% of these deaths specifically involved synthetic opioids (primarily fentanyl and its derivatives) (O'Donnell et al., 2021). Indeed, an estimated 80% of fatal opioid overdoses in the United States now involve synthetics (Skolnick, 2021). Figure 10.2 illustrates this trend in opioid-involved deaths over the years 1999–2020.[5]

An estimated 50.2 million adults in the United States have chronic pain, and 22.1% of those with chronic pain have used prescription opioids (Groenewald et al., 2022).

[4]In 1999–2018, more than 700,000 Americans died from drug overdoses, a number about equal to the population of Boston.

[5]In 2022, the federal Commission on Combating Synthetic Opioid Trafficking offered a multilevel response to this crisis, including expansion of access to evidenced-based treatments for opioid use disorder.

DR. J'S MUSINGS 10.2

Fentanyl

During the period when I practiced clinical anesthesia, from 1977 through 2005, my go-to opioid analgesic for both surgical and postsurgical use was fentanyl, administered at a sufficient dose to relieve most pain. To this day, I wonder if I might have been contributing to the development of continuing use (after hospital discharge) and opioid dependence in some of my patients. Could I have done differently and still accomplished my major goal of alleviating pain? I will likely never know.

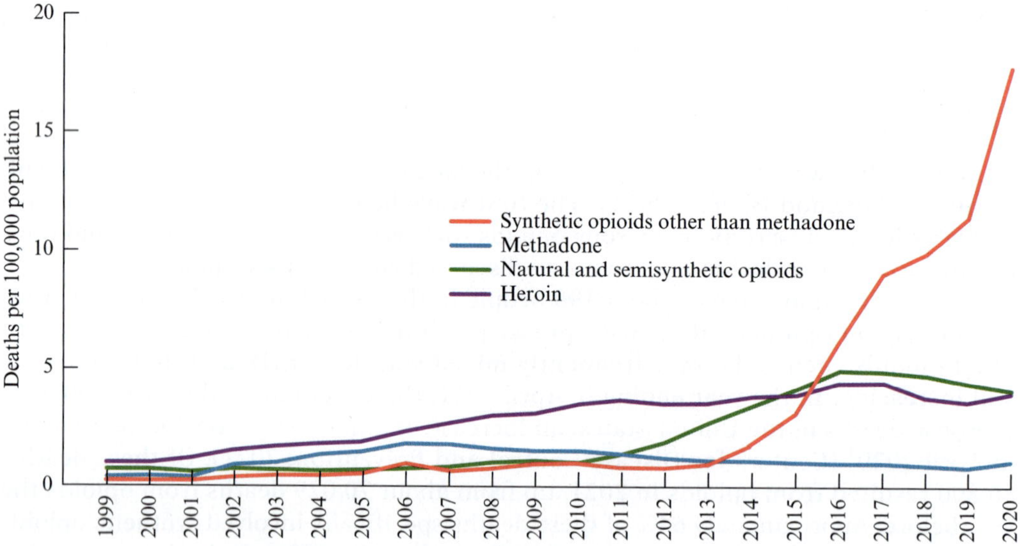

FIGURE 10.2 Overdose Deaths Involving Opioids, 1999–2020. Since 2013, the proportion of U.S. deaths involving synthetic opioids (mainly fentanyl and its derivatives) has risen sharply. Only the proportion of deaths involving methadone has remained relatively constant. [Data from National Center for Health Statistics, 2021.]

Anywhere from about 10% to 29% of patients prescribed opioids for chronic pain misuse them, and 8–10% of those who misuse them develop opioid use disorder (OUD; Singer et al., 2019). No U.S. geographic or demographic community is immune to these trends; the Midwest has seen a remarkable 70% yearly increase in overdoses, many involving fatalities from heroin adulterated with fentanyl derivatives. The national consequences have been horrific, with significant increases in overdoses and associated deaths in every group from the unborn to older adults. In 2017, this epidemic was declared a public health emergency, a health emergency overshadowed only by the COVID-19 coronavirus global pandemic (and perhaps exacerbated by that pandemic, as discussed next[6]). However, the publication of guidelines for reducing opioid use has had minimal effect, with only a 14% reduction in oxycodone prescriptions and no reductions in the prescription of other Schedule II opioids 18 months after publication of the guidelines (Scherrer et al., 2020). In addition, researchers have noted that even short-term and low-dose opioid prescriptions to youths and young adults who had never used opioids were associated with an increased risk of persistent use (Wilson et al., 2021).

These disturbing opioid-related statistics are paired with equally disturbing statistics for overdose deaths overall, not just related to opioids but also to the COVID-19 pandemic. A San Francisco study found that overdose deaths in the eight months after a COVID-19 shelter-in-place order had increased by 50% compared with the eight months prior to the order, with a record 537 drug overdose deaths during the later period (vs. just 169 deaths due to COVID-19 in the same period) (Appa et al., 2021). Another study reported similar increases in Ontario, Canada, with deaths largely due to fentanyl and stimulants (Gomes et al., 2021).

Beginning around 1999, the increased potency of heroin, the drop in the price of the drug, and its combination with synthetic opioids such as fentanyl eventually resulted in a dramatic rise in the annual number of heroin-involved overdose deaths in the United States over the period 2010–2018, after which this second wave of the opioid epidemic began leveling off (see Figure 10.3).

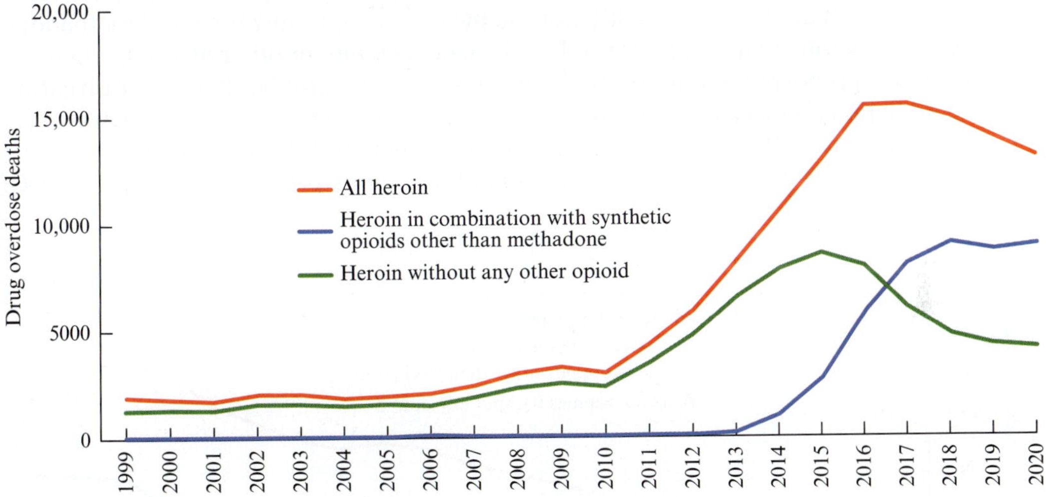

FIGURE 10.3 Overdose Deaths Involving Heroin, 1999–2020. Heroin-involved overdose deaths in the United States began rising dramatically in 2010, spurred after 2013 by a rise in deaths due to combinations of heroin with synthetic opioids. Such combinations have kept the total of heroin-involved deaths high despite a significant drop in the number of deaths due to heroin alone. [Data from National Institute on Drug Abuse, 2022b.]

[6]In the words of one group of researchers: "Opioid overdoses in the US likely reached a record high in 2020 because of COVID-19 increasing substance use, exacerbating stress and social isolation, and interfering with opioid treatment" (Fairley et al., 2021).

Another aspect of this heroin-impacted second wave was the relationship between high rates of prescription opioid use and subsequent heroin use, with increasing numbers of people then alternating between prescription opioids and heroin, depending on which was more easily available (Cicero et al., 2015). This progression from prescription opioid use to heroin use appeared to be a new phenomenon. In the 1960s, more than 80% of opioid abusers noted that they started with heroin, but this was nearly reversed by the 2000s, when 75% of heroin users noted that they started with prescription opioids (Compton et al., 2016). Only a few studies have been performed, but it appears that heroin use increased before policies were in place that made opioid prescriptions more difficult to obtain. As noted, the increased purity and accessibility of heroin, and its lower cost, are considered important reasons for the increased use, especially in a subgroup of people with opioid dependence who frequently misuse prescribed opioids.

Currently, there is additional concern about the concomitant use of opioids and other types of medications that depress the CNS, especially benzodiazepines. In 2020, the U.S. Food and Drug Administration (FDA) issued a warning about this combination, noting that it greatly increases the risk of unintentional overdose and death. The agency added their strongest alert—the "boxed warning"—to the labeling of prescription opioid pain and cough medications, as well as to the labeling of benzodiazepines, in an effort to reduce this combined use. Subsequently, after additional review (Lanham et al., 2022), the FDA published a revision intended to ensure that the warning was not interpreted in a way that would interfere with the treatment of opioid addictions. This revision stated that "the opioid addiction medications buprenorphine and methadone should not be withheld from patients taking benzodiazepines or other drugs that depress the CNS" (buprenorphine and methadone are synthetic opioids; their use in treating opioid addictions is discussed later in this chapter). It appears now that these warnings have had minimal effect on co-prescribing, and overdose fatalities involving combinations of opioids and benzodiazepines remain a serious problem (see Figure 10.4).

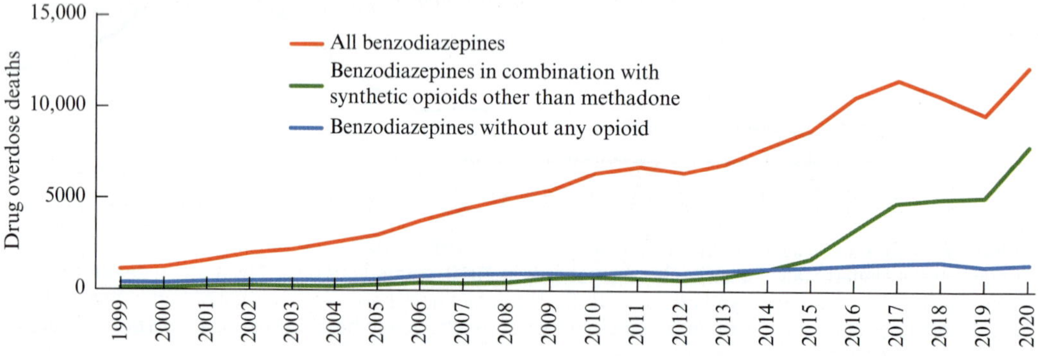

FIGURE 10.4 Overdose Deaths Involving Benzodiazepines, 1999–2020. Relatively few overdose deaths result from the use of benzodiazepines alone. The majority of benzodiazepine-involved deaths result from the combined use of benzodiazepines and opioids other than methadone. (Methadone is excluded from this assessment because of its frequently prescribed use in combination with benzodiazepines in treating opioid addictions.) [Data from National Institute on Drug Abuse, 2022b.]

DR. J'S MUSINGS 10.3

Boy, Was Something About to Change!

One morning in 1978, soon after I had passed my licensure examination allowing me to practice medicine in Oregon, I and others who had passed the exam were being addressed by a member of the Oregon Board of Medicine, welcoming us into the profession as licensed physicians. He made a special point of telling us that too many opioid prescriptions were being written (mainly for hydrocodone, oxycodone, and morphine) and that we would be closely monitored by the board for any sign of overprescribing. Underprescribing was encouraged. Moderate amounts of pain were OK.

BOY, WAS SOMETHING ABOUT TO CHANGE!

In 2001, pain was declared "the fifth vital sign." Four vital signs are easily measured (heart rate, blood pressure, respiratory rate, and temperature). Pain, however, is subjective and not easily measured. Regardless, the Joint Commission on Hospital Accreditation passed a new standard emphasizing that pain should be eliminated whenever possible. Hospitals were required to closely monitor and promptly treat pain, including performing a pain assessment with every patient on every 8-hour shift. The idea (now known to be mistaken) was that pain medication is capable of rendering all patients completely pain-free. Pain clinics prospered and patient expectations of being without pain skyrocketed. So did opioid prescriptions, reaching 200 million yearly. By 2020 an average of 44 people died each day from overdoses involving prescription opioids, totaling more than 16,000 deaths. Prescription opioids were involved in nearly 24% of all opioid overdose deaths in 2020 (Centers for disease Control and Prevention (2022). What a failure!

BOY, WAS SOMETHING ABOUT TO CHANGE!

In 2006, an important study documented that calling pain a fifth vital sign did not improve pain care (Mularski et al., 2006). By 2016, with the opioid epidemic raging, the American Medical Association had rejected the "fifth vital sign" concept and begun urging a more rational approach to pain care. In 2018, when the epidemic was finally confronted, the Joint Commission on Hospital Accreditation relented, and the pendulum began swinging back to appropriate levels of opioid prescribing, along with a call for better treatment of people addicted to opioids.

BOY, WAS SOMETHING ABOUT TO CHANGE!

In 2019, the FDA approved a nasal formulation of naloxone (an opioid antagonist) to be widely distributed to help reverse overdoses, and today we are in a new era of pain management based on the principles of responsible and compassionate care without overuse of opioids, recognition that not all pain can be relieved, and more reliance on nonaddicting medications and complementary treatments (Groenewald et al., 2022).

Over the past few years, for example, U.S. overdose deaths involving benzodiazepines have averaged almost 11,000 annually, and in 85% of these deaths an opioid was also involved (Agarwal et al., 2019; Azad et al., 2020; Zhang et al., 2019). Recently, researchers warned about the increased risk of opioid overdoses from concomitant use of strong opioids (e.g., oxycodone) plus use of certain antidepressants that inhibit drug metabolizing enzymes (especially CYP2D6) (Yunusa et al., 2022).

Finally, there is concern about smoking heroin together with crack cocaine. Although this combination intensifies euphoria, tempers the anxiety and paranoia associated with cocaine, and seems to reduce the depression that typically occurs after the effects of cocaine wear off, it can also lead to a multidrug addiction that is extremely difficult to treat.

PAIN AND PAIN TRANSMISSION

Pain is one of the most common human experiences and one of the most common reasons people seek medical care. Nevertheless, as a sensory phenomenon, pain is very difficult to measure because it is a subjective experience, with assessments of the degree of pain being based mainly on self-report. The International Association for the Study of Pain defines pain as a "highly unpleasant sensory and emotional experience associated with actual or potential tissue damage or described in terms of such damage" (Raja et al., 2020). The Alsatian-German humanitarian and physician Albert Schweitzer (1875–1965) had a more personal and empathetic perspective on pain:

> We must all die. But that I can save him from days of torture, that is what I feel as my great and ever new privilege. Pain is a more terrible lord of mankind than even death itself. (Schweitzer, 2014)

Acute Pain and Chronic Pain

Acute, short-acting pain is biologically useful because it alerts us to actual or potential damage to the body, and it resolves once any injury heals.

In contrast, chronic pain—generally defined as pain lasting more than three months and not caused by cancer—is typically not useful, causes suffering and disability, restricts the activities of daily living, and increases the costs of health care. It is perhaps the single most common complaint that prompts people to see a doctor. Chronic pain can take the form of migraine, back pain, neuropathic pain (pain produced by damage to the nervous system, such as that which occurs in diabetes), and the pain associated with arthritis, AIDS, postherpetic neuralgia, multiple sclerosis, and fibromyalgia, among other disorders. Chronic pain is commonly treated with nonopioid analgesics, either alone or with behavioral treatments such as exercise, weight loss, physical therapy, psychological interventions, and so forth (Centers for Disease Control and Prevention, 2022d). However, people with unremitting pain due to cancer and other terminal conditions should not be denied opioids, despite the inevitable development of tolerance and dependence as well as the potential for hastening the end of life.

Did You Know?

Absence of Pain

For most people, pain is usually an unpleasant sensation. But pain has the crucial function of alerting us to dangerous situations; without, it we would be at risk of serious, life-threatening injuries. In fact, that is exactly the situation for a small group of individuals who, for various reasons, are not capable of feeling pain. For example, 16-year-old Ashlyn Blocker has been unable to sense any kind of physical pain since the day she was born (Costandi, 2015). When her milk (baby) teeth started coming out, she nearly chewed off part of her tongue. Growing up, she once ran around on a broken ankle for two days before her parents noticed the injury. When fire ants swarmed over Ashlyn's body and left hundreds of bites, she did not feel a thing. Nor did she feel any pain when she dipped her hands into boiling water—and when she injured herself in countless other ways.

Ashlyn is one of a small group of people who are born with an insensitivity to pain. Scientists have found that this condition can occur as a result of several possible genetic mutations. By comparing the genomes of such pain-free individuals, researchers have discovered at least three different genes and identified almost two dozen different mutations among them, any one of which may cause this anomaly. Two of the genes provide the code for sodium channels on nerve fibers. A mutation in one of these genes produces a nonfunctional sodium channel such that although the pain fibers can detect painful stimuli, they cannot send signals about them to the brain. Another mutation produces overactive sodium channels that interfere with the ability of the fiber to produce and transmit the signals. People with a third mutation fail to develop pain-sensing neurons and nerve fibers. Understanding these rare conditions should increase our understanding of pain sensation and may provide new options for people suffering from chronic pain.

Pain Transmission

Normal pain transmission is triggered when a harmful or unpleasant stimulus activates primary afferent nociceptive sensory neurons that innervate a structure in the body, such as the skin, a joint, or an internal organ. As shown in Figure 10.5, the cell bodies of these primary afferents are located in the dorsal root ganglia, which lie parallel to the spinal cord. Primary afferents synapse with neurons in the dorsal horn of the spinal cord, which send information about pain stimuli to the brain—first to the thalamus and then to the forebrain, where the subjective and emotional experience of pain arises, as well as to other areas throughout the brain, which modulate responses to pain inputs from the thalamus. In this way, a wide range of brain structures inhibit, facilitate, or otherwise influence the experience of pain (Thien, 2021).

All the parts of the pain transmission pathway illustrated in Figure 10.5 can be targets for different types of analgesic medications:

- NSAIDs (nonsteroidal anti-inflammatory drugs) such as aspirin and ibuprofen work by reducing the firing of the primary afferent neurons at the site of the pain-producing stimulus.

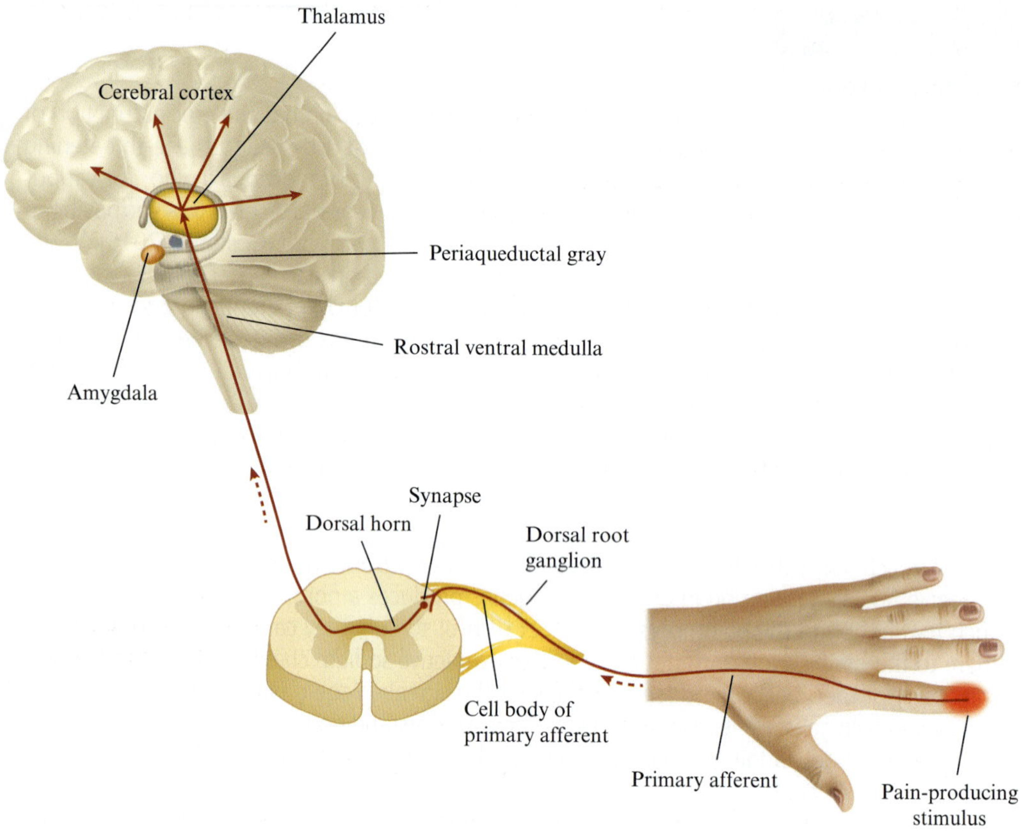

FIGURE 10.5 Pain Transmission. Pain signals arise when certain types of stimuli activate nociceptive (pain-sensing) primary afferent neurons. These neurons have their cell bodies (not shown) in the dorsal root ganglia (DRG) of the spinal cord. The pain signal is transmitted along the axons of the primary afferents into the dorsal horn of the spinal cord, where they synapse with spinal cord neurons that relay the pain signals to structures that include the rostral ventral medulla in the hindbrain, the periaqueductal gray in the midbrain, and the thalamus, which sends the signals to areas in the cortex where pain perception is ultimately experienced. Inhibitory and excitatory pathways (not shown) descend from the brain back to the spinal cord, modulating the same sites that were activated by the ascending pathways. Opioid drugs affect the pain signal and reduce the perception of pain through opioid receptors located at each of these sites, as well as at sites involved in emotional reactions to pain, such as the amygdala. Other drugs, such as antidepressants, anticonvulsants, and ion channel blocking agents, can also reduce pain by acting on other mechanisms involved in the transmission of pain signals.

- Anticonvulsants such as gabapentin and pregabalin reduce the degree of excitation of the primary afferents and thereby decrease the intensity of the signal transmitted to the spinal neurons.
- Topical local anesthetics (in patches) reduce the intensity of the pain signal transmitted from the spinal neurons to the brain. Most recently, a bupivacaine implant

has been marketed for the relief of pain following hernia surgery (Leiman et al., 2021).

- Antidepressant medications (especially the tricyclic antidepressants—see Chapter 12) increase the release of serotonin and norepinephrine in descending pathways from the brain to the spinal cord, which reduces the intensity of ascending pain signals.
- Opioids act on higher brain structures, altering the emotional reaction to pain and reducing its unpleasantness, as well as altering the sensory phenomenon itself to make it more bearable.

The five classes of medications in this list can be used in a balanced approach to treating pain, including to reduce and sometimes even eliminate the use of opioids (Krebs et al., 2018). Relying on opioids only is often unnecessary and can put the patient at risk of opioid dependence. In addition, the types of nonmedication interventions already mentioned (exercise, weight loss, physical therapy, and psychological therapy) must be included as part of a treatment plan (Volkow and McLellan, 2016).

OPIOID RECEPTORS

There is general agreement on the existence of at least three types of opioid receptors—mu, kappa, and delta[7]—all of them G-protein-coupled receptors (GPCRs, discussed in Chapter 3). Each of these three receptor types is specified by its own gene, and each is a chain of approximately 400 amino acids (the amino acid sequences are about 60% identical to one another and 40% different). Some studies indicate the existence of subtypes of these receptors, but this is not universally accepted. The three types are distributed widely throughout the CNS and, to a lesser extent, in the periphery. Soon after the opioid receptors were discovered, their natural neurotransmitters were also identified, as shown in Table 10.2.

TABLE 10.2 Opioid Receptors and Their Natural Neurotransmitters

Receptor	Neurotransmitters
mu	β-endorphin, endomorphin-1, endomorphin-2
kappa	dynorphin-A, dynorphin-B
delta	[met]-enkephalin, [leu]-enkephalin

Information from Pathan and Williams, 2012.

[7]Mu derives from *morphine*, which acts at this type of receptor; kappa derives from *ketocyclazocine*, the first agent known to act at this type of receptor; and delta derives from *vas deferens*, the tissue in which this type of receptor was first identified.

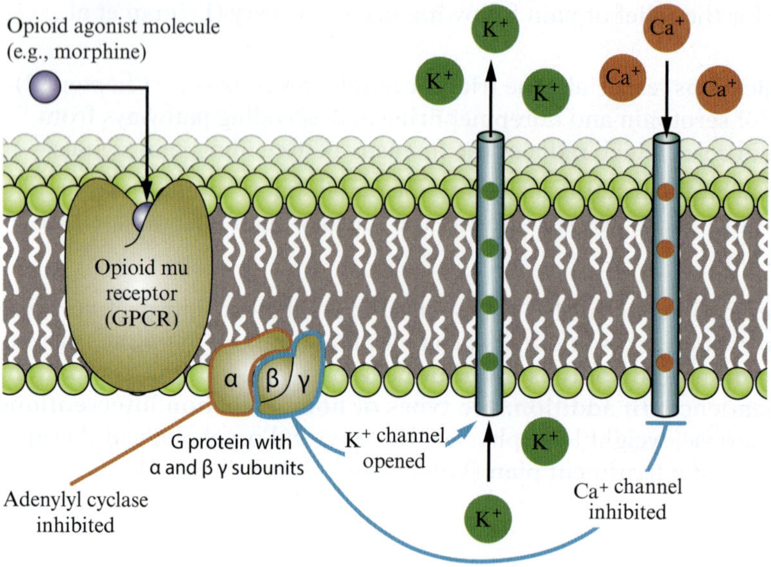

FIGURE 10.6 An Opioid Mu Receptor. The opioid receptor is a G-protein-coupled receptor (GPCR). When a molecule of an opioid such as morphine attaches to its binding site on a mu receptor, it activates the G protein, causing it to dissociate into its α component and its dual βγ component. The α component inhibits the activity of the enzyme adenylyl cyclase, reducing the amount of cyclic AMP inside the neuron. The βγ component opens channels in the membrane through which positively charged potassium ions (K^+) flow out of the neuron, and it inhibits channels through which positively charged calcium ions (Ca^+) would otherwise flow into the neuron. Both of these effects make the inside of the neuron more negative, which reduces neurotransmitter release by making the neuron less likely to fire. All of these processes help reduce the transmission of pain.

Figure 10.6 summarizes the process initiated by the binding of an opioid agonist molecule (e.g., a molecule of morphine) to a mu receptor. As is generally the case with GPCRs, the G-protein subunits dissociate from the rest of the receptor; the subunits then separate into two parts, an α (alpha) component and a βγ (beta-gamma) component. The α component inhibits the enzyme adenylyl cyclase, thereby reducing the amount of cyclic AMP inside the neuron; the βγ component activates potassium ion (K^+) channels and inhibits calcium ion (Ca^+) channels. These actions hyperpolarize the neuron by making the inside of the neuron more negative—that is, activating K^+ channels allows positively charged potassium ions to leave the neuron, and inhibiting Ca^+ channels prevents positively charged calcium ions from entering the neuron. This hyperpolarization has an analgesic effect resulting from a decreased amount of neurotransmitter released when the neuron is stimulated.

Activation of opioid receptors, whether by opioid drugs or by the natural neurotransmitters, has effects throughout the body, including on the primary afferents (outside of the CNS), on spinal neurons in the dorsal horn, and within various brain sites. When opioid receptors on the presynaptic terminals of the primary afferents are activated, the release of substances such as glutamate and substance P is blocked, and this reduces the intensity of ascending pain signals to the brain.

In the brain, high densities of mu opioid receptors are found on neurons in the periaqueductal gray in the midbrain and on neurons in the medulla in the hindbrain. When these mu receptors are activated, a result is indirect activation of descending pathways that release serotonin, norepinephrine, and enkephalin onto the spinal neurons, which further suppresses the transmission of pain signals.

PHARMACOLOGICAL EFFECTS OF OPIOIDS

Opioids have many and varied bodily and behavioral effects (see Figure 10.7), most prominently pain relief (analgesia) and a sense of well-being (euphoria), but also respiratory depression, sedation, anxiety reduction (anxiolysis), constipation, endocrine effects, and pregnancy-related effects. In addition, genetic factors can affect the rate at which opioids are metabolized, which influences the timing and intensity of opioids' other effects.

Finally, it is important to note that interactions between opioids and other psychotropic drugs are common and can be dangerous, even fatal. Many of the enzymes involved in opioid metabolism are either inhibited or induced by other medications, especially antidepressants and benzodiazepines, which means that these interactions must be considered when prescribing opioids for pain.

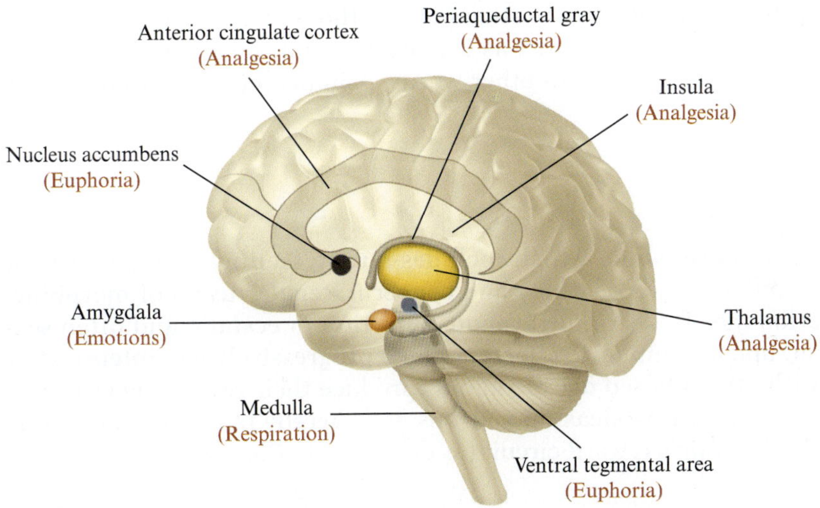

FIGURE 10.7 Morphine in the Brain. The prominent analgesic and euphoric effects of a full opioid agonist such as morphine depend on activation of opioid receptors at multiple sites in the brain. Emotional reactions to pain are modulated by the amygdala, and the respiratory depression associated with opioid use is controlled by the medulla.

DR. J'S MUSINGS 10.4

Drug-Induced Impairment

As a pharmacologist, I am often called by defense attorneys to review toxicology results on blood samples taken from persons stopped for traffic violations and found to be impaired on tests performed by police officers. In many of these cases, where the test results indicate greater than therapeutic levels of an opioid such as oxycodone, along with a benzodiazepine such as alprazolam (Xanax) and an antidepressant such as paroxetine (Paxil), the person claims to have been taking the medications as prescribed, a claim that is often supported by prescription records and pill counts. What is the probable explanation? The answer is straightforward: benzodiazepines and antidepressants inhibit the action of drug-metabolizing hepatic enzymes, with the result that blood concentrations of the opioid increase to impairing levels. This is often unrecognized by the person, and the result can be a traffic stop and a charge of driving under the influence of drugs.

Analgesia

Opioids produce analgesia and indifference to pain—that is, they reduce the intensity of pain and the associated distress by modulating the central processing of pain. Analgesia occurs without loss of consciousness and without affecting other sensory modalities. The pain may actually persist as a sensation, but the person feels more comfortable and is able to tolerate it. In other words, pain perception is significantly altered.

Euphoria

Opioids produce a euphoric state, which includes strong feelings of contentment and well-being, as well as a lack of worry and concern. Regular users of morphine, for example, describe the effects of intravenous injection in ecstatic and often sexual terms. However, opioids' euphoric effects become progressively less intense after repeated use. As with other abused drugs, opioids produce their rewarding effects at least partly by inhibiting GABA-releasing neurons and thereby indirectly increasing dopamine release in the brain's reward circuit (as described in Chapter 4).

Sedation and Anxiolysis

Opioids produce sedation and reduce anxiety, but the level of sedation is not as deep as that produced by other CNS depressants. People who take an opioid such as morphine typically become drowsy and doze, but they can usually be awakened readily. During this sedated state, cognitive slowing is prominent, accompanied by a lack of concentration, apathy, complacency, lethargy, and a sense of tranquility. However, tolerance develops to this effect with continued use.

Respiratory Depression

Opioids cause a profound depression of respiration by decreasing the respiratory center's sensitivity to higher levels of carbon dioxide in the blood (as indicated in Figure 10.7, the respiratory center is in the medulla, in the brain stem). Respiratory rate is reduced even at therapeutic doses, and at higher doses, the rate slows even further, respiratory volume decreases, and breathing patterns become shallow and irregular. At sufficiently high doses, breathing ceases and death follows (this is the usual cause of death in cases of opioid overdose). Fortunately, this respiratory depression can be reversed by the drug naloxone; however, naloxone also reverses the other effects of opioids and precipitates acute withdrawal (for more detailed discussion, see the section on pharmacotherapy with naloxone later in this chapter).

Tolerance to respiratory depression develops at a relatively slow rate, which means that people with a long history of opioid use remain at increased risk for respiratory depression and overdose death. People who are dependent on opioids and then undergo withdrawal (perhaps while incarcerated) and then resume opioid use at their former usual doses (perhaps after release) are especially at risk.

Gastrointestinal Effects

Opioids cause intestinal tone to increase, motility to decrease, and feces to dehydrate, as well as causing intestinal spasms and cramping. This combination of effects hardens the stool and further retards the advance of fecal material. Such opioid-induced constipation is a common adverse consequence of chronic opioid use, estimated to occur in 40–90% of patients. The positive side of this is that nothing more effective than opioids has yet been discovered for treating severe diarrhea, which is perhaps the most important action of opioids outside the CNS (see Dr. J's Musings 10.1 on the traditional use of paregoric, or tincture of opium, to treat diarrhea). In recent years, several medications that only very minimally cross the blood–brain barrier into the CNS have been developed for treating opioid-induced constipation (see Table 10.3).

Endocrine Effects

Opioids exert subtle but important effects on the functioning of the endocrine system, mainly due to drug-induced reductions in the release of sex hormones from the hypothalamus and the pituitary. Lower levels of testosterone in males result in reduced libido, and lower levels of luteinizing and follicle-stimulating hormones in females lead to menstrual irregularities and infertility. In people taking an opioid for chronic pain, both the chronic pain and the reduction in sex hormones may result in loss of sexual

TABLE 10.3 Medications for Treating Opioid-Induced Constipation

Medication	Notes
Diphenoxylate (Lomotil)	—
Loperamide (Imodium)	—
Methylnaltrexone (Relistor)	For use in adults with advanced illnesses who are receiving opioids on a continuous basis.
Alvimopan (Entereg)	For use in hospitalized patients who have undergone bowel surgery.
Naloxegol (Movantik)	For use in adult patients with chronic noncancer pain.
Naldemedine (Symproic)	—
Naloxone (Narcan)	Not officially approved for treatment of opioid-induced constipation. Naloxone crosses the blood–brain barrier, reversing the analgesic effect of opioids and precipitating withdrawal symptoms.*

*The other medication agents listed in this table were developed as "bulkier" molecules that will not cross the blood–brain barrier, thus limiting their effects to the periphery (primarily the GI tract).

desire and impaired performance, fatigue, mood alterations, and loss of muscle mass and strength.

Effects in Pregnancy

In pregnant parents, opioids cross the placental barrier and reach the fetus. Infants born to addicted parents are physically dependent on opioids and exhibit withdrawal symptoms. Opioids are not considered to be teratogenic, as their habitual use during pregnancy does not seem to increase the risk of congenital anomalies; however, their use does seem to increase the risks of fetal growth retardation and birth-related problems (Rausgaard et al., 2020). About 40% of opioid-affected newborns require neonatal intensive care, primarily for treatment of respiratory depression and neonatal withdrawal (Corsi et al., 2020). Moreover, research noted increasing rates of neonatal abstinence syndrome (withdrawal symptoms) and maternal opioid use disorder in the United States over the preceding decade (Hirai et al., 2021). Researchers studied neonatal opioid withdrawal syndromes and noted the severity of withdrawal correlated with intrauterine exposure to strong agonists and long half-life prescription opioids during the last three months of pregnancy (Esposito et al., 2022). Codeine and tramadol had relatively lower risk of neonatal withdrawal, compared with oxycodone, morphine, and other stronger, longer-acting opioids.

Unfortunately, treatment of opioid-abusing pregnant parents is also problematic. For nearly 50 years, methadone was a mainstay of such treatment because it was thought to be relatively safe, with few adverse effects, especially compared with the effects of using heroin or prescription opioids. Recently, however, methadone use (as well as buprenorphine use) by pregnant parents in opioid-maintenance therapy has been correlated with worse outcomes than those seen in pregnant parents who have not been exposed to opioids, including worse cognitive, psychomotor, behavioral, attentional, and executive functions, as well as visual problems (Andersen et al., 2020). Despite the results of a large meta-analysis in which the researchers advocated buprenorphine over methadone as a first-line therapy (Rausgaard et al., 2020), the results of another study indicate that infants born of parents who had been maintained on buprenorphine or methadone should be expected to display a neonatal withdrawal syndrome (Jones and Kraft, 2019). It seems clear that, in addressing the issues of opioid abuse during pregnancy, multiple issues involving the parent, fetus, infant, and family need to be considered (Jarienski et al., 2020).

Other Effects

Opioids can cause the following other effects as well:

- *Pupillary constriction.* Opioids cause pupillary constriction (miosis) by activating the pupillary sphincter muscle. Indeed, pupillary constriction in the presence of analgesia is characteristic of opioid ingestion. As noted later in this chapter, one opioid drug that does not elicit this effect is meperidine (Demerol).
- *Suppression of cough.* Opioids suppress the cough center in the hindbrain and have historically been used as cough suppressants. This is termed an antitussive action. Codeine is particularly popular for this purpose. Today, however, less-addicting drugs (e.g., dextromethorphan) are used as cough suppressants, and opioids have become inappropriate choices for treating persistent cough.
- *Nausea and vomiting*. Opioids stimulate receptors in an area of the medulla called the *chemoreceptor trigger zone.* Stimulation of this area produces nausea and vomiting, which are characteristic and unpleasant side effects of morphine and other opioids, but they are not life-threatening. Like drowsiness, tolerance develops with continued use.
- *Immunological effects*. Opioids can release histamine from its storage sites in mast cells in the blood, which may elicit localized itching or more severe allergic reactions, including bronchoconstriction. Opioids also affect white blood cell function, producing complex alterations in the immune system. It is advisable, perhaps, to avoid the use of morphine in patients with compromised immune function.

Effects of Genetic Influences on Opioid Metabolism

With the current dramatic increase in opioid prescription abuse and concern about the accidental overdose of these medications, the phenomenon of genetic influences on opioid metabolism is receiving increasing attention. The primary pathways for opioid metabolism involve the cytochrome P450 (CYP) 2D6 and 3A4 enzymes. These two enzymes account for over 90% of opioid metabolism, with the CYP-3A4 accounting for 40–60%. Although the evidence is somewhat indirect, estimates are that 20–30% of pain patients have a genetic opioid metabolic defect in one of these enzymes. One exception is the metabolism of methadone. Here, "although CYP3A4 is conventionally considered the principal methadone metabolizing enzyme, more recent data have identified CYP2B6 as the principal enzyme" (Talal et al., 2020).

In some cases, the enzyme is too active. Such patients are termed "rapid" or "ultrarapid" metabolizers in whom the opioid is rapidly metabolized, and pain returns much quicker than usual. These patients require a higher-than-normal dosage of opioid, which may cause them to be mislabeled as addicts and undertreated (Singa, 2016). In other patients, the metabolic enzyme is either inactive or absent, which results in slower-than-normal rates of drug metabolism, causing the opioid to accumulate in the blood and increasing its toxicity from drug-induced respiratory depression. Certainly, this could predispose persons to be at increased risk of opioid overdose deaths. One approach might be to use opioids that bypass the CYP450 system and are metabolized by glucuronidation. These include oxymorphone, hydromorphone, and tapentadol (Tennant, 2016).

SPECIFIC OPIOIDS

As noted earlier and in Chapter 3, *agonist drugs* are those that bind to receptors, activating them to produce a biological response. In the case of opioids, the main targets are the mu opioid receptors in the brain, which are activated when the opioid drug attaches to them. This opens up reward pathways in the brain, resulting in the release of *endogenous endorphins* to reduce pain and produce senses of pleasure and relaxation.

Endorphins are our naturally occurring opioid-like neurotransmitters, which can be produced to respond to certain stimuli by blocking them or signaling other neurological responses. The name is made up of two parts: endo (from within) and orphin (from morphine, meaning morphinelike substances produced naturally in our bodies). An opioid agonist will have the same influence on the opioid receptors and their resulting endorphin responses with a high degree of intensity.

Conversely, *opioid antagonists* specifically block opioid receptors, preventing access to the receptor by either endorphin or pure agonists. Instead of controlling withdrawal and cravings, pure opioid antagonists treat opioid use disorder by preventing any opiate from producing rewarding effects such as euphoria. In the following sections we discuss full agonists, partial agonists, mixed agonist–antagonists, and opioid antagonists in more detail.

Full Opioid Agonists

A full or *pure opioid agonist* is a chemical that produces effects similar to those produced by morphine (Edinoff et al., 2021). Morphine, itself, is a pure agonist to the naturally occurring endorphins in our body that are released in response to stimuli such as pain and emotions. Opioids essentially target mu opioid receptor sites wherever such receptors occur in the body and the brain. With increasing doses of a pure opioid agonist, there is increasing analgesia. Aside from morphine, there are many types of full opioid agonists.

Morphine

There are three sources of morphine:

1. Extraction from the opium poppy[8]
2. Metabolite of heroin (diacetyl morphine), discussed later in the chapter
3. Prescription-based, semisynthetic morphine[9]

Among the analgesics found in the opium poppy, morphine is the most potent and represents about 10% of the crude exudate. Despite decades of research, no other drug has been found that exceeds morphine's effectiveness as an analgesic, and no other drug is clinically superior for treating severe pain.

Morphine can be administered by injection, by inhalation, or orally (as pills) or rectally (as a suppository). Orally, morphine is available in immediate-release formulation and as a long-acting, time-release product (MS Contin). In general, absorption of morphine from the gastrointestinal (GI) tract is slow and incomplete compared to absorption following injection or inhalation. Only about 20% of orally administered morphine reaches the CNS. Absorption through the rectum is adequate, and several opioids (morphine, hydromorphone, and oxymorphone) are available in suppository form.[10]

The risk of an overdose increases in a dose-response manner. It will nearly double at 50 to 99 morphine milligrams equivalents per day and will increase by ninefold at 100 mg or more per day compared with doses of less than 20 mg per day.

The presence of opioid receptors in the spinal cord means that administration of morphine directly onto the spinal cord, an intrathecal route through small surgically implanted catheters, is effective. This route places the drug right at its site of action and may avoid its effects both on higher CNS centers (maintaining wakefulness and avoiding respiratory depression) and in the periphery (avoiding drug-induced constipation). A variation of this approach is the epidural route, where the drug is introduced within the spinal canal and just outside the spinal fluid. The morphine then diffuses into the spinal fluid, where it binds with spinal opioid receptors. In medicine, this technique is used to control the pain of obstetric labor and delivery, to treat postoperative pain, and (for long-term use) to relieve terminal cancer and other forms of intractable pain. In the latter situation, a surgically implanted programmed pump for intraspinal infusion is available.

[8]For thousands of years, the only way to obtain morphine was by harvesting the milky exudate of the opium poppy. However, drug companies and drug traffickers can now synthesize it.

[9]Some common trade names for morphine are Roxanol (morphine sulfate) and MS Contin.

[10] This kind of preparation might be indicated for patients suffering from muscle-wasting diseases who cannot tolerate other routes of administration.

Morphine crosses the blood–brain barrier fairly slowly, as it is more water soluble than lipid soluble. Other opioids cross the blood–brain barrier much more rapidly.

The liver metabolizes morphine, and as much as 40–60% of the drug may not reach the systemic circulation because of first-pass metabolism. One of morphine's metabolites (morphine-6-glucuronide) is 10 to 20 times more potent as an analgesic than morphine itself, and much of morphine's analgesic action is mediated by this active metabolite. The half-lives of morphine and morphine-6-glucuronide are both about 3 to 5 hours. Patients with impaired kidney function tend to accumulate the metabolite and thus may be more sensitive to morphine administration.

Urine screening tests can be used to detect morphine as well as its glucuronide metabolite.

Codeine

Codeine is much less potent than morphine and constitutes only 0.5% of the crude exudate from the opium poppy. Codeine is a prodrug that must be metabolized by the enzyme CYP-2D6 in the body to morphine, the pharmacologically active drug. Hence, the efficacy and safety of codeine are governed by CYP-2D6 activity. Codeine used to be widely prescribed as a low-potency opioid, but in recent years has fallen out of favor because of more reliable and stronger opioids such as hydrocodone and oxycodone. Codeine was usually combined with aspirin or acetaminophen for the relief of mild to moderate pain. These combination products were frequently sought drugs of abuse. Because it has been used for so long, codeine never underwent the safety studies required for new drugs. The plasma half-life and duration of action are about 3 to 4 hours, but codeine's pharmacokinetics are unpredictable. Moreover, almost one in ten Americans have a genetic variation that causes very rapid metabolism of codeine. As a result, abnormally high levels of morphine may accumulate, leading to drowsiness and respiratory depression. Furthermore, morphine may also be passed to infants through breast milk. In 2013, the FDA warned that products containing codeine should not be used for pain relief in children after tonsillectomy or adenoidectomy because of the risk for adverse effects or death. This was based on medical reports of three deaths and one life-threatening case of respiratory depression in children with sleep apnea given codeine after one of the aforementioned surgeries.

In addition to its inherent pharmacokinetic disadvantages, four of the six selective serotonin reuptake inhibitor (SSRI) antidepressants (fluoxetine, fluvoxamine, sertraline, and paroxetine; see Chapter 12) can block the pain relief of codeine because they block the conversion of codeine to morphine (Cazet et al., 2018). For patients taking an SSRI, an analgesic drug other than codeine may be necessary.

Hydrocodone

Hydrocodone is one of the most commonly prescribed and abused opioid medications. Like codeine, hydrocodone is a relatively weak analgesic. CYP-2D6 converts much of the hydrocodone to the more active compound *hydromorphone* (Dilaudid). Short-acting hydrocodone is commonly found in combination with acetaminophen in formulations such as Vicodin, Norco, and Lortab. In 2014, these compounds, because of their high abuse risk, were rescheduled from Schedule III to Schedule II, which is a more restricted category. In the first year following the rescheduling, there were 26.3 million fewer prescriptions (a 22% decline) and 1.1 billion fewer tablets sold (a 16% decline).

In 2018, a drug trade-named Apadaz was approved. Instead of containing the active drug hydrocodone, Alpadaz is a combination of a prodrug (an inactive precursor molecule), benzhydrocodone, and acetaminophen. When ingested, stomach enzymes cleave the benzhydrocodone prodrug and release the active parent drug hydrocodone (Mustafa et al., 2018).

Oxycodone

Oxycodone (Percodan, OxyContin) is another semisynthetic opioid similar in action to morphine. The short-acting, generic preparation was, until recently, widely prescribed for the treatment of acute pain. The enzyme CYP-3A4 metabolizes oxycodone to the opioid agonist noroxycodone, which is not very potent, and the enzyme CYP-2D6 metabolizes oxycodone to oxymorphone, which is more potent. Beginning about 25 years ago, "super poppies" containing high concentrations of *thebaine* were planted in Tasmania. Thebaine is a chemical precursor for making oxycodone

Over the past decade, oxycodone became widely abused as part of the opioid crisis. Manufacturers responded to this by developing long-acting, slow-release "abuse-deterrent" products containing much more oxycodone per pill. Not surprisingly, this only compounded the abuse and overuse problem, with many transitioning to heroin. The long-acting, high-dose formulations of oxycodone (such as OxyContin) contain oxycodone in doses up to 80 milligrams (normal acute doses are about 5 to 10 milligrams). Abusers crushed the pill, destroying the time-release mechanisms, and snorted the powder, smoked the drug, or diluted it in water and injected it. OxyContin has contributed to thousands of overdose deaths, resulting in ongoing legal consequences.

Hydromorphone and Oxymorphone

Hydromorphone (Dilaudid) and **oxymorphone** (Numorphan) are both structurally related to morphine and are six to ten times more potent. They produce somewhat less sedation but equal respiratory depression. Palladone (not to be confused with *paliperidone*; see Chapter 11) and Exalgo are trade names for two long-acting formulations of hydromorphone that are taken once daily for treatment of chronic pain in patients who have developed a tolerance to opioids and thus can tolerate the high doses of 10 to 32 milligrams per day (the dose of short-acting hydromorphone is about 1 to 2 milligrams).

As might be expected, long-acting formulations of oxymorphone were developed and have been controversial. Several of these have been removed from commercial sale.

Propoxyphene

Propoxyphene (Darvon) is an analgesic compound that is structurally similar to methadone; it is less potent than codeine but more potent than aspirin. Darvon was marketed in 1957 when there were few alternatives for treating pain, except aspirin and strong opioids. In 2010, the FDA determined that the drug should be removed from commercial sale because of concerns about potentially fatal heart rhythm abnormalities, drug overdose suicide, and overdoses.

Meperidine

Meperidine (Demerol) is a synthetic opioid whose structure differs from that of morphine. Because of this structural difference and because it was not derived from opium, meperidine was originally thought to be free of many of the undesirable properties of the opioids. However, like most opioids, it is a potent stimulant of mu opioid receptors. Meperidine is addictive and it can be substituted for morphine or heroin in addicts. It is one-tenth as potent as morphine, produces a similar type of euphoria, and is equally likely to cause dependence. Meperidine's side effects differ from morphine's and include more excitatory effects, such as tremors, delirium, hyperreflexia, and convulsions. These excitatory actions are produced by a metabolite of meperidine (normeperidine). Unlike other opioids, meperidine does not cause pinpoint pupils, but it may dilate the pupils. Meperidine and normeperidine can accumulate in people who have kidney dysfunction or who use only meperidine for their opioid addiction. Following cessation of use, withdrawal symptoms develop more rapidly than with morphine because of meperidine's shorter duration of action.

Fentanyl and Its Derivatives

Fentanyl (Sublimaze) and three related compounds, sufentanil (Sufenta), alfentanil (Alfenta), and remifentanil (Ultiva), are FDA approved and commercially available short-acting, intravenously administered mu opioid agonists that are structurally related to meperidine. They were originally marketed to be used by injection during and after surgery to relieve surgical pain. Currently, multiple formulations are commercially available to treat varying types of pain:

- *Lollipops.* Fentanyl lollipops were originally developed for use in treating postsurgical pain in children. This use was rapidly abandoned. More recently, lollipops have been used in critically ill patients who cannot tolerate other routes of drug administration.
- *Transdermal patches.* These vary in absorption levels from 12.5 to 100 micrograms per hour of fentanyl. Transdermal patches are used for continuous drug absorption in patients with chronic pain.
- *Tablets.* These are intended for absorption of fentanyl across the mucous membranes of the mouth.
- *Lozenges.* As above, lozenges are used for absorption of fentanyl across mucous membranes of the mouth.
- *Nasal spray.* The nasal spray is intended for absorption through the mucous membranes of the nose.
- *Buccal film.* Uses of buccal film are the same as for tablets and lozenges.
- *Intravenous liquid (usually injected in a hospital setting).* The intravenous liquid is intended for treatment of intraoperative and postsurgical pain.

However, in recent years fentanyl and its analogues have been widely synthesized in laboratories and adulterated with illicit supplies of heroin, cocaine, methamphetamine, and counterfeit pills, contributing to the exponential growth in the number of drug-related overdose deaths, a topic we will discuss in more detail later (Han et al., 2019; National Institute on Drug Abuse, 2022a).

Methadone

Methadone (Dolophine) is a synthetic mu agonist opioid very similar to morphine. Methadone was first shown to block the effects of heroin withdrawal in 1948. In 1965, it was introduced as a substitute treatment for opioid dependency (discussed later in the chapter). The outstanding properties of methadone are its effective analgesic activity, efficacy by the oral route, long half-life (10–60 hours) by oral administration, extended duration of action in suppressing withdrawal symptoms in physically dependent people, and tendency to show persistent effects with repeated administration.

Today, methadone has two primary legitimate uses: (1) as noted, as an orally administered substitute for heroin in methadone maintenance treatment programs, and (2) as a long-acting analgesic for the treatment of chronic pain syndromes.

Multiple CYP hepatic enzymes are required to metabolize methadone. Therefore, methadone is the opioid most susceptible to serious drug interactions resulting from drug-induced enzyme inhibition. For example, some sedatives and antidepressants inhibit methadone's metabolism, resulting in large elevations in blood concentrations, often leading to unexpected fatalities.

Oliceridine

Oliceridine (Olinvyk) is a newly FDA-approved mu opioid receptor agonist used intravenously in the treatment of acute pain severe enough to require intravenous opioid therapy (Markham, 2020). Analgesic efficacy is presumably comparable to that exerted by morphine, supposedly without morphine's reductions in gastrointestinal motility (constipation) and respiratory depression (Dahan et al., 2020; Figura and Atkinson, 2020; Gan and Wase, 2020). Further trials to verify its possible reduced side effects are warranted.

Partial Opioid Agonists

Partial agonists can have similar effects to full agonists; however, they lose effectiveness at higher doses. Medications that belong to the partial agonist category include two related drugs, tramadol and tapentadol, buprenorphine, and one drug currently under development, cebranopadol. In general, these drugs have utility in the management of chronic pain (Gress et al., 2020; Webster et al., 2020) as well as in the treatment of opioid dependence and withdrawal (Coe et al., 2019; Srivastava et al., 2020).

Tramadol

Tramadol (Ultram) is considered a mixed-mechanism opioid drug that exerts analgesic effects through inhibition of ascending pain pathways (closest to a partial mu agonist), leading to an altered perception of pain. It also inhibits the reuptake of serotonin and norepinephrine, with components of a descending inhibitory pain pathway and contributing antidepressant activity (this is considered beneficial since chronic pain is also associated with depression) (Edinoff et al., 2021).

Tramadol is a synthetic analogue of codeine. Like codeine, tramadol is a prodrug that is converted (metabolized) to an active drug (desmethyltramadol). Patients with deficiencies in drug metabolism (i.e., poor metabolizers) will tend to get reduced analgesic effects from tramadol. Those who produce increased quantities of drug-metabolizing enzymes (rapid metabolizers) may experience increased pharmacological and unexpected adverse effects. Compared with codeine, tramadol seems to be associated with a higher risk of adverse cardiovascular reactions and mortality (Xie et al., 2021). It had been generally assumed that tramadol was less liable to abuse than opioid painkillers. With an increase in tramadol prescriptions, however, came an increase in reported problems with abuse and addiction. In 2014, the DEA reclassified tramadol from Schedule V to Schedule IV, which was comparable to the scheduling of benzodiazepines. In addition, because it was thought to be safer than other opioids, tramadol was often prescribed to older patients. This cohort, however, accounted for the largest number of emergency room visits associated with the drug, possibly because older adults are often prescribed multiple medicines that can negatively interact with tramadol (Chapter 12). Nevertheless, the extended-release formulation of tramadol was recently found to be effective in suppressing opioid withdrawal in a small clinical trial (Dunn et al., 2017). It was also reported that tramadol was effective in a three-day detoxification program for opioid-dependent patients (Radcliff et al., 2018). Despite this, currently, tramadol has no FDA-approved indication for medication-assisted treatment of opioid withdrawal. In late 2021, the FDA approved a combination product of celecoxib (a nonsteroidal analgesic) and tramadol. This product is marketed under the trade name Seglentis.

The active metabolite of tramadol, *O*-desmethyltramadol (*O*-DSMT), has been synthesized; it is not a prescribed substance but is available from Internet sources. It is presently a legal alternative to illegal opioid drugs, packaged as a powder or combined with other agents. One example is marketed as the blend "Krypton," which consists of powdered kratom leaf (*Mitragyna speciosa*) in combination with *O*-DSMT. It has been linked to several accidental overdose deaths (Chapter 8).

Tapentadol

Tapentadol (Nucynta) is a partial opioid agonist, similar to tramadol. It has two types of action: first, it activates the mu opioid receptor (analgesic action) and second, it inhibits the reuptake of norepinephrine (antidepressant action) (Basu et al., 2018; Romualdi et al., 2019). Unlike tramadol, tapentadol is (by itself) biologically active, not a prodrug, and has no known active metabolites. As a result, it does not have to be metabolized to elicit its therapeutic effects. Consequently, there is less risk of drug interactions. This characteristic is advantageous for its use in patients who are poor metabolizers of other opioids (Faria et al., 2018). Both immediate-release and extended-release forms of tapentadol are available. Because of the increased amount of drug in the extended-release product, it is accompanied by an increased risk of abuse and dependence (Fudin, 2020; Peacock et al., 2020).

Buprenorphine

Buprenorphine is widely used today in the treatment of opioid dependence (Substance Abuse and Mental Health Services Administration, 2021b). In addition, as a partial opioid agonist, buprenorphine has also found use as an analgesic (Davis et al., 2018; Londhe et al., 2020) with analgesic effects proportional to its blood concentration (Guarnieri, 2021). In its chemical structure, buprenorphine is related to several other opioid agents, including oxycodone, hydromorphone, and oxymorphone. But buprenorphine works in a different way. It is both a partial agonist at mu opioid receptors and an antagonist at kappa receptors. While therapeutic doses provide mild to moderate analgesic effect, there is a ceiling that limits respiratory depression, and the partial agonistic action plateaus with an increase in dose. It can be used to reverse respiratory depression following methadone overdose (Zamani et al., 2020).

Recently, opioids' known anxiolytic effects have prompted interest in using buprenorphine in the treatment of comorbid posttraumatic stress disorder (PTSD) and chronic pain (Madison and Eitan, 2020), which are often accompanied by anxiety and depression, placing people at high risk of suicide. The high degree of interest in this treatment possibility is due to the fact that the SSRI-type antidepressants typically used in such cases have a success rate of 30% at best (Kind and Otis, 2019; Lake et al., 2019). Studies of buprenorphine plus an SSRI in the treatment of PTSD are critically needed.

Buprenorphine is now available in multiple preparations, each under a different trade name:

- Buprenex was marketed in the United States in 1985 for the treatment of moderate to severe pain as an injectable buprenorphine formulation.
- Subutex, a sublingual tablet, was approved in 2002 as a treatment for opioid dependence, especially during the initial therapeutic period. Additionally, it has an off-label application in chronic pain patients who cannot tolerate long-acting, full agonist opioids or for whom such agents are inappropriate. Because of abuse problems, the manufacturer discontinued sale in 2011, but not for reasons of safety or effectiveness. Therefore, it is still available in generic form.
- Bunavail, Suboxone, and Zubsolv: These three trade-named products are transmucosal films or small dissolvable tablets to be placed under the tongue from where the medication is absorbed. Each product is formulated in conjunction with the opioid antagonist naloxone. These are treatments for dependence on any opioid, both at the beginning of opioid withdrawal and for maintenance therapy.
- Butrans is a transdermal patch, which is approved for pain treatment that is not sufficiently alleviated by other drugs and therefore warrants around-the-clock, long-term opioid administration. Available doses range from 5 to 20 micrograms per hour; however, for opioid-naive patients, only the 5 micrograms per hour dose is recommended. This formulation is also indicated for maintaining opioid abstinence. Butrans patches should remain on for a week before they are removed.
- Belbuca is a formulation of buprenorphine indicated for around-the-clock treatment of pain that is not sufficiently relieved with alternative drugs. It is a newer formulation, available as a buccal film in doses of 75 to 900 micrograms, each lasting about 12 hours. This formulation was developed to adhere to the buccal mucosa and

dissolve completely within 30 minutes. The time to peak concentration is 2.5 to 3 hours and the elimination half-life is 27.6 hours.

- Probuphine is the first buprenorphine implant for maintenance treatment of opioid dependence. It releases a constant, low-level amount of the drug for six months in patients who have been stabilized on low to moderate doses of another buprenorphine agent. Probuphine consists of four 1-inch rods that are implanted under the skin on the inside of the upper arm.
- Sublocade is a new injectable formulation of buprenorphine. It is a viscous liquid injected subcutaneously and, as a depot, the drug is released slowly over a period of one month (Ling, et al., 2020).

The most common side effects of buprenorphine are flulike symptoms, including headache, sweating, sleeping difficulties, nausea, vomiting, and mood swings. It appears that the depot formulation of buprenorphine may be more acceptable to patients than the daily sublingual preparation (Compton and Volkow, 2021; Lintzeris et al., 2021). Overdose deaths with buprenorphine have been reported, most (94%) involving concomitant use of benzodiazepines (Mariottini et al., 2021).

Tens of thousands of opioid-dependent persons are now being treated with various buprenorphine products. Regarding one's ability to drive, it is imperative to know to what extent buprenorphine affects one's ability to operate an automobile. Researchers evaluated the effects of methadone and buprenorphine on driving performance and neurocognitive function (Strand et al., 2019). Experiments were performed in non-opioid-dependent volunteers. Analgesic doses of buprenorphine produced mild impairments on driving performance and related cognitive skills. Methadone only affected cognitive performance. Effects on opioid-dependent persons receiving buprenorphine were not studied, but are thought to be minimal. Real-world studies on opioid-dependent persons receiving buprenorphine therapies are urgently needed. These studies should include results obtained by officers trained in field sobriety testing and related drug recognition training. The use of buprenorphine in the treatment of opioid abuse disorder is discussed later in this chapter.

Cebranopadol

Another type of opioid receptor that shares analgesic actions with mu opioid receptor agonists is the NOP receptor (nociception receptor; Kiguchi and Ko, 2019). It is another member of the opioid family of GPCR that also includes kappa, delta, and mu receptors. The human gene encoding the NOP receptor has been localized to chromosome 20. Nociceptin is the endogenous ligand of this nociceptin receptor.

Mixed NOP/mu opioid receptor agonists are currently being developed that elicit similar effects to pure mu agonist opioids but potentially with reduced side effects (Coluzz, et al., 2022; Kiguchi et al., 2022; Pacifico et al., 2021). One such agent under development is **cebranopadol**. The drug has been shown to have analgesic efficacy similar to that of morphine in a variety of pain states (Figure 10.8). Researchers reported that, in patients with moderate to severe cancer-related pain, the drug was comparable or superior to morphine with tolerable side effects (Eerdekens et al., 2019). Future development and FDA approvals are as yet unclear.

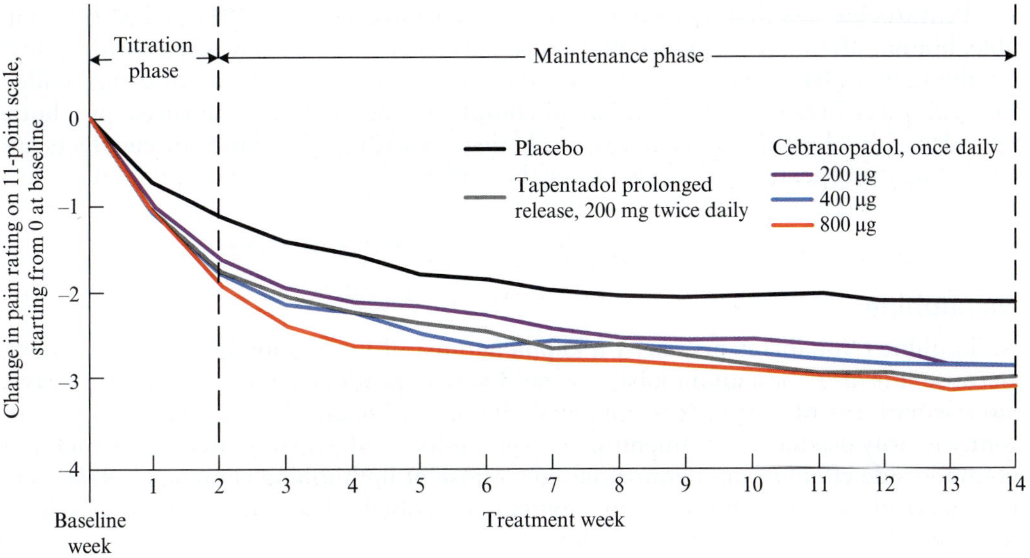

FIGURE 10.8 Pain Relief with Cebranopadol. Change from baseline pain level in weekly average 24-hour pain scores during an initial 2-week initial titration period and 12-week maintenance phase in treating chronic low back pain. Patients received daily doses of cebranopadol, 200, 400, or 600 mg/day, or tapentadol 200 mg twice daily. [Data from: Christoph et al., 2017]

Mixed Agonist–Antagonist Opioids

Three drugs classified as mixed agonist–antagonist opioids remain available in the United States: **butorphanol**, **pentazocine**, and **nalbuphine**. Each of these drugs binds with varying affinity to the mu and kappa receptors. The drugs are weak mu antagonists; most of their limited analgesic effectiveness results from their stimulation of kappa receptors (refer to Table 10.1). Low doses cause moderate analgesia; higher doses produce little additional analgesia. In opioid-dependent people, these drugs precipitate withdrawal. A high incidence of adverse psychotomimetic side effects (dysphoria, anxiety reactions, hallucinations, etc.) is associated with these agents, limiting their therapeutic use.

Butorphanol and Pentazocine

Butorphanol (Stadol) and pentazocine (Talwin) are prototypical mixed agonist–antagonist analgesics. Neither has much potential for producing respiratory depression or physical dependence. In 1993, butorphanol, previously available for use by injection, became available as a nasal spray (the first opioid analgesic so formulated). After it is sprayed into the nostrils, peak plasma levels (and maximal effect) are achieved in 1 hour, with duration of 4 to 5 hours. Use of the nasal spray can result in euphoria, and abuse of butorphanol spray can occur but has not been a major problem. Doctors recommend against using butorphanol during pregnancy, as a neonatal withdrawal syndrome may result following delivery. Today the use of butorphanol is generally limited to veterinary medicine.

Pentazocine was first approved for use in the United States in 1967 and is still available, but not often used. Pentazocine abuse developed, particularly when the drug was combined with tripelennamine, an antihistamine. This combination of drugs, called "Ts and blues," caused serious medical complications, including seizures, psychotic episodes, skin ulcerations, abscesses, and muscle wasting. (The latter three effects are caused by the repeated injections rather than by the drugs themselves.) Following recognition of this abuse, pentazocine was combined with naloxone to prevent injection misuse, and the reported incidence of misuse declined precipitously.

Nalbuphine

Nalbuphine (Nubain) is primarily a kappa agonist of limited analgesic effectiveness. Because it is also a mu antagonist, it is not likely to produce either respiratory depression or patterns of abuse. It is only available in an injectable formulation. It is currently mainly used as a treatment for morphine-induced pruritus (itching), which is a common side effect of mu agonist opioids. Abuse of nalbuphine is unusual. Researchers successfully used nalbuphine in a patient-controlled intravenous technique to limit postoperative pain after colon resection (Jiang et al., 2020).

Other Agonist–Antagonist Combinations

One option for addressing opioid addiction is to make opioid pain medications resistant to tampering. The development of abuse-deterrent formulations is an ongoing effort, and there are numerous approaches under evaluation. One solution is to combine an agonist with an antagonist. In late 2009, the FDA approved the first of these types of medications, a combination of morphine and naltrexone (Embeda ER), a drug discussed later in the chapter in more detail. Embeda extended-release capsules are for oral use and contain pellets of morphine sulfate that surround a core of naltrexone. The naltrexone does not interfere with the analgesic action of morphine, but morphine's abuse potential is considerably reduced. Different dosing regimens are commercially available, all with a morphine-to-naltrexone ratio of 100:4.

As discussed earlier in this chapter, an abuse-deterrent version of OxyContin was introduced in 2010, which, when combined with water, produced a gel-like substance that was hard to inject. Misuse by injecting, snorting, and smoking fell by two-thirds within two years. Another combination product using extended-release oxycodone and naloxone was marketed in 2014 under the trade name Targiniq ER. With this formulation, the oxycodone provides analgesic action, but the naloxone remains in the intestine (not being absorbed when taken orally) and blocks the constipating effect of the oxycodone. When crushed and subsequently injected, the oxycodone remains active, but some naloxone is absorbed, which antagonizes the opioid.

A combination of oxycodone and low-dose naltrexone was developed by the same company that made Embeda. The new drug, Troxyca, was approved in 2016. The capsules contain pellets in which a core of naltrexone is surrounded by extended-release oxycodone hydrochloride. When used as directed, the oxycodone is released as intended while the naltrexone remains sequestered. If the pellets are crushed in an effort to abuse the opioid, naltrexone is released and blocks the effect of the oxycodone. If the dose of naltrexone in the product is sufficient and if the drug is abused by injection, the antagonist would precipitate withdrawal symptoms.

Opioid Antagonists

As stated earlier, opioid antagonists can be and are used in the treatment of opioid overdose, addiction, and dependence. Three pure opioid antagonists are currently clinically available: naloxone, naltrexone, and nalmefene. Each is a structural derivative of oxymorphone, a pure opioid agonist. All three have an affinity for opioid receptors (especially the mu receptor); however, after binding, they exert no agonistic effects of their own. Therefore, they antagonize the effects of opioid agonists, blocking access to the receptor for both endogenous transmitter (e.g., endorphin) and exogenous opioid medicines (e.g., morphine). Such action can reverse any analgesic or respiratory depressant effects and precipitate an acute withdrawal syndrome. Specific agents are discussed later in this chapter.

Novel Opioid-Based Compounds Under Development

Here, we describe a few novel options for pain relief, claimed to have lower side effects, good analgesic effects, and possibly less abuse potential than currently available opioids.

- HS665 is a pure kappa agonist (Guerrieri et al., 2015). Clinical trials with HS665 have not yet been reported. Being devoid of mu receptor agonism, abuse liability should be low, although analgesic activity may also be low. As a kappa agonist, this drug appears to resemble nalbuphine, an older, mixed agonist–antagonist with prominent kappa agonist activity. A 2018 review updates the current status of kappa agonist analgesics and describes experimental agents that have greater selectivity, and potency and presumably less risk of dependence, abuse, and respiratory depression (Zhu et al., 2018).
- Difelikefalin (Korsuva) was FDA approved in late 2021 as another kappa receptor agonist that appears to possess both analgesic and antipruritic (anti-itch) activity. It poorly crosses the blood–brain barrier, and thus its analgesic and antipruritic actions are restricted to the periphery, bypassing many of the abuse and side effect issues of centrally acting agents. Difelikefalin has been shown to reduce severe itching in hemodialysis patients, improving their quality of life (Fishbane et al., 2020).
- Since 2009, nalfurafine, yet another kappa receptor agonist, has been marketed in several countries to treat uremic itching. Currently, the therapeutic potential of nalfurafine is being examined (Meariman et al., 2022; Mores et al., 2019).
- Oxycodegol (Olinvo) is a mu opioid agonist analgesic with a very slow rate of entry into the CNS, presumably limiting its abuse potential. Its analgesic effect

DR. J'S MUSINGS 10.5

More Efficacy with Fewer Side Effects

I remember reading and teaching that when heroin was synthesized, it was purported to be safer than morphine, with less respiratory depression. What a crock!

Virtually all opioids that are effective in relieving severe pain come with a myriad of side effects, some of which are bothersome but can be overcome (itching, nausea, vomiting, constipation), and some of which can be deadly (respiratory depression). As the conflict between the FDA and the manufacturer of Olinvo shows, safety must be unequivocally shown.

What really is needed are new approaches to treating chronic pain with minimal reliance on opioids. This calls for a revolution in thinking. It involves cooperation of prescribers, counselors, and therapists, all working to minimize (not totally eliminate all) pain. With medication, I urge a multilayer approach to treatment:

- Layer 1 is an NSAID (e.g., ibuprofen to maximal doses).
- Layer 2 adds to the NSAID a tricyclic antidepressant (e.g., imipramine; Chapter 12).
- Layer 3 adds to the NSAID and TCA an analgesic mood stabilizer (e.g., gabapentin; Chapter 14).
- Layer 4 adds to the NSAID, TCA, and a cannabinoid mood stabilizer (e.g., CBD or CBD/THC combination; Chapter 9).
- Layer 5 considers use of an opioid for short-term use only IF some pain persists. Of note, Benzodiazepines should be avoided (additive sedation, lack of analgesic action, risks of additive impairment, risks of overdose deaths, risks of elevating levels of other drugs; Chapter 13). In addition, alcohol as well as bedtime sedatives should be discouraged (Chapter 13).

is purportedly similar to that of oxycodone and morphine, with a 90% slower delivery rate into the brain. Its respiratory depression should be low compared to other mu agonists (Gan and Wase, 2020). Manufacturer-sponsored clinical trials have been published (Bergese et al., 2019; Gudin et al., 2020). However, while the drug has been shown to reduce moderate to severe low back pain (Henningfield et al., 2020), as of 2022, its new drug application has been denied by the FDA.

- PF614 is an extended-release oxycodone prodrug, for which fast-tract status from the FDA was granted in 2018. Animal studies with PF614 were reported (Joshi et al., 2019), but human studies have not been published (although Phase 1 clinical studies are underway).
- UMB 425 is a mixed mu agonist–delta antagonist that theoretically results in potent analgesic effects without tolerance liabilities (Healy et al., 2013). Clinical studies have not been reported.

ILLICIT OPIOIDS OF ABUSE

All opioids can be misused. This applies not only to prescription pain products, but also to many substances that are not prescribed medications. Here we review a few notable illicit drugs that have been abused. Some of these have been discussed earlier in this chapter (e.g., heroin and synthetic fentanyl derivatives), and some opioidlike drugs were discussed in Chapter 8 as psychedelic agents (e.g., Kratom).

Heroin

In 1895 the drug company Bayer synthesized diacetylmorphine and branded it **heroin**. Bayer originally claimed heroin was a nonaddictive replacement for morphine. Now, however, it's clear that the nonaddictive claims were delusional. Heroin is a semisynthetic opioid because it is not directly made from the opium poppy, but from morphine, which, as discussed earlier, is directly extracted from the poppy.

Heroin is three times more potent than morphine. The increased lipid solubility of heroin leads to rapid penetration of the blood–brain barrier, producing an intense rush when the drug is injected intravenously. Heroin is metabolized to monoacetylmorphine, which is eventually metabolized and excreted. Because of this, heroin use is suspected when monoacetylmorphine, morphine, and codeine are present in either blood or urine.[11] Of note, urinalysis cannot accurately identify the source of morphine. The morphine metabolite morphine-6-glucuronide may be detected in a patient's urine for two to four days.

Heroin is rarely used medicinally or clinically except, as in the case of the United Kingdom, under restricted clinical guidelines. In the United States, heroin remains illegal.

Synthetic Fentanyl Derivatives

Fentanyl is one of the cheaper drugs sold on the street and is frequently used to mix with more expensive drugs such as heroin and cocaine to increase the potency. However, many people are unaware of the dangerous mix and overdose, as noted earlier. Even prescribed fentanyl medication can prove to be lethal; a speck of powder fentanyl equaling a few grains of salt can kill an adult man. Reviving overdose victims has grown increasingly difficult. Fentanyl overdose victims sometimes require double the amount of naloxone[12] to recover than a heroin overdose victim. Antifentanyl vaccines that block lethal fentanyl doses are under investigation in animals (Baehr et al., 2022), although the number of fentanyl analogues hinders development.

[11]Even poppy seeds contain small amounts of morphine.

[12]As discussed later in this chapter, Kloxxado, a 8-mg nasal spray formulation of naloxone, has been marketed for this purpose.

DR. J'S MUSINGS 10.6

Heroin + Illicit Fentanyl = Death!

I have recently been consulting on several overdose deaths involving injections of heroin contaminated with illicit fentanyl. In one of my reviews, I found it necessary to call and interview a coroner in rural Pennsylvania where one of the deaths occurred. When asked about it, he stated that he had just completed his 150th autopsy in an otherwise totally healthy young person whose only injury was a heroin/fentanyl overdose. What a tragedy!

To that end, several fentanyl analogues have been synthesized. Carfentanyl is a fentanyl derivative approved for use to immobilize large animals, such as elephants, in veterinary practice. Carfentanyl is 10,000 times more potent than morphine and 20 times more potent than fentanyl (Leen and Juurlink, 2019). There have been numerous reports of deaths around the world as a result of carfentanyl, including terrorism attacks and exposure of first responders (Zawilska et al., 2021).

Acetyl fentanyl is another widely found and abused fentanyl analogue responsible for hundreds of deaths. Reasons are unclear, but it is postulated that acetyl fentanyl is less potent, but no less lethal, than fentanyl (Finkelstein et al., 2019).

Another analogue known as alpha-methylfentanyl was identified in heroin that was found in users who had overdosed. Although alpha-methylfentanyl was placed into the Schedule I category in the United States in 1981, it can be detected in contaminated amounts of heroin, often accompanied by another, even more potent analogue, 3-methyl-fentanyl (TMF). TMF was made illegal in 1986 but continued to show up intermittently for a number of years.

Besides carfentanyl, acetyl fentanyl, and alpha-methylfentanyl, perhaps 17 other synthetic fentanyl analogues have been identified, with furanylfentanyl, 4-ANPP, and carfentanyl being most frequently identified in postmortem toxicology (Daniulaityte et al., 2019). Furanylfentanyl was identified in 44% of fatalities, 4-ANPP[13] in 56%, and carfentanyl in 25% (Moody et al., 2018).

Desomorphine

Desomorphine (dihydrodesoxymorphine) is an opioid-derived compound, developed in the United States in 1932. It can be synthesized from codeine with other ingredients such as gasoline, paint thinner, hydrochloric acid, iodine, and red phosphorus (from the striking pads of matchboxes), in a manner similar to the production of methamphetamine

[13]4-ANPP is apparently an active metabolite of furanylfentanyl (Martucci et al., 2018).

from pseudoephedrine. This designer drug began to appear in Russia after first showing up in Siberia in 2002, perhaps because codeine is commonly sold over the counter in Russia. Unfortunately, this homemade mixture has many contaminants, is very toxic, and, when injected, can produce severe tissue damage. The user's skin becomes coarse and scaly at the injection sites, leading to the street name of "krokodil."

U-47700

U-47700 (3,4-dichloro-*N*-[2-(dimethylamino)cyclohexyl]-*N*-methylbenzamide) is a synthetic opioid that was patented in 1978 as an analgesic, although studies in humans had not been published. U-47700, which is known on the street as "pink," "pinky," and "U4," has 7.5 times greater binding affinity for mu opioid receptors than morphine. Effects are said to be very similar to those of morphine and heroin. Citing "an imminent hazard to the public safety," the DEA classified U-47700, which was freely available on the Internet, as a Schedule I substance in 2016. Researchers reviewed the pharmacology and toxicology of U-47700 and analogues (Baumann et al., 2020).

W-18 and W-15

In 2016, police in Florida confiscated 2.5 pounds of a potent, albeit legal, synthetic fentanyl-like opioid called *W-18*. This substance is approximately 10,000 times more potent than morphine and 1000 times more potent than fentanyl. Although it was developed in Canada as an alternative painkiller, it was not manufactured and sold until a Chinese chemist discovered the formula. There is no medical use of W-18 or related drugs such as W-15. Researchers reported that these drugs lack appreciable opioid activity at opioid receptors (Huang et al., 2017; Walker et al., 2021). W-18 and W-15 are potentially fatal at high dosages, and even opioid-tolerant users are at high risk for overdoses. Because of their extreme potency, it is unclear if naloxone also blocks their lethal effects.

Ibogaine

Ibogaine is a naturally occurring substance found in the roots of the iboga tree, *Tabernanthe iboga*, located on the west coast of Central Africa in Gabon and Cameroon. For centuries it has been used for psychedelic and divination purposes. In the 1930s it was used in France under the trade name Lambarene as a stimulant and antidepressant. Anecdotal reports on the drug identified antiaddictive properties, predominantly against opioid and alcohol dependence, reducing withdrawal symptoms, drug cravings, and relapse prevention (Corkery, 2018). Unfortunately, it was removed from the market in 1967 and its use has been limited because of major issues including poor drug availability (for research and clinical use) and a poor safety profile, including cardiotoxicity and resultant deaths. The cardiotoxicity is thought to be the result of QT interval prolongation (Rubi et al., 2017). It also produces long-lasting hallucinations. Currently, ibogaine is classified as a Schedule I compound in the United States.

Mechanistically, ibogaine is metabolized to an active metabolite (noribogaine). Ibogaine's antidepressant effect seems to follow from increases in brain-derived neurotropic factors in the hippocampus (Guez et al., 2020), while its antiaddictive property may follow from its action as a competitive antagonist at cholinergic nicotinic receptors (functioning as a NMDA receptor antagonist) (Corkery, 2018). Despite its toxicities, several ibogaine clinics have been established throughout the world.

Analogues of ibogaine have been developed and examined in order to seek a nonhallucinogenic and noncardiotoxic variant with antiaddictive properties (Cameron et al., 2021). One such compound, *tabernanthalog*, or TBG, has been identified and is under further evaluation. Should initial hopes be realized, TBG may be a significant advance in the treatment of both depression and addiction.

OPIOID TOLERANCE, DEPENDENCE, AND ADDICTION

The development of tolerance and dependence with repeated use is a characteristic feature of all opioid drugs. This reflects a progressive reduction in the ability of opioid receptors to initiate a signal after long-term opioid intake, a phenomenon termed receptor desensitization. The process is thought to involve the uncoupling of the receptors from the G protein, after which the receptors are taken inside the neuron until they are eventually returned to the membrane and resensitized to opioid binding (usually with drug abstinence). Binding of endogenous endorphins is short lived. In contrast, when opioid analgesics are administered for long periods of time, they facilitate tolerance because they are constantly attached to the receptors and interfere with receptor recycling and resensitization.

In other words, when morphine or other opioids are used only intermittently, little if any tolerance develops and the opioids retain their initial efficacy. When administration is repeated, tolerance becomes so marked that very large doses have to be administered to either maintain a degree of euphoria or prevent withdrawal discomfort. The degree of tolerance is illustrated by the fact that the dose of morphine can be increased from clinical doses (50 to 60 milligrams per day) to 500 milligrams per day over as short a period as 10 days.

Tolerance to one opioid leads to cross-tolerance for all other natural and synthetic opioids, even if they are chemically dissimilar. Cross-tolerance, however, does not develop between the opioids and the sedative hypnotics. In other words, a person who has developed a tolerance for morphine will also have a tolerance for other opioid agonists, but not for alcohol or benzodiazepines.

An important point concerning opioid tolerance involves persons who have opioid use disorder and who have become incarcerated. These individuals do not receive opioid maintenance treatment while in prison, lose their tolerance to opioids, and upon release relapse to former levels of opioid use. Such persons are 120 times more likely than persons in the general population to die of an overdose (Berk, 2020), a point made earlier in the chapter.

Physical dependence is an altered physiological state induced by a drug, whereby withdrawal of a drug elicits biological reactions typical for that class of drugs. Generally, symptoms of withdrawal are the opposite of pharmacological effects (Table 10.4).

TABLE 10.4 Pharmacological Effects of Opioids and the Associated Withdrawal Symptoms

Pharmacological Effects	Associated Withdrawal Symptoms
Analgesia	Pain, irritability, hyperalgesia
Respiratory depression	Rapid breathing
Euphoria	Dysphoria, depression
Relaxation, tranquilization, sleep	Agitation, anxiety, insomnia
Constipation	Diarrhea
Pupillary constriction	Pupillary dilation
Peripheral vasodilation; flushed and warm skin	Chilliness and goosebumps
Decreased sex drive	Spontaneous ejaculation
Drying of secretions	Lacrimation, runny nose

Information from Feldman et al., 1997.

The magnitude of these acute withdrawal symptoms depends on the dose of opioid that had been used, the frequency of previous drug administration, and the duration of drug dependence. Acute opioid withdrawal, while extremely uncomfortable and excruciating, is not considered life-threatening. Nevertheless, merely stopping prescribed opioid therapy is generally not an option; as noted, such cessation is often followed by drug seeking, a relapse, and an increased risk for heroin use (Binswanger et al., 2020).

To help alleviate the symptoms of acute withdrawal, several pharmacological approaches have been tried, most of which we will discuss in more detail in the next section. These approaches include methadone (pure agonist) maintenance, buprenorphine (partial agonist) maintenance, and naloxone (pure antagonist) maintenance. Withdrawal discomfort can be further attenuated by use of alpha-2 agonists such as clonidine or lofexidine (Renfro et al., 2020). While use of medications in the treatment of opioid use disorder is cost-effective (Fairley et al., 2021), most persons with this disorder, especially adolescents and older persons, receive no treatment. Indeed, only about 27% of persons requiring treatment received medication assistance in 2019 (Mauro et al., 2022). Despite calls for expanded care, to date little progress has been made (Stephenson, 2022).

In an unusual treatment called rapid anesthesia-aided detoxification (RAAD), a pure opioid antagonist, such as naloxone or naltrexone (covered in the next section), and the sympathetic blocker clonidine are administered intravenously to the opioid-dependent person while they are asleep under general anesthesia. The procedure is appropriate for withdrawal from any opioid. The procedure continues for about 72 hours, during which time the withdrawal signs are blunted. The objective is to enable the patient to tolerate high doses of an opioid antagonist and thus undergo complete detoxification while asleep. After awakening, the patient is maintained on naltrexone and undergoes supportive psychotherapy and group therapies for relapse prevention and to address the underlying causes of addiction. The RAAD technique is controversial, in part because it is expensive, involves the risks of anesthesia, and focuses only on short-term dependence rather than on long-term cravings and social adjustments. Thus, this technique for treating opioid addiction is infrequently used now.

Regardless of the method, there is a protracted opioid abstinence syndrome following acute withdrawal that can persist as long as six months. Symptoms include depression, abnormal responses to stressful situations, drug hunger, anxiety, and other psychological disturbances, as well as other psychiatric disorders. Risk of relapse and overdosing is high, even following release from prison or from a detoxification program (Volkow and McLellan, 2016).

PHARMACOTHERAPY FOR OPIOID OVERDOSE, DEPENDENCE, AND ADDICTION

Most of the long-term effects of opioid abuse can be addressed through treatment, although the damage done can last for years. Additionally, some psychological or physical functioning might be permanently altered; a team of counselors and support groups can help the patient accommodate for their new reality.

For people who have been using opioids for a long time, simply taking acute detoxification ("cold turkey") will cause harmful withdrawal symptoms, which themselves can be dangerous if left untreated. The accepted option is medication-assisted treatment (MAT), in which patients are put on a course of buprenorphine or methadone (as noted earlier) for a period of months. This will allow them to avoid the worst of the withdrawal symptoms while gradually reducing their psychological dependence on stronger opioids such as oxycodone or heroin.

We've mentioned the role of physicians' prescribing patterns in the opioid crisis, and one goal of opioid prevention has been to limit physicians' reliance on opioids for the treatment of noncancerous pain. As stated by researchers:

> Although overprescription of opioid medications triggered the opioid crisis, improving opioid prescription practices for pain management, though important for addressing the opioid crisis, is no longer sufficient. (Volkow et al., 2019a)

In 2022, the, FDA released a draft guidance for the development of nonopioid treatments for acute pain, including trauma and surgery (U.S. Department of Health and Human Services, Food and Drug Administration, 2022). The modest efficacy of opioids in chronic pain management has been discussed as well (Barnett, 2020). Again, while methadone and buprenorphine alone are effective in reducing opioid abuse, do these drugs render psychotherapy or cognitive-behavioral therapy obsolete? Likely not. Most doctors believe that medication treatment on its own is not sufficient for a complete recovery; therapy is needed to address the emotional and mental health damage done by opioid dependence. Mental health programs can also help clients repair relationships with friends and family members and rebuild bridges of trust and communication that were destroyed because of the addiction. Even if medications work in getting a person to stay away from powerful opioids, the mental health processing of therapy and counseling is invaluable for recovery.

When formalized treatment is completed, a person in recovery can join a peer-support program, like Narcotics Anonymous. Based on the 12-step model, these groups provide accountability and support for former opioid addicts who are learning how to live without the constant presence of opioid drugs or medication. The people in these groups know what long-term opioid use looks like, and this solidarity is invaluable for those in the early stages of recovery. Recovering from long-term opioid use is not easy, and some of the changes the abuse brings about could last for years or even a lifetime. However, recovery is always possible. With diligent treatment, hard work, and support, it is possible to live a balanced life after an opioid problem.

Other ways of dealing with opioid addiction continue to be explored. As mentioned, one approach now employed is to try to mitigate the likelihood of overdose death by distributing nasal formulations of naloxone (4- to 8-milligram products are currently available) to heroin users.

Opioid Agonists

Methadone maintenance reduces and/or eliminates the use of heroin, reduces death rates and criminality associated with heroin use, and allows patients to improve their health and social productivity (Joseph et al., 2000). What makes methadone unique as a pure agonist, opioid, or a heroin replacement? In brief, methadone (and a similar drug, levo-alpha acetylmethadol) are well absorbed with oral administration and have long half-lives.

Methadone

Physicians who do not practice in federally licensed methadone treatment programs may not prescribe the drug for the maintenance of opioid dependency; the drug may be prescribed only through licensed methadone maintenance treatment program centers. Currently, efforts are being made to improve patient access and reduce driving times to obtain the drug (Joudrey et al., 2020; Kleinmann, 2020).

The main objectives of methadone maintenance treatment programs are rehabilitation of the dependent person and reduction of diseases associated with needle use, illicit drug use, and crime. Randomized controlled trials have shown that these aims are generally accomplished. Moreover, long-term use is relatively safe; for example, it does not impair cognitive function. Comparison between methadone patients, opioid users, and normal control persons in laboratory tests showed that cognitive function in methadone maintenance patients improved compared to those dependent on illicit opioids.

Although there are a number of predictors of the success of a program, the most important is the magnitude of the daily methadone dose. Programs that prescribe average daily doses exceeding 100 milligrams have higher retention rates and lower illicit drug use rates than those in which the average dose is lower. However, with difficulties posed by COVID-19 restrictions, for stable methadone patients, take-home doses increased markedly without undue increases in diversion and with an average daily dose of about 105 milligrams (Amram et al., 2022; Figgatt et al., 2021).

Even where liberal doses are used (sometimes up to 160 milligrams per day or higher), about one-third of the clients regularly experience withdrawal (known as "nonholders") and two-thirds (known as "holders") do not experience withdrawal on a once-daily dosing schedule. The generally accepted half-life of methadone is 24 hours. The Substance Abuse and Mental Health Services Administration (2021a) published a useful guide to medications for opioid (especially methadone and buprenorphine) use disorder.

Levo-Alpha Acetylmethadol

Levo-alpha acetylmethadol (LAAM) is related to methadone. It is an oral opioid analgesic that was approved in mid-1993 for the clinical management of opioid dependence in heroin addicts. LAAM has a slow onset and a long duration of action (about 72 hours), the latter being a primary advantage over methadone. In maintenance therapy it is administered by mouth three times a week. LAAM is generally considered a second-line treatment for the management of opioid dependence, sometimes used in patients who fail to respond to methadone or buprenorphine.

In general, LAAM and methadone are of equal efficacy as measured by opioid-free urine samples in heroin-dependent persons. Higher doses of methadone (60 to 100 milligrams) and 75- to 115-milligram doses of LAAM both substantially reduced the use of heroin. LAAM is rarely used today due to possible serious cardiac complications.

Buprenorphine

As mentioned, buprenorphine has emerged as a new mainstay of opioid dependence treatment, usually through authorized medical office locations. Indeed, medical practitioners who undergo modest training can prescribe buprenorphine and a buprenorphine–naloxone (Suboxone) combination product for use in the treatment of opioid addiction. Such treatment has been shown to be cost-effective (Fairley et al., 2021), and legislative barriers to treatment are slowly receding (Olsen et al., 2021; Weimer et al., 2021).

In 2021, the Substance Abuse and Mental Health Services Administration (SAMHSA) announced regulations that increased access to buprenorphine and the combination buprenorphine and naloxone (Suboxone) medications in office-based settings. The new rules permitted practitioners to dispense or prescribe Schedule III, IV, or V controlled substances already approved by the FDA without requiring a separate registration to dispense narcotic maintenance and detoxification drugs. Qualified practitioners who filed an initial notification of intent were also allowed to treat a maximum of 30 patients at a time. After one year, practitioners may file a revision indicating an intent to treat up to 100 patients at a time, while a later rule expanded this access to medication-assisted treatment for up to 275 patients. The final rule also incorporates efforts to provide all aspects of evidence-based treatment and to reduce the likelihood that the drugs are misused or diverted. These rules mean that, unlike with methadone, a physician in his or her office can prescribe buprenorphine and buprenorphine/naloxone products for the treatment of opioid dependence.[14] The buprenorphine/naloxone

[14]In April 2021, buprenorphine regulations were altered such that the drug may be prescribed by physicians, physician assistants, and nurse practitioners who have received a waiver allowing them to prescribe the drug to up to 30 patients without first meeting statutory certification requirements.

combination is less liable to abuse, not only because buprenorphine is a partial agonist, but also because the naloxone causes withdrawal if Suboxone is crushed and injected. When used correctly, however, the naloxone is not well absorbed through the GI tract or mucosa and has a minimal withdrawal effect.

Since the introduction of buprenorphine for opioid dependence, its use is increasing (Figure 10.9) at a rate of about 9% per year. The drug can be diverted and is not without problems. Buprenorphine itself can be abused by intravenous injection. It was thought that adding naloxone to the tablet would precipitate withdrawal if it were crushed and injected. However, it turns out that the effect of naloxone is short-lived, and the overall effect is more like taking buprenorphine alone. Likewise, when illicitly injected, both can cause death from overdose. Moreover, even though buprenorphine alone has a ceiling effect, the risk of death with buprenorphine overdose is increased if either benzodiazepines or alcohol is taken at the same time (Wightman et al., 2021). The data from a review of the long-term success with buprenorphine therapy for opioid use disorder were concerning (Williams et al., 2020). The drug is currently dispensed to more than 700,000 persons annually, but the majority of patients who initiate the drug are not retained in care. Between 50% and 80% discontinue the medication within several months of starting treatment. The American Psychiatric Association recommends treatment duration of 180 days (six months), based solely on consensus rather than on empirical evidence. It was reported that buprenorphine abuse is decreasing even as prescriptions for the drug to treat opioid abuse is increasing (Han et al., 2021); the researchers call for expansion of programs to use buprenorphine to treat opioid abuse disorder. Other researchers discussed the efficacy of telemedicine, noting that

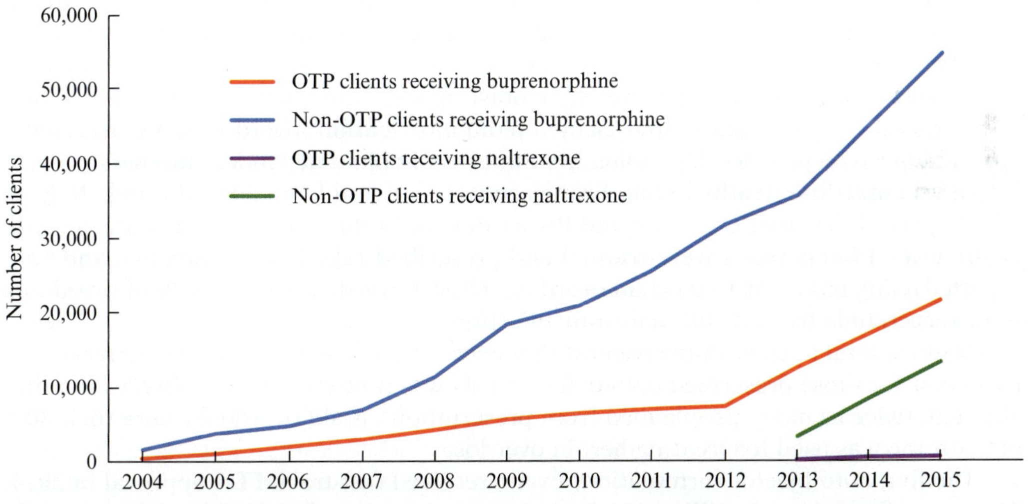

FIGURE 10.9 Opioid Use Disorder Treated with Naltrexone or Buprenorphine. Total number of clients with opioid-use disorder treated yearly from 2004 to 2015 with either naltrexone or buprenorphine. Extended-release naltrexone counts were first collected in 2013. OPT = Opioid treatment program. [Data from "Medications for Opioid Use Disorder." Treatment Improvement Protocol, TIP 63, Substance Abuse and Mental Health Services Administration (SAMUSA), updated 2020.]

remote medicine can be used to treat opioid disorder; diversion of buprenorphine did not appear to be a problem (Barsky et al., 2022). Indeed, lack of access to treatment programs remains a major obstacle to treatment (Morris, 2022; Nguyen et al., 2022; Thakrar, 2022).

Opioid Antagonists

As stated earlier, three pure opioid antagonists are used in the treatment of opioid overdose, addiction, and dependence. These three opioid antagonists, naloxone, naltrexone, and nalmefene, are clinically available. Each is a structural derivative of oxymorphone, a pure opioid agonist. All three have an affinity for opioid receptors (especially the mu receptor); however, after binding, they exert no agonistic effects of their own. Therefore, they antagonize the effects of opioid agonists, blocking access to the receptor for both endogenous transmitter (e.g., endorphin) and exogenous opioid medicines (e.g., morphine). Such action can reverse any analgesic or respiratory depressant effects and precipitate an acute withdrawal syndrome.

Naloxone

Naloxone (Narcan) is the prototype pure opioid antagonist: it has no effect when injected into people who do not use opioids, but it rapidly precipitates withdrawal when injected into opioid-dependent people. Naloxone is neither analgesic nor subject to abuse. Because naloxone is absorbed from neither the GI tract nor the oral mucosa, it must be given by injection. (It can also be administered via nasal spray.) Naloxone injection was first approved for use by clinicians in 1971, and generic versions have been available since 1985 in two doses: 0.4 milligram per milliliter and 1 milligram per milliliter. Naloxone's duration of action is very brief, in the range of 15 to 30 minutes. Thus, for continued opioid antagonism, it must be reinjected at short intervals to avoid return of the depressant effects caused by the longer-acting agonist opioid. Naloxone is used to reverse the respiratory depression that follows acute opioid intoxication (overdoses) and to reverse opioid-induced respiratory depression in newborns of opioid-dependent mothers.

Opioid overdose deaths in San Francisco were studied from 2003 through 2009 as well as part of the Drug Overdose and Prevention and Education project (Enteen et al., 2010). Over 1900 persons were trained and prescribed take-home naloxone, and 11% reported using naloxone to treat an overdose. Of 399 overdose events, 89% of overdoses were successfully treated with naloxone injection.

Many federal agencies now suggest that access to naloxone should be increased, in particular for those prescribed opioid drugs. This was prompted by the observation that although twice as many people died from prescription opioid overdose, more than 80% of naloxone was used for treating heroin overdose.

The first autoinjector formulation, Evzio, received fast-track FDA approval in 2014. This was a fixed-dose, 2-milligram, single-injection product developed to automatically inject the dose into the thigh muscle so that people without medical expertise could reverse an opioid overdose (Harris et al., 2020). Naloxone doses are generally increased and necessary for opioid overdoses involving illicit fentanyl-contaminated products (Carpenter et al., 2020).

The first nasal spray formulation (a 4-milligram dose) was fast-tracked in 2015, followed by a second 2-milligram dose (also marketed as Narcan) in January 2017. Currently available are several formulations of FDA-approved nasal sprays containing naloxone to treat opioid overdose: (1) naloxone nasal spray, 4 milligrams, (2) Zimhi, a prefilled syringe containing 5 milligrams of naloxone, and (3) Kloxxado nasal spray, containing 8 milligrams of naloxone. The latter can deliver a higher dose of naloxone and may be more effective in treating overdoses that are more difficult to reverse, specifically from polydrug reactions involving synthetic fentanyl or its derivatives.

Researchers published a comparative study of various intramuscular and intranasal naloxone products (Strang et al., 2019). Blood concentrations following drug administration are illustrated in Figure 10.10. Note the rapid rise and fall in the naloxone concentration following intravenous administration and the slower rise and prolonged duration following intramuscular administration. Intranasal administration results in a rise almost as fast as intramuscular injection. The graph shows blood concentrations following a 2-milligram nasal spray. Narcan nasal spray commonly administers 4 milligrams. Had that 4-milligram dose been studied, it is likely that the concentration in blood would have approached 4 milligrams by the intramuscular route. The development of the nasal product and the necessary patient instruction labeling for use of the product have been described (B. R. Cohen and coworkers (2020)).

Naltrexone

Naltrexone (Revia) became clinically available in 1985 as the first orally absorbed, pure opioid antagonist approved for the treatment of heroin dependence. An extended-release injectable formulation taken once a month is marketed under the trade name Vivitrol. The actions of naltrexone resemble those of naloxone, but naltrexone is well

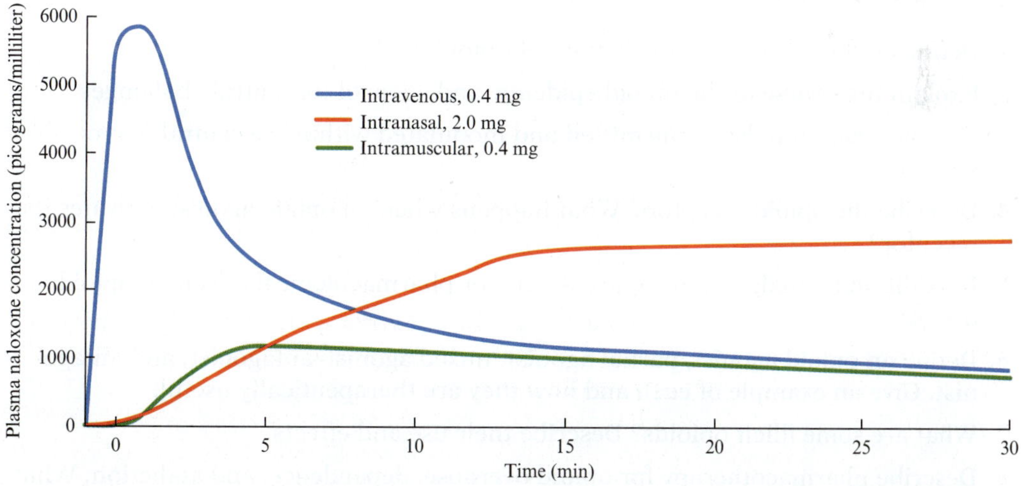

FIGURE 10.10 Plasma Concentrations of Naloxone. In healthy volunteers over a 30-minute period following intranasal, intramuscular, or intravenous administration. Concentrations shown in picograms per liter. [Data from Strang et al., 2019.]

absorbed orally and has a long duration of action, necessitating only a single oral daily dose of about 40 to 100 milligrams. In people who take naltrexone daily, injection of an opioid agonist such as heroin is ineffective. Naltrexone can cause nausea (which can be quite severe in some people) and dose-dependent liver toxicity. One problem with naltrexone is that the drug must be taken in order to be effective. Trite as that sounds, the opioid-dependent person must choose between taking naltrexone or returning to heroin use.

Today, naltrexone is used primarily to treat alcoholism. Naltrexone reportedly decreases heavy drinking, the number of days that alcohol is consumed, and the total amount of alcohol consumed, although the overall benefit has been described as "modest." The mechanism is believed to be due to antagonism of endorphin, elicited by drinking alcohol, rather than from an as-yet-unidentified action outside the opioid system.

Naltrexone has also been reported to have benefits in some other medical conditions, for example, a preventive role in reducing self-injurious behaviors. Effects, however, are weak.

Nalmefene

Nalmefene (Selincro) is a third pure opioid antagonist. Developed in the early 1970s, it is used mainly to treat alcohol dependence and has been investigated for the treatment of other addictions such as pathological gambling. Compared to naltrexone, the advantages of nalmefene include longer half-life, greater oral bioavailability, and few cases of liver toxicity. If given to people who are dependent on opioids or postoperatively for reversal of surgically administered opioids, nalmefene can precipitate acute withdrawal symptoms.

CHAPTER REVIEW

1. Define an opioid. What is the history of opioid use?
2. Explain the course of the opioid epidemic and some of its central challenges.
3. How are pain impulses transmitted and modulated within the central nervous system?
4. Describe the opioid receptors. What happens when an opiate agonist activates its receptor?
5. In addition to analgesia, what are the major pharmacological effects of opioid drugs?
6. Define an opioid agonist, partial agonist, mixed agonist–antagonist, and antagonist. Give an example of each and how they are therapeutically useful.
7. What are some illicit opioids? Describe their use and effects.
8. Describe pharmacotherapy for opioid overdose, dependence, and addiction. What are the various options for management of dependence and relapse? Explain the opioid agonists that are used as well as the antagonists that are used.

KEY TERMS

buprenorphine
butorphanol
ceiling effect
cebranopadol
codeine
desomorphine
fentanyl
heroin
hydrocodone
hydromorphone
ibogaine
levo-alpha acetylmethadol (LAAM)
meperidine
methadone
morphine
nalbuphine
nalmefene
naloxone
naltrexone
oliceridine
opioid
opioid receptors
opium
opium poppy (*Papaver somniferum*)
oxycodone
oxymorphone
pain
paregoric
pentazocine
propoxyphene
tapentadol
tramadol
U-47700

PART 3

Psychotherapeutic Drugs

The four chapters in this part introduce the drugs that are used to treat psychological disorders. These medications include the first-generation and second-generation ("atypical") antipsychotics (Chapter 11), the antidepressants (Chapter 12), the medications used classically to treat anxiety and insomnia (Chapter 13), and the medications for treating bipolar disorder (Chapter 14).

Since the 1950s, important advances have been made in the pharmacological treatment of psychological disorders, allowing affected people to lead much more "normal" lives than ever before in human history. Progress began with the first wave, or first generation, of antipsychotic drugs (for the treatment of schizophrenia), the first two categories of antidepressant drugs, anxiolytics, and mood stabilizers. The first modern precursor of all these psychiatric medications was discovered prior to the 1970s. The next wave of development occurred in the late 1980s with the advent of the second-generation drugs for the treatment of schizophrenia and treatment-resistant depression. Nevertheless, since those early periods of rapid development of successful drugs to treat schizophrenia, depression, anxiety, and bipolar disorder, further progress has stalled. There have been few real advances in the treatment of schizophrenia, depression, anxiety, and bipolar disorder since the advent of the second-generation agents. The goals of these next four chapters are to impart a sense of the historical development of therapeutics for each of these disorders, to describe the pharmacology of drugs currently being used to treat these disorders, to convey the disappointment in the lack of current progress in these areas, but to also show that research is still ongoing to find new and better treatment options.

The drugs are organized in these chapters under descriptive headings (antidepressants, mood stabilizers, antipsychotics, and so forth), but their application is much broader than indicated by these headings. For example, besides being used to relieve major depression, antidepressants are used as antianxiety drugs and analgesics. Many of the mood stabilizers, besides being used to treat bipolar disorder, are used to treat chronic pain syndromes, psychological disorders associated with agitation and aggression, and even substance abuse. Antipsychotic drugs, besides being used to treat schizophrenia, are being used to treat bipolar disorder, explosive and aggressive disorders, autism, and other pervasive developmental disorders. Newer antipsychotic agents are being used to treat depression and dysthymia. Nevertheless, the artificial distinctions are maintained to present the pharmacology of the drugs in a logical manner.

CHAPTER 11

Antipsychotic Drugs

CHAPTER OUTLINE

The **antipsychotic drugs** discussed in this chapter can be used to treat a variety of psychiatric disorders, particularly those disorders that present with psychotic, hallucinogenic, or delusional symptoms. But, as you will see later in this chapter, many of the newer drugs can be used to treat other psychiatric disorders, even if no psychotic symptoms are present.

SCHIZOPHRENIA

Schizophrenia is one of the most severe mental diseases. It presents as a psychiatric syndrome characterized by psychotic symptoms of hallucinations, delusions, and disorganized speech and behavior; by negative symptoms such as decreased motivation and diminished expressiveness; and by cognitive deficits involving impaired executive functions, memory, and speed of mental processing (Marder and Cannon, 2019). Researchers (Jonas et al., 2022) discuss the time course of cognitive decline in schizophrenia. The onset of schizophrenia occurs primarily in late adolescence to early adulthood. It affects about 1% of the world's population and is a major cause of disability (Goff, 2021).

The cause—or causes—of schizophrenia are currently unknown. At present, schizophrenia is considered a polygenetic disorder with genetics playing a large role. When one parent has the disorder, the probability of any child having the disorder is 7%; when both parents have the disorder, the probability that any child will have the disorder increases to 27%. In fraternal twins, if one twin has the disorder, the risk the other twin will also have the disorder is 6–14%. In identical twins, the risk that if one twin has the disorder, the other twin will also have the disorder rises to 33–60% (Hilker et al., 2018). Large-scale genetic studies have identified 108 genetic markers that are associated with an increased risk for developing schizophrenia. However, at present, genetic testing cannot be used to diagnosis a disorder, select treatment medications, or predict response to treatment (Geschwind and Flint, 2015). Ethical issues have also been raised about the use of these tests to predict that an individual will eventually develop disorders such as schizophrenia and base treatment upon the findings (DeLisi, 2014).[1]

Much of the recent research has suggested the influence of an array of risk factors, including early-life environmental and genetics, for developing schizophrenia (McCutcheon et al., 2020b). These risk factors occur during the prenatal, perinatal, and postnatal periods and include maternal stress, maternal infections, nutritional deficiencies, and pregnancy and birth complications. Socioeconomic factors such as childhood poverty, other childhood adversities, immigration status, a late winter or early spring birth, and having an older father have also been linked to an increased risk for developing schizophrenia (Owen et al., 2016). Lastly, adolescents who are frequent users of

[1]For example, there could be potential harm to the individual if antipsychotic medications are used as preemptive treatment based on the results of the test, without knowing if the individual would actually develop the disorder; exposing the individual to the stigma of attaching a diagnostic label based on a genetic test could affect their ability to get a job or health insurance.

marijuana may be at risk for developing psychotic symptoms or experiencing worsening of symptoms:

> Once schizophrenia has developed, patients should be advised that use of marijuana or synthetic cannabinoids has the potential to worsen the course of the illness and to provoke violence and suicidality. (Marder and Cannon, 2019)

Schizophrenia is associated with a life expectancy of 10–25 years shorter than that of the general population as well as a large increase in mortality from suicides (Huang et al., 2021). This mortality risk is related more to lifestyle and comorbidity risk factors than to the genetic aspects of the disorder. These risk factors include higher rates of smoking, higher rates of substance use disorders, poor diets, lack of exercise, lack of access to primary health care, poor attention to treatment for chronic medical conditions, and increased cardiovascular diseases. Some of these risk factors may be related to or exacerbated by the side effects of the treatment medications for schizophrenia. An interesting study from Finland suggests that use of antipsychotic medications regularly, in particular, the long-acting depot formulations, can actually reduce mortality rates of individuals with schizophrenia by up to 40–50% compared to individuals with schizophrenia who do not take their medications regularly (Taipale et al., 2018). In a 20-year follow-up study of over 62,000 patients in Finland with schizophrenia (Taipale et al., 2020), researchers found that long-term use of antipsychotic medication "did not increase severe physical morbidity and is associated with substantially decreased mortality, especially among patients treated with clozapine (a classic antipsychotic)."

Neurochemistry

The most frequently studied neurotransmitters in schizophrenia have been dopamine and glutamate (McCutcheon et al., 2020a). The focus on these neurotransmitters has stemmed from observations that stimulant drugs such as amphetamine release dopamine and may produce some symptoms similar to schizophrenia in normal individuals. Also, stimulants may exacerbate underlying positive symptoms (hallucinations and delusions) in individuals who have schizophrenia. Finally, drugs such as phencyclidine (PCP) and ketamine can exacerbate positive symptoms in individuals who have schizophrenia. Therefore, based on these observations and the synaptic relationship among these neurotransmitter systems, there continues to be interest in understanding if any of these neurotransmitters or combinations of neurotransmitters can be involved in the pathophysiology of schizophrenia. However, although there have been numerous hypotheses or theories about neurochemical disturbances that would explain the development of schizophrenia, none of the neurochemical models completely explain the phenotypic presentation of behaviors associated with the disorder.

Dopamine Involvement

The dopamine system is, in some way, involved in the pathophysiology of schizophrenia. All drugs that have efficacy as antipsychotics block dopamine receptors. Furthermore, of all the different types of dopamine receptors (D_1, D_2, D_3, D_4, and D_5),

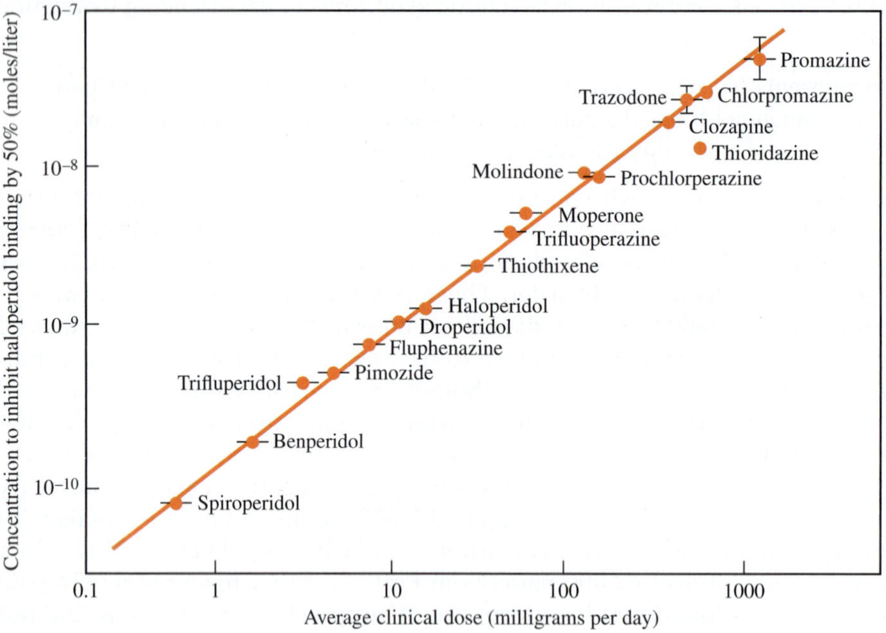

FIGURE 11.1 Dopamine Receptor Blockage and Clinical Dose of Antipsychotic Drugs. Correlation between the clinical potency and receptor-binding activities of neuroleptic drugs. Clinical potency is expressed as the daily dose used in treating schizophrenia, and binding activity is expressed as the concentration needed to produce 50% inhibition of haloperidol binding. Haloperidol binds to dopamine D_2 receptors; other antipsychotic drugs compete for the same receptors. Thus, measuring the competitive inhibition of haloperidol binding correlates with potency of an antipsychotic drug.

all effective antipsychotic drugs block the D_2 receptor. Not only do all antipsychotic drugs have an affinity for the D_2 receptor, but this affinity is also the single best predictor of the effective clinical dose of an antipsychotic (Figure 11.1). Using SPECT (single photon emission computed tomography), researchers found that amphetamine caused an increased release of dopamine in one area of the brain, the striatum, and also caused a worsening of symptoms. This effect was only observed at the beginning of the person's illness, when they had acute symptoms, or at times when there was an exacerbation of symptoms to the point that the person was considered acutely ill (Chang et al., 2020). No such changes were found when the individual was stable and not expressing symptoms. These results suggest that the expression of schizophrenic symptoms in individuals with the disorder is related in part to an underlying dysregulation in dopamine transmission that may be state related, that is, acutely ill versus stable.

Dopamine, released by neurons in the basal ganglia of the brain, is crucial for maintaining normal coordination of movement. In fact, the loss of these neurons in the basal ganglia is responsible for the neurological disorder called **Parkinson's**

disease. Similarly, by blocking dopamine receptors, antipsychotic drugs produce neurological side effects similar to Parkinson's disease, known as **extrapyramidal symptoms** (EPS), because the drugs affect the dopamine neurons in the extrapyramidal motor system. Long-term antipsychotic administration may also elicit another syndrome of abnormal motor function called **tardive dyskinesia** (TD). A more detailed description of extrapyramidal symptoms and tardive dyskinesia is presented later in this chapter.

All drugs that block the dopamine D_2 receptor have the potential to produce both extrapyramidal symptoms and tardive dyskinesia. Clinical experience has shown that the risk of producing these side effects is greatly reduced, but not eliminated, when using the second-generation antipsychotic medications discussed later in this chapter.

Glutamate Involvement

While dopamine is certainly involved in the pathogenesis of schizophrenia, that involvement may be downstream from other processes. Certainly, the wide variety of expressions of symptoms of schizophrenia suggest the involvement of other neurotransmitter systems, one of which is glutaminergic neurotransmission.

As we discussed in Chapter 2, glutamate is the major excitatory neurotransmitter in the brain, involved in learning and memory. And as we discussed in Chapter 8, PCP and ketamine act as antagonists at NMDA-type glutamate neurons and mimic many of the symptoms seen in schizophrenia. As stated by researchers (McCutcheon et al., 2020a):

> The administration of NMDA-glutamate receptor antagonists, such as phencyclidine and ketamine, has been repeatedly shown to induce manifestations similar to the positive, negative, and cognitive symptoms of schizophrenia. It has been demonstrated that NMDA receptor blockade by these compounds is both necessary and sufficient for their psychotomimetic effects.

Based on this and other evidence, it has been hypothesized that NMDA receptor hypofunction results in downstream effects on striatal dopamine, glutamate, and gamma aminobutyric acid (GABA) that may underlie the deterioration seen in patients with schizophrenia.

Serotonin Involvement

Besides dopamine and glutamate, other neurotransmitter dysfunctions may contribute to the pathogenesis of schizophrenia and provide targets for medication therapy. Early investigations into the possible role of serotonin in schizophrenia followed from observations that the psychedelic drugs such as lysergic acid diethylamide (LSD) can produce hallucinations. Therefore, drugs such as LSD were initially proposed to be involved in the clinical syndrome seen in schizophrenia. LSD is one of a group of hallucinogenic drugs that are thought to exert their psychedelic effect as agonists at $5\text{-HT}2_A$

receptors. For this reason, it was hypothesized that 5-HT2 receptor antagonism might be responsible for some of the beneficial actions of antipsychotics. Although it has since been concluded that serotonin does not play an important role in the etiology of schizophrenia, antagonism of serotonin at 5-HT2 receptors may be involved in the improved neurological side effect profile of the newer antipsychotic medications.[2] Recently, a drug that exerts inverse agonist and antagonistic effects at 5-HT2_A receptors, pimavanserin (Nuplazid), has been marketed for the treatment of hallucinations and delusions that occur in some patients with Parkinson's disease and dementia-related psychosis (Tampi et al., 2019; Yunusa et al., 2020).

Cannabinoid Involvement

As we have discussed, the main psychoactive component of cannabis is tetrahydrocannabinol (THC). THC acts as a partial agonist of cannabinoid-1 receptors, and use of THC can induce psychotic symptoms and cognitive deficits seen in patients with schizophrenia (Borgan et al., 2019; Hasan et al., 2020). Synthetic cannabinoid agonists are more potent pure agonists and even more likely to induce schizophreniclike behaviors and symptoms. Cannabidiol (CBD), on the other hand, acts as a cannabinoid antagonist; the drug exerts antipsychotic beneficial effects with cognitive improvements (Kozela et al., 2020). These data suggest that cannabinoid-1 receptors may be a potential target for treatment of psychotic disorders.

TAARS Involvement

Beyond traditional neurotransmitters, many other intracerebral chemicals affect brain function. Recently, attention has been focused on trace amine-associated receptors (TAARs) and drugs that activate or block their actions. These TAARs are predominantly intracellular and have a role in body homeostasis (Dodd et al., 2021). They interact with the catecholamine system and are involved in regulating AMP signaling and potassium channels. There are nine subfamilies of TAARs, and at least one of these is postulated to be involved in schizophrenia (TAAR1), substance abuse, obesity, and the metabolic syndrome (Dodd et al., 2021). Others seem to be involved in addiction, depression, and anxiety. One of these (SEP-363856, Ulotaront) has received FDA Breakthrough Therapy designation for the treatment of schizophrenia (Correll et al., 2021; Dedic et al., 2019; Koblan et al., 2020a, 2020b). SEP-363856 is thought to be an agonist at the TAAR1 and serotonin 5-HT1_A receptors. This mechanism of action is unique among available antipsychotics, which generally antagonize dopamine D_2 receptors.

[2]For a detailed discussion of the relationship of the various serotonin receptors to the symptoms observed in schizophrenia, see Meltzer (2012). This review also discusses the differences between the first-generation antipsychotics and the newer second-generation antipsychotics based on the differences in their mechanism of action at the various dopamine and serotonin receptors.

Did You Know?

Genetic Involvement

As discussed, there has been substantial advancement in the technology for studying genetics. In particular, genome-wide association studies (GWASs) have been employed to examine the human genome in an effort to detect the genetic locus of the major psychiatric disorders such as schizophrenia and link a disease risk with a specific area of the genome. This is a highly technical and complex process that searches the genome for evidence of variations that are called single-nucleotide polymorphisms (SNPs) or copy number variants (CNVs). GWAS technology is used to identify which SNPs or CNVs occur more frequently in individuals who have a particular disorder compared to individuals without the disorder. Using this information, researchers attempt to pinpoint genes or sections of genes that may increase the risk for having the disorder. Using GWAS, researchers report that genes that code for the dopamine receptor, such as the DRD_2 gene, are involved in the pathophysiology of schizophrenia, as are genes associated with the glutamate neurotransmitter system. These findings are important because they continue to support the role of the neurotransmitter dopamine in schizophrenia and drugs that block the dopamine receptor, particularly the D_2 receptor, as effective antipsychotic drugs. In addition, recent clinical trials have focused on testing drugs that affect the glutamate system. Although these trials have not yielded positive results, glutamate remains an area for continued examination for its involvement in the treatment for schizophrenia.

Another study has pointed to the major histocompatibility complex (MHC), a region of the genome containing genes associated with the body's immune system, as also playing a role in the pathophysiology of schizophrenia. More recently, researchers have shown that within the major histocompatibility complex, the risk of schizophrenia is most closely linked to the C4 gene, such that the higher the expression of the C4A subtype, the greater the risk of developing schizophrenia. The relationship of the C4A gene to the developmental process of synaptic pruning makes this finding especially intriguing. Humans are born with redundancies in synaptic connections, and as the brain develops, it goes through a process of eliminating unneeded or unused synapses. The C4 gene is thought to be involved in this pruning process. Researchers (Sekar et al., 2016) found that an upregulation of the expression of the C4 gene results in a greater degree of synaptic pruning. Since there is evidence of loss of cortical gray matter or cortical thinning in individuals with schizophrenia (Chung et al., 2017), this finding of an abnormally energetic pruning process may help explain the neuroanatomical findings. This loss of neuronal connections due to excessive pruning may also relate to the expression of both negative symptoms and cognitive deficits in schizophrenia.

None of these genetic or neurochemical models completely explain the phenotypic presentation of behaviors associated with schizophrenia. Schizophrenia is understood to be multiple related disorders involving multiple genetic markers. Furthermore, serotonin antagonists alone are not effective in the treatment of schizophrenia, nor are GABA or glutamate antagonists effective antipsychotics. The only consistent finding thus far is that any drug shown to be effective in the treatment of schizophrenia has to block dopamine receptors, primarily the D_2 receptor.

HISTORICAL BACKGROUND AND CLASSIFICATION OF ANTIPSYCHOTIC MEDICATIONS

The first drug to be used as a treatment for schizophrenia was developed from a class of compounds known as *phenothiazines*. The first phenothiazine was derived from antihistamines. Antihistamines were being used at the time to reduce the agitation of patients experiencing postsurgical shock due to their sedative effect and the understanding that histamine release was involved in the shock reaction. In 1951, Paul Charpentier, working for a French pharmaceutical company, synthesized a new phenothiazine, **chlorpromazine.** Once released to the market in 1952, the French anesthesiologist and surgeon Henri Laborit used chlorpromazine in his "lytic cocktail," an anesthetic mix of drugs administered prior to surgery to deepen anesthesia and reduce body temperature with the goal of preventing postsurgical shock. Laborit found that adding chlorpromazine to his anesthetic cocktail had several beneficial effects: reducing the number of anesthetic drugs a patient needed; producing sedation without clouding of consciousness; and producing a state of indifference, analgesia, and hypothermia, which we now know are characteristic of these drugs.

Later the same year, based on Laborit's report of the effect of chlorpromazine on his surgical patients, the French psychiatrists Jean Delay and Pierre Deniker began to use it to treat their agitated patients at Sainte-Anne's Hospital in Paris. Although chlorpromazine did not provide a permanent cure, it was found to be remarkably effective in alleviating the clinical manifestations of psychosis in psychiatric patients. Chlorpromazine was marketed in France under the trade name Largactil in 1952 and in the United States as Thorazine in 1954. Unfortunately, chlorpromazine had many side effects (discussed later), so research continued for equally effective medications with fewer side effects. These early drugs, in which antipsychotic actions could not be separated from neurological side effects (e.g., drug-induced Parkinsonism and tardive dyskinesias), are now referred to as **first-generation antipsychotics**.

DR. J'S MUSINGS 11.1

The Greatest Advance in Psychopharmacology?

Prior to 1955, effective drugs for treating schizophrenia were virtually nonexistent, with schizophrenic patients usually permanently or semipermanently hospitalized. By 1955, more than half a million people were residing in psychiatric hospitals. With the introduction of chlorpromazine shortly thereafter, the numbers of hospitalized schizophrenic patients began a rapid downward trend, reaching a current level of about 170,000 beds. This decline occurred despite a doubling in admission rates and coincided with the introduction of antipsychotic drugs, most notably chlorpromazine. Today, inadequate community-based funding and care remains a continuing problem. Regardless, the introduction of chlorpromazine and other phenothiazines remains as perhaps one of the single greatest achievements in psychopharmacology (Ban, 2007; Pow et al., 2015).

Clozapine was discovered in 1959, and in 1966 it was found to have antipsychotic efficacy without the disabling neurological side effects that were seen with chlorpromazine and other phenothiazine antipsychotics. As a result, clozapine became the first of the **second-generation antipsychotics**. Interestingly, the fact that clozapine did not produce neurological side effects dampened enthusiasm for it. This was due to the mistaken notion at the time that in order for a drug to be an effective antipsychotic, it had to produce neurological side effects. In addition, during clinical trials using clozapine in Finland in 1975, 18 subjects developed a blood disorder known as agranulocytosis, and nine of them died. Agranulocytosis occurs when the body does not produce enough white blood cells to fight off infections. This side effect was attributed to clozapine, and, as a result, restrictions were placed on its use in Europe beginning in 1975, and the development and testing process in the United States was halted indefinitely in 1976. The restrictions imposed in Europe included the requirement for regular laboratory blood work to measure white blood cells. Between 1976 and 1982, the use of clozapine in Europe actually expanded, and by measuring white blood cell levels during treatment, the onset of agranulocytosis was detected early enough to stop the medication and avoid mortality. Furthermore, during this time, researchers and clinicians were reporting remarkable outcomes in those patients who were able to continue treatment with clozapine without developing agranulocytosis. Based on these continued reports of positive outcomes coming out of Europe, work on the drug resumed in the United States, and in 1990 the FDA approved clozapine, subject to continued monitoring for agranulocytosis. Under these conditions, the clinical trials demonstrated clozapine's effectiveness as an antipsychotic and the absence of neurological side effects. In 1990, clozapine was approved for the U.S. market.

Confusingly, the second-generation antipsychotics are also widely referred to as *atypical antipsychotics* when compared to the first-generation antipsychotics. This is so because these atypical agents have a much lower risk of producing neurological (Parkinsonian) and metabolic side effects (such as obesity and diabetes, discussed later). Following clozapine's approval, pharmaceutical companies began marketing other drugs that had properties similar to clozapine but without the risk of developing agranulocytosis, Parkinsonian, and metabolic side effects. Success varies between individual agents.

The distinguishing characteristic of the second-generation antipsychotic medications' mechanism of action is that, although they still block the dopamine D_2 receptors, they also block one additional and specific serotonin receptor, the 5-HT2 receptor. Also, their potency at blocking these serotonin receptors needs be greater than their potency at blocking the dopamine receptor. For some (unknown) reason, greater affinity for the serotonin receptor over the dopamine receptor allows a separation between antipsychotic efficacy and induction of extrapyramidal symptoms or other movement disorders.[3]

[3]Ramachandraiah et al., 2009 discuss the history of antipsychotic drugs from their serendipitous discovery in the 1950s through development of the "atypical" antipsychotics in the 1990s. Other researchers (De Risio and Lang, 2014) follow this with the history and development of the long-acting antipsychotic agents.

FIRST-GENERATION ANTIPSYCHOTICS

The first-generation antipsychotics are drugs that were, and often continue to be, widely used to treat schizophrenia (Table 11.1), even though today they may seem out-of-date and used less often than the second-generation antipsychotics. Some of them also have a few other FDA-approved indications such as in the treatment of bipolar disorder, behavioral problems, hyperactivity, agitation, and anxiety (Table 11.2). Furthermore, these antipsychotics are also used "off-label" (see Dr. J's Musings 11.2 later in the chapter) for other disorders in which psychotic symptoms, such as hallucinations, delusions, and severe thought disorder, are present. The **phenothiazines** are the prototypes of these first-generation agents.

Pharmacokinetics

First-generation antipsychotics are lipid soluble and highly bound to protein and tissue, with large volumes of distribution. Oral absorption is unpredictable, and several of them undergo first-pass metabolism in the liver, which means that oral bioavailability is low or variable. Most first-generation antipsychotics have long half-lives (20–40 hours), which allows doses to be given only once or twice a day after reaching steady-state levels. All first-generation antipsychotics are extensively metabolized by the liver,

TABLE 11.1 First-generation Antipsychotic Drugs

Generic name	Trade name	Dose equivalent (mg)[a]	Formulation[b]	Age group[c]
Chlorpromazine	Thorazine	100	PO; Sol; IM	C; A; AD
Prochlorperazine	Compazine	15	Suppository	C; A; AD
Fluphenazine	Prolixin	2	PO; Elixir; IM; Sol; LAI	AD
Trifluoperazine	Stelazine	5	PO; IM; Sol	C; AD
Perphenazine	Trilafon	8	PO	C; A; AD
Thioridazine	Mellaril	100	PO	C; A; AD
Thiothixene	Navane	4	PO	A; AD
Haloperidol	Haldol	2	PO; IM; LAI	C; A; AD
Loxapine	Loxitane	10	PO	A; AD
Molindone	Moban	10	PO	A; AD
Pimozide	Orap	2	PO	A; AD

[a]Dose equivalence: all drug doses are equated to 100 milligrams of chlorpromazine.
[b]Formulation: PO = oral, usually tablets or capsules; Sol = oral solution; Elixir = oral solution in suspension; IM = intramuscular injectable solution; LAI = long-acting injectable solution, usually one injection every 2 to 4 weeks.
[c]Age group: C = children (1–9 years old); A = adolescent (10–17 years old); AD = adult (≥18 years old).

TABLE 11.2 FDA Indications for First-generation Antipsychotic Drugs

Generic name	Trade name	Indications
Chlorpromazine	Thorazine	Schizophrenia; nausea; presurgical sedation; bipolar disorder, manic phase; intractable hiccups; hyperactivity; severe behavior problems
Prochlorperazine	Compazine	Schizophrenia; generalized anxiety; severe nausea and vomiting
Fluphenazine	Prolixin	Psychosis
Trifluoperazine	Stelazine	Schizophrenia; generalized anxiety disorder
Perphenazine	Trilafon	Schizophrenia; nausea and vomiting
Thioridazine	Mellaril	Schizophrenia
Thiothixene	Navane	Schizophrenia
Haloperidol	Haldol	Psychosis; Tourette syndrome; hyperactivity; severe childhood behavior problems
Loxapine	Loxitane	Schizophrenia
Molindone	Moban	Schizophrenia
Pimozide	Orap	Tourette syndrome

and some have active metabolites. Metabolites of some of the phenothiazines can be detected for several months after the drug has been discontinued.

Pharmacological Effects

As noted earlier in this chapter, the effectiveness of the first-generation antipsychotics as antipsychotic agents is related to their ability to block the dopamine D_2 receptor. But, as we shall discuss, blocking dopamine receptors also contributes to some of the side effects of these drugs. Other side effects occur because these drugs also block acetylcholine (muscarinic), histamine, serotonin, and norepinephrine receptors. Cholinergic blockade produces dry mouth, dilated pupils, blurred vision, cognitive impairments, constipation, urinary retention, and tachycardia. Histaminergic blockade produces sedation as well as beneficial antiemetic effects. Blockade of the serotonin receptors is related to part of the therapeutic efficacy as well as side effects of sedation and weight gain. Noradrenergic blockade can result in hypotension and sedation. Lastly, through actions on the brain stem, antipsychotics suppress the centers involved in behavioral arousal, the ascending reticular activating system and inhibit vomiting by affecting dopamine receptors in the chemoreceptor trigger zone. These drugs do not depress respiration, nor are they analgesic (pain relieving).

All of the first-generation antipsychotics are equally effective in reducing the psychotic (positive) symptoms related to schizophrenia and the other disorders that can also present with psychotic symptoms, such as bipolar disorder and severe major depressive disorder. Although they have been shown in the short term to reduce positive symptoms, they have not been shown to consistently reduce either the negative or cognitive symptoms of schizophrenia.

Negative Symptoms

Dopaminergic neurons of the central midbrain portion of the brain stem project to limbic structures (mesolimbic pathway), which regulate emotional expression, as well as to forebrain areas (mesocortical pathway), where emotion and cognition are integrated. It is believed that antipsychotics, by blocking dopamine D_2 receptors in the mesolimbic or mesocortical pathways, reduce the intensity of schizophrenic delusions, hallucinations, and thought disorder, that is, the **positive symptoms** of schizophrenia. Besides positive symptoms, individuals who have schizophrenia may also display negative symptoms and cognitive impairment. **Negative symptoms** of schizophrenia include deficits in communication skills, emotion, or affect; social or interpersonal skills; motivation; and psychomotor activity. As stated by researchers (Correll and Schooler, 2020):

> . . . primary negative symptoms generally do not respond well to currently available antipsychotic treatment with dopamine D_2 antagonists or partial D_2 agonists.

Side Effects and Toxicity

To more easily describe the typical side effects associated with the first-generation antipsychotics, we can divide these agents into two broad categories: low-potency drugs and high-potency drugs (Table 11.3). The low-potency agents are those drugs that require higher oral doses to achieve a certain level of occupancy of the dopamine receptors. The prototypical drug in this class is chlorpromazine (Thorazine). Drugs in the low-potency category usually require doses of hundreds of milligrams orally to produce a therapeutic effect. By comparison, the high-potency group of antipsychotic drugs are those for which the oral dose necessary to occupy a sufficient number of receptors to produce an antipsychotic effect is in the range of only tens of milligrams or less. The prototypical drug in this latter category is haloperidol (Haldol). The potency level of first-generation antipsychotics can be compared by setting chlorpromazine at an oral dose of 100 milligrams as the base. Then all other drugs can be compared to this dose to determine what dose of the comparison drug will produce the same effect as 100 milligrams of chlorpromazine. For example, the dose equivalent of 100 milligrams of chlorpromazine (low-potency antipsychotic) would be 2 milligrams of haloperidol (a high-potency antipsychotic; Table 11.1). Note that the high-potency antipsychotics, such as haloperidol, are no different in efficacy from the low-potency antipsychotics. All of the first-generation agents, regardless of their potency, effectively treat the acute positive symptoms of schizophrenia if dosed properly. For example, the

TABLE 11.3 Side Effects of the First-generation (Typical) Antipsychotic Medications

Low-potency drugs (such as chlorpromazine)
Sedation
Anticholinergic symptoms (dry mouth, urinary retention, constipation, disorientation, confusion, memory problems)
Cardiovascular symptoms (orthostatic hypertension, arrhythmias)
Endocrine symptoms (gynecomastia, galactorrhea, weight gain, dysmenorrhea/amenorrhea)
Skin (photosensitivity reaction/pigmentation changes, sunburn)
Sexual dysfunction (anorgasmia, decreased libido, inhibition of ejaculation, retrograde ejaculation, priapism)
Ocular symptoms (retinitis pigmentosa)
High-potency drugs (such as haloperidol)
Acute dystonia
Parkinsonian symptoms (resting tremor, cogwheel-type rigidity, bradykinesia)
Akathisia
Tardive dyskinesia (TD)
Neuroleptic malignant syndrome (NMS) risk (both low- and high-potency drugs):
Fever (>40°C [140°F])
Severe muscle rigidity ("lead pipe" type)
Altered consciousness (clouding of the sensorium, stupor, coma)
Autonomic changes (fluctuating blood pressure, tachypnea, diaphoresis)

response rates of individuals with schizophrenia who are treated with antipsychotic medications during their first episode range anywhere from 40% to 80%, with an average response rate between 60% and 70%. Why discuss the difference between high-potency and low-potency antipsychotic agents then?

Drugs in the low-potency category have an extensive array of side effects. These include sedation; dry mouth, blurred vision, urinary retention, constipation, disorientation, confusion, and memory impairment (caused by acetylcholine receptor blockade); hypotension (caused by adrenergic receptor blockade); a variety of hormonal alterations[4] (caused by dopamine receptor blockade); and weight gain (caused by serotonin and histamine receptor blockade). Other side effects include photosensitivity, a skin reaction to sunlight, and worsening of glaucoma. Since these drugs primarily block dopamine D_2 receptors, they also produce a higher rate of neurological side effects like extrapyramidal symptoms (similar to that seen in Parkinsonism), akathisia, and

[4]Amenorrhea or disruption of the menstrual cycle, gynecomastia or breast development in males, galactorrhea or milk production in females, blockade of ovulation leading to infertility, and decreased sexual libido, anorgasmia, inhibition of ejaculation.

tardive dyskinesia, which will be discussed later in conjunction with the high-potency drugs. Management of these potential side effects includes (1) starting with low doses of the medication and slowly increasing the dose over time and (2) treating the specific side effect with drugs that will counter the effect of the receptor blockade, such as giving drugs that are acetylcholine agonists to treat the effects of cholinergic receptor blockade.

There may be no other way to totally eliminate side effects other than stopping (discontinuing) the offending antipsychotic drug. In this case, switching to another antipsychotic drug from a different chemical class may provide the necessary control of psychotic symptoms with less risk of unwanted side effects. The high-potency first-generation drugs can produce some of the same autonomic and physiological side effects as the low-potency drugs. But the high-potency drugs are more often noted for producing an array of neurological side effects related to their blockade of dopamine receptors.

Blockade of dopamine receptors in the hypothalamic-pituitary pathway cause an increase in systemic prolactin levels that can produce the side effects listed in footnote 4. Blockade of dopamine receptors in the nigrostriatal pathway (as soon discussed) produces extrapyramidal side effects including dystonia, Parkinsonian movements, akathisia, and tardive dyskinesia.

Dystonia presents as involuntary muscle contractions and sustained abnormal, bizarre postures of the limbs, trunk, head, and tongue. Dystonias are the earliest of the extrapyramidal symptoms to occur. Ninety-five percent of dystonias occur within the first four days. Individuals most at risk for developing dystonia are young males. The most effective treatment for dystonia is an intramuscular (IM) injection of a cholinergic agonist such as benztropine (Cogentin) or trihexyphenidyl (Artane).

Parkinsonian symptoms include the classic Parkinsonian triad of bradykinesia, tremor, and rigidity (Chapter 16). These symptoms can appear within 5–30 days after the initiation of treatment. Bradykinesia is a generalized slowing of movements. The tremor is a resting tremor, which means that when a person engages in some voluntary movement, such as writing with a pencil or touching their finger to their nose, the tremor appears to decrease in intensity or is absent. The rigidity is what is called a cogwheel-type rigidity. This refers to the ratchetlike resistance an examiner can feel when they passively move the arm of affected persons. Due to the slowness and stiffness of movements, individuals can display a stiff, shuffling gait. They may also lack normal fluidity of movements such as an arm swing while walking; have a decreased blink rate; and lose a degree of postural reflexes such that they are at risk of falls.

Akathisia is a syndrome characterized by the subjective internal feeling of anxiety, manifested externally by restlessness, pacing, constant rocking back and forth, and other repetitive, purposeless, actions. These external movements are attempts by the individual to reduce the uncomfortable feeling of internal anxiety that they experience. Because it can be extremely upsetting to the patient, akathisia is a common cause of nonadherence to psychotropic treatment and may lead to an increased risk for suicide. Akathisia occurs slowly over time and is quite subtle at its outset. Many patients do not realize that they are becoming more restless until the behavioral manifestations are quite pronounced. Although its cause is not well established, a decrease in dopaminergic activity appears to be an important etiological factor. Treatments include reducing the dose of the offending antipsychotic medication, switching to a low-potency FGA, or switching to one of the newer second-generation antipsychotics with low risk for this side effect.

Tardive dyskinesia is an even more serious form of movement disorder. This side effect develops later in the course of treatment, hence the name *tardive*, meaning tardy or late onset. Usually, tardive dyskinesia develops after a minimum of six months or more of continuous treatment with antipsychotic medications. Affected persons exhibit involuntary hyperkinetic, choreiform (dancelike) movements in single or multiple locations of the body, including the head, neck, lips, tongue, jaw, arms, fingers, feet, toes, and trunk. The prevalence of tardive dyskinesia has been estimated to be 20% of patients who are treated with first-generation agents. The risk of developing tardive dyskinesia depends on a number of variables, including the particular drug (such as first-generation vs. second-generation agents; low-potency vs. high-potency; oral vs. injectable form); the dosage; gender (females are at higher risk than males); and the age of the patient (for older individuals, the incidence rate for developing tardive dyskinesia is about 20–30% per year of treatment).

Although the incidence of tardive dyskinesia is much less with the second-generation agents, it is not zero. Overall, lifelong prevalence rates of tardive dyskinesia with the second-generation agents is estimated to be about 15% compared to 30% with first-generation agents (Carbon et al., 2017).

Options for the treatment of tardive dyskinesia are limited. The first choice is to discontinue treatment with the offending antipsychotic agent. But this may not always be possible if it results in the reemergence of severe psychotic symptoms that affect the health, safety, and functional capacity of the individual. Other options for treatment include switching to a drug with a lower risk of producing tardive dyskinesia, such as a second-generation agent. In 2017, the FDA approved two medications, deutetrabenazine (Austedo) and valbenazine (Ingrezza), for the treatment of tardive dyskinesia. The aim of both drugs is to provide sustained, low levels of dopamine to minimize side effects associated with excessive dopamine depletion. Results of the clinical trials demonstrated a reduction in dyskinesia scores with both drugs (Citrome, 2020), although treatment with valbenazine was more cost-effective compared with deutetrabenazine (Ganz et al., 2021). Head-to-head studies comparing the two drugs have not been reported (Artukoglu et al., 2020).

Although rare, one potentially lethal side effect of treatment with antipsychotic medications is **neuroleptic malignant syndrome** (NMS). This is an acute reaction that may occur in response to a variety of agents that increase dopaminergic transmission. The risk of developing NMS is present for any of the currently available antipsychotic medications, whether first- or second-generation. The incidence of NMS in first-generation-treated patients is 0.02–2.4%, and it has been reported to occur, albeit at lower levels, with second-generation agents such as clozapine, risperidone, and olanzapine. The most common symptoms include fever; severe muscle rigidity of the "lead pipe" type; autonomic changes, such as fluctuating blood pressure; and altered consciousness that may progress to stupor or coma. Eighty percent of the cases of NMS occur within the first two weeks of treatment, but it can arise at any time. NMS develops rapidly over the course of 24–48 hours and can last for 7–14 days. If NMS develops, it is considered a medical emergency, because without treatment, there is a 20% mortality risk. The most important aspects of effective treatment are early recognition, immediate withdrawal of the responsible agent, and initiation of supportive measures including treatment with anticholinergic drugs; treatment with dopaminergic agents, such as bromocriptine (Parlodel); treatment with muscle relaxants, such as dantrolene sodium (Dantrium); and cooling the body with ice packs.

SECOND-GENERATION ANTIPSYCHOTICS: SPECIFIC AGENTS

Second-generation (atypical) antipsychotics are drugs that block dopamine D_2 receptors, just like the first-generation antipsychotics. The distinguishing characteristic of the second-generation agents is that their potency for blocking serotonin receptors—$5\text{-HT}1_A$ and $5\text{-HT}2_A$, specifically—is as great or greater than their potency for blocking dopamine D_2 receptors. This is mechanistically different than the first-generation agents, whose potency for blocking dopamine receptors is greater than their potency for blocking serotonin receptors. It is believed that this ratio of 5-HT > dopamine potency is related to the general finding that the second-generation agents are less likely to produce neurological side effects, such as extrapyramidal symptoms and tardive dyskinesia, compared to the first-generation agents.

Table 11.4 lists the currently available second-generation antipsychotics. In general, these drugs are as therapeutically effective as the first-generation antipsychotics for treating the symptoms of schizophrenia. Also, like the first-generation agents, the newer second-generation agents have FDA-approved indications to treat other disorders (Table 11.5). "Off-label" uses of the second-generation antipsychotics (nonantipsychotic uses) are discussed later in this chapter (see also Dr. J's Musings 11.2). In general, the second-generation agents produce lower rates of extrapyramidal symptoms and tardive dyskinesia when compared to the first-generation antipsychotics, a significant clinical advantage and allowing exploration of such uses. Adversely, many of the second-generation agents have been associated with a risk of producing what is known as a metabolic syndrome, which is described later in this chapter.

Although drugs such as aripiprazole (Abilify), brexpiprazole (Rexulti), and lumateperone (Caplyta) are sometimes referred to as third-generation antipsychotics due to their unique mechanism of action at dopamine receptors, they will be considered here as the most recently approved, newer antipsychotics. The second-generation antipsychotics will not be presented in their entirety because they are all similar in efficacy. Instead, we will highlight specific agents and side effects of drugs that may be of importance when considering which drug to use for treatment.

Clozapine

As discussed earlier, clozapine (Clozaril) was the first clinically available atypical (second-generation) antipsychotic, therapeutically superior to the older first-generation antipsychotics, effective in about one-third of patients who are resistant

TABLE 11.4 Second-generation Antipsychotic Drugs

Generic name	Trade name	Dose equivalence (mg)[a]	Formulation[b]	Age group[c]
Clozapine	Clozaril; Fazaclo	50–100	PO; Sol; ODT	A; AD
Risperidone	Risperdal; Consta	1–2	PO; IM; ODT; LAI	C; A; AD
Olanzapine	Zyprexa; Zydis; Relprevv	3–5	PO; IM; ODT; LAI; Combo	A; AD
Quetiapine	Seroquel	60–75	PO	C; A; AD
Ziprasidone	Geodon	50–60	PO; IM	C; A; AD
Aripiprazole	Abilify; Discmelt; Maintena	4–7	PO; Sol; IM; ODT; LAI	C; A; AD
Paliperidone	Invega; Sustenna; Trinza	1–2	PO; LAI	A; AD
Iloperidone	Fanapt	2–5	PO	AD
Asenapine	Saphris	2–5	PO-SL	A; AD
Lurasidone	Latuda	10–20	PO	A; AD
Brexpiprazole	Rexulti	1	PO	AD
Cariprazine	Vraylar	1	PO	AD

[a]Dose equivalence: All drug doses are equated to 100 milligrams of chlorpromazine.
[b]Formulation: PO = oral, usually tablets or capsules; Sol = oral solution; ODT = orally disintegrating tablet; PO-SL = oral sublingual film; Combo = combination tablet: olanzapine + fluoxetine; IM = intramuscular injectable solution; LAI = long-acting injectable solution, usually 1 injection every 2 to 4 weeks or 3 months (Trinza).
[c]Age group: C = children (1–9 years old); A = adolescent (10–17 years old); AD = adult (≥ 18 years old).

to first-generation medications. Importantly, clozapine lacks the extrapyramidal side effects associated with the first-generation drugs (Masuda et al., 2019). In patients with Parkinsonism who demonstrate psychotic symptoms (such as hallucinations and delusions), clozapine can effectively treat their psychosis without exacerbating the underlying movement disorder (Chang and Fox, 2016). Also, clozapine can reduce the risk of suicide in schizophrenic patients, a fact that led the FDA to approve clozapine for both treatment-resistant schizophrenia and the treatment of suicidal behavior in schizophrenia. Side effects (soon discussed) limit its wider use. Researchers (Chan et al., 2018) compare clozapine and ketamine for use in treatment-resistant depression with suicidal behaviors.

Aripiprazole

Aripiprazole (Abilify) was approved in 2002 as perhaps the first of a new "third-generation" antipsychotic drug. It has a different mechanism of action from first-generation agents and other second-generation agents. Aripiprazole is a partial

TABLE 11.5 Indications for Second-generation Antipsychotic Drugs

Generic name	Trade name	Indications
Clozaril	Clozapine	Schizophrenia (not first-line agent); suicide risk
Risperidone	Risperdal	Schizophrenia; BPD (mania/mixed); Tourette syndrome; irritability/aggressive behavior in autism
Olanzapine	Zyprexa	Schizophrenia; BPD (mania/depressed/mixed); treatment-resistant depression; agitation in schizophrenia or bipolar disorder
Quetiapine	Seroquel	Schizophrenia; BPD (mania/depressed/mixed)
Ziprasidone	Geodon	Schizophrenia; BPD (manic/mixed); agitation in schizophrenia or bipolar disorder; Tourette syndrome
Aripiprazole	Abilify	Schizophrenia; BPD (manic/mixed); depression; agitation in schizophrenia or bipolar disorder; irritability/aggression in autism
Paliperidone	Invega	Schizophrenia; schizoaffective disorder
Iloperidone	Fanapt	Schizophrenia
Asenapine	Saphris	Schizophrenia; BPD (manic/mixed/maintenance)
Lurasidone	Latuda	Schizophrenia; BPD (depression)
Brexpiprazole	Rexulti	Schizophrenia; MDD (adjunct)
Cariprazine	Vraylar	Schizophrenia; BPD (manic/mixed)

agonist at D_2 and 5-HT1$_A$ receptors as well as an antagonist at 5-HT2 receptors (de Bartolomeis et al., 2015). This dopaminergic partial agonism is meant to stabilize the dopamine system because, although the drug binds with high affinity to D_2 receptors, it has lower intrinsic activity (less efficacy). This means that in areas of the brain where dopamine levels are normally high (e.g., in the limbic and nigrostriatal systems), aripiprazole may displace dopamine from the dopamine receptor, but it will not produce as strong an effect as the natural transmitter. This effect in the limbic and nigrostriatal systems is thought to be responsible for aripiprazole's antipsychotic effect and potentially lower risk of extrapyramidal signs and tardive dyskinesia. Conversely, in areas of the brain where dopamine concentration is low (e.g., in the frontal lobes and/or mesocortical dopamine system), aripiprazole can produce a net increase in dopaminergic action. This is thought to be related to aripiprazole's lower risk for producing cognitive impairment and exerting positive effects on the negative symptoms of schizophrenia.

Aripiprazole's partial agonism at 5-HT1$_A$ receptors confers anxiolytic and antidepressant actions. Indeed, aripiprazole has been reported to augment the effect of antidepressants in patients with depression and anxiety disorders who were only partial responders to selective serotonin reuptake inhibitors (SSRIs) alone; however, using an antipsychotic drug in treatment-resistant depression remains very controversial. In 2017, the FDA approved a new technology to monitor whether a person actually swallows their medication as directed. Abilify *MyCite* is a pill containing aripiprazole and a sensor that sends out an electrical signal when the pill reaches the stomach and contacts the stomach acid. The signal is transmitted to a wearable patch on the user's wrist that can link to a mobile application that allows patients to track whether they have taken their medication. Despite its novelty, Abilify MyCite is about 80 times more expensive than generic aripiprazole tablets and superior efficacy is meager at best (Cosgrove et al., 2019).

Other clinical uses of aripiprazole include bipolar disorder (Nestsiarovich et al., 2021), treatment-resistant depression (Cantu et al., 2021), and schizoaffective disorder (Munoz-Negro et al., 2021; Quan et al., 2021). A long-acting injectable dosage formulation is available and is well-tolerated (Mason et al., 2021). In line with current research on depression (Chapter 12), aripiprazole reduces hippocampal atrophy, preserving hippocampal volume and reducing central inflammation (Wang et al., 2021).

Since aripiprazole has now become available in less expensive, generic formulation, two other dopamine partial agonist antipsychotics have been developed and approved by the FDA, albeit at a much higher price: cariprazine (Vraylar) and brexpiprazole (Rexulti).

Cariprazine

Cariprazine (Vraylar) is unique among second-generation agents because it has a higher affinity for D_3 receptors than D_2 receptors. It is thought that by favoring D_3 over D_2 receptors and being a partial agonist at those receptors, cariprazine would have the necessary D_2 effects as an antipsychotic and, due to its partial agonism at D_3 receptors, it would have fewer side effects and produce less cognitive impairment. (For a comparison of three newer antipsychotic drugs, see Keks et al., 2020; Leucht et al., 2020.) Cariprazine was approved by the FDA in 2015 for the treatment of schizophrenia as well as the acute treatment of mania in persons with bipolar disorder, bipolar depression, and major depressive disorder (Citrome, 2018; Pinto et al., 2020; Ragguett and McIntyre, 2019).

Brexpiprazole

Brexpiprazole (Rexulti) was developed by the manufacturer of aripiprazole. It is a new atypical antipsychotic drug (perhaps considered another third-generation antipsychotic drug), FDA-approved for the treatment of schizophrenia, treatment-resistant major depression, and anxiety (Edinoff et al., 2021; Fornaro et al., 2019a; Ward and Citrome, 2019). The use of brexpiprazole in treating major depression is discussed in Chapter 12.

Asenapine

In 2009, **asenapine** (Saphris) was approved in a sublingual formulation for the treatment of schizophrenia and manic or mixed episodes of bipolar disorder in adults. Asenapine received an additional indication in 2010 for the acute treatment of bipolar disorder manic or mixed episodes as an adjunct to either lithium or valproic acid. In 2015, the FDA approved asenapine for the treatment of schizophrenia and bipolar disorder in adolescents. Most recently, asenapine was approved as a transdermal patch, with each patch lasting 24 hours. This was the first approval of a transdermal patch for treating schizophrenia (Zhou et al., 2020).

Asenapine is a second-generation antipsychotic with 5-HT2_A antagonist and 5-HT1_A/1_B partial agonist properties, which provides *a* favorable profile in targeting schizophrenic symptoms, while reducing motor side effects and improving mood and cognition.

Lumateperone

Lumateperone (Caplyta) was approved by the FDA in December 2019 for the treatment of schizophrenia and other neuropsychiatric disorders (Blair, 2020; Syed and Brasic, 2021). It is also useful in treating bipolar depression (D'Souza et al., 2021), behavioral disorders associated with dementia and Alzheimer's disease (Blair, 2020), and major depressive disorder (Vyas et al., 2020). Lumateperone has a unique profile of receptor effects: (1) only about 40% of dopamine D_2 receptors require occupancy, unlike the usual 60–80% required of other antipsychotics; (2) the 5-HT2_A occupancy is greater than the D_2 receptor occupancy; (3) it is a presynaptic partial agonist at D_2 receptors as well as a postsynaptic D_2 antagonist; (4) it inhibits serotonin reuptake (an antidepressant action); and (5) it indirectly enhances glutamate neurotransmission. Some claim that all this occurs without metabolic or endocrine alterations (Correll et al., 2020). It remains to be seen whether or not lumateperone offers unique therapeutic benefits.

PROMINENT SIDE EFFECTS OF SELECTED SECOND-GENERATION ANTIPSYCHOTICS

As noted previously, while the second-generation antipsychotic agents generally have a lower risk of producing early-onset extrapyramidal side effects and late-onset tardive dyskinesia than the first-generation antipsychotics, the risk is not zero, and the second-generation agents can still produce extrapyramidal signs and tardive dyskinesias in some proportion of the population of individuals who are treated with these agents. In addition, the second-generation agents can also produce many of the physiological, endocrine, and cardiovascular side effects that are associated with treatment with the first-generation agents. Furthermore, the second-generation agents are most often associated with producing an array of side effects that are collectively referred to as the **metabolic syndrome** (Table 11.6). This syndrome is composed of weight gain, dyslipidemia, and glucose intolerance, which can lead to diabetes. The most characteristic side effects of specific second-generation agents are summarized in Table 11.7.

TABLE 11.6 Symptoms of Metabolic Syndrome

Abdominal obesity (waist circumference):
- Men: >102 cm (>40 in.)
- Women: >88 cm (>35 in.)

Triglyceride level (mg/dL): >150

HDL cholesterol (mg/dL):
- Men: >40

Blood pressure (mm Hg): ≥130/≥85

Fasting blood glucose (mg/dL): >100

TABLE 11.7 Side Effects of the Second-generation (Atypical) Antipsychotic Drugs

Clozapine	Orthostatic hypotension, anticholinergic symptoms, myocarditis, sedation, seizures, hypersalivation, neuroleptic malignant syndrome (NMS), agranulocytosis, metabolic syndrome, possible hematological malignancies
Risperidone	Extrapyramidal symptoms (EPS), tardive dyskinesia (TD), hyperprolactinemia, NMS
Olanzapine	Orthostatic hypotension, anticholinergic symptoms, sedation, NMS, metabolic syndrome, drug reaction with eosinophilia and systemic symptoms (DRESS), a serious dermatological reaction also affecting other internal organ systems with risk of mortality
Quetiapine	Sedation, orthostatic hypotension
Ziprasidone	Sedation, EPS, TD, increase in QT_c interval, metabolic syndrome, DRESS; Stevens–Johnson syndrome (SJS), a serious dermatological reaction with risk of mortality
Aripiprazole	Orthostatic hypotension, nausea, tremor, insomnia, headache, agitation, akathisia, risky compulsive behaviors (gambling, shopping, sexual behavior, etc.)
Paliperidone	Akathisia, EPS, tachycardia, hyperprolactinemia, QT_c prolongation
Iloperidone	Dizziness, dry mouth, fatigue, nasal congestion, somnolence, tachycardia, orthostatic hypotension, some elevation in prolactin, weight gain, hypersensitivity reactions (including anaphylaxis, angioedema, throat tightness, oropharyngeal swelling, swelling of the face, lips, mouth, and tongue, urticaria, rash, and pruritus)
Asenapine	Dizziness, EPS, TD, NMS, akathisia, oral hypoesthesia, dysgeusia, somnolence, weight gain
Lurasidone	Somnolence, akathisia, nausea, EPS, TD
Brexpiprazole	Weight gain, akathisia
Cariprazine	EPS, akathisia, TD, vomiting, dyspepsia, somnolence

Clozapine

Common side effects of clozapine include sedation, significant weight gain, decrease in seizure threshold, sialorrhea (increased saliva production), and constipation, with rare instances of agranulocytosis. Recently, researchers (Tiihonen et al., 2022), in a Finnish study, reported that long-term use of clozapine was associated with increased odds of developing hematological malignancies, including lymphoma, leukemia, and myeloma. This risk was not associated with use of other antipsychotic drugs.

Sedation occurs in about 40% of patients, can be severe, and may be dose limiting and have a negative impact on medication compliance. Taking the drug at bedtime may help. Weight gain is a problem for up to 80% of patients; it can be severe, with gains of 20 pounds or more not unusual (Musil et al., 2015). Of all the second-generation agents, clozapine is the drug most likely to cause significant weight gain (see Figure 11.2). Researchers concluded that "most antipsychotics led to a significantly higher risk for clinically-relevant weight gain equal to or greater than 7% compared to placebo" (Barton et al., 2020).

Seizures occur at a greater rate with clozapine than with other antipsychotics, especially at high doses. Sialorrhea occurs in one-third to one-half of patients, not only during the day but often much more extensively at night, with patients complaining of waking up with a wet pillow. The mechanism is believed to be due to an impaired ability to swallow, which causes saliva to accumulate. It may be severe and difficult to treat, although it can resolve over time. Constipation occurs in about 30% of patients and can be quite bothersome.

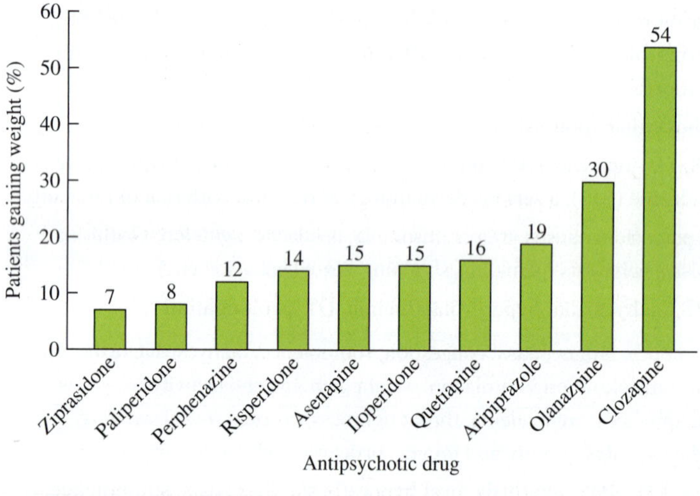

FIGURE 11.2 Weight Gain with Antipsychotic Drugs.
Percentage of patients who gained 7% or more of their baseline body weight while being treated with the indicated antipsychotic drugs. The 7% threshold is the accepted measure for determining a significant effect.
[Data from Ellinger et al., 2010.]

The greatest concern with clozapine is the risk of developing severe, life-threatening (although reversible) agranulocytosis (reduction in white blood cell levels), with an incidence of about 1–2%. In 2015, the FDA determined that that the risks of agranulocytosis were being well managed and established criteria to ensure that signs of agranulocytosis are detected as early as possible (Kar et al., 2016). These criteria require that the prescriber, the pharmacy dispensing the clozapine, and the patient receiving clozapine be enrolled in a Clozapine registry (Clozapine Risk Evaluation and Mitigation Strategy program with patients enrolled by a certified doctor). This program tracks prescriptions and whether patients have had blood samples drawn to detect for early signs of agranulocytosis. The program has been controversial, but the FDA has recently restated program requirements (U.S. Food and Drug Administration, 2021b).

Clozapine is also associated with risk for metabolic syndrome, which includes abnormalities of blood pressure, lipids, glucose utilization, and, as noted earlier, body mass index (BMI). These abnormalities contribute to an increased risk for cardiovascular disease and diabetes. It is recommended that body weight and blood glucose be monitored while taking the drug. In addition, Clozapine is highly anticholinergic, producing dry mouth, urinary retention, constipation, blurred vision, and, in some individuals, cognitive impairment.

Clozapine also has warnings for cardiac muscle irritation (myocarditis) and, like all antipsychotic agents, for an increased risk of death in older patients with dementia. This last warning has been extremely controversial since the FDA first published it in 2005. Antipsychotic drugs are very effective in calming agitation and aggression in older patients with dementia displaying these symptoms. While the warning did reduce the prescribing of antipsychotics (e.g., risperidone) for dementia-associated behavioral control, there were adverse consequences, such as increased prescribing of opioids (Rubino et al., 2020). One research group (Marcinkowska et al., 2020) published an extensive review of the controversy and of possible alternative medications to treat behavioral problems in older adults with dementia.

Currently, because of potentially serious side effects, clozapine is the least prescribed of all the second-generation antipsychotics, despite the fact that it is one of the most effective antipsychotic medications, reducing mortality and both aggressive behavior and suicide risk (Meltzer, 2012). Some advocate for combining clozapine with a second antipsychotic agent, such as aripiprazole (Correll et al., 2019; Tiihonen et al., 2019), although combination therapy with two antipsychotic agents is unusual.

Risperidone

Among all second-generation agents, **risperidone** is most likely to produce extrapyramidal symptoms. Further, risperidone, compared to the other similar agents, is most likely to be associated with increased prolactin levels, which can markedly affect body hormones and sexual functioning. On the plus side, risperidone has not been associated with need for white blood cell monitoring and has been quite effective in treating nonpsychotic disorders such as autism (Chapter 16).

Olanzapine

Olanzapine is chemically similar to clozapine, and both are similar to the first-generation agent chlorpromazine. Therefore, they share a similar array of side effects. Olanzapine carries a risk of producing significant weight gain (Figure 11.2) and the metabolic syndrome comparable to that seen with clozapine. Olanzapine is highly sedating and also highly anticholinergic, producing cognitive impairment in at risk individuals. Olanzapine does not carry a risk for producing agranulocytosis and therefore does not require white blood cell monitoring.

A rare side effect of olanzapine is a skin rash that can be serious and even fatal if not recognized and treated. Another rare side effect, with an incidence rate of 2%, is related only to the long-acting depot injectable form of the drug with the trade name of *Relprevv*. Postinjection delirium/sedation syndrome is a syndrome of intense sedation than can lead to ataxia and abrupt onset of sleep. Thus, the FDA requires that anyone who receives a Relprevv injection must stay in the clinic for a minimum of 3 hours post-injection and be driven home by an escort.

Quetiapine

The most prominent side effects of **quetiapine** are sedation, postural hypotension, and, rarely, a potentially fatal increase in the QT interval of the electrocardiogram (ECG). Quetiapine is the most implicated of several drugs that has the potential to increase the QT interval and place one at risk. It should be used with caution or not at all in individuals who have existing cardiac rhythm disturbances or who are taking other medications that could prolong the QT interval. Finally, while medium or high doses of quetiapine have been associated with increased risk of type 2 diabetes, low doses commonly used clinically do not appear to be associated with this risk (Højlund et al., 2021).

Ziprasidone

Ziprasidone can be sedating, but it generally does not produce a significant risk for weight gain. It does carry a risk of producing a metabolic syndrome and may also carry a very slight risk for extending the QT interval. Thus, it should be used with caution in individuals who have existing cardiac disturbances, similar to what was noted for quetiapine.

Ziprasidone also carries a risk for inducing two serious and potentially fatal dermatological reactions. One, Stevens–Johnson syndrome, is a rare form of toxic skin necrolysis, in which cell death causes the epidermis to separate from the dermis, thereby destroying the skin. The other reaction is the serious skin rash described previously in the section on olanzapine. Fortunately, both risks are rare occurrences, but the person being treated should be closely monitored.

Aripiprazole

Aripiprazole is relatively nonsedating and possesses minimal risk of weight gain. Its most common side effects include orthostatic hypotension, nausea, tremor, insomnia, headache, and agitation. Of all the second-generation agents, it is the drug most likely to produce the side effect of akathisia. In May 2016, the FDA issued a warning that aripiprazole may also produce an increased risk for pathological gambling and other compulsive behaviors, such as binge eating, shopping, or having sex (Wolfschlag and Hakansson, 2021).

Paliperidone

Paliperidone is one of the major metabolites of risperidone. Therefore, it can produce the same side effects as the parent drug, namely, increased risk for extrapyramidal symptoms, tardive dyskinesia, and akathisia in higher doses. Paliperidone can also increase prolactin levels, producing the same sexual side effects as risperidone.

Iloperidone

Iloperidone can produce dizziness, dry mouth, fatigue, nasal congestion, somnolence, tachycardia, orthostatic hypotension, some elevation in prolactin, and weight gain. It may also produce hypersensitivity reactions, including anaphylaxis; angioedema; throat tightness; oropharyngeal swelling; swelling of the face, lips, mouth, and tongue; rash; and pruritus.

Cariprazine

Similar to aripiprazole (and brexpiprazole, discussed next), cariprazine's most common side effects include somnolence, dyspepsia (indigestion), vomiting, extrapyramidal symptoms, and akathisia. Cariprazine does not appear to adversely impact metabolic variables, prolactin, or the electrocardiogram (ECG) QT interval.

Brexpiprazole

Brexpiprazole appears to have less sedative effect than many other antipsychotic medications, and may produce less restlessness and akathisia (Pahwa et al., 2021). As mentioned, it seems to be comparable in efficacy and side effects with aripiprazole (Kishi et al., 2020a) and more effective than paliperidone (Yan et al., 2020). Unfortunately, because brexpiprazole is metabolized by CYP-3A4, genetic variances in this enzyme result in wide variability in a person's responses to the drug, leading to unpredictable side effects and even therapeutic failure.

Asenapine

Asenapine has been reported to produce a variety of side effects, including extrapyramidal symptoms, tardive dyskinesia, akathisia, and neuroleptic malignant syndrome. It also can produce dizziness, somnolence, and weight gain. Because of its method of administration (as noted, it is embedded on a film strip that is placed under the tongue), it can produce numbing of the mouth and tongue and abnormal taste sensations.

Lurasidone

Lurasidone's most common side effects include somnolence, nausea, extrapyramidal symptoms, and akathisia.

Lumateperone

Sedation is a prominent side effect and can be minimized by taking the drug at bedtime (Kane et al., 2020). One researcher stated (Knable, 2020):

> It is encouraging that lumateperone did not appear to effect body weight, lipids, blood sugar, prolactin, or to produce involuntary movements.

CATIE AND CUTLASS STUDIES

Over the years, a number of studies have measured the effectiveness of antipsychotic drugs. Two of the most notable and classic are the CATIE and CUtLASS studies. The **Clinical Antipsychotic Trials of Intervention Effectiveness (CATIE) study** was conducted in the United States between January 2001 and December 2004 at 57 clinical sites for up to 18 months or until treatment was discontinued for any reason. In the first of three phases, 1493 patients were randomly assigned to receive either one of three second-generation agents (olanzapine, risperidone, or quetiapine) or the first-generation agent perphenazine under double-blind conditions. Ziprasidone was added later following its FDA approval. Results showed that patients discontinued antipsychotic medications at a high rate, 64–82% across all the drugs, primarily because of lack of efficacy, intolerable side effects, or lack of insight into their disease (Kim et al., 2020).

In general, clozapine treatment was found to be more effective than the other agents. Olanzapine and risperidone were more effective than quetiapine or ziprasidone in "time until discontinuation" for any reason.

Unfortunately, using data from the CATIE study, Rhee and Rosenbeck (2019) noted that reductions in patient symptoms and quality of life did not lessen the family burden of caring for a family member with schizophrenia.

A British comparison between antipsychotics—**Cost Utility of the Latest Antipsychotic Drugs in Schizophrenia Studies (CUtLASS 1)**—was reported in October 2006 (Jones et al., 2006). It evaluated 227 people with a diagnosis of schizophrenia who had an inadequate response or adverse reaction to their previous medication. Prescriptions for an antipsychotic (excluding clozapine) were monitored for one year, with blind assessments at 12, 26, and 56 weeks. Like the CATIE trial, the results of the CUtLASS 1 study showed that patients with schizophrenia did just as well on antipsychotic drugs from either category, with patients taking first-generation agents actually showing a trend toward greater improvement on the quality-of-life scale and symptom-severity scores.

Although antipsychotic drugs remain the "cornerstone of treatment for schizophrenia" (Lieberman et al., 2005), the results of the CATIE and CUtLASS 1 trials have prompted a reassessment of the perceived advantages of the second-generation antipsychotics. The initial optimism generated by second-generation antipsychotics has been tempered by evidence that they may not improve clinical outcomes as much as anticipated. And it may be the case that antipsychotics differ among themselves based on what factor is being examined. For example, one drug may produce fewer extrapyramidal symptoms than another, but the newer agent may produce more weight gain. So comparisons between antipsychotics are not simple and may depend on a broader analysis of desired outcomes than enter into any risk–benefit analysis. Essentially, it is now understood that every antipsychotic medication is unique in its efficacy and side effects (as I hope this chapter has demonstrated). Newer second-generation agents do not always produce better outcomes than older drugs; and the merits of each drug must be determined independently. In situations where the risk of extrapyramidal symptoms may preclude the use of first-generation agents, such as autism, bipolar disorder, borderline personality disorder, and aggressive disorders, newer second-generation agents may be the first choice. The transition to less expensive generic status of specific drugs (reducing their cost) will most likely affect such considerations as well.[5]

It is also important to note that at least 20% of persons with schizophrenia do not adequately respond to monotherapy with antipsychotics. As stated by one set of researchers (Lahteenvuo and Tiihonen, 2021):

> . . . . 70% of patients with schizophrenia require long-term medication to control their symptoms and do not achieve complete recovery. Different combinations of treatments, polypharmacy, have been tried, but have been shown to cause more side effects than monotherapy, which is the main reason why most treatment guidelines caution against it.

ADDITIONAL USES FOR SECOND-GENERATION ANTIPSYCHOTICS

The use of antipsychotic drugs in disorders that do not present with psychotic symptoms has continued to advance. For many of these disorders, the use of these drugs is considered off-label since they have not received formal FDA approval for such use (see Dr. J's Musings 11.2).

Having a more favorable neurological profile, second-generation agents are most tried in these off-label uses. At present, it should be kept in mind that most of the available evidence comes from evaluations of these drugs as adjuncts to other psychotropic medication treatments, that few direct comparisons between antipsychotic agents have been published, and that there is a growing, but not necessarily adequate, body of high-quality information on their long-term safety. This expansion of off-label usage continues despite FDA warnings about risks concerning the use of atypical antipsychotics in certain vulnerable populations, especially in older adults with dementia.

[5]Kane and Correll (2010) provide a comprehensive summary of the history of the role of drug treatments for schizophrenia, the evolution from first-generation to second-generation antipsychotics, successes and lack of success for novel interventions, and future directions for research.

DR. J'S MUSINGS 11.2

Why Off-Label?

What does off-label mean? In essence, it means that the FDA has not formally approved the use of a specific medication for that particular use. The questions are: (1) where does that use come from, and (2) does it mean that the medication is not appropriate for that use? To answer those questions, we ask, "Where does FDA designation come from?"

A manufacturer develops a new drug, patents the compound, and, starting from that date, receives exclusive marketing rights for the drug for 20 years, after which time other manufacturers may market the drug, usually at a lower price. In essence, the drug "goes generic." To receive initial FDA approval, the manufacturer conducts extensive preclinical and clinical research into the drug's efficacy and safety. An application is sent to the FDA, requesting approval for marketing the drug for a specific indication. If approval is granted, the drug is marketed under patent exclusivity for a specific indication. If medical literature, following initial marketing, indicates that the drug is also effective in treating another nonindicated indication, medical prescribers are legally able to prescribe that medication for another use, provided of course that they take responsibility for that use. The FDA does not look at such use and approve it for that use unless the manufacturer submits a formal application so it can promote the drug for that use. Usually there is no financial incentive for them to do that.

Once the drug goes generic (20 years after patenting), there is absolutely no financial incentive for anyone to request the FDA to approve the drug for further use for that off-label use (which has already been well defined in the literature), and such use will always be off-label. If a manufacturer develops another drug for that specific off-label use, does the research, submits a request, and gains approval, it can then promote that new drug for that use and it will become an approved use (usually at a much higher price). All this is complicated and confusing to the consumer!

These second- and third-generation drugs are being used for multiple disorders, including bipolar disorder, treatment-resistant depression, schizoaffective disorder, and dysthymia, as well as behavioral problems associated with dementia, autism spectrum disorders, severe treatment-resistant anxiety disorders, and borderline personality disorder. These drugs are also being used symptomatically to treat anger, aggression, and tantrums in various behavioral dyscontrol disorders.

Given the broad use of antipsychotics across a range of disorders that display no psychotic symptoms, it is somewhat of a misnomer to refer to them as antipsychotic medications. However, since antipsychotic is generally accepted as the class of medications in this group, we will continue to refer to them as such.

Bipolar Disorder

For the last 15+ years, atypical antipsychotic agents have been widely used to treat the mood swings and depression associated with bipolar disorder. In such situations, the patient's moods swings will typically become less frequent and less intense. There are currently seven commonly prescribed atypical antipsychotic medications also used for treating bipolar disorder: Abilify (aripiprazole), Risperdal (risperidone), Zyprexa (olanzapine), Seroquel (quetiapine), Geodon (ziprasidone), Clozaril (clozapine), and Symbyax (olanzapine/fluoxetine).

In addition, we can add the newer second-generation agents lurasidone, brexpiprazole, and cariprazine, which can be used either as adjuncts to other antibipolar medications (such as the mood stabilizers; Chapter 14), and all can be used as monotherapy. Several of these agents have been approved to treat bipolar disorder in children (6–10 years old) and/or adolescents (10–17 years old).

Treatment-Resistant Depression

Only about one-third of patients with major depressive disorder who receive initial antidepressant treatment actually achieve remission (see STAR*D study in Chapter 12). Many second-generation antipsychotics are used to augment treatment-resistant major depression (Bailey and Panjwani, 2018; Earley et al., 2018; Fornaro et al., 2019s). At this time, only aripiprazole and brexpiprazole have an FDA indication for the treatment of major depressive disorder as adjunctive treatment to antidepressant therapy. However, any second-generation agent can be used for this purpose. Indeed, the use of atypical antipsychotic drugs as adjunctive treatments has also become part of clinical guidelines for the treatment of individuals who suffer from major depression and who have not responded or not responded sufficiently to treatment with antidepressant medication alone.

Reviews of the use of different antipsychotics as adjunctive treatment to antidepressants for major depressive disorder report few significant differences in efficacy among them; this includes the newer atypical antipsychotic drug, cariprazine, when added to antidepressant treatment (Durgam et al., 2016; Nunez et al., 2022).

Dementia

Along with cognitive decline, 90% of patients with dementia experience behavioral and psychological symptoms of dementia, such as psychosis, aggression, agitation, and depression (Marcinkowska et al., 2020). Atypical antipsychotics are commonly prescribed off-label to manage certain symptoms, despite warnings from the regulatory agencies regarding a purported increased risk of mortality associated with their use in older patients. Indeed, antipsychotic medications are not approved by the FDA for the treatment of neuropsychiatric symptoms, including psychosis, in older adults with dementia. The FDA maintains a black box warning (its highest level of warning) to notify prescribers of the increased risk of death related to their use in such persons. To that end, their use to control abnormal behaviors in older persons with

DR. J'S MUSINGS 11.3

My Mother

About 15 years ago, my parents retired to an assisted living center, where they thrived. However, as my mother became progressively more disabled, my father was unable to care for her. She was developing Parkinsonian symptoms and signs of dementia. As they struggled more and more, the family moved them to an excellent Romanian-run residence with three or four other similar older adults. Again, they thrived. Eventually, my father passed away, leaving my mother a widow. In her state of dementia, she could not understand why he was not there, thinking perhaps he had run away with another woman. She became more and more confused, agitated, and even combative, wandering the house during the night. The caregivers became unable to offer her the care and monitoring she required, stating that she might have to move out to a more formal nursing home. Very concerned, I suggested that her prescriber give her a trial of quetiapine (Seroquel), at a very low dose (25 mg at bedtime), despite the controversial black box warning. The quetiapine calmed her remarkably, and she was able to stay in the home, living in dignity, until her natural death two years later. No dose increases were made during this period. We can see in my mother's case and elsewhere how prescribing medication can sometimes be like an art form where we use our professional expertise to assist a specific individual, and no two situations are ever the same.

dementia is controversial. Here there is conflict between the drugs' effectiveness, their claimed potential to cause harm, their lack of universal efficacy, and the lack of other alternatives.

In general, meta-analytic studies have demonstrated that there is a slightly increased risk of death attached to the use of antipsychotic medications in individuals who have dementia, and that risk seems to be dose dependent, that is, higher doses of the antipsychotic result in increased risk of mortality. Further, antipsychotic polypharmacy, that is, using two or more antipsychotics, also increases the risk of mortality compared to monotherapy. Based on these results, antipsychotic medications should be used sparingly, and not in combination, in the treatment of behavioral and psychological symptoms of dementia.

In 2017, the FDA granted Breakthrough Therapy designation to the new antipsychotic **pimavanserin** (Nuplazid) for the treatment of hallucinations and delusions in Parkinson's disease. Researchers (Ballard et al., 2018; Yunusa et al., 2020) reviewed the pharmacological activity, clinical efficacy, and safety of pimavanserin as a novel atypical antipsychotic with potential to address the unmet needs of older adults with dementia-related psychosis. In 2020, the FDA approved the use of pimavanserin for the treatment of hallucinations and delusions associated with dementia-related psychosis. Researchers (Tariot et al., 2021) reported on a trial of pimavanserin in over 300 patients with dementia-related psychosis, noting that the trial was stopped early because of superior efficacy over placebo. Another group (Cummings et al., 2022) reviewed the beneficial effects of pimavanserin in "treating the hallucinations and delusions without worsening cognitive or motor function."

Beyond this, there are reasons to be cautious in using antipsychotic agents in older adults with or without dementia-related behavioral problems: (1) Older patients are prescribed many medications to treat a variety of chronic medical conditions. Adding an antipsychotic medication increases the risk for drug interactions. (2) Older adults are more sensitive to the effects and side effects of medications. The lowest possible doses must always be used. (3) Anticholinergic side effects can and do appear, leading to blurred vision, urinary retention, constipation, and further memory impairments. (4) Neurological side effects including Parkinsonian-like extrapyramidal symptoms and tardive dyskinesia (upon drug discontinuation) are all possible.

The American Geriatrics Society (AGS) publishes a list of drugs that would cause increased risk when used in older adults. This list, known as the Beers Criteria, is periodically updated by the AGS (American Geriatrics Society, 2019). In the latest update, the AGS states that antipsychotic drugs should not be generally used to treat "for behavioral problems of dementia/delirium unless other options have failed or are not possible and patient is threat to self/others." This is certainly reasonable. Lastly, their criteria specifically state that all drugs high in anticholinergic side effects should be avoided in older patients regardless of whether or not they suffer from dementia.

Autism Spectrum Disorders, Agitation, and Aggression

According to the Center for Disease Control's Autism and Developmental Disabilities Monitoring Network (Centers for Disease Control and Prevention, 2020c), the prevalence of autism spectrum disorder is 1 in 54 children. Risperidone (Risperdal) and aripiprazole (Abilify) are FDA-approved for autism-related irritability. In addition, these drugs also may reduce behaviors such as aggression, deliberate self-injury, and "lashing out" or temper tantrums about 30–50% of the time; however, these drugs don't address all behavior issues, and psychiatric problems are common in children with autism.

In 2018 the FDA granted its Breakthrough Therapy designation for the development of balovaptan, a drug with potential to improve "core social interaction and communication" in those with autism (Schnider et al., 2020). Results from early trials in adults with autism were encouraging, but results from a recent study indicated that balovaptan did not improve socialization and communication difficulties (Jacob et al., 2022).

Posttraumatic Stress Disorder

In addition to antidepressants, atypical antipsychotics may be effective in veterans with posttraumatic stress disorder (PTSD) (Huang et al., 2021). Older clinical case reports support the use of risperidone, olanzapine, quetiapine, ziprasidone, and aripiprazole in combat veterans for reducing such symptoms as hyperarousal, reexperiencing, avoidance, nightmares, and flashbacks. Similarly, risperidone monotherapy was found useful for women with a current diagnosis of PTSD as a result of domestic violence or sexual abuse. Nevertheless, based on negative studies elsewhere, risperidone and other antipsychotics are generally not recommended for the treatment of PTSD (Williams et al., 2022). Antipsychotic medications, however, may still be useful to treat those individuals who have posttraumatic stress disorder and are expressing psychotic symptoms (Friedman and Bernardy, 2017).

Obsessive-Compulsive Disorder

Studies have examined using risperidone, olanzapine, quetiapine, and aripiprazole to augment the clinical response of patients with severe obsessive-compulsive disorder (OCD) refractory to SSRI treatment. In general, there is limited evidence for the effectiveness of risperidone and aripiprazole and only in short-term use. Indeed, the use of antipsychotic agents increases the risk of side effects such as weight gain, metabolic disorder, extrapyramidal symptoms, and tardive dyskinesia. Researchers (Goodman et al., 2021; Tundo et al., 2022b) conclude that up to 60% of patients with OCD do not respond to antidepressant therapy, cognitive-behavioral therapy, or exposure therapies, and therefore augmentation with a second-generation antipsychotic may be needed. As noted, "beyond SSRI monotherapy, antipsychotic augmentation is the only medication approach for OCD with substantial empirical support" (Goodman et al., 2021).

Borderline Personality Disorder

Borderline personality disorder (BPD) is a psychological disorder characterized by a pervasive pattern of instability in affect regulation, impulse control, interpersonal relationships, and self-image.

As stated by researchers (Mendez-Miller et al., 2022):

> Individuals with borderline personality disorder have an underlying vulnerability to emotional hyperarousal states and social and interpersonal stressors. Clinically these patients may have high health care utilization, health-sabotaging behaviors, chronic or vague somatic concerns, aggressive outbursts, high-risk sexual behaviors, and substance use.

Surveys have estimated the prevalence of BPD to be 1.6% in the general population and 20% of the psychiatric in-patient population. Patients with BPD have been shown to utilize extensive treatment resources and are at increased morbidity and mortality compared with the general population (Chapman et al., 2022).

There is no drug or class of drugs that have been shown to be globally effective in treating BPD, and no medications are FDA-approved for its treatment. Most pharmacological interventions target some of the specific symptoms of the disorder. Antipsychotic agents reduce affective instability, impulsivity, psychosis, and interpersonal dysfunction. As stated by one research group (Del Casale et al., 2021):

> Specific second-generation antipsychotics (SGAs) or serotonergic antidepressants can be effective for different core symptoms of BPD, mainly including mood symptoms, anxiety, and impulse dyscontrol. Some atypical antipsychotics can also be effective for psychotic and dissociative symptoms.

Evidence-based treatment for BPD remains the psychotherapeutic intervention known as dialectical behavior therapy, which is a specific form of cognitive-behavior therapy (Keefe et al., 2021).

Parkinson's Disease

We begin with a paradox: while all antipsychotic drugs (especially the first-generation agents) potentially produce extrapyramidal side effects that closely resemble the symptomatology seen in Parkinsonism (due to D2 receptor blockade), some of these drugs can be used to treat psychotic symptoms seen in patients with Parkinson's disease.

Up to 60% of individuals with Parkinson's disease develop psychotic symptoms, primarily hallucinations and delusions (Dashtipour et al., 2021). Successful treatment of psychotic symptoms in Parkinson's disease would rely on the use of an agent that has low to no affinity for the D_2 receptor. Two older second-generation agents, quetiapine and clozapine, have shown some efficacy, but, because of clozapine's undesirable side effect profile, quetiapine is the preferred treatment.

As discussed earlier, in 2016, the FDA approved a new drug for the treatment of psychotic symptoms in Parkinson's disease. Pimavanserin (Nuplazid) is a 5-$HT2_A$ inverse agonist with no significant dopaminergic, histaminergic, or cholinergic activity. It has been shown to be effective in reducing the severity of psychosis and caregiver burden without exacerbating the movement disorder in Parkinson's disease (Friedman, 2018). However, in a Phase 3, double-blinded study, researchers (Tariot et al., 2021) ceased the trial early because of lack of efficacy. Other researchers (Hwang et al., 2021) noted that the use of pimavanserin in older adults was associated with an increased rate of hospitalization and mortality. To date, SEP-363856 (Ulotaront), another investigational non-D2 antipsychotic agent, has not been evaluated for use in Parkinson's disease psychosis.[6]

THE ART OF PRESCRIBING ANTIPSYCHOTIC MEDICATIONS

Perhaps nowhere in psychopharmacology are more dilemmas, contradictions, multiple uses, and trade-offs apparent than in the use of antipsychotic medications. Many of these should be clear to the reader after studying this chapter. Here there is a fine line between art and science in the prescriber's approach to a patient.

[6]In 2021, Ulotaront was awarded a Breakthrough Therapy designation due to its increased efficacy and reduced side effects compared to current treatments. The drug is undergoing clinical trials for the treatment of schizophrenia and Parkinson's disease psychosis.

Much of the art of using antipsychotic medications to treat individuals with schizophrenia lies first in making a correct diagnosis. Then it is important to document objectively the major symptoms being expressed. Choice of medication is based on a risk–benefit analysis, whereby an attempt is made to choose a medication that will provide the greatest benefit to the patient based on symptom reduction and functional improvement while minimizing risk-inducing side effects. This selection process should be a joint effort in which the prescriber, the patient, and their caregivers participate as equal members of a team. Outcomes to treatment are improved when the patient feels that they have some control over choices and the course of treatment. As discussed in the chapter, the side effects of antipsychotic medications can be related to a particular drug's ability to block various transmitter receptors. Knowing this information can help the prescriber make treatment choices that will address the specific needs of a given individual while possibly avoiding unnecessary exposure to the side effects, or at least understanding what side effects to expect and then how to manage them. For example, for individuals who may be agitated or having difficulty sleeping, choosing a medication that is more sedating, like a low-potency first-generation agent, may be desired. If anticholinergic side effects limit adherence, a high-potency first-generation agent drug may be more appropriate, and drug-induced movement disorders, if elicited, may be controlled with anticholinergic agents.

The historical discovery and development of the first-generation antipsychotics in the 1950s was a major advance in the treatment of schizophrenia, allowing many persons with schizophrenia to be released from in-patient institutions back to the community. Equally important was the introduction of the second-generation agents. As noted, the pluses and minuses of each agent must be delineated before definitive roles in treating schizophrenia and other nonpsychotic disorders can be evaluated. Finally, tapering of antipsychotic medication is an art unto itself (Horowitz et al., 2020). Hence the art of prescribing!

CHAPTER REVIEW

1. What are the symptoms of schizophrenia? What are the risk factors?
2. Which neurotransmitters are most involved in the pathogenesis of schizophrenia?
3. What are the primary clinical differences between first-generation and second-generation (atypical) antipsychotic drugs?
4. Discuss the mechanisms of action of first- and second-generation antipsychotics.
5. Discuss the side effects of first- and second-generation antipsychotics.
6. Name the currently available atypical antipsychotic drugs. How are they alike? How do they differ? What appears unique about ziprasidone, aripiprazole, and brexpiprazole?
7. Why might antipsychotic drugs induce weight gain and/or diabetes?
8. Compare and contrast the newer atypical antipsychotics in terms of their efficacy, diabetes potential, effect on weight gain, QT effects, and other side effects.

KEY TERMS

antipsychotic drugs
aripiprazole
asenapine
brexpiprazole
cariprazine
Clinical Antipsychotic Trials of Intervention Effectiveness (CATIE) study
chlorpromazine
clozapine
Cost Utility of the Latest Antipsychotic Drugs in Schizophrenia Studies (CUtLASS) study
extrapyramidal symptoms
first-generation antipsychotics
iloperidone
lumateperone
lurasidone
metabolic syndrome
negative symptoms (of schizophrenia)
neuroleptic malignant syndrome
olanzapine
paliperidone
Parkinson's disease
phenothiazines
pimavanserin
positive symptoms (of schizophrenia)
quetiapine
risperidone
schizophrenia
second-generation antipsychotics
tardive dyskinesia
ziprasidone

CHAPTER 12

Antidepressant Drugs

CHAPTER OUTLINE

> Happiness was articulated as a fundamental right by the founding fathers of the United States. Few illnesses interfere with the pursuit of happiness more than depression. . . . Depression is common in primary care with up to one third of patients having depressive symptoms and 10% meeting criteria for major depression (Jackson, 2021).

In the almost 70 years since **antidepressant drugs** were first introduced into medicine, these drugs have been heavily promoted by the pharmaceutical industry and prescribed by physicians in the hope that they might:

- Alleviate the signs, symptoms, and distress associated with clinical depression
- Relieve anxiety either as a single diagnosis or as part of a simultaneous diagnosis of anxiety and depression
- Improve the quality of life of persons with debilitating depression
- Repair the neuronal damage associated with depression

Given these promising expectations, however, to what extent have they been accomplished?

- Depression is only modestly improved by the use of antidepressant medication. This implies these drugs have only limited efficacy.
- Side effects of the antidepressant drugs can be very bothersome and may cause individuals to prematurely discontinue their treatment.

Questions about the true efficacy of antidepressant medication have been asked almost as long as these drugs have been marketed (Cipriani et al., 2016). As stated some years ago by researchers (Fournier et al., 2010):

> The magnitude and benefit of antidepressant medication compared with placebo increases with severity of depression symptoms and may be minimal or non-existent, on average, in patients with mild to moderate symptoms. For patients with very severe depression, the benefit of medications over placebo is substantial. (Figure 12.1)

Unfortunately, in patients with mild to moderate depression, antidepressants remain frequently prescribed despite their poor efficacy and bothersome side effects, including sexual dysfunction, weight gain, possible adverse cognitive effects, and even increased risk for suicidal ideation. This lack of response is frequently termed **treatment-resistant depression** and additional medications are added, often with little improvement but with the burden of additional side effects (Cantu et al., 2021). There is little consensus on how to improve treatment outcomes. Combinations of antidepressants and psychotherapy may help, but outcomes may differ only slightly from either alone. Perhaps the type of treatment offered is less important than getting depressed patients involved in an "active therapeutic program" (or personalized treatments for depression) (Sanacora, 2020). Researchers performed a meta-analysis of 87 controlled studies of antidepressant medications, concluding that there are marked individual differences in responses, lending support for identifying moderators and personalizing antidepressant treatment (Maslej et al., 2020). Such treatment is often "trial-and-error" (Maj, 2020). Other researchers, using a World Health Organization survey database, found that the probability that patients with *major depressive disorder* obtain treatment that they consider

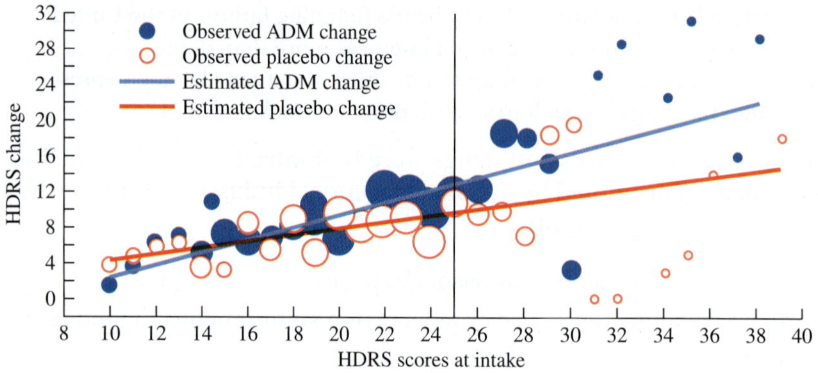

FIGURE 12.1 Efficacy of Antidepressant Medication and Depression Severity. Shown are the positive changes in the Hamilton Depression Rating Scale (HDRS, ordinate) after treatment versus the HDRS at the beginning of treatment (abscissa) in patients taking antidepressant medication (ADM, solid circles) or placebo (open circles). As illustrated, higher levels of depression at the start of treatment predicted greater medication response. The size of each circle is proportional to the number of patients at each HDRS score at intake. As illustrated, the few patients with very severe depression (HDRS scores >30) taking placebo pills exhibited wide variability in response. [Data from Fournier et al., 2010.]

helpful might increase, perhaps markedly, if they persisted in help-seeking after unhelpful treatments with up to nine prior professionals (Harris et al., 2020). This is quite discouraging, as most patients will not go through nine professionals for a shot at success! It is certainly a call for early individualization. It is also reason for the recent surge in the use of psychedelic medicines (e.g., ketamine, psilocybin) as aids to psychological therapies in the treatment of treatment-resistant depression.

As another form of treatment, researchers advocate activity scheduling and planning activities that enhance mood (such as exercise) (Taquet et al., 2020). Others expand on the beneficial effects of even modest physical exercise in alleviating depression (Pearce et al., 2022). In this light, especially in the shadow of COVID-19-induced isolation during which rates of depression skyrocketed, treatment for depression remains a significant challenge.

DEPRESSION

Depression, or **major depressive disorder (MDD)**, is a highly prevalent, chronic, recurring, and potentially life-threatening illness. Depression has become the second leading cause of disability worldwide (following ischemic heart disease) and the largest cause of disability in developing regions. Depression can worsen the health of people with other chronic illnesses, although associations remain elusive (Dragioti et al., 2019).[1]

[1]Indeed, the use of antidepressants has since grown steadily: by the late 1990s nearly 3% or more persons were taking one or another antidepressant for depression or for diseases assumedly on the depressive spectrum. That 3% number has grown to an estimated 4.3% as of 2022.

Formerly referred to as "melancholia," descriptions of what we now call depression can be found in many ancient documents including the Old Testament, the Book of Job, and Homer's *Iliad*. However, little or no information existed on the frequency of melancholia until the mid-19th century (Kendler, 2020), and it was not until the period of 1940 to 1955 that several reports indicated that the prevalence of depression in the general population was below 1%, statistics that drastically underestimate current estimates. More recent figures estimate that that 8.4% of U.S. adults (21 million people) suffered from at least one major depressive episode, with females experiencing a major depressive episode at a rate about 50% higher than males. The highest age group with depression was persons aged 18–25 years (17%) (SAMHSA, 2020). As indicated, the COVID-19 pandemic drastically increased the incidence of depression, especially in persons with moderate to severe disease, although some authors report more modest increases (Kessler et al., 2022). Persons with lower resources and economic status reported a greater burden of depression symptoms (Ettman et al., 2020).

Depression is an affective disorder, characterized by sometimes profound alterations of emotion or mood. Beside mood alterations, there may be decreased interest in pleasurable activities and in the ability to experience pleasure, sleep difficulties, fatigue or loss of energy, feelings of worthlessness or excessive guilt, and possible thoughts of death or suicide. Symptoms may be mild, moderate, or severe, depending on the extent of impairment in daily social and occupational functioning. Severe depression may be associated with symptoms of psychosis or loss of touch with reality. According to the DSM-V-TR, individuals who experience ongoing symptoms of depression of any severity for a period of two years or more can be considered to have **persistent depressive disorder (dysthymia)** (American Psychiatric Association, 2022).

Symptoms of anxiety are also seen in many people with depression. In fact, comorbidity between anxiety and depression can be found in 34% of adults (Spijker et al., 2020). Although many of the anxiety disorders have historically been (inappropriately) treated with benzodiazepine anxiolytics (Chapter 13), currently antidepressant drugs are also used for treatment of many of the anxiety disorders.[2] Not only are the antidepressant drugs efficacious for treating anxiety, they are less prone to induce dependence and less likely to impair learning, memory, and concentration than the benzodiazepines. In addition to anxiety, individuals with depression may also frequently have co-occurring obsessive-compulsive symptoms and substance abuse. Treating comorbid anxiety and depression can be a challenging clinical situation.

Pathophysiology of Depression

Historically, depression was conceptualized as a deficiency in the levels of various neurotransmitters, particularly the catecholamines or monoamines serotonin, norepinephrine, and dopamine (Pereira and Hiroaki-Sato, 2018). It was thought that restoring the levels of these neurotransmitters to "normal," usually by sustaining their presence

[2]According to current diagnostic criteria, anxiety disorders include separation anxiety disorder, selective mutism, specific phobias, social anxiety disorder (social phobia), panic disorder (PD), agoraphobia, and generalized anxiety disorder (GAD).

in the synaptic cleft by blocking their degradation and/or presynaptic reuptake, was responsible for their efficacy in restoring a normal mood state. In 2022, this monoamine theory is being expanded to include glutamate dysfunction in the pathophysiology of depression as well as several other psychiatric disorders such as schizophrenia (Henter et al., 2021). In other words, depression continues to be viewed as being the result of a chemical imbalance in the brain, and antidepressants work by correcting the imbalance.

One of the weaknesses of this chemical imbalance theory has been that there is no consistent evidence to show that there is any deficiency of any of the neurotransmitters in individuals with depression compared to individuals without depression (Moncrieff et al., 2022). Another weakness of this model is that the neurotransmitter changes occur soon after drug administration, but the clinical antidepressant effect develops much more slowly (Bourin, 2021). This delay in response was hypothesized to be due to changes in receptor sensitivity caused by the chronic increase in synaptic levels of neurotransmitter. In the past few years, however, this view has broadened, and attention has shifted to the study of the long-term actions of antidepressant treatments on intracellular processes, such as second messengers, and their functions in the neuron.

Two of these second-messenger functions are (1) to protect neurons from damage due to injury or trauma and (2) to promote and maintain the health and stability of newly formed neurons. Research into these processes has led to a new way of thinking about depression (and the effect of antidepressant treatment) called the **neurogenic theory of depression**.

The neurogenic theory is a result of the relatively recent discovery that, contrary to what we once believed, (1) existing neurons are able to "repair" or "remodel" themselves and (2) the brain is capable of making new neurons (Abbott and Nigussie, 2020; Owji and Shoja, 2020; Planchez et al., 2020). In particular, it is now known that new neurons are produced throughout life in the hippocampus and the frontal cortex of several species, including humans (Escalante-Alcalde and Chimal-Monroy, 2021). The birth of new neurons is called **neurogenesis**. This finding is especially relevant to understanding depressive disorders because the hippocampus influences many functions that are impaired in a depressed person, such as attention, concentration, and memory. At the same time, we know that the hippocampus is also very vulnerable to the effects of trauma, such as hypoglycemia, lack of oxygen, toxins, infections, and especially stress, and to the hormones that are activated by stressful situations (Fares et al., 2019). In fact, stressful situations are known both to reduce hippocampal and frontal cortical neurogenesis and to damage existing neurons.

Among the stressful conditions that can damage the hippocampus is a state of depression—not surprising, as stress is believed to be one of the most significant causes of depression. Moreover, hippocampal nerve cells are among the most sensitive to stress-induced damage and may shrink in volume when under recurrent stressful conditions. Remarkably, hippocampal shrinkage is reversible with antidepressant treatment, consistent with a role of neurotrophic factors in neuronal plasticity in the hippocampus (Yang et al., 2020). Consequently, depression is now viewed as a neurodegenerative disorder involving atrophy of neurons in the hippocampus and frontal cortex (Duman et al., 2021).

Just as a variety of stimuli can damage neurons and decrease neurogenesis, several factors are known to repair neurons and increase neurogenesis—among them, antidepressant drugs. It has been proposed that the therapeutic delay in the clinical effect of classical monoamine antidepressants occurs because of the time required for new neurons to develop, mature, and become functional. This hypothesis is supported by the observation that the increase in neurogenesis requires chronic antidepressant administration, which is consistent with the time course for the therapeutic action of these medications. This classical theory is currently under review as certain drugs that exert antidepressant action (such as esketamine, discussed later) act through the amino acid neurotransmitter system, including glutamate (the primary excitatory neurotransmitter (Hecking et al., 2021). Agents acting through this mechanism produce much more rapid-onset antidepressant effects.

A major focus of current research is to identify the cellular processes in the hippocampus and frontal cortex that are responsible for the protective effects of antidepressants. Most current studies are directed toward the second-messenger systems, as noted, which are activated by the synaptic action of neurotransmitters. This action in turn stimulates production of intracellular proteins that control the expression of certain genes (Miller and Raison, 2016; Wohleb et al., 2016).

One of the intracellular targets of second-messenger systems is called **cAMP response-element-binding protein (CREB)**. The fact that the amount of CREB protein increases in the hippocampus during chronic antidepressant treatment provides additional evidence for the neurogenic hypothesis. In turn, it is known that CREB activates genes that control the production of a protein called **brain-derived neurotrophic factor (BDNF)**. BDNF is one of a group of substances called *neurotrophins*, produced by many brain structures, which are important for the normal development and health of the nervous system (de Martin et al., 2021; Yang et al., 2020). Of particular significance, blood levels of BDNF are decreased in depressed patients, and antidepressant treatment can reverse this effect (de Martin et al., 2021).

If BDNF is deficient in the brains of depressed persons and if this deficiency leads to depressive symptomatology, might there be genetic influences that predispose a person to depression and perhaps offer new insights into therapy? Much has been done to elucidate candidate genes associated with major depression. The heritability of depression is approximately 40% but increases to approximately 70% when twins with recurrent and severe major depression are examined. Likewise, the majority of studies suggest a relative risk of approximately threefold among siblings of patients with major depression. Indeed, as many as 40% of patients with depression can trace it to a genetic link. Environmental and other factors make up the other 60%. Researchers have updated the genetic and environmental influences on the etiology of major depression (Pitsillou et al., 2020).

In summary, multiple lines of evidence gathered over the past 20 years suggest that depression is a consequence of stress, which, like any injury, disease, and physical trauma, damages the brain and weakens its ability to recover (Malberg et al., 2021). Antidepressants relieve depressed mood by acting at the cellular level to promote neuronal survival and reverse stress-induced neuronal damage (Figure 12.2). Although the immediate effect of antidepressants is to modulate synaptic levels of neurotransmitters,

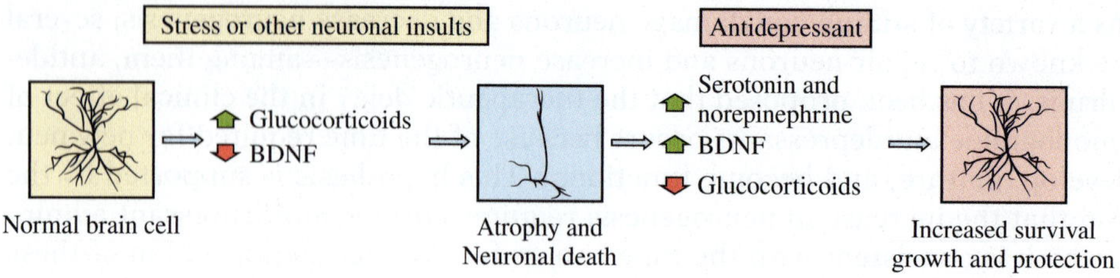

FIGURE 12.2 Hippocampal Neurons in Health and Disease. The figure shows a normal brain cell in the hippocampus on the left panel. In the middle panel, stress or other neuronal insults like hypoxia-ischemia, hypoglycemia, neurotoxins, and viruses can cause an increase in glucocorticoids and a decrease in the expression of BDNF. This combination causes atrophy of the brain cells in the hippocampus, which in turn leads to hippocampal shrinkage. Antidepressants and even electroconvulsive therapy (ECT), by elevating levels of serotonin and norepinephrine, can increase the expression of BDNF and, by reducing stress, can reduce the circulating levels of glucocorticoids, thus allowing for cell growth and increased cell survival. This leads to increased hippocampal volumes.

their ultimate targets are the intracellular molecules responsible for maintaining neuronal health and plasticity (S-C. Park, 2019). This reconceptualization of depressive disorder has broadened the search for new drug treatments, including agents that block the effect of stress hormones or that directly stimulate neurotrophic processes or directly block inflammatory responses.

Evolution of Antidepressant Drug Development

In about 1950, the antidepressant properties of the drug **imipramine** were discovered accidentally. Since then, it has been learned that imipramine and other structurally related drugs, called **tricyclic antidepressants** (TCAs, discussed next), block the presynaptic transporter protein receptors for the neurotransmitters norepinephrine and serotonin (Table 12.1). Note that the term tricyclic antidepressant refers to a commonality in chemical structure, in contrast to newer antidepressants (such as the selective serotonin reuptake inhibitors), which are defined by their mechanism of action. This is because when the antidepressant effect of imipramine was discovered, its mechanism of action was unknown so its structural classification had to suffice; the classification persists to this day.[3]

At about the same time the tricyclic antidepressants were discovered, another class of early antidepressant drugs, called the **monoamine oxidase inhibitors** (MAOIs, discussed in more detail in the next section), was identified. These drugs (Table 12.1) bind to and block the enzyme monoamine oxidase. This enzyme normally metabolizes and regulates the amount of the biogenic amine transmitters in the presynaptic nerve terminal. Therefore, when a monoamine oxidase inhibitor is administered, the levels of these neurotransmitters increase, and more transmitter is available for

[3]This same classification, by structure rather than actions on specific neurotransmitters, occurs for many older classes of drugs, including the benzodiazepines, barbiturates, and antipsychotics.

TABLE 12.1 First-Generation Antidepressant Drugs

Drug name: *Generic* (Trade)	Sedative Activity	Anticholinergic Activity[a]	Reuptake Inhibition		
			Norepinephrine	Serotonin	Dopamine
TRICYCLIC COMPOUNDS					
Imipramine (Tofranil)	Moderate	Moderate	+++	+++	+
Desipramine (Norpramin)	Low	Low	++++	++	+
Trimipramine (Surmontil)	High	Moderate	++	+	+
Protriptyline (Vivactil)	Moderate	Moderate	++++	++	+
Nortriptyline (Pamelor, Aventyl)	Moderate	Low	++++	++	+
Amitriptyline (Elavil)	High	High	+++	+++	+
Doxepin (Adapin, Sinequan, Silenor)	High	Moderate	+++	++	+
Clomipramine (Anafranil)	High	High	+++	++++	+
ATYPICAL COMPOUNDS					
Amoxapine (Asendin)[b]	Moderate	Moderate	++++	++	+
Maprotiline (Ludiomil)	High	Moderate	++++	+	=
Trazodone (Desyrel, Oleptro)	Moderate	Low	0	++	0
MAO INHIBITORS					
Phenelzine (Nardil)	Moderate	Moderate	0	0	0
Isocarboxazid (Marplan, Enerzer)	Low	Low	0	0	0
Tranylcypromine (Parnate)	Moderate	Low	0	0	0
Selegiline (Deprenyl, Emsam)	Low	Low	0	0	0

[a]Anticholinergic activity is reflected in symptoms such as dry mouth, blurred vision, urinary retention, tachycardia, and constipation.
[b]Also has antipsychotic effects due to blockade of dopamine receptors.

release when stimulated by an action potential reaching the nerve terminal. Both the tricyclic antidepressants and the monoamine oxidase inhibitors are effective in the treatment of major depression, but both possess adverse side effects discussed later in this chapter. Together, these two classes of drugs are referred to as **first-generation antidepressants**.

Problems with the first-generation agents prompted the search for new antidepressants that were equally effective and better tolerated, but less toxic. First was the development of several drugs that were slight modifications of the basic tricyclic structure but that still exhibited antidepressant efficacy. These drugs were termed **atypical antidepressants** (see Table 12.1).

During the late 1980s, newer classes of antidepressants were developed that are grouped according to their proposed mechanism of action. These **second-generation antidepressants** have varying degrees of monoamine uptake blocking properties as well as specific presynaptic receptor blocking properties. The first class of such second-generation drugs were the **selective serotonin reuptake inhibitors (SSRIs)**, the first of which was fluoxetine (Prozac) (Table 12.2). Five more selective serotonin reuptake inhibitors were eventually marketed. Because of the limitations and side effects of these drugs, antidepressant drug research is ongoing to identify compounds that act by different mechanisms. These drugs are not necessarily more clinically efficacious than the older drugs, but they may have a more favorable profile of side effects.[4] Three main therapeutic improvements still must be met: (1) superior efficacy, especially for treatment-resistant depression, (2) faster onset of action, and (3) improved side effect profile. Newer drugs, such as ketamine and psilocybin (discussed later in the chapter), both of which act through glutaminergic action, appear to be effective in reducing onset of action and improved efficacy (DeGregorio et al., 2021), but side effects still remain a problem. The following discussion of specific antidepressant drugs is subdivided into categories according to the chronology of their introduction into medicine and the neurotransmitters upon which each group is thought to act.

FIRST-GENERATION ANTIDEPRESSANTS

The first two classes of antidepressants, tricyclic antidepressants and monoamine oxidase inhibitors (Table 12.1), primarily increased the levels of norepinephrine and serotonin in the brain, which led the medical community to infer that depression resulted from a relative deficiency of these neurotransmitters and that depression could be treated by restoring these neurotransmitters to "normal" levels (although deficiencies were never demonstrated). That concept arose from an observation that reserpine (a drug that lowers blood pressure) causes depression and depletes brain monoamines. Conversely, amphetamine releases monoamines in the brain and can cause antidepressant and stimulatory effects. The correlation between monoamine levels and mood led to the *catecholamine theory of mania* (too much catecholamine) (Chapter 2) and

[4] Most importantly, the selective serotonin reuptake inhibitors are not fatal in overdose (as in a suicide attempt), as are the tricyclic antidepressants.

TABLE 12.2 Second-Generation Antidepressant Drugs

Drug Name: *Generic* (Trade)	Sedative Activity	Anticholinergic Activity[a]	Reuptake Inhibition		
			Norepinephrine	Serotonin	Dopamine
SELECTIVE SEROTONIN UPTAKE INHIBITORS (SSRIS)					
Fluoxetine (Prozac, Sarafem)	Low	Low	+	++++	0
Sertraline (Zoloft)	None	Low	+	+++++	++
Paroxetine (Paxil)	None	Low	+++	+++++	++
Fluvoxamine (Luvox)	None	None	++	++++	0
Citalopram (Celexa)	Moderate	Low	+	++++	0
Escitalopram (Lexapro)	Low	Low	+	++++	0
NOREPINEPHRINE + DOPAMINE REUPTAKE INHIBITORS (NDRIS)					
Bupropion (Wellbutrin, Zyban, Aplenzin, Forfivo)	Low	None	+	0	++
SEROTONIN + NOREPINEPHRINE REUPTAKE INHIBITORS (SNRIS)					
Venlafaxine (Effexor)	None	None	+	+++	+
Duloxetine (Cymbalta)	Low	Low	++++	++++	++
Desvenlafaxine (Pristiq, Khedezla)	None	None	+	+++	+
Levomilnacipran (Fetzima)	None	None	+++	+++	0
SEROTONIN-2 ANTAGONISTS/REUPTAKE INHIBITORS (SARIS)					
Nefazodone (Serzone)	None	None	++	++	++
NORADRENERGIC/SPECIFIC SEROTONERGIC ANTIDEPRESSANTS (NASSAS)					
Mirtazapine (Remeron)	High	Moderate	+	0	0
ATYPICAL ANTIDEPRESSANTS (SSRI +)					
Vilazodone (Viibryd)	Low	Low	+++	++++	+++
Vortioxetine (Trintellix)	None	None	++	++++	+

[a]Anticholinergic activity is reflected in symptoms such as dry mouth, blurred vision, urinary retention, tachycardia, and constipation.

DR. J'S MUSINGS 12.1

Catecholamines and Depression

I have been taught for 60 or 70 years that there was an inverse relationship between the levels of catecholamines in the brain and the continuum of mania and depression. As noted, low levels of catecholamines were associated with depression and, conversely, excessive levels were associated with a state of mania. One group of researchers wrote long ago that reserpine, an antihypertensive and antipsychotic drug, causes depression (Baumeister et al., 2003). The discovery that reserpine depletes brain monoamines was an important factor in the development of the monoamine hypothesis of depression, and it continues to be widely cited in support of this hypothesis. Conversely, catecholamine hyperfunctioning results in behavioral stimulation, hypomania, and mania. Only in very recent years has this hypothesis been reexamined if not overturned. As this chapter delineates, new transmitter targets (from orexin antagonists to certain antipsychotics to psychedelic-glutaminergic agents) also demonstrate antidepressant effects, necessitating reexamination of the catecholamine hypothesis.

depression (too little catecholamine). This theory continues to be widely cited in support of the use of monoamine drugs in the treatment of depression.

Tricyclic Antidepressants

The term *tricyclic antidepressant* describes a class of drugs that all have a characteristic three-ring molecular core. Tricyclic antidepressants (TCAs) not only effectively relieve symptoms of depression but also possess significant anxiolytic and analgesic actions. Historically, the TCAs were drugs of first choice for the treatment of major depression. The selective serotonin reuptake inhibitors, now being widely prescribed, are no more effective than the older tricyclic antidepressants, but they are less toxic, and their use is promoted by having a higher rate of patient comfort and compliance.

As noted, imipramine (Tofranil) is the prototype tricyclic antidepressant, but another clinically available tricyclic, desipramine (Norpramin), is the pharmacologically active intermediate metabolite of imipramine. Likewise, amitriptyline (Elavil) has an active intermediate metabolite, nortriptyline (Pamelor, Aventyl). In fact, these two active intermediates may be responsible for much of the antidepressant effect of both imipramine and amitriptyline, respectively.[5]

[5]It is not unusual for a manufacturer, as the patent runs out on a drug (that has an active metabolite), to market the metabolite to maintain sales.

Mechanism of Action

Tricyclic antidepressants exert two significant pharmacological actions that are presumed to account for both the therapeutic effects and most side effects of these drugs:

1. They block the presynaptic reuptake transporter for norepinephrine and serotonin.[6]
2. They block postsynaptic receptors for histamine and acetylcholine. Such blockade accounts for most of the side effects of this class of drugs.

In addition to blocking receptors for histamine and acetylcholine, many of the TCAs also block epinephrine and norepinephrine receptors on peripheral blood vessels, leading to a fall in blood pressure, especially evident when a person transitions from a supine or seated position to standing. The subsequent abrupt drop in blood pressure can cause dizziness, increased heart rate (palpitations), and fainting (orthostatic hypotension).

The therapeutic effects of the TCAs were historically thought to result from blockade of presynaptic serotonin and norepinephrine reuptake transporters. We now know that the therapeutic effects follow actions on brain-derived neurotrophic factors and subsequent improvements in synaptic plasticity in the brain. Blockade of histamine receptors results in drowsiness and sedation, an effect similar to the sedation seen after administration of the classic antihistamine diphenhydramine (Benadryl). Blockade of acetylcholine receptors can result in confusion, memory and cognitive impairments, dry mouth, blurred vision, increased heart rate, constipation, and urinary retention. These drugs should be avoided in older people.

In general, nortriptyline and desipramine are reasonable choices for initial treatment of depression when therapy with a tricyclic antidepressant is chosen. These two drugs cause less sedation and exert fewer anticholinergic side effects than other tricyclic antidepressants. More common today is the use of these drugs for their analgesic effects, as part of a pain management program for such disorders as fibromyalgia (Farag et al., 2022).

Pharmacokinetics

The tricyclic antidepressants are well absorbed when administered orally. Because most of them have relatively long half-lives, taking them at bedtime can reduce the impact of unwanted side effects, especially daytime sedation. These drugs are metabolized in the liver. As discussed earlier, two tricyclics, imipramine and amitriptyline, are converted into pharmacologically active intermediates, that is, desmethylimipramine and nortriptyline. This combination of a pharmacologically active drug (e.g., imipramine and amitriptyline) and active metabolite results in a clinical effect lasting up to four days, even longer in older patients, who can be adversely affected by the detrimental cognitive and other anticholinergic and sedative effects of these drugs.

[6] They were therefore the first "dual action" antidepressants, decades before venlafaxine (Effexor) and duloxetine (Cymbalta).

Tricyclic antidepressants readily cross the placental barrier. However, in utero exposure does not affect global IQ, language development, or behavioral development in preschool children. No fetal abnormalities from these drugs have yet been reported.

Pharmacological Effects

All the tricyclic antidepressants attach to and inhibit the presynaptic transporter proteins for both norepinephrine and serotonin, an action that is thought to account for their therapeutic efficacy. The tricyclic antidepressants, however, have three clinical limitations:

1. Tricyclic antidepressants in clinical practice have a slow onset of action, although overall, they seem to start acting as fast as any other antidepressant drug, provided that comparable dosage strategies can be tolerated.
2. The tricyclic antidepressants exert a wide variety of effects on the CNS, causing numerous adverse side effects that the serotonin antidepressants do not cause.
3. In overdose (as in suicide attempts), tricyclic antidepressants are cardiotoxic and potentially fatal in overdose because they can cause cardiac arrhythmias.

Because tricyclic antidepressants do not produce euphoria, they have no recreational or addictive liability. Therefore, abuse and psychological dependence are not concerns. The clinical choice of drug is determined by effectiveness, tolerance of side effects, prior good response, family history of good response, and duration of action of the particular agent.

In depressed patients, tricyclics elevate mood, increase physical activity, improve appetite and sleep patterns, and reduce morbid preoccupation. They are useful in treating acute episodes of major depression as well as in preventing relapses. Some patients resistant to other antidepressants respond favorably to a tricyclic. In addition, tricyclic antidepressants are clinically effective in the long-term therapy of persistent depressive disorder and in treating bipolar depression as an adjunct to a mood stabilizer, although the selective serotonin reuptake inhibitors are equally efficacious and better tolerated.

Importantly, tricyclic antidepressants are effective analgesics in a variety of clinical pain syndromes, and they are consistently superior to placebo in the treatment of chronic pain. Uses include treatment of diabetes-associated peripheral neuropathies, postherpetic neuralgia, migraine headache, fibromyalgia, chronic back pain, myofascial pain, and chronic fatigue. The antidepressant action may not only provide analgesic relief but also promote well-being and improve affect as it reduces physical discomfort. One review compared the analgesic effect of three types of antidepressants and concluded that the tricyclic antidepressants were more analgesic than the selective serotonin reuptake inhibitors (Sindrup et al., 2005).

Side Effects

Side effects follow from the anticholinergic, antihistaminic, and antiadrenergic actions that can be attributed to tricyclic antidepressants. In the patient on long-term tricyclic therapy, tolerance may develop to many of these side effects, but some will persist. Often, choosing a particular TCA with an awareness of its side effects can turn a disadvantage into a therapeutic advantage. For example, amitriptyline and doxepin (Silenor) are the most sedating of the tricyclics, making them useful in treating people with comorbid depression and insomnia. Administering one of these drugs at bedtime would provide both the antidepressant effect and any needed sedation.

Doxepin is available in inexpensive formulation as 10- to 150-milligram tablets. Silenor is formulated in a very low dose tablet (3 or 6 milligrams), priced 10–20 times the price of 10-milligram preparations of generic doxepin. The expensive formulation has little or no advantage over the lower cost generic.

The effects of TCAs on memory and cognitive function are significant. The direct adverse effects on cognition are related to the anticholinergic and antihistaminic properties of the drugs, which may be partly compensated for by the improvement in mood. Relatively nonsedating compounds with minimal anticholinergic side effects may be advantageous in persons not needing the sedative effect for sleep.

As already noted, cardiac side effects of the tricyclic antidepressants can be life-threatening when an overdose is taken. Cardiac arrhythmias caused by the drug can lead to ventricular fibrillation and cardiac arrest. Thus, all tricyclic antidepressants can be lethal in doses that are commonly available to depressed patients. For this reason, it is unwise to dispense more than a week's supply of a tricyclic antidepressant to an acutely depressed patient who is a potential suicide risk.

Because of side effects and limited efficacy, tricyclic antidepressants are not recommended for use in treating depression in children and there is limited efficacy for such use in adolescents (Hofmann, 2020).

Monoamine Oxidase Inhibitors

Monoamine oxidase (MAO) is an enzyme that regulates the amount of monoamine neurotransmitters (norepinephrine, dopamine, and serotonin) in the body and the brain.[7] Drug-induced inhibition of monoamine oxidase by MAO inhibitors (MAOIs) allows monoamine transmitters to accumulate within the axon terminals of neurons. Such blockade of monoamine metabolism causes transmitter molecules to build up in the terminal, which means that more transmitter than usual is released into the synaptic cleft upon activation. Such accumulation results in robust antidepressant action through a different mechanism of action than the tricyclic antidepressants. But the efficacy of MAOIs has been limited by potentially serious, even fatal, side effects. The risk of these side effects and potential fatalities has limited the widespread clinical utility of these drugs, although they remain a very effective treatment option for individuals who do not respond to other classes of antidepressant drugs or who may present with what is termed *atypical depression*.

---

[7]*Monoamine oxidase* is primarily found associated with the mitochondria and metabolizes catecholamines after they are taken back up into the presynaptic neuron from the synaptic cleft. Thus, monoamine oxidase prevents excess catecholamines from being repackaged into synaptic vesicles for re-release. There are two monoamine oxidase isoenzymes: (1) MAO-A generally metabolizes tyramine, norepinephrine, serotonin, and dopamine; and (2) MAO-B mainly metabolizes dopamine. MAO-B is found primarily in the brain. MAO-A is found throughout the body and especially in the gastrointestinal tract, where it may serve to limit the absorption and physiological effect of dietary monoamines.

Three monoamine oxidase inhibitors (irreversibly blocking both MAO-A and MAO-B) were developed in the mid-1950s for treating major depressive illnesses (Table 12.1). Because of toxicity, the need for dietary restrictions, and the lack of prescriber training in the use of MAO inhibitors, they are not used very frequently in clinical practice. Monoamine oxidase inhibitors are currently used as third-line antidepressants (nonselective MAO-A inhibitors) or as adjuvants for neurodegenerative diseases. Selective, MAO-B inhibitors are increasingly being studied in depression and neurodegenerative disorders (Carradori et al., 2018).

The use of the three classic, nonselective, and irreversible monoamine oxidase inhibitors is limited by potentially fatal interactions when taken with certain foods and medicines. Medicines include adrenalinelike drugs found in nasal sprays, antiasthma medications, and cold medicines. Foods include those that contain tyramine, a byproduct of fermentation, such as in many aged cheeses, wines, beers, liver, and some beans. Tyramine induces release of monoamine neurotransmitters, elevating mood[8] but also increasing blood pressure. Too much tyramine release can elevate blood pressure to extreme levels, potentially resulting in a heart attack or rupture of an aneurysm or vascular malformation, possibly resulting in death. Because monoamine oxidase is also found in the gastrointestinal tract, inhibition of the enzyme there blocks the metabolism of dietary tyramine, resulting in increased absorption of the compound. In the absence of monoamine oxidase, tyramine may modestly elevate blood pressure; in patients on monoamine oxidase inhibitors, such elevation may be extreme. Nevertheless, although they are potentially dangerous, monoamine oxidase inhibitors can be used safely with strict dietary restrictions.[9] In general practice, there have been few instances of true adrenergic crises or serotonergic crises related to use of monoamine oxidase inhibitors, so the dietary risk may be less concerning than many prescribers believe. In the past decade, dietary restrictions have been revised to minimize the inconvenience of avoiding foods that have little risk of producing deleterious effects.

Interest in monoamine oxidase inhibitors has remained strong because (1) they can be as safe as selective serotonin reuptake inhibitors or other second-generation antidepressants; (2) they can work in many patients who respond poorly to both tricyclic antidepressants and second-generation antidepressants; and (3) they are particularly effective drugs for the treatment of atypical depression, masked depression (such as hypochondriasis), anorexia nervosa, bulimia, bipolar depression, persistent depressive disorder, depression in older adults, panic disorder, and phobias.

The original three classic monoamine oxidase inhibitors are *irreversible* in their effects, since they form a chemical bond with the monoamine oxidase enzyme that cannot be broken; enzyme function returns only as new enzyme is slowly biosynthesized. For this reason, patients who need to switch from a monoamine oxidase inhibitors to another type of antidepressant must still observe the dietary restrictions and other precautions for approximately 10–14 days, until new enzyme is produced.

In the late 1990s, a specific monoamine oxidase A inhibitor, moclobemide, was developed that was reversible in action; it did not bond as tightly to the enzyme as the classic monoamine oxidase inhibitors. When detachment occurred, the drug was able

[8]Do we "feel better" after drinking red wine and eating tyramine-containing meats and cheeses?

[9]Multiple sites on the Web detail tyramine-free diets for use when *monoamine oxidase inhibitors* are prescribed.

be metabolized. Unfortunately, although this was a logical approach for developing a better monoamine oxidase inhibitor, moclobemide was not a very efficacious antidepressant and is no longer commercially available.

Interest in the monoamine oxidase inhibitors has undergone recent resurgence because of the availability of three new selective, reversible monoamine oxidase B inhibitors. Specific drugs (generic and trade names) and formulations include:

Selegiline

- Eldepryl (tablets)
- Zelapar (dissolvable tablets)
- Emsam (transdermal skin patch)

Rasagiline

- Azilect (tablets)

Safinamide

- Xadago (tablets)

All three drugs increase dopamine neurotransmission in the brain, making them useful in the treatment of Parkinson's disease, depression, and perhaps other neurodegenerative disorders such as the dementias (Ozdemir et al., 2021; Tabi et al., 2020). The first of these, selegiline (Emsam), became available as a transdermal patch that allows for slow, continuous absorption of drug. At the lowest dose of 6 milligrams, food and drug interactions were not a concern because transdermal administration bypasses the gastrointestinal tract and does not achieve blood concentrations sufficient to seriously elevate blood pressure. At higher doses, some potential exists for drug/food interactions. As initially reported by Amsterdam (2003), selegiline, as a 6-milligram patch, was robustly effective in reducing moderate to severe depression, with onset of effect in only a few days. Sexual functioning was not impaired, and compliance was excellent. Therefore, for refractory patients with severe depression, transdermal selegiline may be a reasonable choice.

ATYPICAL ANTIDEPRESSANTS

Efforts from the late 1970s to the mid-1980s to find structurally different agents that might overcome some of the disadvantages of the tricyclic antidepressants, such as slow onset of action, limited efficacy, and significant side effects, resulted in development of the so-called atypical antidepressants (refer back to Table 12.1).

Maprotiline (Ludiomil), developed in the early 1980s, was one of the first clinically available antidepressants that modified the basic tricyclic structure. It has a long half-life, blocks norepinephrine reuptake, and is as efficacious as imipramine, which is considered the gold standard of tricyclic antidepressants. However, it offers few, if any, therapeutic advantages. A major limitation of maprotiline is that, depending on the dose, it can potentially cause seizures, presumably because of the accumulation of active metabolites that excite the CNS. It is generally not an antidepressant of first choice.

Amoxapine (Asendin), also introduced in the early 1980s, is the second atypical antidepressant, structurally different from the tricyclic antidepressants. It is primarily a norepinephrine reuptake inhibitor but is also a potent blocker of serotonin 5-HT2_A receptors. It is clinically as effective as imipramine, although it may be slightly better at relieving accompanying anxiety and agitation. Amoxapine may produce Parkinsonian-like side effects as a result of postsynaptic dopamine receptor blockade. The drug is metabolized to an active intermediate, 8-hydroxy-amoxapine, which may be responsible for the dopamine receptor blockade. As with the tricyclic antidepressants, overdose can potentially result in fatality. For this reason, amoxapine is also not considered to be an antidepressant of first choice.

Trazodone (Desyrel), approved by the FDA in 1981, is the third atypical antidepressant, therapeutically as efficacious as the tricyclic antidepressants. However, it is not a potent reuptake blocker of either norepinephrine or serotonin, although its active metabolite is a serotonin agonist. Drowsiness is the most common side effect. This property makes this drug an attractive sleep aid for depressed patients with comorbid insomnia (Cuomo et al., 2019; Yi et al., 2018). Taken at bedtime, trazodone essentially blocks 5-HT2_A, alpha-1 adrenergic receptors and histamine receptors, producing sedation. A new extended-release formulation of trazodone (Oleptro) appears to be effective for a 24-hour period. Daytime sedation may be problematic with this extended-release formulation. Trazodone is also used to treat aggressive behaviors, panic disorder, and alcoholism. Trazodone can occasionally produce priapism (prolonged and painful penile erection). This side effect requires appropriate screening and, if priapism occurs, prompt attention (Shah et al., 2021).

Clomipramine (Anafranil) is structurally a tricyclic, but it has a greater effect on serotonin reuptake than the classic tricyclic antidepressants. It is an effective antidepressant and anxiolytic. In addition, it and its active metabolite, desmethyl-clomipramine, also inhibit norepinephrine reuptake. Thus, it is classified as a *mixed serotonin-norepinephrine reuptake inhibitor*, similar to venlafaxine (soon discussed). Clomipramine is approximately equal to the tricyclic antidepressants in both its efficacy and its profile of side effects.

Clomipramine has long been used to treat obsessive-compulsive disorder (OCD) (Del Casale et al., 2019), even cases resistant to SSRI therapy. The drug has also been used in the treatment of anxiety disorders. Historically, it was the first antidepressant medication to be appreciated as having efficacy in the treatment of anxiety disorders, an observation later applied to the selective serotonin reuptake inhibitor-type antidepressants.

Psychostimulants, such as the amphetamines and methylphenidates, release the neurotransmitters dopamine and norepinephrine from nerve terminals in the brain. They are occasionally examined for antidepressant efficacy (McIntyre et al., 2017). Psychostimulants promote alertness and reduce fatigue, both important features of depression. In low doses, their action is of rapid onset, and they are well tolerated with only modest side effects. Despite potential for abuse and dependence, psychostimulants are being reexamined for short-term use in treatment-resistant depression. As stated by researchers (McIntyre et al., 2017):

> Psychostimulants may be more appropriately tested in select domains of psychopathology (e.g., cognitive emotional processing) rather than as "broad spectrum" antidepressants.

They may also be useful in treating depression in older patients. For example, methylphenidate added to the second-generation antidepressant citalopram was shown to produce a faster onset of antidepressive effect and a higher rate of remission compared to treatment with citalopram alone or methylphenidate alone in an older population (Lavretsky et al., 2015). With amphetamines, the potential for tolerance and dependence must be remembered as a concern.

SELECTIVE SEROTONIN REUPTAKE INHIBITORS

Starting with fluoxetine, selective serotonin reuptake inhibitors (SSRIs) have been available since 1988. The latest two are *vilazodone* (Viibryd), released in 2011, and *vortioxetine* (Trintellix), released in late 2013 (Table 12.2). These two drugs, although blocking the reuptake of serotonin like the other SSRIs, have other effects on norepinephrine and dopamine and thereby have a different mechanism of action compared to the earlier SSRIs. In this book, these two drugs will be discussed in their own section as being atypical "SSRI +" drugs (Table 12.2). The earlier SSRIs include fluoxetine (Prozac), sertraline (Zoloft), paroxetine (Paxil), fluvoxamine (Luvox), citalopram (Celexa), and escitalopram (Lexapro).

These six drugs are all potent and selective blockers of the presynaptic transporter for serotonin reuptake. As a class, they are considered "first-line" antidepressants in the treatment of depression (Fugger et al., 2022). The degree to which they block reuptake of other neurotransmitters, primarily norepinephrine, varies greatly, with more than a twelvefold difference between citalopram, the most selective for serotonin, and paroxetine or sertraline, the least selective for serotonin. More selectivity implies a more severe discontinuation syndrome and greater potential for inducing serotonin syndrome (both discussed later in this chapter).

These SSRIs do not block postsynaptic serotonin receptors. Therefore, the primary acute neuronal effect of SSRIs is to make more serotonin available in the synaptic cleft, which activates all of the many postsynaptic receptors for serotonin. The action of serotonin at all its postsynaptic receptors is responsible for both their therapeutic actions and their serotonergic side effects.

The current view is that increased serotonin availability at $5\text{-HT}1_A$-type receptors is associated with antidepressant and anxiolytic effects, whereas increased serotonin availability at 5-HT_2-type and 5-HT_3-type receptors produces adverse effects. Increased 5-HT_2 receptor activity is associated with insomnia, anxiety, agitation, sexual dysfunction, and the production of serotonin syndrome at higher doses. Increased 5-HT_3 receptor activity is responsible for the nausea that these drugs can cause. Because of their receptor selectivity, SSRIs exert few anticholinergic or antihistaminic side effects. Most importantly, these drugs are not fatal in overdose because they are devoid of the cardiac toxicity that can be produced by TCAs.[10]

As a general statement, the clinical differences among individual SSRIs are modest; all are equally effective and about as effective as older antidepressants (Andrade, 2018a; Cipriani et al., 2018). As a class, they have an efficacy of about 17% over placebo in

[10]It is important to note that the SSRIs were never claimed to be more efficacious than the TCAs, they have fewer side effects, and they are not considered to be fatal in overdose.

TABLE 12.3 Ability of Selective Serotonin Reuptake Inhibitors to Inhibit Various Subtypes of CYP Liver Enzymes

Drug name: *Generic* (Trade)	CYP-450 1A2	CYP-450 2C9	CYP-450 2C19	CYP-450 2D6	CYP-450 3A4
Citalopram (Celexa)	0	+	+	+	0
Escitalopram (Lexapro)	0	+	+	+	0
Fluoxetine (Prozac)	++	+	++	+++	+
Paroxetine (Paxil)	+	+	++	+++	+
Sertraline (Zoloft)	+	+	+++	+	+
Fluvoxamine (Luvox)	+++	++	+++	++	+
Vilazodone (Viibryd)				+	
Vortioxetine (Trintellix)	–	–	–	–	–

clinical trials. This is not a huge improvement, but their popularity appears to be due to their perceived safety despite side effects, ease of use, and broad clinical utility for both anxiety and depression, rather than to well-demonstrated superior efficacy.

It has long been recognized that if a patient fails to respond to one SSRI, another might be tried, sometimes with improved response. This suggests some differences between drugs; the six traditional SSRIs and the atypical SSRI + drugs are not necessarily interchangeable. Differences lie in individual pharmacokinetics (half-lives), receptor selectivity, and their potency at inhibiting cytochrome P450 (CYP) drug-metabolizing enzymes in the liver (Table 12.3). Different SSRIs inhibit hepatic drug-metabolizing enzymes differently and thereby differentially affect the metabolism of other drugs the patient may be taking. For example, fluoxetine and paroxetine are potent inhibitors of CYP-2D6, while fluvoxamine markedly inhibits CYP-1A2 and 2C19. Citalopram and escitalopram are very weak inhibitors of drug-metabolizing enzymes and may be safer to use when a patient is on multiple medications.

Approved therapeutic indications for SSRI therapy include major depression, persistent depressive disorder, and multiple anxiety disorders (panic disorder, OCD, generalized anxiety disorder [GAD], posttraumatic stress disorder [PTSD], phobias). The conditions for which each of the newer drugs is currently FDA-approved are summarized in Table 12.4.

Before discussing individual SSRIs, we address several concerns associated with all SSRI medications:

- The treatment-resistant patient
- Serotonin syndrome
- SSRI discontinuation syndrome
- SSRI-induced sexual dysfunction

TABLE 12.4 FDA-Approved Indications for Antidepressant Medication

	ADHD	MDD	GAD	OCD	Panic	PTSD	Social Anxiety	Bulimia	Premenstrual Dysphoria	Smoking Cessation	Diabetic Neuropathy	Fibromyalgia
SELECTIVE SEROTONIN REUPTAKE INHIBITORS (SSRIs)												
Fluoxetine		✓		✓	✓			✓				
Sertraline		✓		✓	✓	✓	✓		✓			
Fluvoxamine		✓		✓			✓(CR)					
Paroxetine		✓	✓	✓	✓	✓	✓		✓(CR)			
Citalopram		✓		✓								
Escitalopram		✓	✓									
Vilazodone		✓										
Vortioxetine		✓										
SELECTIVE SEROTONIN NOREPINEPHRINE REUPTAKE INHIBITORS (SSNRIs)												
Duloxetine		✓	✓								✓	✓
Venlafaxine		✓	✓(XR)		✓(XR)		✓(XR)					
Mirtazapine		✓										
Desvenlafaxine		✓										
Milnacipran												✓
SELECTIVE NOREPINEPHRINE REUPTAKE INHIBITORS (SNRIs)												
Atomoxetine	✓											
NOREPINEPHRINE DOPAMINE REUPTAKE INHIBITORS (NDRIs)												
Bupropion		✓								✓		

CR = controlled-release formulation
XR = extended-release formulation

The Treatment-Resistant Patient

Many, if not most, patients only partially respond to a trial of SSRI medication. This can be due to several reasons, including inadequate dose or inadequate length of treatment. It might also be the result of administration of the drug to an individual who, based on a genetic polymorphism of their CYP liver enzymes, is considered a "rapid metabolizer," such that therapeutic blood concentrations of the drug are not achieved at normally sufficient oral dosages (Milosavljevic et al., 2021). Guidelines to improve the efficacy of SSRIs or any other antidepressant in partial or nonresponders include (this topic will also be covered later in the chapter):

1. Increasing the dose of antidepressant
2. Switching to a different antidepressant
3. Augmenting with a non-antidepressant, such as a mood stabilizer or atypical antipsychotic drug
4. Adding a second antidepressant to the original drug

None of these strategies, however, has been found to be consistently effective, and there is evidence that simply continuing treatment with the original antidepressant for a longer period of time may be more effective in the long run than switching antidepressants (Bschor et al., 2018). Conversely, researchers, in a meta-analysis of 39 clinical trials of antidepressants concluded that "Combination treatment in patients with acute depression was superior to monotherapy" (Henssler et al., 2022). Further, "Combining reuptake of an antagonist of presynaptic alpha-2-autoreceptors was superior to other combinations." An example of a presynaptic alpha-2-autoreceptors is mirtazapine (Remeron), discussed later in this chapter.

Some researchers discuss the management of treatment-resistant depression (Voineskos et al., 2020), while others discuss the use of an experimental agent (esmethadone) as an add-on agent for resistant depression (Fava et al., 2022). The four approaches listed above are discussed along with somatic therapies[11] and psychotherapeutic strategies. For example, some researchers advocate sequential preventive cognitive therapy or mindfulness-based cognitive therapy during and/or after tapering antidepressants used to help prevent relapse of depression (Breedvelt et al., 2021).

Serotonin Syndrome

High doses of an SSRI or the combination of an SSRI plus another serotonergic can induce the disturbing reaction termed serotonin syndrome (Francescangeli et al., 2019). Accumulation of serotonin leads to a cluster of responses (Figure 12.3), including cognitive disturbances (disorientation, confusion, and hypomania), behavioral agitation and restlessness, autonomic nervous system dysfunctions (fever, shivering, chills, sweating, diarrhea, hypertension, and tachycardia), and neuromuscular impairment (ataxia, increased reflexes, and myoclonus). Visual hallucinations have even been reported. Some of these symptoms might result from excess serotonin at

[11]Such therapies include electroconvulsive therapy, transcranial magnetic stimulation, vagus nerve stimulation, magnetic seizure therapy, and deep brain stimulation. These will not be discussed in this text.

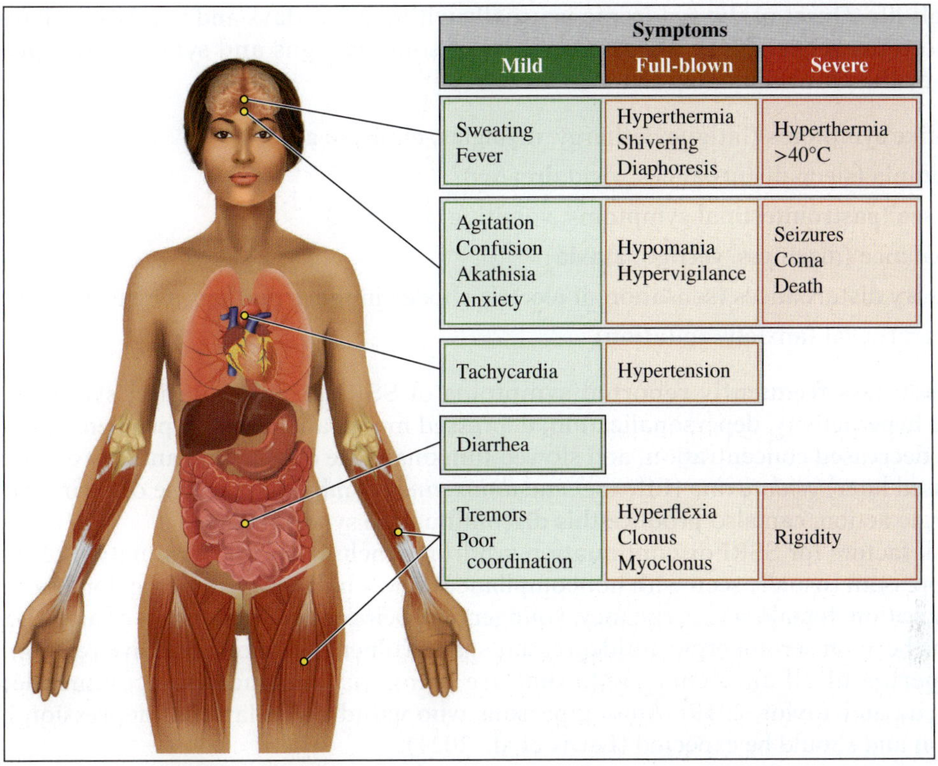

FIGURE 12.3 Signs and Symptoms of the Serotonin Syndrome. Signs and symptoms of the serotonin syndrome occur along a spectrum of severity. Mild symptoms may easily be overlooked as little more than diarrhea and flu-like symptoms. Unless the syndrome is recognized and the causative drugs discontinued, it can progress to muscle rigidity, hyperthermia, and death. [Data from Francescangeli et al., 2019.]

5-HT$_2$ receptors, which is the same site of action for the psychedelic drug LSD. The syndrome can even occur when SSRIs are combined with herbal substances such as St. John's wort or valerian. Once the SSRIs are discontinued, the syndrome usually resolves within 24–48 hours; during this time, supportive treatment for the presenting symptom(s) is indicated.

There is a positive relationship between the specificity of the SSRI in blocking the 5-HT transporter and the likelihood of producing serotonin syndrome. Therefore, SSRIs, such as citalopram or escitalopram, that have a high degree of specificity for blocking the serotonin transporter may pose the highest risk for causing the syndrome. But in clinical practice, any drug or combination of drugs potentiating levels of serotonin can increase the risk for producing serotonin syndrome.

Discontinuation Syndrome

Discontinuation syndrome occurs in perhaps 60% of SSRI-treated patients following abrupt cessation of drug intake. This syndrome can occur following discontinuation of any SSRI, although it is least likely with fluoxetine because of its active metabolite's long half-life. Onset of the syndrome is usually within a few days and persists perhaps three to four weeks. There are six core sets of somatic signs and symptoms, represented by the mnemonic FINISH:

1. Flu-like symptoms (fatigue, lethargy, myalgias, chills, headache)
2. Insomnia (sleep disturbances, vivid dreams)
3. Nausea (gastrointestinal symptoms, vomiting, diarrhea)
4. Imbalance (dizziness, vertigo, ataxia)
5. Sensory disturbances (sensation of electric shocks in the arms, legs, or head)
6. Hyperarousal (anxiety, agitation)

Other, less frequently reported symptoms of SSRI discontinuation syndrome include hyperactivity, depersonalization, depressed mood, and memory problems (confusion, decreased concentration, and slowed thinking). The dual-action antidepressants (discussed later) *venlafaxine* (Effexor) and *duloxetine* (Cymbalta), because of their serotoninergic action, can also produce this discontinuation syndrome.

Risk factors for SSRI discontinuation syndrome include abrupt termination of the antidepressant (usually seen with noncompliance), short half-life of the drug, long treatment duration, female sex, pregnancy, younger age, being a newborn infant of a mother who has been on serotonergic antidepressants, and vulnerability to depressive relapse.

Tapering of all antidepressants that are being discontinued is recommended (Horowitz and Taylor, 2019). Among persons who withdraw, relapse of depression is common and should be expected (Lewis et al., 2021).

SSRI-Induced Sexual Dysfunction

Sexual dysfunction is often associated with major depressive disorder, and SSRI medications can further compound it (Clayton et al., 2014) in both women (Lorenz et al., 2016) and men (Segraves and Balon, 2014). Up to 80% of depressed patients treated with SSRIs exhibit sexual dysfunction, including problems with orgasm, erection, sexual interest, desire, and psychological arousal. In males, ejaculatory dysfunction seems most prominent. Loss of desire and sexual dysfunction can affect medication compliance and impair interpersonal relationships. Treatment of sexual dysfunction may involve discontinuation of the SSRI and switching to an antidepressant in another class, such as bupropion or vortioxetine (Clayton et al., 2015; Jacobsen et al., 2019). Sildenafil (Viagra) and tadalafil (Cialis) are useful for some patients (Luft et al., 2021) as is bupropion (Jing et al., 2016). It may be the case that with successful treatment of the underlying depression with these antidepressants, the impairment in sexual function will coincidentally improve.

Additional Side Effects of SSRIs

In addition to the specific issues described in the previous section, there are several other notable consequences of long-term SSRI use:

- *Suicidality*. A review of FDA trials in pediatric and adolescent patients indicated that antidepressants increased the risk of suicidal ideation and behavior. In 2005,

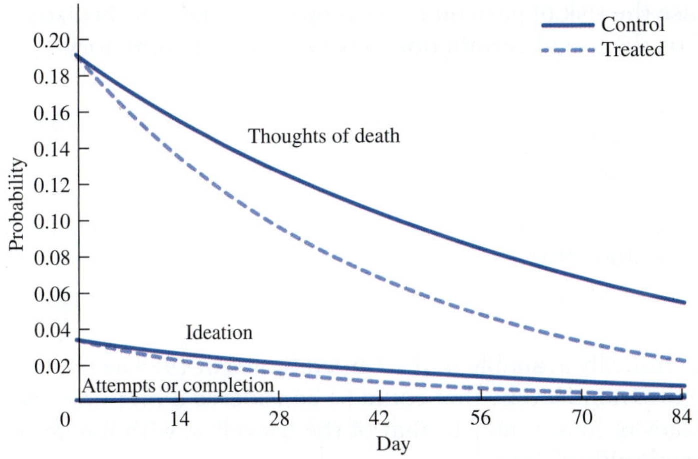

FIGURE 12.4 Suicidal Risk Decreases with Time in Patients Receiving Fluoxetine or Venlafaxine. Probabilities of suicide risk in adults receiving fluoxetine and venlafaxine. Dark blue lines indicate estimated probabilities for control patients receiving placebo; light blue lines, estimated probabilities for treated patients; thoughts of death curves, "wishes he or she were dead or any thoughts of possible death to self" or worse; ideation curves, "suicide ideas or gestures" or worse; and attempts or completion curves, "suicide attempts or suicides." [Data from Gibbons et al., 2012.]

the FDA required that manufacturers include a warning in product labeling, recommending that young patients be monitored for the occurrence of suicidality. After that, the number of prescriptions for youth fell dramatically, followed by an *increase* in adolescent suicide. In 2007, the FDA extended the suicidality warning to young adults aged 18–24, with the emphasis that depression itself may lead to suicide and that anyone started on antidepressants should be monitored for worsening symptoms. Researchers noted that in children and adolescents, SSRIs doubled the risk of suicide (Sharma et al., 2016). This was not the case in older adults. In these patients, suicidal risk lessens as depression severity decreases, and so the use of antidepressants reduces suicide risk as well as the severity of depression (Figure 12.4).

- *Sleep disturbance*. SSRIs interfere with sleep function, although these difficulties vary among the agents. They may produce insomnia with sleep fragmentation (episodes of awakening).
- *Apathy*. Although uncommon, lack of motivation and apathy have been reported in children and adults treated with SSRIs.
- *Physiological symptoms*. A variety of physiological symptoms have been reported with SSRIs. *Hyponatremia* (reduced serum sodium concentrations) may occur within the first few weeks of treatment but will resolve after discontinuation. Symptoms include nausea, headache, lethargy, muscle cramps, seizures, coma, and possibly respiratory arrest. In adults over 50 years of age, SSRI use may slightly increase the risk of sustaining fractures in a fall and of osteoporosis (Warden and

Fuchs, 2016). SSRIs increase the risk of gastrointestinal bleeding and easy bruising, although this is magnified by the use of certain nonsteroidal anti-inflammatory agents, such as aspirin.

Specific SSRIs

Following is a discussion of some individual SSRIs: fluoxetine, sertraline, paroxetine, fluvoxamine, citalopram, and escitalopram.

Fluoxetine

Fluoxetine (Prozac) became clinically available in the United States in 1988 as the first SSRI antidepressant and the first nontricyclic that could be considered a first-line antidepressant. Fluoxetine's efficacy is comparable to that of the tricyclics, with few or no anticholinergic or antihistaminic side effects.

Besides major depression, fluoxetine has been used in the treatment of persistent depressive disorder, bulimia, alcohol withdrawal, and virtually all the various subtypes of anxiety disorders. Specific formulations of fluoxetine, sertraline, and paroxetine have been shown to be effective in relieving the symptoms of a controversial syndrome termed *premenstrual dysphoric disorder.* For this use, the manufacturer of Prozac marketed fluoxetine under the trade name Sarafem.

Fluoxetine has a half-life of about two to three days, but its active metabolite norfluoxetine, which is an even stronger reuptake inhibitor than fluoxetine, has a half-life of about six to ten days. This prolonged action distinguishes fluoxetine from other SSRIs, which have half-lives of about one day and no active metabolite. Also because of its long half-life, fluoxetine need not be administered every day; it can be taken as infrequently as once a week, and a once-weekly oral formulation of fluoxetine was marketed under the trade name *Prozac Weekly*. That formulation of fluoxetine has now been discontinued.

As with all SSRIs, fluoxetine's antidepressant action is of slow onset, taking four to six weeks. Therefore, the drug and its metabolite tend to accumulate with repeated doses over about two months, presumably because levels of both compounds continue to increase. This action can explain not only the slow onset of peak therapeutic effect but also the late onset of side effects and the prolonged duration of action following drug discontinuation. Therapeutic trials with fluoxetine should continue for at least eight weeks before the drug is determined to be ineffective. Significant and important side effects of fluoxetine include anxiety, agitation, insomnia, and serotonin syndrome. In addition, sexual dysfunction is common.

Fluoxetine, sertraline, paroxetine, and fluvoxamine inhibit certain of the drug-metabolizing enzymes in the liver (Table 12.3). Therefore, coadministration of any of these four drugs can increase the level of other drugs that the patient might be taking.

In 2004, the FDA approved Symbyax, a combination of fluoxetine and olanzapine, an atypical antipsychotic (Chapter 9), for the treatment of depressive episodes associated with bipolar disorder. One review supports the benefit of this combination in treatment-resistant depression, although it produced greater increases in body weight, prolactin, and total cholesterol than either of the two agents independently or a combination of fluoxetine plus an atypical antipsychotic, such as aripiprazole, with less potential for weight gain. The olanzapine–fluoxetine combination drug has also been shown to enhance remission rates and promote better survival from relapse in individuals with treatment-resistant depression compared to treatment with fluoxetine alone (Brunner et al., 2014).

Sertraline

Sertraline (Zoloft) was the second SSRI approved for clinical use in the United States. Clinically, like all SSRIs, it is as effective as TCAs in the treatment of major depression and persistent depressive disorder, and it has fewer side effects and improved patient compliance.

Sertraline is four to five times more potent than fluoxetine in blocking serotonin reuptake but also may block the uptake of dopamine. Because of increased potency, serotonin-associated side effects (serotonin syndrome and discontinuation syndrome) may be more intense than with fluoxetine. Steady-state levels of the drug in plasma are achieved within four to seven days, and its metabolites are much less pharmacologically active. Like all SSRIs, sertraline has few anticholinergics, antihistaminic, and adverse cardiovascular effects, as well as a low risk of toxicity in overdose.

Paroxetine

Paroxetine (Paxil) was the third SSRI to become available in the United States for clinical use in treating major depression, persistent depressive disorder, various anxiety disorders, and premenstrual dysphoric disorder. The FDA has also approved paroxetine for treating generalized anxiety disorder, although this capability is probably shared by all SSRIs. Like sertraline, paroxetine is more potent than fluoxetine in blocking serotonin reuptake. The drug's metabolic half-life is about 24 hours and steady state is achieved in about seven days; its metabolites are relatively inactive.

Paroxetine is perhaps the SSRI most associated with serotonin syndrome. Furthermore, because it has the shortest half-life of the SSRIs, it is most associated with discontinuation syndrome, new onset or precipitation of psychosis, paranoid ideations, temper dyscontrol, delusions, and even visual hallucinations upon abrupt discontinuation. It is also the most likely of the SSRIs to produce an increase in prolactin levels that would increase the risk for sexual dysfunction in both men and women. It has been reported that the use of paroxetine was associated with a small but statistically significant increase in the risk of cleft lip and palate deformities and cardiac malformations in newborns of women who took the drug during their pregnancy (Berard et al., 2017). In 2006, the American College of Obstetricians and Gynecologists (ACOG) published a position statement that paroxetine probably should not be used during pregnancy. In addition, the FDA moved paroxetine from a pregnancy risk category C to category D based on the evidence of increased risk of birth defects associated with the drug.[12]

---

[12]The FDA Pregnancy Risk Categories of A, B, C, D, and X have been replaced by the Pregnancy and Lactation Labeling Rule as of 2015. Drugs approved after June 30, 2015, have this new labeling information that is more detailed and provides more specific researched-based information on (1) risk in the areas of pregnancy (including labor and delivery), (2) lactation (including nursing mothers), and (3) females and males of reproductive potential. Drugs approved after 2001 will be phased in, and drugs approved prior to 2001 are not included (Pernia and DeMaagd, 2016).

Fluvoxamine

Fluvoxamine (Luvox) is a structural derivative of fluoxetine. Like all SSRIs, fluvoxamine has well-described antidepressant properties, comparable in efficacy to the TCA imipramine, but fewer serious side effects. It has been shown effective in the treatment of all anxiety disorders. The FDA approved an extended-release formulation of this drug (Luvox CR) in 2008 for the treatment of social anxiety disorder and OCD in adult patients.

Citalopram

Citalopram (Celexa) is an SSRI available in Europe since 1989 and introduced into the United States in 1998 as the fifth SSRI. Citalopram was claimed to have a more rapid onset of action than fluoxetine, but this observation was probably overstated. Efficacy was also likely overstated, with the drug being only modestly more effective than placebo treatment. Efficacy of the antidepressants, including citalopram, may in part be dependent on which depressive symptoms are being used as outcome variables. In an analysis of results from the STAR*D study (soon discussed) to establish three symptom clusters, researchers (Chekroud et al., 2017) applied regression analysis to the data from the CO-MED study (discussed later in this chapter), using those symptom clusters to see if there were any differences in the efficacy of the antidepressants used. Although there were no overall differences among the antidepressants, when symptom clusters were examined, some antidepressants were more effective against certain symptoms than others. For example, citalopram was found to be more effective at treating the core emotional symptoms of depression than sleep symptoms or atypical symptoms, such as psychomotor or suicidal symptoms.

Citalopram is well absorbed orally; peak plasma levels are reached in about 4 hours. Steady state is achieved in about one week, and maximal effects are seen in about five to six weeks. The elimination half-life is about 33 hours, enabling once-per-day dosing. Older people have a reduced ability to metabolize citalopram. For this reason, a 33–50% reduction in dose is necessary in this population.

Citalopram has been reported to moderately reduce alcohol craving in people with alcoholism (Zorick et al., 2019). Citalopram might be expected to exert anxiolytic effects similar to those exerted by other SSRIs. Adverse effects of citalopram resemble those of other SSRIs. Citalopram likely should be avoided during pregnancy (Berard et al., 2017).

Escitalopram

Escitalopram (Lexapro) was released in the United States in 2002 for the treatment of major depression. It is also approved for the treatment of generalized anxiety disorder. The drug is the therapeutically active isomer (mirror-image molecule) of citalopram. As an active isomer, the major difference is potency: escitalopram is twice as potent as citalopram, so the prescribed dose is 50% of the dose of citalopram. In other words, 10 milligrams of escitalopram are equivalent to 20 milligrams of citalopram (Long et al., 2021). Researchers noted that doses to 50 milligrams were very effective, with 40–50% of patients eventually reaching remission over a 12-week study period (Wade et al., 2011).

One observation that has occurred with long-term treatment of SSRIs and other drugs that interact with the serotonin system is that over time, depressive symptoms that were once well controlled begin to re-emerge. This phenomenon has been termed the *poop-out effect* or *antidepressant tachyphylaxis* (Fornaro et al., 2019b; Sharma, 2019). Although this phenomenon was thought to have evolved with the administration of the SSRIs, historically it was recognized with the first-generation antidepressants and with the MAOIs. Other causes for loss of antidepressant effect must be ruled out, including medication noncompliance, recurrence of symptoms of the underlying disorder related to the natural course, or use of alcohol or illicit drugs. The frequency of tachyphylaxis may approach rates varying from 9% to 57%, depending on the patient population studied and the duration of follow-up (Kinrys et al., 2019). It has also been reported that those individuals who experience tachyphylaxis to their initial antidepressant treatment may also be less responsive to subsequent treatments (Targum, 2014). Like serotonergic antidepressants, strategies for addressing tachyphylaxis include raising the dose of the SSRI, providing a drug holiday, decreasing the dose of the medication, switching to a different class of antidepressant drug, or augmenting treatment with another psychotropic drug, such as lithium or an antipsychotic (Targum, 2014.)

NOREPINEPHRINE-DOPAMINE REUPTAKE INHIBITORS

Bupropion (Wellbutrin, Zyban) is a weak reuptake inhibitor of the neurotransmitters dopamine and norepinephrine, potentiating the synaptic effects of these transmitters (Table 12.2). In other words, it blocks the reuptake of both norepinephrine and dopamine, increasing the levels of both monoamines in the synaptic cleft (Patel et al., 2016). Therefore, clinically it has effects similar to those exerted by the psychostimulants discussed earlier, but with a lower potential for abuse. Bupropion has no effect on serotonin neurons and, therefore, does not have the side effects associated with the use of serotonin antidepressants (discussed next).

Bupropion has several uses in medicine. It has been used to treat children with attention deficit/hyperactivity disorder, although efficacy is not very robust. Under the trade name Zyban, it is FDA-approved for use in smoking cessation programs (Chapter 6). Bupropion is also useful for the treatment of depression as monotherapy, seasonal affective disorder, an add-on (augmenting) therapy in patients only partially responsive or nonresponsive to other antidepressants, and in patients with difficult-to-treat bipolar depression. Like the psychostimulants, bupropion may also reduce the fatigue associated with depression. Its therapeutic efficacy is comparable to that of the selective serotonin reuptake inhibitors. Compared with SSRIs, bupropion appears to have procognitive effects (Blumberg et al., 2020).

Bupropion has a very low rate of the sexual side effects frequently associated with use of the SSRIs (Patel et al., 2016). Treatment with long-acting bupropion (Wellbutrin SR) may result in weight loss, an advantage in patients for whom weight gain is a problem, although tolerance to this action appears to develop.

Perhaps the most bothersome side effects of bupropion include production of or increasing anxiety, restlessness, tremor, and insomnia. These are due to the dopaminergic-augmenting action of the drug. Older research indicated that seizures might occur at doses exceeding 450 milligrams per day. Therefore, doses rarely exceed 300 mg/day. Also, due to its risk of producing seizures, bupropion should not be used for treating individuals who may be in alcohol withdrawal or who may be bulimic, since these conditions, in and of themselves, increase the risk for seizures. Bupropion is not very effective in the treatment of panic disorder. Since it also increases levels of dopamine, bupropion also increases the risk for producing or exacerbating psychosis in individuals who present with disorders such as schizophrenia that include psychosis as a symptom.

Because bupropion and cocaine share similar mechanisms of action (blockade of dopamine reuptake), it is possible that bupropion exerts a reinforcing or dependency-inducing action. Although there are a few reports of snorting this drug, it does not seem to have a large potential for abuse (Naglich et al., 2019). Lastly, since bupropion enhances dopaminergic neurotransmission, it has been tried in the treatment of abuse of other reinforcing drugs such as cocaine, methamphetamine, and especially nicotine. Researchers (Ahmadi et al., 2019) compared bupropion and buprenorphine (discussed later) in the treatment of methamphetamine dependence; buprenorphine was considered the more effective choice.

Pramipexole (Mirapex) is a dopaminergic agonist used to treat symptoms in Parkinsonism and in restless legs syndrome (Martins et al., 2022). It also has antidepressant efficacy (Tundo et al., 2022) and is being studied for efficacy in treatment-resistant depression in both unipolar and bipolar depression. The drug is also discussed in Chapter 16.

SEROTONIN-NOREPINEPHRINE REUPTAKE INHIBITORS

Historically, the TCAs were the first dual-action antidepressants: blocking the presynaptic reuptake of both norepinephrine and serotonin. They also block other receptors such as cholinergic and adrenergic receptors that contribute to a wide variety of side effects, limiting their widespread use. The more limited action of the **serotonin-norepinephrine reuptake inhibitors** (herein called *SNRIs*) provided efficacy against a wide variety of anxiety and depressive disorders, with side effects associated with serotonin overactivity. Four SNRIs will be discussed in this section.

Venlafaxine

Venlafaxine (Effexor) is classified as a mixed SNRI approved for the treatment of major depressive disorder. The serotonin blockade occurs at lower doses than does the norepinephrine blockade, and at higher doses venlafaxine also inhibits the reuptake of dopamine. Venlafaxine lacks anticholinergic or antihistaminic effects, a distinct advantage. Like the serotoninergic antidepressants, venlafaxine may produce sexual dysfunction (Shelton, 2019). Some evidence also suggests that venlafaxine may be more likely than other antidepressants to trigger a manic state in people who are taking the drug as treatment for bipolar depression (Patel et al., 2015). This suggests a possibility that venlafaxine might precipitate agitated or aggressive behavior in some patients.

Concern was raised about venlafaxine's known association with blood pressure elevation in some 3–4% of patients using the sustained-release formulation and 2–13% of those taking the immediate-release preparation. Essentially, higher overdose fatality rates were seen according to studies using population datasets. In December 2006, the U.S. manufacturer issued a warning stating that prescriptions for venlafaxine should be written for the smallest quantity of capsules consistent with good patient management in order to reduce the risk of overdose. In 2010, a large population study from the United Kingdom looked at the sudden cardiac death, or near-death, rate of new users (18–89 years old) of several antidepressants. The results found no association of venlafaxine, used for either depression or anxiety, with increased cardiac risk over a period of 3.3 years (Martinez et al., 2010).

An extended-release formulation venlafaxine (Effexor XR) was approved by the FDA for the treatment of generalized anxiety as well as panic and social anxiety. Venlafaxine appears to have only minimal effects on drug-metabolizing enzymes, and drug interactions are few. Venlafaxine's primary metabolite, desvenlafaxine, is pharmacologically active; the half-lives of the parent compound and the primary metabolite are 5 hours and 11 hours, respectively.

An important review examined the adverse fetal effects (birth defect risks) of early maternal use of antidepressants (Anderson et al., 2020). Of all antidepressants studied, venlafaxine was associated with the highest number of birth defects with "meaningfully elevated associations with many specific birth defects." This implies that venlafaxine should likely be avoided in depressed individuals who have the potential or desire to become pregnant. In an accompanying editorial (Wisner et al., 2020), the authors state:

> One must balance the risks and benefits of pharmacotherapy with maternal and fetal risks of untreated mental illness. . . . avoidance of medication is not an option for some women. . . . The risk for birth defects associated with antidepressants seems acceptable compared with the risks of undertreated maternal depression.

Desvenlafaxine

In 2008, **desvenlafaxine** was approved for the treatment of major depressive disorder under the brand name Pristiq (for an immediate-acting preparation) and for generic extended-release formulations of desvenlafaxine. As stated previously, desvenlafaxine is the active metabolite of venlafaxine. Therefore, it has the antidepressant efficacy, safety, and tolerability of venlafaxine (Ferguson et al., 2012). With an 11-hour half-life, it requires only once-daily dosing. Desvenlafaxine has also been shown to reduce the frequency and severity of hot flashes in postmenopausal women, but in 2011 the FDA refused approval for this use. Desvenlafaxine was not included in the birth defect study noted earlier, but likely should be considered as perhaps teratogenic, at least until proven otherwise. The extended-release formulations do not appear to offer any advantages over the immediate-acting generic formulation.

Duloxetine

Duloxetine (Cymbalta) is another dual-action antidepressant that binds to and blocks the reuptake transporters for norepinephrine and serotonin. The blockade seems to be more complete than that of venlafaxine (Bymaster et al., 2005). Duloxetine seems to be mildly effective in the treatment of both depression and anxiety, and it has FDA indications for major depressive disorder and generalized anxiety disorder. Researchers (Cipriani et al., 2018), however, found evidence of superiority over other antidepressants to be underwhelming. Other researchers (Hellerstein et al., 2012) reported duloxetine useful in the acute treatment (10-week) of chronic mild depressions, including persistent depressive disorder.

Duloxetine has been reported to significantly reduce physical symptoms of pain, such as backaches, headache, muscle and joint pain, and back and shoulder pain; that is, it reduces interference with daily activities as well as the time in pain while awake. This drug has been approved for the management of neuropathic pain associated with diabetic peripheral neuropathy and fibromyalgia. There is also evidence that this agent may induce a manic or hypomanic episode in patients with bipolar disorder (Peritogiannis et al., 2009).

The half-life of duloxetine is about 12 hours, allowing once-daily dosing. Nausea is the most common side effect. Weight gain and sexual dysfunction have not yet been problems with the drug. Elevations in blood pressure (hypertension), theorized to be possible with duloxetine, have not yet been a major problem in clinical studies.

Levomilnacipran

Levomilnacipran (Fetzima) is another drug that blocks norepinephrine and serotonin reuptake and is approved by the FDA for the treatment of major depressive disorder. Levomilnacipran is comparable in efficacy to other antidepressants (Citrome, 2016). Its typical side effects include sexual dysfunction, tachycardia, palpitations, hypertension, and vomiting. Unlike other drugs in this class, the dose of levomilnacipran may need to be adjusted in individuals who have renal impairment. It has been postulated to reduce fatigue cluster symptoms of major depressive disorder (Gautam et al., 2019).

All four of these SNRIs can produce sexual dysfunction, produce blood pressure changes, trigger a switch to mania if used alone to treat bipolar depression, and produce tachyphylaxis (poop-out) with extended treatment.

SEROTONIN-2 ANTAGONIST/REUPTAKE INHIBITOR

Nefazodone is a dual-action antidepressant that is chemically related to trazodone, but with some important pharmacological distinctions. Nefazodone's strongest pharmacological action is 5-HT_2 receptor blockade, which distinguishes it from the SSRIs, and it also inhibits *both* serotonin and norepinephrine reuptake at therapeutic doses.

Unfortunately, nefazodone can produce liver failure at a rate of nearly three to four times greater than that which occurs in the general population not taking the drug, sometimes necessitating liver transplantation. The branded drug was removed from the market, and though it is still available in generic formulation, it is seldom used because of its toxicity and the availability of many alternatives.

NORADRENERGIC/SPECIFIC SEROTONERGIC ANTIDEPRESSANT

Mirtazapine (Remeron) was introduced into clinical use in the United States in 1997 and is approved for the treatment of major depressive disorder. The drug is clinically effective, and its antidepressant action may be more rapid than that achieved with other antidepressants. Overall, mirtazapine is a dual-action antidepressant that increases the presynaptic release of both norepinephrine and serotonin through several actions:

- It blocks central $alpha_2$-adrenergic autoreceptors. By blocking adrenergic autoreceptors, it causes an increase in the release of norepinephrine.
- It blocks adrenergic receptors located on the terminals of serotonin-releasing neurons, where they normally inhibit the release of serotonin. When these adrenergic receptors are blocked, 5-HT neurons release more serotonin.
- The increased release of serotonin stimulates only 5-HT_1 receptors because 5-HT_2- and 5-HT_3-type receptors are specifically blocked by mirtazapine.

Although complicated, this mechanism explains how mirtazapine enhances both norepinephrine and serotonin neurotransmission. Because mirtazapine is a potent antagonist of postsynaptic 5-HT_2 and 5-HT_3 receptors, it does not produce the side effects of SSRIs, especially anxiety, insomnia, agitation, nausea, and sexual dysfunction.

Mirtazapine is also a potent blocker of histamine receptors, and drowsiness is a prominent and often therapeutically limiting side effect. Sedation may be advantageous in depressed patients with symptoms of anxiety and insomnia, a common occurrence. Because of the drowsiness, the drug is best taken at bedtime and probably should not be combined with alcohol or other CNS depressants.

Other side effects of mirtazapine include increased appetite and weight gain. The drug may therefore be advantageous in certain situations, such as in the treatment of patients with anorexia, in patients with diseases such as cancer and AIDS, and in older patients, where bedtime sedation and maintenance of body weight are a goal. The drug may produce constipation and dry mouth. Abrupt discontinuation should likely be discouraged in favor of tapering (McGowan et al., 2021).

Mirtazapine is rapidly absorbed orally; peak blood levels occur 2 hours after administration. The elimination half-life is 20–40 hours, allowing once-a-day administration.

OTHER ATYPICAL ANTIDEPRESSANTS

The following are other atypical antidepressants (SSRI+). These show varying sedative activity, anticholinergic activity, and reuptake inhibition.

Vilazodone

Vilazodone (Viibryd), FDA-approved in 2011 for the treatment of major depressive disorder, is a blocker of presynaptic serotonin reuptake that is also a weak stimulant at 5-HT1_A receptors (dual serotonin action). In addition, it may have some effect on blocking the presynaptic reuptake of both norepinephrine and dopamine. Researchers performed a study comparing vilazodone, escitalopram, and placebo in 375 patients, noting comparable efficacy of vilazodone to escitalopram and superior efficacy over placebo (Sinha et al., 2021). Claims of more rapid onset of action and fewer sexual side effects have not been verified. The most frequent side effects reported for vilazodone were nausea, vomiting, diarrhea, and insomnia.

Vortioxetine

Vortioxetine (Trintellix) is a multimodal serotoninergic antidepressant, approved for the treatment of major depressive disorder. The drug exerts several different actions at various serotonin receptor subtypes. Short-term, noncomparative trials have been reported. Low doses (2.5–5.0 milligrams daily) are generally considered to be ineffective (Jain et al., 2013) and higher doses (10–20 milligrams daily) likely effective (Kotzalidis et al., 2021). The usual starting dose is 10 mg once daily (Gonda et al., 2019). Like other SSRIs, vortioxetine was effective in the treatment of generalized anxiety disorder (Rothschild et al., 2012) and in the treatment of neuropathic pain (Adamo et al., 2021). Vortioxetine inhibits the serotonin transporter with a high affinity, antagonizes the 5-HT_3, 5-HT1_D and 5-HT_7 serotonin receptors, and activates the 5-HT1_A and 5-HT1_B receptors (Adamo et al., 2021).

How each action translates into antidepressant action is unknown. However, it is the first antidepressant to exhibit this combination of actions at multiple serotonin receptors. In a double-blind, placebo-controlled study comparing vortioxetine to venlafaxine-XR in patients with major depressive disorder, vortioxetine was as good as but not superior to venlafaxine-XR in reducing scores on a depression rating scale (Wang et al., 2015). Citrome (2016) did not find any differences between vortioxetine and duloxetine, escitalopram, levomilnacipran, sertraline, venlafaxine, or vilazodone. The most likely side effects of vortioxetine are constipation, nausea, and vomiting. Interestingly, vortioxetine can improve mild cognitive dysfunction in depressed patients (Tan and Tan, 2021) and does not impair sexual functioning (Jacobsen et al., 2019).

Brexpiprazole

As discussed in Chapter 11, brexpiprazole (Rexulti) has been FDA-approved for the treatment of both schizophrenia (Frampton et al., 2019; Reyad et al., 2020) and treatment-resistant major depressive disorder (Fornaro et al., 2019a). Brexpiprazole is a dopamine/serotonin receptor partial agonist (D_2, 5-HT1_A) and antagonist (5-HT2_A).

Researchers reviewed six randomized studies of brexpiprazole in the treatment of major depression in patients with inadequate response to antidepressant medication (Hobart et al., 2019). All six studies compared brexpiprazole plus antidepressant to brexpiprazole plus placebo. In all studies reviewed, brexpiprazole was superior to placebo in improving several measures of daily functioning. Brexpiprazole provides yet another atypical antipsychotic to consider. Brexpiprazole may also have usefulness in treating bipolar mania (Vieta et al., 2021).

COMPARATIVE STUDIES

In 2018, researchers published a meta-analysis of the efficacy and acceptability of 21 clinically available (FDA-approved) antidepressants used to treat major depression in adults (Cipriani et al., 2018). In terms of efficacy, all antidepressants were more effective than placebo. For acceptability, only fluoxetine was associated with fewer dropouts than placebo, whereas clomipramine was worse than placebo. In head-to-head studies, amitriptyline, escitalopram, mirtazapine, paroxetine, venlafaxine, and vortioxetine were more effective than other antidepressants, whereas fluoxetine, fluvoxamine, reboxetine, and trazodone were the least efficacious drugs. For acceptability, citalopram, escitalopram, fluoxetine, sertraline, and vortioxetine were more tolerable than other antidepressants, whereas amitriptyline, clomipramine, duloxetine, fluvoxamine, reboxetine, trazodone, and venlafaxine had the highest dropout rates.

Recently, researchers reported an unusual (and controversial) finding with antidepressants: while they might be efficacious in short-term studies, their efficacy in improving health-related quality of life over a longer time was much less or nonexistent (Almohammed et al., 2022). While their report did not differentiate the many antidepressants, the authors stated that practitioners must remember the importance of nonpharmacological interventions (e.g., psychotherapy) as perhaps more efficacious than medication therapy. The authors concluded, "The real-world effect of using antidepressant medications does not continue to improve patients' health-related quality of life over time." Future studies should focus not only on short term effects of medications, but also on their long-term impact on quality of life. Next, we discuss other notable studies conducted over the years.

STAR*D Study

While basic research continues to improve our understanding of the pathophysiology of depressive disorders and the mechanisms of action of antidepressants, progress has been much slower in the clinical management of depression. An older, but still the largest and most consequential, antidepressant clinical trial, the **Sequenced Treatment Alternatives to Relieve Depression (STAR*D) study**, was conducted over a six-year period ending in 2006 (Pigott, 2015). The aim was to identify specific treatment strategies that would improve the long-term outcome of people with depressive disorder. The study started with almost 3000 patients at 41 clinical sites. Patients were started on citalopram at standard doses. The primary outcome was remission; patients not responding were offered a medication switch, combination, or augmentation strategies. No placebo group was included, and augmentation strategies did not include the atypical antipsychotics that are today approved by the FDA for the treatment of resistant depression (olanzapine, aripiprazole, brexpiprazole, and quetiapine-extended release). Switch options included sertraline, bupropion-SR, or venlafaxine-XR; add-on options were either bupropion-SR or buspirone. Participants who became symptom-free continued with the treatment in a follow-up period; participants who did not or who experienced intolerable side effects could continue on to other options, including mirtazapine or nortriptyline, a tricyclic antidepressant, for up to 14 weeks.

Finally, participants who had not become symptom-free were taken off all other medications and randomly switched to one of two treatments, the MAOI tranylcypromine or the combination of extended-release venlafaxine with mirtazapine.

Results

Only about 30% of patients placed on citalopram reached "remission," and about 10–15% more were "responders," who did not achieve remission but whose symptoms decreased to at least half of what they had been at the start of the trial. On average, it took nearly six weeks for a participant to respond and nearly seven weeks to achieve remission. With a historical response to placebo usually around 20–25%, these results were very discouraging because they documented the poor efficacy of the chosen SSRI to achieve significant therapeutic benefits.

Of the nonresponders, 51% agreed to switch their medication and 39% agreed to receive medication augmentation; the rest received cognitive-behavioral therapy (CBT). About 25% of the participants who switched became symptom-free. This result was the same for each of the three medication groups: no one drug was best, none worked more quickly than another, and there was no difference in side effects or serious problems. About one-third of the participants in the augmentation group achieved remission. Among patients who did not respond adequately to citalopram, CBT produced outcomes comparable to those of medications; antidepressant therapy was more rapidly effective than CBT, but CBT was better tolerated than were the antidepressants.

Researchers updated the STAR*D study, addressing what to expect when switching from a failed trial of a SSRI (citalopram) to a second antidepressant (Rush et al., 2020). Results were disappointing: following nonefficacy of citalopram, only about 20% of patients remitted while 58% had no benefit from the second drug (bupropion XL, sertraline, or venlafaxine). Other researchers propose a new STAR*D study incorporating new treatments and study design (Perlis and Fava, 2022).

Conclusions

Over the course of all four treatment levels (a total of 48 weeks), about two-thirds of participants were able to achieve remission if they did not withdraw from the study. Dropout rates, however, were high: 21% after level 1, 30% after level 2, and 42% after level 3. The data show that, overall, many patients with treatment-resistant depression can get better, but the odds of remission diminish with every additional treatment strategy needed. Overall, there appeared to be no antidepressant that was superior to all the others, and clinical decisions currently need to be based not only on effectiveness but also on side effects, cost, and patient preference.

CO-MED Study

Another large-scale study, the **Combining Medications to Enhance Depression Outcomes (CO-MED) trial**, was a prospective, randomized, single-blind, multicenter, placebo-controlled trial comparing the efficacy of escitalopram monotherapy versus two-antidepressant combinations, bupropion SR plus escitalopram or venlafaxine ER plus mirtazapine, for both acute (12 weeks) and long-term (28 weeks) treatment of major depressive disorder. Researchers (Rush et al., 2011) describe that the results of this study indicated no difference between monotherapy and the combination

Did You Know?

Genetic Influences

Cost-effective genetic testing is available to identify genetic deficits in drug metabolism, such as CYP enzymes, that predict drug interactions with many antidepressants. These interactions are important as they inhibit the action of these enzymes and increase the blood concentrations of other drugs. Recent interest, however, has centered on how genetic alterations may influence the clinical response—or lack of response—to these medications. We have also discussed how the neurotrophin brain-derived neurotrophic factor (BDNF) serves as a transducer, acting as the link between the antidepressant drug and the neuroplastic changes that result in the improvement of the depressive symptoms, and how increases in hippocampal and cortical expression of BDNF mRNA parallel the antidepressantlike response of conventional antidepressants such as SSRIs (Bjorkholm and Monteggia, 2018; Park et al., 2019).

One group of researchers studied polymorphisms on five genes: (1) cytochrome P450 2D6 gene (CYP-2D6); (2) cytochrome P450 2C19 (CYP-2C19); (3) cytochrome P450 1A2 gene, (CYP-1A2); (4) the serotonin transporter gene (SLC-6A4); and (5) the serotonin 2A receptor gene (HTR2A) (Hall-Flavin et al., 2012). Using therapy guided by these results, remission of depression was significantly improved.

Other researchers studied genetic variation of a glucocorticoid receptor protein (FKBP51) with a genotype–phenotype association between rs352428 being associated with positive responses in the STAR*D study (Ellsworth et al., 2013). Another group examined similar genomic variations possibly involved in the side effects of citalopram, again from the STAR*D study (Adkins et al., 2012). With the marketing of several genetic tests for clinical practice, the use of such testing is becoming more common not only for providing data-based decisions when initial treatments fail, but also to guide initial medication selection hopefully to maximize the probability of a good response and avoid side effects and costly delays in recovery related to treatment failures. An examination of 22 available genetic tests for clinical practice concludes that although there may be value to these tests for clinical decision making, there is a need for more research to establish reliability, validity, clinical usefulness, and cost effectiveness before such value can be established (Bousman and Hopwood, 2016; Lyman and Moses, 2016). The Veterans Administration reviewed the use of genetic testing within their system and found insufficient data to support the use at the present time (McCarthy et al., 2021). Finally, researchers note that antidepressant prescribing along guidelines for pharmacogenetic principles resulted only in "small nonpersistent effects on symptom remission" (Oslin et al., 2022).

therapies at either 12 weeks or 28 weeks of treatment; there was no difference among the therapies in overall quality of life or work function; and the side effect burden was greater with one of the combination therapies than with the monotherapy. The conclusion from this study was that there was no advantage in efficacy to adding another antidepressant for individuals who fail to respond fully to a single antidepressant and that the combination leads to greater risk of side effects. As discussed in a prior section, a subsequent analysis of the data from the STAR*D study using symptom clusters derived from the CO-MED study found that although the overall outcomes were disappointing, if certain drugs could be matched to certain symptom clusters, greater efficacy might be achieved (Chekroud et al., 2017).

NONCATECHOLAMINE ANTIDEPRESSANTS

The history of antidepressant drugs now encompasses over 70 years. As is apparent in the descriptions of current drugs, we still seek the "perfect" antidepressant, and the search continues for either new medications or new antidepressant uses for older drugs. This search focuses on compounds that possess antidepressant actions independent of actions on the catecholamine or serotonin systems. A few such compounds are now available and several more are under development. Many of these center on the glutamate and opioid systems (Pappagallo et al., 2022). Some notable examples include GABA-targeting drugs such as brexanolone and zuranolone as well as buprenorphine/samidorphan, dextromethorphan/buprenorphine, REL-1017, ketamine, esketamine, psilocybin, LSD, and nitrous oxide. Before discussing these, however, we first cover two other drugs, agomelatine and seltorexant.

Agomelatine

Agomelatine is a novel antidepressant which acts as a melatonin MT_1 and MT_2 receptor agonist and serotonin 5-HT_{2C} receptor antagonist. The combined action at these receptors appears necessary for antidepressant efficacy (Norman and Olver, 2019).

In the acute treatment of depression, agomelatine seems to be more effective in patients with severe anxiety symptoms or disturbed circadian rhythms (Konstantakopoulos et al., 2020). It can improve sleep in depressed patients (Mi et al., 2020). As will be discussed in Chapter 13, it is useful in the treatment of moderate to severe anxiety (Stein et al., 2021). Due to a potential for liver problems, the drug is not available in the United States.

Seltorexant

Adults with insomnia have a high risk of experiencing depression (Jha, 2022). Unfortunately, most of the available medications used for treating insomnia (discussed in Chapter 13) inhibit cognitive functioning and can actually worsen depression (e.g., benzodiazepines). Chapter 13 will introduce a class of drugs known as orexin receptor antagonists that function as hypnotic drugs in the absence of cognitive impairment.

Two dual orexin (orexin-1 and orexin-2) receptor antagonists are commercially available for the treatment of insomnia (Muehlan et al., 2020), and one, **seltorexant** (a specific orexin-2 receptor antagonist), is under investigation for the treatment of insomnia and major depression. The antidepressant effects appear to be greatest in those with the highest insomnia ratings (Jha, 2022; Savitz et al., 2021).

Brexanolone

Brexanolone (Zulresso) is a newly marketed intravenous formulation of allopregnanolone, the first of a new class of neuroactive steroid drugs and a modulator of gamma aminobutyric acid ($GABA_A$) receptors, for the treatment of postpartum depression, a serious condition that, when severe, can be life-threatening. Postpartum depression can be persistent, lasting for months or years. Women may experience thoughts about harming themselves or harming their child. It is estimated that postpartum depression affects one in nine women nationally. Postpartum depression historically has been treated with counseling and SSRI medication that can take weeks to work, if at all. Brexanolone may hopefully improve that outlook.

Brexanolone is delivered as a continuous infusion over the course of 60 hours under medical supervision. The drug works quickly, usually within one to two days, and costs $20,000 or more. In a manufacturer-sponsored study, this expenditure was deemed to be cost-effective (Eldar-Lissal et al., 2020).

Brexanolone is a synthetic formulation of the hormone allopregnanolone, a progesterone derivative. This hormone increases throughout a woman's pregnancy and then falls drastically after she gives birth, a possible contributor to postpartum depression. The mechanism by which neurosteroid $GABA_A$ receptor modulators like brexanolone have antidepressant effects is unknown (Antonoudiou et al., 2022). Other $GABA_A$ receptor modulators, such as benzodiazepines, are not known to have antidepressant effects. Neurosteroid $GABA_A$ receptor modulators are known to interact with $GABA_A$ receptors and subpopulations differently than benzodiazepines.[13] Several reviews of brexanolone in postpartum depression are available (Edinoff et al., 2021; Leader et al., 2019; Luscher and Mohler, 2019; Payne, 2021; Powell et al., 2020; Zheng et al., 2019).

Zuranolone

The manufacturer of brexanolone is developing another compound called **zuranolone** for the treatment of major depressive disorder in general and postpartum depression in particular (Deligiannidis et al., 2021; Walkery et al., 2021). Zuranolone was developed as an improvement to brexanolone for the treatment of postpartum depression. Zuranolone has better bioavailability and can be administered orally, whereas brexanolone is administered via intravenous injection. In a Phase 2 study, zuranolone

[13]As examples, $GABA_A$ receptor-potentiating neurosteroids may preferentially target δ subunit-containing $GABA_A$ receptors and enhance both tonic and phasic inhibition mediated by $GABA_A$ receptors. It is also possible that neurosteroids like allopregnanolone may act on other targets, all of which is currently poorly understood.

(89 patients received 30 milligrams zuranolone for two weeks and were followed for four more weeks) was considered effective not only in reducing depression scores but also in improving quality-of-life scores (Gunduz-Bruce et al., 2019; Suthoff et al., 2022). Side effects consisted of headache, dizziness, nausea, and somnolence.

Zuranolone is rapidly effective, and one course of treatment is only 14 days long. This may allow for episodic rather than continuous treatment. In 2022, the manufacturer reported positive results of a Phase 3 study of zuranolone in the treatment of unipolar depression (Arnaud and Bonthapally, 2022). The drug received FDA Fast Track and Breakthrough Therapy designation in 2018 and may soon be marketed.

Buprenorphine/Samidorphan

In another departure from the traditional monoamine hypothesis of depression, one focus has been on modulating the opioid system (Ragguett et al., 2018, 2019). Of current interest is a combination product consisting of the opioid kappa receptor antagonist and mu opioid partial agonist buprenorphine with samidorphan, the latter drug being a naloxone derivative and a mu opioid receptor antagonist (Chaudhary et al., 2019). In clinical studies, this combination product was found to have beneficial effects in patients with treatment-resistant depression (Fava et al., 2020; Thase et al., 2019). The combination product was well tolerated, with low risk of abuse, and discontinuation led to minimal withdrawal effects. Conversely, researchers (Dinoff et al., 2020) found the antidepressant effectiveness of buprenorphine (with or without samidorphan) to be underwhelming. Unfortunately, the barriers to physicians' prescribing buprenorphine persist and limit the prescription of this medicine (Lanham et al., 2022).

Dextromethorphan/Buprenorphine

A combination of dextromethorphan and bupropion (DXM/BUP) was recently FDA approved for the treatment of depression under the trade name *Auvelity*. The **DXM/BUP** combination was effective in clinical trials with minimal relapse over at least six months of double-blind treatment (Tabuteau et al., 2022). DXM is an antagonist of the NMDA receptor, an ionotropic glutamate receptor, and a sigma-1 receptor agonist. These actions modulate glutamatergic neurotransmission. The bupropion component of Auvelity inhibits the metabolism of dextromethorphan by inhibiting the enzyme CYP2D6, the major enzyme responsible for the bioavailability of DXM, prolonging its half-life. Auvelity is generally superior to both placebo and bupropion (Losifescu et al., 2022; Majeed et al., 2021; Tabuteau et al., 2022). Auveity is also being examined for the treatment Alzheimer's disease agitation.

A related drug, deudextromethorphan (AVP-786), is being studied as another glutaminergic antagonist rapid-onset antidepressant. It is being studied in combination with a low dose of quinidine, another potent inhibitor of CYP2D6. That combination is also being evaluated for the treatment of Alzheimer's disease agitation (Khoury, 2022).

REL-1017 (Esmethadone or Dextromethadone)

Racemic methadone is an opioid agonist most commonly used in the treatment of opioid dependence, primarily dispensed through methadone clinics (Chapter 10). **REL-1017** is a glutaminergic NMDA channel blocker that preferentially targets hyperactive channels while maintaining physiological glutaminergic neurotransmission. As stated by researchers, this "allows for improvement in depressive symptoms in the absence of cognitive side effects typical of NMDA channel blockers" (de Martin et al., 2021). In this case, REL-1017 resembles ketamine, a NMDA receptor antagonist with rapid antidepressant effects in humans (de Martin et al., 2021). In animal studies, "REL-1017 did not produce initial or cumulative neurotoxic effects or other evidence of damage to cortical neurons" (Bifari et al., 2022). In studying esmethadone, researchers (Fava et al., 2022) concluded:

> This trial showed favorable safety, tolerability, and pharmacokinetic profiles and suggests that REL-1017 may have rapid and sustained antidepressant effects compared with placebo in patients with inadequate response to antidepressant treatments.

Ketamine

Chapter 9 presented the pharmacology of ketamine and its close relative phencyclidine as psychedelic (dissociative) drugs, use and abuse of which can be accompanied by out-of-body effects (Wei et al., 2020). Specifically, the actions of both drugs were characterized by amnesia, analgesia, and psychotomimetic effects; these made the two drugs useful as anesthetics and analgesics. Other off-label uses of ketamine have been explored, including use of ketamine-assisted psychotherapy (Botteranne et al., 2022; Mathai et al., 2022). By about the year 2000, the first controlled, double-blinded, placebo-controlled use of ketamine as an antidepressant was reported (Hashimoto, 2019). In 2013, researchers had demonstrated the antidepressant effects of repeated ketamine infusions in the treatment of resistant major depression (Murrough et al., 2013) (Figure 12.5). As a glutamate NMDA-type antagonist, this was a significant demonstration of antidepressant action *independent* of actions of the catecholamine systems (Jaso et al., 2017; Kalmoe et al., 2020).

Since that demonstration, many other studies have investigated the antidepressant actions of ketamine as well as its active isomer (mirror-image molecule) S-ketamine (also named esketamine), resulting in FDA approval in 2019 of an esketamine nasal spray (Spravato) for the treatment of major depression in adults (Andrade, 2017; Kryst et al., 2020; Zheng et al., 2020). Researchers compared intravenous ketamine (0.5 mg/kg body weight over 40 minutes of infusion) with intranasal esketamine (56 or 84 mg) and concluded that data favored ketamine over esketamine (Nikayin et al., 2022). Regardless, esketamine nasal spray is FDA-approved for depression treatment while ketamine has no such approval (Yavi et al., 2022). Esketamine is administered in a certified facility with the patient observed for at least 2 hours before discharge. Dosing is twice weekly for four weeks, then once weekly. Patients are not to drive until after a restful

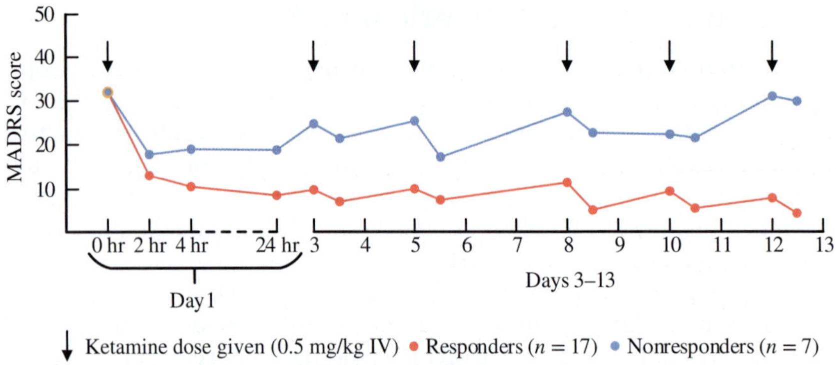

FIGURE 12.5 Effect of Ketamine Infusions on Depression Severity in Treatment-Resistant Major Depression. The MADRS score is a measure of depression severity on the Montgomery-Asberg Depression Rating Scale. Ketamine was administered intravenously on days 1, 3, 5, 8, 10 and 12. Baseline depression severity was measured prior to the first ketamine infusion at 0 hours on day 1 and then at subsequent times corresponding to the data points in the graph (on days 3–13, measurements were taken in the morning prior to any ketamine infusion and then 4 hours later). At every measurement after the baseline measurement, responders showed a significantly decreased MADRS score compared to baseline, and there was a significant difference between the MADRS scores of responders and nonresponders. (Three of the nonresponders did not receive all six ketamine infusions.) [Data from Murrough et al., 2013.]

night's sleep. Sedation, cognitive impairment, and dissociative reactions are major side effects. Researchers (Daly et al., 2019) reported that patients with treatment-resistant depression who responded or remitted with esketamine treatment and were continued on esketamine plus an oral antidepressant maintained clinical improvement over a 90-week study period. Other researchers reported that both younger and older patients with treatment-resistant depression responded equally well to esketamine over a one-year study period (Ochs-Ross et al., 2021).

Researchers (Andrade et al., 2022; Ekstrand et al., 2021) compared racemic ketamine with electroconvulsive therapy (ECT) (see Espinoza and Kellner, 2022, for a review of ECT in treating depression). ECT was generally superior to ketamine in hospitalized, depressed patients. Older patients were more responsive to ECT, while younger patients seemed to respond as well to ketamine as to ECT.

With knowledge of the antidepressant activity and the marketing of the active isomer of racemic ketamine, many other psychedelic drugs are being reexamined for antidepressant activity. These drugs include psilocybin, ayahuasca, ibogaine, 5-methoxy-N-N-dimethyltryptamine (5-MeO-DMT), and LSD, some of which we cover next.

Psilocybin

Like ketamine, psilocybin was discussed in Chapter 9. In a small study in 2016, researchers reported the efficacy and safety of psilocybin (two doses) in 12 patients with moderate to severe unipolar treatment-resistant major depression

(Carhart-Harris et al., 2016). Other researchers reviewed four studies of the efficacy of psilocybin, confirming efficacy with few serious side effects (Goldberg et al., 2020). In 2020, the FDA granted Breakthrough Therapy designation (with clinical trials ongoing) to psilocybin for major depression (Heifets and Malenka, 2019). Researchers compared psilocybin with escitalopram in a Phase 2, double-blinded, six-week controlled trial in 59 patients with long-standing severe depression (Carhart-Harris et al., 2021). Psilocybin patients received two doses, three weeks apart; escitalopram patients received daily doses of the drug. In general, the two agents exerted comparable effects on depression scores, with psilocybin exerting greater effect of scores for psychological well-being. The authors concluded that "larger and longer trials are required to compare psilocybin with established antidepressants." Other researchers reviewed the receptor pharmacology and neuronal mechanisms underlying the antidepressant properties of psilocybin, primarily agonism at 5-HT2_A receptors and "downstream changes in gene expression" (Ling et al., 2022). One research group studied the mechanism of action of psilocybin, whereby "5-HT2_A receptor-rich higher-order functional networks became more functionally interconnected and flexible after psilocybin treatment" (Daws et al., 2022). They concluded, "Consistent efficacy-related brain changes, correlating with robust antidepressant effects across two studies, suggest an antidepressant mechanism for psilocybin therapy: global increases in brain network integration."

In essence, psilocybin (and likely other psychedelic drugs) may rewire the brain, briefly disrupting neuronal connections, allowing them to "reform in new ways in the days and weeks following treatment" (Carhart-Harris, 2022).

LSD

Like psilocybin and ketamine the resurgence of psychedelic psychopharmacology, LSD has been examined for antidepressant activity and for use in drug and alcohol dependence (Lowe et al., 2022). Such trials are in their infancy (Fuentes et al., 2020). Researchers discuss the current status of psychedelic drugs as antidepressants and other potentially clinical uses (Gonda et al., 2021; Henter et al., 2021; Siegel et al., 2021). Likely, psychedelic therapy will be most effective when combined with psychological therapies, such as mindfulness training (Eleftheriou and Thomas, 2021) and CBT (Thase et al., 2020; Wright et al., 2022).

Nitrous Oxide

The discovery of ketamine's action as an antidepressant initiated a search for additional drugs that act via similar glutamate antagonistic effects (Demchenko et al., 2022) and that might be devoid of ketamine's side effects (memory impairments and psychosis). **Nitrous oxide** (used as an anesthetic for many years) is also an NMDA receptor antagonist and has shown promise as a rapid-acting antidepressant in patients with treatment-resistant depression (Kalmoe et al., 2020; Nagele et al., 2018). Nitrous oxide is a gas that must be administered through a blender mixed with 50% oxygen to avoid hypoxic reactions. Because of this, the drug must be administered in a medical setting and in the presence of trained administrators of the drug.

ADDITIONAL AND ALTERNATIVE APPROACHES TO TREATMENT-RESISTANT DEPRESSION

Because it is so important, we return to the topic of treatment-resistant depression. In general, the response to initial treatment with an antidepressant medication is in the range of 35% (Demchenko et al., 2022). Although individuals may have a reduction in symptoms, they may not reach a point in their recovery where an examination, using a standardized rating scale of the presence and severity of depressive symptoms, would indicate that they no longer meet the criteria for the diagnosis of major depressive disorder. For these individuals with treatment-resistant depression, a careful investigation into the reasons for lack of full response or remission is needed (Voineskos et al., 2020). As noted earlier in the chapter, potential reasons for not achieving a good response include (1) not receiving an adequate dose of the antidepressant drug for an adequate period of time; (2) not being given the correct diagnosis and then being treated with the wrong drug; (3) the individual, feeling that he or she is better, voluntarily stops medication and relapses; or (4) the individual is having too many uncomfortable side effects and he or she stops the medication. All these factors, if present, should be corrected before declaring that a person has treatment-resistant depression.

In the face of resistant depression, several options have been explored. Mentioned previously, one option is to simply switch to a different antidepressant medication in the same class or different class. Studies have not found much benefit in switching drugs as opposed to simply maintaining treatment for a longer period of time using the drug that was first administered. In addition, it should not be forgotten that some individuals may do best on the first-generation antidepressant drugs, especially those with comorbid pain and insomnia.

Another approach to treatment-resistant depression mentioned earlier is to combine antidepressant drugs (Ruberto et al., 2020). This may include combining an SSRI with an SNRI. However, this may not always improve outcome. For example, adding mirtazapine to an SSRI or SNRI did not improve response rates over placebo (Kessler et al., 2018). In some cases, additional approaches must be considered.

Augmentation

Lithium has been shown to be an effective agent when combined with an antidepressant to enhance antidepressant efficacy. Lithium augmentation appears to be more effective in older patients compared to younger patients (Buspavanich et al., 2019). Historically, triiodothyronine (T_3) has also been used as an augmenting agent, although it has not been shown to be consistently effective in controlled studies (Haddad et al., 2015).

As discussed, four atypical antipsychotics, aripiprazole, olanzapine, brexpiprazole, and quetiapine extended release, have been approved by the FDA for treatment-resistant depression. There does seem to be some evidence for the efficacy of combining an atypical antipsychotic with an antidepressant for treatment-resistant depression. But this combination has been shown to increase the likelihood of side effects.

One group of researchers (Casey et al., 2012) included review of three studies in patients with inadequate response to a selective serotonin reuptake inhibitor; aripiprazole accelerated early response and this predicted maintenance of response through the end point (Figure 12.6). Another group (Richardson et al., 2011) noted that aripiprazole potentiated inadequate SSRI response in treating comorbid military-related posttraumatic stress disorder and depression. Other researchers (Han et al., 2013) noted that aripiprazole potentiated escitalopram in both improving antidepressant response and reducing alcohol dependence. Similarly, quetiapine was found to be an effective antidepressant as a sole agent and for improving both depression and poor sleep quality.

Researchers demonstrated augmentation of the antidepressant action of fluoxetine by the addition of modafinil (Provigil), a nonstimulant wakefulness-promoting drug used to combat daytime fatigue in patients with narcolepsy (Abolfazli et al., 2011). It does not produce typical psychostimulant-induced side effects, and, in narcoleptic patients, modafinil may also improve subjective well-being, reduce fatigue, and enhance cognition and concentration. Several randomized controlled trials and a meta-analysis support the efficacy of modafinil as an augmenting agent to antidepressant treatment of unipolar depression (Haddad et al., 2015).

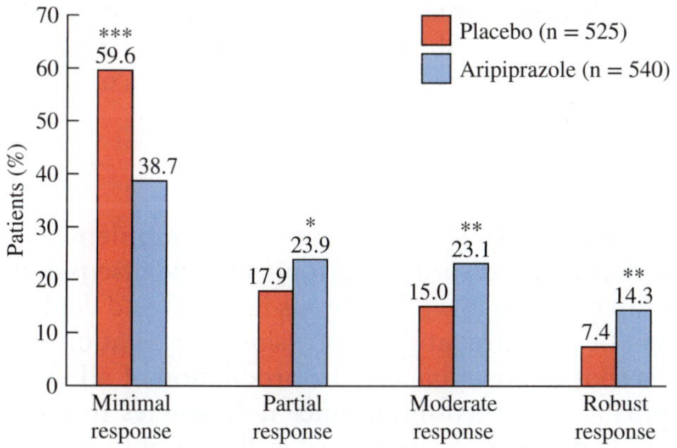

FIGURE 12.6 Efficacy of Aripiprazole in Treating Depression. Shown is the percentage of 1065 patients exhibiting minimal to maximal response to aripiprazole (blue bars) or placebo (red bars) as measured by the Massachusetts General Hospital Antidepressant Treatment Response Questionnaire. Patients were classified as nonresponders to standard medication treatment, and aripiprazole or placebo was added for a six-week trial of combination therapy. Asterisks indicate a statistical difference between the two treatments. [Data from Casey et al., 2012.]

Modafinil has two isomers, each of which is active. Armodafinil (Nuvigil) is the longer-acting isomer formulation of modafinil now FDA-approved for the treatment of narcolepsy and shift-work sleep disorders.

Lamotrigine (Lamictal) is an effective anticonvulsant and mood stabilizer. It is unique as an anticonvulsant in that it has clearly stated antidepressant properties. Therefore, it has become a staple in the treatment of bipolar depression. However, it has not proven to be effective as an augmenting agent for the treatment of unipolar depression and is considered as second-line augmentation to SSRIs in treatment-resistant patients (Goh et al., 2019).

Complementary and Alternative Medicine Approaches

Beyond augmentation, alternative approaches to treatment-resistant depression include the following.

Omega-3 Fatty Acids

Two types of omega-3 fatty acids are found in fatty fish such as salmon, sardines, and mackerel: eicosapentaenoic acid (EPA) and docosahexaenoic acid (DHA), also known as *polyunsaturated fatty acids* (PUFA). The American Heart Association recommends eating at least two servings of fatty fish each week, suggesting that the omega-3 fats found in the fish help protect against cardiovascular disease. Omega-3 oils are also essential during pregnancy for brain maturation in the neonate. Much speculation has developed about the potential efficacy of omega-3 oils in the treatment of depression. Here, evidence for efficacy is weak and conflicting (Deacon et al., 2017). Researchers (Deane et al., 2021; Okereke et al., 2021; Thesing et al., 2020) concluded the polyunsaturated fatty acids are of little use in preventing relapses of major depressive disorder.

Folate and Vitamin B_{12}

Folate is a B vitamin that occurs naturally in food and in nutritional supplements. The possible significance of folate in depressive disorder is a topic of wide discussion. Indeed, there seems to be a relationship between low folate levels in blood and depressive disorder. Thus, replacement might be a treatment for depression. The relationship between folate and antidepressants is that folate enhances the production of all three monoamines, dopamine, norepinephrine, and serotonin. Since deficiencies in these neurotransmitters are theoretically linked to depressive disorder, this might underlie the etiology of some cases of depression. It has been postulated that some people have a genetic defect in folate metabolism that might increase the risk of depression. There is ongoing controversy whether, in depressed patients with folate deficiency who have not responded to antidepressants, augmentation with a new, expensive folate metabolite, L-methylfolate (Deplin) or delta methylfolate (EnLyte), which is considered a medical food under FDA regulations, might be more effective than dietary folate.

Researchers (Bender et al., 2017) performed a meta-analysis of folate in depression. Not surprisingly, they reported that persons with depression have lower serum folate levels than persons without depression. They conclude by stating, "Clinicians may wish to consider folate supplementation for patients with depression." Other researchers took this a step further by including analysis of vitamin B_{12} (Khosravi et al., 2020). They concluded their study by stating:

> The healthy dietary pattern was associated with a reduced risk of depression via increased serum levels of folate and vitamin B_{12}. However, the unhealthy diet pattern was associated with increased risk of depression via decreased serum levels of folate and vitamin B_{12}.

Much of what can be said of folate can be said of vitamin D: low vitamin D levels can be associated with depression (Hoang et al., 2011) and dietary replacement may be therapeutically effective as an adjunct to SSRI therapy (Khoraminya et al., 2013). Researchers reported on a series of 22 children and adolescents to whom EnLyte (a B-vitamin-based coenzyme monotherapy) was administered and some of whom received other antidepressant medication. Side effects were minimal and no patient reported suicidal thoughts (Farah and Madan, 2021).

S-Adenosylmethionine

S-Adenosylmethionine (SAM-e) is a naturally occurring molecule present in all body cells. It catalyzes methylating reactions, including L-methylfolate. There is some evidence for deficiency in depression, with supplementation perhaps assisting to relieve mild depression, but the evidence does not support use in severely depressed persons (Sarris et al., 2020). Part of this difficulty may be due to the fact that oral absorption of SAM-e is poor and less than 1% of the ingested drug reaches the bloodstream.

St. John's Wort

St. John's wort is an extract of *Hypericum perforatum*, a perennial herb. It has been used to treat mild to moderate depression (Ng et al., 2017). In most studies, the compound was superior to placebo and equivalent to standard drugs, although most studies have been methodically flawed. Mechanistically, St. John's wort mimics the neurotrophic effect of BDNF in the hippocampus. St. John's wort likely should not be combined with most other antidepressants (especially SSRIs) because of its potential to induce serotonin syndrome. The drug also induces drug-metabolizing enzymes such that other drugs taken by an individual may become more toxic at usual doses. Other side effects, such as gastrointestinal distress, photodermatitis, elevated thyroid-stimulating hormones, hypertensive crisis, induction of mania, and fatigue, may further reduce its therapeutic utility.

CHAPTER REVIEW

1. What is the relationship between depression and the biological amine transmitters in the brain?
2. List and differentiate the major classes of antidepressants.

3. Describe the probable mechanism of tricyclic antidepressants and monoamine oxidate inhibitors. What are their clinical limitations and possible side effects?
4. Discuss some of the major atypical antidepressants. How are they different from the tricyclic antidepressants, and what are their side effects?
5. Discuss the side effects of SSRIs. What is serotonin syndrome? What is SSRI discontinuation syndrome? Discuss the effects of these drugs on sexual function.
6. Which drug or class of drugs do you think is the "best" antidepressant? Why?
7. Which antidepressants are used in the treatment of anxiety disorders? Why? How do these drugs differ from the benzodiazepine-type anxiolytics?
8. Discuss the strategies being used to discover the next generation of antidepressant drugs and the types of drugs that are being developed from those approaches.
9. Discuss the reasons for not achieving a good response to medication in individuals with treatment-resistant depression. What are some alternative approaches for treatment?
10. Outline the drugs being considered as psychedelics used in the treatment of depression.

KEY TERMS

agomelatine
amoxapine
antidepressant drugs
atypical antidepressants
brain-derived neurotrophic factor (BDNF)
brexanolone
bupropion
cAMP response-element-binding protein (CREB)
citalopram
clomipramine
Combining Medications to Enhance Depression Outcomes (CO-MED) trial
depression (major depressive disorder; MDD)
desvenlafaxine
duloxetine
DXM/BUP
escitalopram
first-generation antidepressants
fluoxetine
fluvoxamine
imipramine
levomilnacipran
maprotiline
mirtazapine
monoamine oxidase inhibitors (MAOIs)
nefazodone
neurogenesis
neurogenic theory of depression
nitrous oxide
paroxetine
persistent depressive disorder (dysthymia)
pramipexole
REL-1017
second-generation antidepressants
selective serotonin reuptake inhibitors (SSRIs)
seltorexant
Sequenced Treatment Alternatives to Relieve Depression (STAR*D) study
serotonin-norepinephrine reuptake inhibitors (SNRIs)
sertraline
trazodone
treatment-resistant depression
tricyclic antidepressants (TCAs)
venlafaxine
vilazodone
vortioxetine
zuranolone

CHAPTER 13

Sedative-Hypnotic Drugs: Treatment of Anxiety, Insomnia, and Epilepsy; Induction of Anesthesia

CHAPTER OUTLINE

Sedative-hypnotic drugs are a chemically diverse group of substances that act on the CNS to depress brain activity, principally by increasing the inhibitory effects of gamma aminobutyric acid (GABA), the major inhibitory neurotransmitter (e.g., by increasing the activity of GABA-releasing neurons). Clinically, these CNS depressants are used to alleviate anxiety, treat insomnia, and manage epilepsy (seizure disorders, or convulsions), as well as to induce general anesthesia or an amnestic state of sedation. Among the drugs of this group is ethyl alcohol, which has no medical use and is subject to widespread misuse (see Chapter 5). Although the drugs discussed in this chapter have many medical uses, they are also subject to misuse, which can not only lead to the development of substance abuse disorders but also result in serious and even life-threatening overdoses.

The term *sedative-hypnotic* derives from the typical effects of lower doses versus higher doses of these drugs: as with ethyl alcohol, lower doses usually have a sedating (calming) effect, whereas higher doses have a hypnotic (sleep-inducing) effect. When used to alleviate anxiety, these drugs may be called **anxiolytic drugs** (or *antianxiety drugs* or *tranquilizers*). When used to manage epilepsy, they are termed **anticonvulsant drugs** (or *antiepileptic drugs*). The biochemical nomenclature of sedative-hypnotic drugs has changed over time: the terms **barbiturates** and **benzodiazepines** reflect an older type of classification, by chemical structure; today, in contrast, drugs are typically classified by the receptors with which they interact. Thus, barbiturates and benzodiazepines are classified as *GABA receptor agonists* or, more specifically, as *barbiturate receptor agonists* or *benzodiazepine receptor agonists*, based on what is now known about binding sites for barbiturates and benzodiazepines on the GABA receptor.

Most of the sedative-hypnotic drugs are relatively nonspecific in their actions and have different uses at different doses, sometimes overlapping with the uses of drugs discussed in other chapters. In general, however, the sedative-hypnotics are not used as antipsychotics or antidepressants and are not analgesic (i.e., unlike opioids, they are not pain relieving).

DR. J'S MUSINGS 13.1

Sedative-Hypnotic Drugs in My Professional Life

As a graduate student in pharmacology, I did research on antiepileptic drugs. This continued during the 1970s when I directed a psychopharmacology research laboratory, including a study of two drugs that were later approved for use in treating epilepsy (valproic acid and carbamazepine). In 1980, I began a long career as an anesthesiologist, which included administering sedative-hypnotics for general anesthesia and for sedation during procedures in which the patient is kept conscious but then has no memory of the procedure. Finally, for the last 20 years, I have consulted and testified on the pharmacology of sedative-hypnotic drugs (from alcohol to zolpidem) in a wide variety of legal cases. This varied career, most of it revolving around sedative-hypnotic drugs, has been both challenging and rewarding and has been filled with personal satisfaction. I can ask for no more!

HISTORY AND EPIDEMIOLOGY

Beginning in the mid-nineteenth century, bromide compounds (e.g., potassium bromide) and chloral hydrate were used clinically to induce sleep, as alternatives to alcohol and opium. Then, in 1912, **phenobarbital**—the first of the barbiturates—was introduced as a sedative drug (the barbiturates are discussed in more detail below). Over the following decades, as the danger of death from barbiturate overdose was increasingly recognized, other types of sedatives were marketed as potentially safer alternatives (discussed in the section on nonbarbiturates, later in this chapter). While the overdose lethality associated with these newer drugs may have been less than that associated with barbiturates, other dangers remained, including dependence and addiction.

In 1960, chlordiazepoxide (Librium)—the first of the benzodiazepines—was brought to market, followed by the development of several other drugs of that class (the benzodiazepines are discussed in detail later in this chapter). The major advantage of the benzodiazepines over the barbiturates was that overdoses of the benzodiazepines were rarely, if ever, fatal unless they were combined with alcohol or opioids. Because of this greater safety, the benzodiazepines became wildly popular for the treatment of anxiety and insomnia. Indeed, through the 1970s, benzodiazepines were the most prescribed class of drugs in the world (Brunetti et al., 2021). Gradually, however, the adverse side effects and toxicities of benzodiazepines were recognized, leading to decreases in benzodiazepine prescriptions. An unfortunate and unintended consequence of this decrease was the development and spread of illicit, "designer" benzodiazepines that are now encountered as "club drugs" or "date rape drugs" and are associated with other forms of abuse, as well as with adverse effects such as driving impairments (Brunetti et al., 2021; Rohrig et al., 2021).

Even though the benzodiazepines are rarely fatal by themselves, they figure prominently in the continuing epidemic of deaths from opioid overdoses discussed in Chapter 10, as shown by a comprehensive study of benzodiazepine-related overdose deaths during the period 2018–2020, which revealed a number of alarming statistics (Liu et al., 2021) (see the more detailed discussion in the section on the abuse of benzodiazepines later in this chapter).

Also of concern are brain dysfunctions that can result from the use of sedative-hypnotic drugs, including blackouts, dysfunctions associated with loss of nerve cell function, and dysfunctions known as *complex sleep-related behaviors*.

Blackouts

A blackout is a state of anterograde amnesia—that is, the person has little or no memory for events that occur or for actions that the person performs while in that state. As discussed in Chapter 5, blackouts often occur when the person's blood alcohol level exceeds about 0.25–0.30 grams% and persists until the blood alcohol level falls below the level that produced the amnesia. However, alcohol is not the only drug that can produce a blackout; in fact, any sedative, in high enough doses, can result in this type of amnesia. Thus, we can describe a blackout as a drug-induced, reversible brain syndrome resulting from the use of a sedative. Note that the amnesia that occurs during a blackout is not due to a loss of consciousness—that is, the person experiencing a blackout is still awake and is capable of performing activities (e.g., see the section below on complex sleep-related behaviors).

Some sedative drugs are used as so-called date rape drugs: a person given such a drug may experience a blackout and, if then induced to participate in sexual activity, will not remember having done so, despite having been awake and active. In medicine, this same state—but in this case referred to as *conscious sedation*—may be induced to keep the patient awake and cooperative yet not later able to remember the medical procedure (e.g., for a colonoscopy, the patient may be given the short-acting benzodiazepine midazolam).

Dysfunctions Associated with Loss of Nerve Cell Function

Older adults and other people who already have some natural loss of nerve cell function are more likely to experience adverse effects from sedative-hypnotic drugs, such as disorientation and clouding of consciousness. Another frequent effect in this population is a state of drug-induced paradoxical excitement, characterized by labile emotions with marked expressions of anger and by delusions, hallucinations, and confabulations (i.e., unconscious fabrications of information to fill memory gaps). This drug-induced condition is treated by stopping administration of the sedative drug and allowing time for the drug to be metabolized and eliminated.

Complex Sleep-Related Behaviors

In March 2007, the FDA released an advisory requesting that manufacturers of certain sedative-hypnotic products[1] for the treatment of insomnia strengthen their product labeling to note the risk that these products may induce various **complex sleep-related behaviors** (or *parasomnias*), which can include "sleep driving," making phone calls, preparing and eating food, having sex, and other activities, all without subsequent memory of having engaged in those behaviors (Pressman, 2011). However, the FDA advisory may not be inclusive enough, as all benzodiazepines (not just the ones specified in the advisory) are associated with the same risks of these behaviors.

Once thought to be rare, the reported incidence of these behaviors has been increasing (likely due to improved awareness and more assiduous reporting). For example, one study noted that 24% of young or middle-aged adult patients (aged 20–55 years) and 17% of older adult patients (aged 65 years or older) reported experiencing some sort of adverse sleep-related effect of the nonbenzodiazepine zolpidem (marketed under various trade names, including Ambien and Edluar) (Chen et al., 2014). The same study noted that the risks of such effects appear to be somewhat related to doses and the

[1]Thirteen products were listed by their trade names on the FDA advisory: the barbiturates Butisol, Carbrital, and Seconal; the benzodiazepines Dalmane, Halcion, ProSom, and Restoril; the nonbenzodiazepines Ambien, Sonata, and Lunesta; the melatonin agonist Rozerem; and the products Doral and Placidyl.

resultant blood concentrations, at least among the young or middle-aged adults (those reporting sleep-related effects had ingested an average dose of 15 milligrams, whereas those who did not report adverse effects had ingested an average dose of 6.8 milligrams); in contrast, older adult patients who reported adverse sleep-related effects had not taken a higher dose on average than those who did not report such effects (all had taken an average dose of 12 milligrams).

SITES AND MECHANISMS OF ACTION

Initially, the barbiturates were thought to produce their sedative-hypnotic actions by a nonselective neuronal depression throughout the brain. For example, the deep coma, cessation of respiration, and death that can follow barbiturate overdose was presumed to result from brain stem depression that increased as dosage increased. Today, we have a much better understanding of how the actions of barbiturates, benzodiazepines, and other types of sedative-hypnotic drugs are mediated by specific receptor–drug interactions, in particular by interactions with $GABA_A$ receptors (see Figure 13.1; drugs that interact with other receptors are discussed later in this chapter).

Benzodiazepines do not directly stimulate the $GABA_A$ receptor; rather, they produce a three-dimensional conformational change in the structure of the receptor that increases the affinity of GABA for the receptor. That effect, in turn, facilitates the flow of chloride ions through the ion channel by increasing the frequency of ion channel opening, and the increased flow of chloride ions into the postsynaptic neuron increases GABA's inhibitory synaptic action.

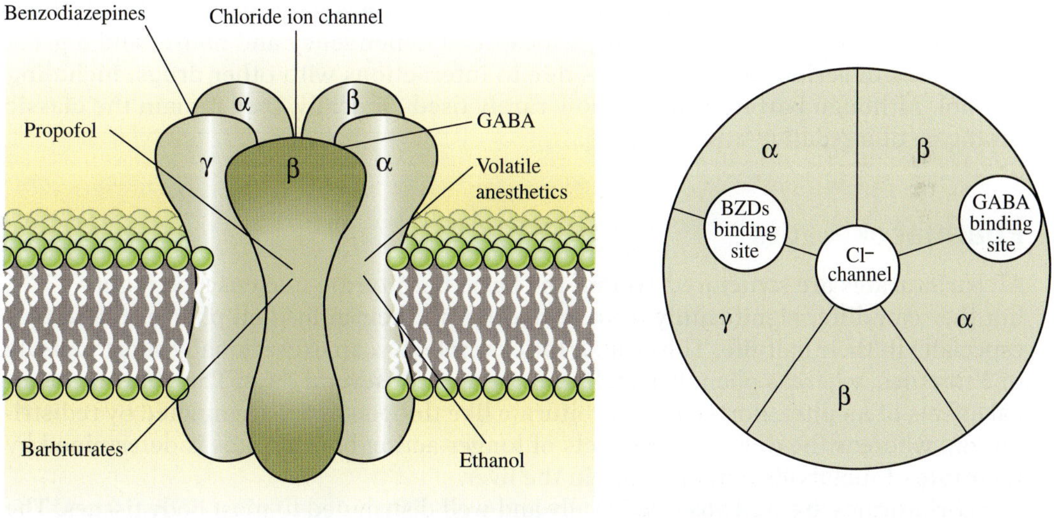

FIGURE 13.1 Interactions of Sedative-Hypnotic Drugs with $GABA_A$ Receptors. The neurotransmitter GABA, the benzodiazepines (BZDs), and various other types of sedative-hypnotic drugs all bind at different sites on the $GABA_A$ receptor complex, which consists of five subunits, shown here schematically in a side view (left) and in cross-section (right). The injectable anesthetic propofol and the barbiturates bind to a β subunit, whereas ethanol and volatile anesthetics bind to an α subunit.

The action of barbiturates at the $GABA_A$ receptor is somewhat different. Whereas benzodiazepines indirectly increase the *frequency* of the ion channel opening via a conformational change, barbiturates directly increase the *duration* of ion channel opening. This direct action explains why barbiturates are more toxic than benzodiazepines in cases of overdose.

The interactions of benzodiazepines with GABA-releasing neurons in regions such as the cerebral cortex and brain stem produce effects such as sedation, increased seizure threshold, cognitive impairment, amnesia, and muscle relaxation, which are generally regarded as side effects when the intended effect is anxiety reduction. The anxiolytic effects of benzodiazepines derive from their interactions with GABA-releasing neurons in the limbic system, especially in the amygdala. The association between GABA, emotional states of anxiety and fear, and the amygdala has been documented in reviews covering both animal and human studies (Delli et al., 2016; Liu et al., 2017). Animal studies have shown that electrical stimulation of the amygdala, orbitofrontal cortex, and insula evokes behavioral and physiological responses associated with fear and anxiety and that electrical lesions of the amygdala can result in an anxiolytic effect; and humans studies with PET scanning of the brain have demonstrated that anxiety is accompanied by increased blood flow in the amygdala, whereas studies with MRI scanning of the brain have found abnormalities of the amygdala in people with panic disorder.

BARBITURATES

Between 1912 and 1950, about 50 different barbiturate formulations were commercially marketed. During their decades of use, barbiturates were associated with thousands of suicides, accidental deaths, widespread dependency and abuse, and a great many cases of serious adverse effects due to interactions with other drugs, including alcohol. Although barbiturates are now rarely used clinically, they remain the classic prototype of a sedative-hypnotic drug.

Pharmacokinetics

All barbiturates are structured around the basic barbiturate nucleus (see Figure 13.2), but they can differ significantly from each other in their individual pharmacokinetics, especially in their half-life. Thiopental, for example, has an exceptionally short half-life of 3 minutes, whereas phenobarbital has a half-life of several days. The pharmacological effects of an ultrashort-acting barbiturate like thiopental are terminated by redistribution, whereas the duration of effects of longer-acting barbiturates is determined by their rate of metabolism by enzymes in the liver.

Barbiturates are well absorbed orally and well distributed to most body tissues. The ultrashort-acting barbiturates are exceedingly lipid soluble, cross the blood-brain barrier rapidly, and induce sleep within seconds following their intravenous injection. The longer-acting barbiturates are more water soluble and less lipid soluble and are slower to cross the blood-brain barrier, which means that sleep induction with these compounds is delayed for 20–30 minutes. Also, the longer-acting barbiturates are associated

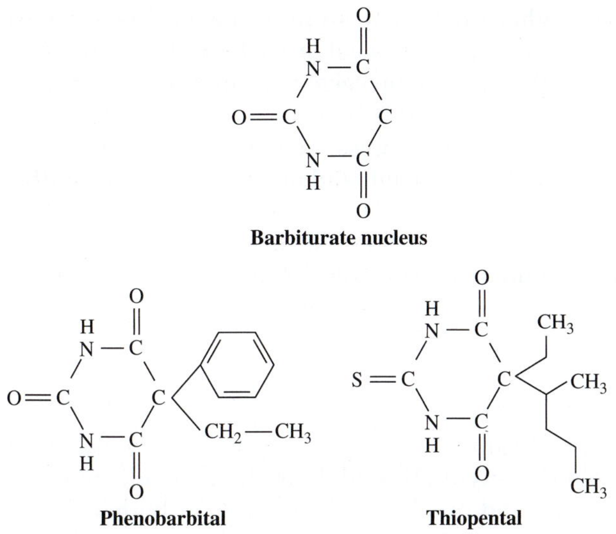

FIGURE 13.2 Chemical Structures of Barbiturates.
The barbiturate nucleus is the basic structure in all the barbiturates, including those with a longer half-life, such as phenobarbital, and those with a shorter half-life, such as thiopental.

with a prominent residual hangover because their half-lives are longer than the 8 hours or so of induced sleep.

Pharmacological Effects

Barbiturates have a low degree of selectivity and so cannot be used to achieve anxiolysis without sedation. Also, because they are not analgesic, barbiturates cannot be relied on to produce sedation or sleep in the presence of even moderate pain. Sleep patterns are decidedly affected by barbiturates, including marked suppression of rapid eye movement (REM) sleep. Because dreaming occurs during REM sleep, barbiturates suppress dreaming. If the person stops taking the drug, dreaming becomes vivid and excessive, a withdrawal effect known as *REM rebound*. The vivid nature of the dreams can lead to insomnia, which can be clinically relieved by restarting the drug.

Barbiturates in less than toxic doses exert few significant effects on the cardiovascular system, the gastrointestinal tract, the kidneys, or other organs. In the liver, barbiturates stimulate the synthesis of enzymes that metabolize other drugs as well as the barbiturates themselves, which produces significant tolerance to the other drugs.

Psychological Effects

The behavioral, motor, and cognitive effects of barbiturates are similar to those of alcohol. At low doses, the person may experience relief from anxiety (the expected effect) but may also experience side effects such as social withdrawal, emotional depression, or aggressive and violent behavior. Higher doses lead to more general behavioral depression and sleep. The person's mental set and physical or social setting can determine which of these effects occur or whether other unexpected or unpredictable effects are experienced.

Barbiturates are also cognitive inhibitors: they depress memory functioning, cause drowsiness, and have subtle effects on judgment, insight, and other aspects of cognitive functioning. They also have physical and behavioral effects (e.g., on motor skills and coordination, including on driving skills) that may persist for hours or days, until the drugs are completely metabolized and eliminated. Overdoses, especially in combination with alcohol, can result in death.

Clinical Uses

Clinical use of barbiturates has declined rapidly for several reasons: they are more lethal in overdose than are other sedative-hypnotics such as the benzodiazepines; they have a narrow therapeutic window and quickly become toxic at higher doses; they have a high potential for inducing tolerance, which can easily result in dependence and abuse; and they interact dangerously with many other drugs, sometimes fatally. Certain short-acting barbiturates are still used in anesthesia (e.g., thiopental and methohexital). Occasionally, barbiturates are used in combination with other medications—for example, the barbiturate butalbital is used in combination with caffeine and aspirin or acetaminophen in medications for the treatment of migraine headache. Finally, barbiturates are also used as part of a lethal cocktail in U.S. jurisdictions where physician-assisted suicide is allowed.

Adverse Effects

Drowsiness is the effect sought when barbiturates are used to produce either daytime sedation or nighttime sleep, but it is an inescapable adverse effect when the intended effect is anxiolysis. Similarly inescapable are the adverse cognitive and behavioral effects described earlier. Finally, it should be emphasized that barbiturates, like all other sedative drugs, are equivalent to alcohol in their effects, and when used with alcohol, the effects are additive and persist longer than when used alone.

Tolerance, Dependence, and Withdrawal

Barbiturates can induce tolerance by either of two mechanisms: the induction of drug-metabolizing enzymes in the liver or the adaptation of neurons in the brain to the presence of the drug. With the latter mechanism, tolerance develops primarily to the sedative effects and much less to the depressant effects on respiration via actions in the brain stem. Tolerance to the sedative effects reduces the margin of safety for the person using the drug, because the person may need to use more of the drug to achieve the desired sedative effect, and this will lead to increasing respiratory depression.

Normal clinical doses of barbiturates can induce a degree of physical dependence, usually manifested by sleep difficulties during attempts at withdrawal. Withdrawal from high doses may result in hallucinations, restlessness, disorientation, and even life-threatening convulsions. No specific treatments or antidotes are available. Treatment is usually aimed at supporting the respiratory and cardiovascular system until the drug is metabolized and eliminated, while slowly tapering off the barbiturate and treating any acute symptoms.

NONBARBITURATES, EXCEPT BENZODIAZEPINES

With recognition of the danger of barbiturate overdoses and prior to the introduction of the benzodiazepines in 1960, the pharmaceutical industry attempted to develop less dangerous alternatives to barbiturates. In the early 1950s, several nonbarbiturate sedatives, such as glutethimide (Doriden), ethchlorvynol (Placidyl), and methyprylon (Noludar), were introduced as anxiolytics, daytime sedatives, and hypnotics. However, it turned out that these drugs offered no advantages over the barbiturates, and neither did other nonbarbiturates that were developed subsequently. Despite being pharmacologically interchangeable with barbiturates, the differences in structure meant they could not legally be marketed as barbiturates. Now considered obsolete for use in medicine, they are occasionally encountered as drugs of abuse. Figure 13.3 shows the chemical structures of the three drugs mentioned above and the other nonbarbiturates discussed below.

Paraldehyde

Paraldehyde, a nonbarbiturate sedative-hypnotic that was introduced into medicine in the late nineteenth century, is a polymer of acetaldehyde, an intermediate by-product in the body's metabolism of ethyl alcohol. Administered either rectally or orally, paraldehyde was historically used to treat the severe alcohol withdrawal symptoms known as *delirium tremens*. It is rapidly absorbed from both rectal and oral routes, and sleep ensues within 10–15 minutes after hypnotic doses. Most of the drug is metabolized in the liver to acetaldehyde, although some is eliminated through the lungs, producing a characteristic unpleasant breath odor.

Chloral Hydrate

Chloral hydrate is, like paraldehyde, a nonbarbiturate drug of historical interest, having been available clinically since the late 1800s. It is rapidly metabolized to trichloroethanol, a derivative of ethyl alcohol, which is the active form of chloral hydrate, with nonselective CNS depressant effects. The drug is an effective sedative-hypnotic, with a half-life of about 4–8 hours, which means that next-day hangover is less likely to occur than with compounds having longer half-lives. Withdrawal of the drug may be associated with disrupted sleep and intense nightmares. The combination of chloral hydrate with alcohol can produce increased intoxication, stupor, and amnesia (this mixture, called a *Mickey Finn*, was an early example of a date rape drug).

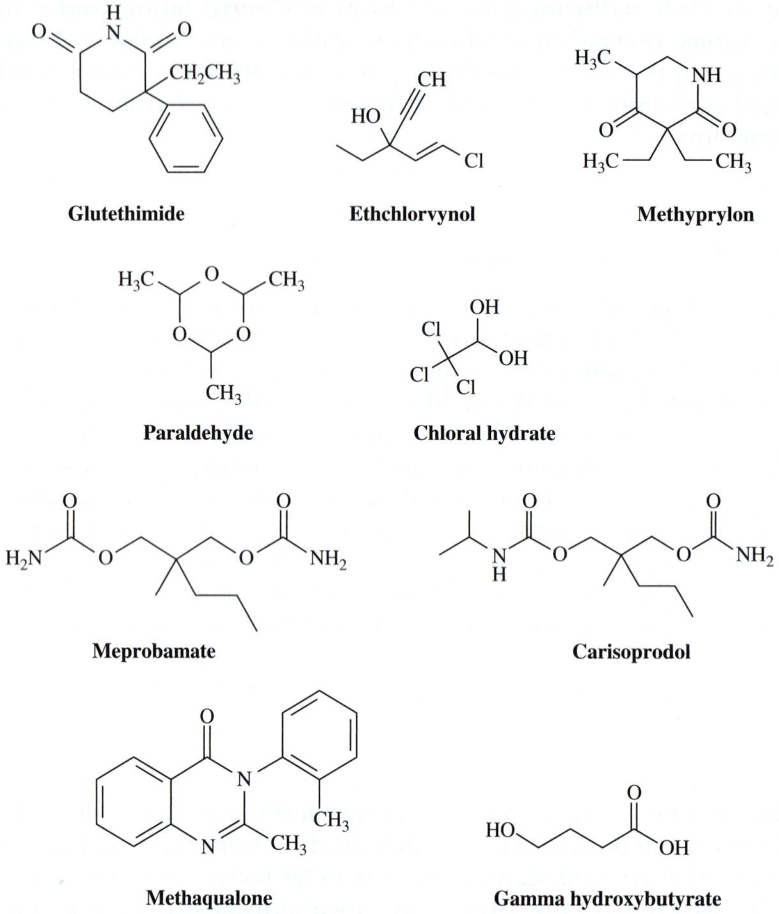

FIGURE 13.3 Chemical Structures of Nonbarbiturates. Despite their differences in structure from each other and from the barbiturates, these sedative-hypnotic drugs are pharmacologically equivalent to the barbiturates.

Meprobamate and Carisoprodol

Meprobamate (Equanil, Miltown) was marketed in 1955 as an alternative to the barbiturates for daytime sedation and anxiolysis. The term *tranquilizer* was used to describe it in a marketing attempt to distinguish it from the barbiturates, a distinction that was not borne out in clinical practice. For a time, it was the best-selling minor tranquilizer, but it has largely been replaced by the benzodiazepines due to their wider therapeutic index (lower risk of toxicity at therapeutically prescribed doses) and lower incidence of serious side effects. Like barbiturates, meprobamate produces long-lasting daytime sedation, mild euphoria, and relief from anxiety. It is a less potent respiratory depressant than the barbiturates, meaning that attempted suicides from overdose are seldom successful unless the drug is mixed with an opioid such as morphine or oxycodone. Despite a steady reduction in clinical use, meprobamate continues to be abused, and dependency is difficult to treat. Another possible risk is that use of meprobamate during pregnancy may be associated with an increased frequency of congenital malformations.

Carisoprodol (Soma) is a precursor compound to meprobamate; after it is absorbed, it is rapidly metabolized to meprobamate, which is the active form of the drug. Without much clinical justification, it continues to be prescribed and is often abused as an intoxicant.

Methaqualone

Methaqualone (Quaalude) was frequently prescribed in the 1960s and 1970s as a nonbarbiturate sedative-hypnotic but with little clinical justification for its widespread use. During the late 1970s, its popularity as a recreational drug peaked, and its level of abuse rivaled that of marijuana and alcohol. This was mainly due to its undeserved reputation as an aphrodisiac; in fact, its sedative properties make it an anaphrodisiac, much like alcohol. However, it also was used as a date rape drug, because its amnestic effect occurred at doses lower than the dose required to produce incapacitation or unconsciousness. Extensive illicit use and numerous overdose deaths led to its being banned in the United States in 1984, although the occasional availability of illicit supplies mean it still shows up as a drug of abuse.

Gamma Hydroxybutyrate

Gamma hydroxybutyrate (GHB) (Xyrem) is an interesting example of a nonbarbiturate sedative-hypnotic drug because it is a natural neurotransmitter. It binds to GHB receptors on both pre- and postsynaptic neurons, with the effect of inhibiting GABA release; in addition, GHB acts both directly as a partial $GABA_B$ receptor agonist and indirectly through its being metabolized to GABA.[2]

GHB has a rapid onset of about 15 minutes and a half-life of about 30 minutes. The drug is rapidly metabolized to carbon dioxide and water and is detectable in urine for only very brief periods of time after ingestion. Overdoses are characterized initially by stupor and, as dosages increase, by delirium, unconsciousness, coma, and death. The drug's toxic potential is greatly magnified by combination with alcohol. Acute withdrawal in a GHB-dependent person results in rapid onset of insomnia, anxiety, hallucinations, tremors, agitation, and other signs (Wolf et al., 2021). GHB withdrawal is usually accomplished by tapering off the drug, with or without use of long-acting benzodiazepines; withdrawal symptoms usually resolve in 3–10 days.

GHB was synthesized in 1960 and developed as a short-acting anesthetic. It later became popular as a recreational drug and a nutritional supplement marketed to bodybuilders.[3] In 1990, it was classified in 1990 as a Schedule I drug due to its recreational abuse, which meant that sales were banned; however, it and its precursors (gamma butyrolactone and 1,4-butanediol) remain available on the Internet. In 2002, sodium

---

[2]For a fuller discussion of the complicated mechanisms of action of GHB, see Busardo and Jones, 2015.

[3]GHB is thought to promote a deep sleep, and because growth hormone is produced during sleep, the drug allegedly increases levels of growth hormone.

Did You Know?

Preventive Measures Against Spiked Drinks

In a study with more than 900 participants, 44% of men and 56% of women reported having had their drinks spiked (American Addiction Centers, 2022). What measures can you take to avoid being slipped a date rape drug? Don't accept an open drink from anyone you don't know and trust completely, don't drink from a communal source like a punch bowl, and if there is a bar, order your own drink and watch the bartender make it. Even if you never leave your drink unattended, you should keep in mind that the bartender who mixed the drink or the server who brought it to you might not be trustworthy.

For extra assurance, you can check whether your drink contains any of a variety of date rape drugs, using a portable test such as the Test My Drink kit, which detects common date rape drugs such as GHB and ketamine.

Regardless of whether you tested your drink, if it has a salty taste or you begin to feel unusually tired or sick after drinking from it, you should suspect that it may have been spiked, and you should go to an emergency room and request a urine screening (Cal Poly Campus Health & Wellbeing; U.S. Drug Enforcement Administration).

oxybate (a formulation of GHB that is also marketed as Xyrem), also classified as a Schedule III drug, was approved by the FDA for the treatment of narcolepsy. In January 2017, the FDA approved the first generic version of sodium oxybate oral solution to treat cataplexy (sudden short attacks of weak or paralyzed muscles) and excessive daytime sleepiness in patients with narcolepsy.

In clinical use, the drug is administered twice nightly as a hypnotic, promoting improved sleep. This tends to decrease daytime sleepiness and also reduce the attacks of cataplexy.

As a sedative, GHB has been abused as a purported aphrodisiac and a euphoriant. It is also encountered in cases of sexual assault, having been used as a date rape drug, usually mixed with alcohol (Berretta and Vari, 2020).[4] As a date rape drug, it produces alcohollike disinhibition and amnesia, without necessarily producing sleep or unconsciousness.

BENZODIAZEPINES

In the years after chlordiazepoxide was brought to market in 1961 as the first benzodiazepine tranquilizer, the benzodiazepines largely replaced the barbiturates and nonbarbiturates as sedatives, hypnotics, and anxiolytics. Benzodiazepines quickly became the most widely used class of psychotherapeutic drugs, and the terms *tranquilizer* and *anxiolytic* soon became synonymous with the various drugs of this class. In the decades that followed, these drugs remained popular. A study covering the years 1996–2013 found that the number of U.S. adults filling at least one benzodiazepine prescription annually increased from about 8 million in 1996 to about 13 million

[4]GHB has been sold illicitly under such names as "RenewTrient," "Revivarant," "Blue Nitro," "Remiforce," "GH Revitalize," "Gamma G," "Nature's Quaalude," and "Liquid Ecstasy."

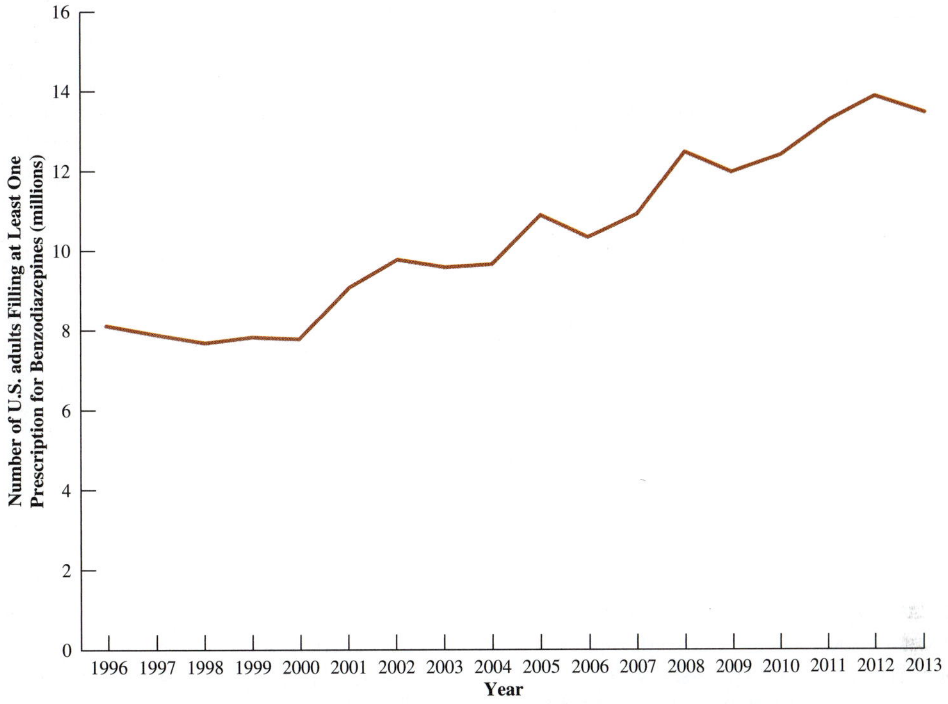

FIGURE 13.4 Adults Receiving Benzodiazepine Prescriptions, 1996–2013. The number of U.S. adults aged 18 years and over who filled at least one benzodiazepine prescription annually during this time period increased both in absolute terms and as a proportion of the adult population. [Data from Bachhuber et al., 2016.]

in 2013 (see Figure 13.4), or from about 4.1% to about 5.6% of the adult population (Bachhuber et al., 2016).

In this section, we will discuss the pharmacokinetics and pharmacological effects of benzodiazepines; we will see why the pharmacological advantages of the benzodiazepines as sedative hypnotics led to their wide use; we will describe the adverse effects associated with their use; and we will see how their wide use has led to overuse, misuse, and abuse, resulting in large and increasing numbers of overdoses and deaths, especially when benzodiazepines are used in combination with opioids and alcohol.

Pharmacokinetics

Figure 13.5 illustrates the chemical structures of the benzodiazepine nucleus, chlordiazepoxide, and five other drugs of this class. Table 13.1 shows some of the characteristics of the 17 benzodiazepines currently available by prescription (several other benzodiazepines are available on the illicit market). The table shows the drugs' routes of administration and their active compounds (the drug itself and/or one of its active metabolites); it also shows the most important pharmacokinetic difference among these drugs—their mean half-life, which varies from as little as 2.5 hours for some of the shorter-acting agents to as long as 60 or even 80 hours for some of the longer-acting agents.

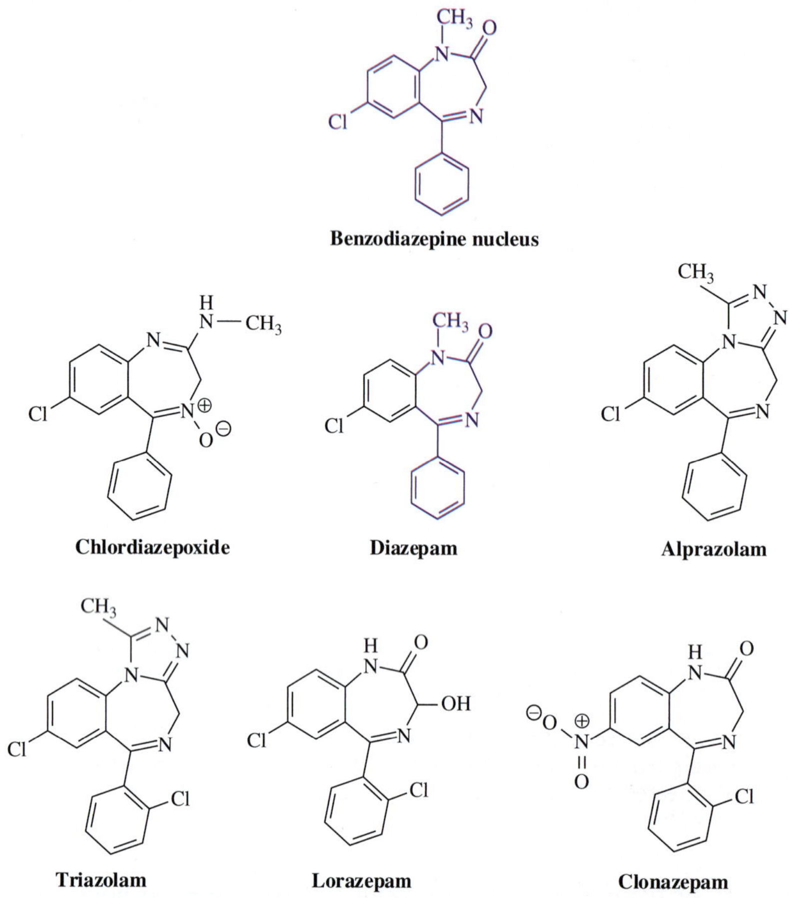

FIGURE 13.5 Chemical Structures of Benzodiazepines. The benzodiazepine nucleus is the basic structure in all the benzodiazepines. Chlordiazepoxide was the first benzodiazepine brought to market; the other five compounds are among the most widely prescribed drugs of this class.

Absorption and Distribution

Benzodiazepines are well absorbed when they are taken orally. Typically, peak plasma concentrations are achieved in about 1 hour, but some are absorbed more slowly (e.g., oxazepam and lorazepam), while others are absorbed more rapidly (e.g., triazolam). All benzodiazepines are well and equally distributed throughout the body.

Metabolism and Elimination

Most psychoactive drugs are metabolized to pharmacologically inactive products, which are then excreted in urine. Although some benzodiazepines behave this way, others are first metabolized to pharmacologically *active* intermediates, which are then metabolized into inactive products that are excreted. As can be seen from Table 13.1 and Figure 13.6, among the benzodiazepines that are metabolized into active

TABLE 13.1 Benzodiazepines

Drug	Dosage Form: Oral	Dosage Form: Parenteral	Active Compounds in Blood (* = metabolite)	Mean Half-Life in Hours (range)
LONG-ACTING AGENTS				
Diazepam	X	X	Diazepam Nordiazepam*	24 (20–50) 60 (50–100)
Chlordiazepoxide	X		Chlordiazepoxide Nordiazepam*	10 (8–24) 60 (50–100)
Flurazepam	X		Desalkylflurazepam*	80 (70–160)
Halazepam	X		Halazepam Nordiazepam*	14 (10–20) 60 (50–100)
Prazepam	X		Nordiazepam*	60 (50–100)
Chlorazepate	X		Nordiazepam*	60 (50–100)
Clobazam	X		N-Desmethyl clobazam*	32 (12–42)
INTERMEDIATE-ACTING AGENTS				
Lorazepam	X	X	Lorazepam	15 (10–24)
Clonazepam	X		Clonazepam	30 (18–50)
Quazepam	X		Quazepam Desalkylflurazepam*	35 (25–50) 80 (70–160)
Estazolam	X		Hydroxyestazolam*	18 (13–35)
SHORT-ACTING AGENTS				
Midazolam		X	Midazolam	2.5 (1.5–4.5)
Oxazepam	X		Oxazepam	8 (5–15)
Temazepam	X		Temazepam	12 (8–35)
Triazolam	X		Triazolam	2.5 (1.5–5)
Alprazolam	X		Alprazolam	12 (11–18)
Remimazolam		X	Remimazolam	0.5 (0.2–0.7)

intermediates are several with the long-acting active intermediate nordiazepam (which is then metabolized into the shorter-acting oxazepam). The half-life of nordiazepam is about 60 hours, and much longer in older adults; this shows why the long-acting benzodiazepines are as long acting as they are, because their pharmacologically active metabolites nordiazepam, desalkylflurazepam, and N-desmethyl clobazam have longer half-lives than the drugs themselves (in fact, two of the long-acting agents—flurazepam and clobazam—are not themselves pharmacologically active). In contrast, the short-acting benzodiazepines are short acting because they have short half-lives and are metabolized directly into inactive products.

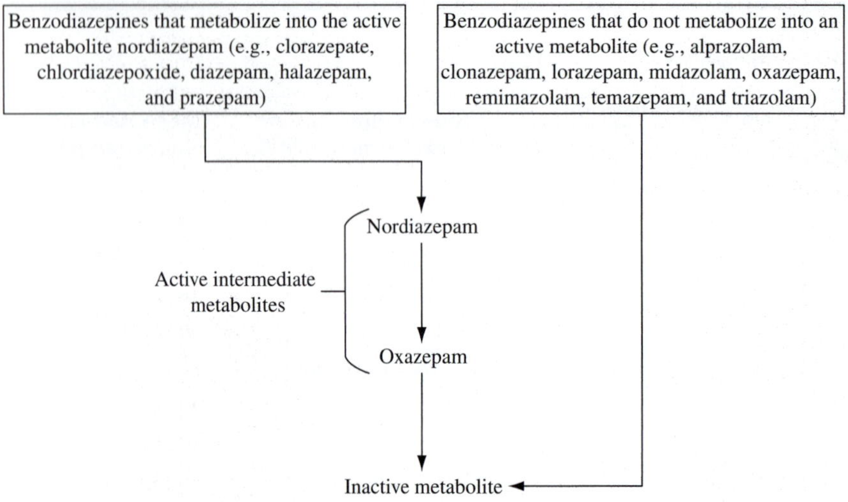

FIGURE 13.6 Metabolism of Benzodiazepines. Several of the benzodiazepines metabolize into the pharmacologically active intermediate nordiazepam, which then metabolizes into oxazepam (itself a prescription benzodiazepine), which in turn metabolizes into inactive products. Other benzodiazepines metabolize directly into inactive products.

Pharmacological Effects

All benzodiazepines are pure GABA agonists because they facilitate GABA binding at $GABA_A$ receptors, which increases the inhibitory influence of GABA in the brain and presumably leads to the benzodiazepines' antianxiety and sedative effects, as described earlier (see Figure 13.2 and the accompanying text).

Low doses of benzodiazepines moderate anxiety, agitation, and fear by their actions on $GABA_A$ receptors in the amygdala, orbitofrontal cortex, and insula, whereas effects such as mental confusion and amnesia result from actions on $GABA_A$ receptors in other areas of the cerebral cortex and the hippocampus. The mild muscle relaxant effects of the benzodiazepines probably result both from their anxiolytic effects and from their effects on $GABA_A$ receptors in the spinal cord, cerebellum, and brain stem. Their anticonvulsant effects seem to follow from their actions on $GABA_A$ receptors in the cerebellum and the hippocampus. Their rewarding effects, and thus their potential for abuse and psychological dependency, probably result from actions on $GABA_A$ receptors in the ventral tegmentum and the nucleus accumbens.

Use and Misuse

In this section, we will discuss the clinical uses of benzodiazepines in the treatment of anxiety and insomnia; their use as anticonvulsants and amnestics; their use in older adults and in pregnant women; their adverse effects; their tolerance, dependence, and withdrawal risks; and their misuse, including overdose and abuse.

Clinical Uses and Limitations

Benzodiazepines have actions that are therapeutically useful as anxiolytics, hypnotics, anticonvulsants, and amnestics. Their major clinical advantages are high efficacy, rapid onset of action, and low toxicity—that is, they work well, they act quickly, and they are safe when used alone (i.e., not in combination with other drugs such as opioids or alcohol). However, as with all psychoactive drugs, their potential benefits have to be weighed against certain risks: the therapeutic effects of benzodiazepines are accompanied by adverse side effects, and long-term or chronic use leads to tolerance and dependence.

Benzodiazepines can also be useful in treating acute symptoms of alcohol withdrawal and in long-term therapy to reduce the risk of relapse to previous drinking habits. Today, however, certain of the anticonvulsant mood stabilizers are viable and perhaps less risky alternatives.

Treatment of Anxiety. In short-term treatment of anxiety that is so debilitating that the patient's lifestyle, work, and interpersonal relationships are severely hampered, benzodiazepines may alleviate the symptoms of nervousness, dysphoria, and psychological distress. More specifically, benzodiazepines have been used to treat panic disorders and phobias; however, the efficacy of benzodiazepines in treating these disorders, as well as generalized anxiety disorder, may be less than that of serotonin-type antidepressants or mood-stabilizing anticonvulsants. (See the section on alternatives to benzodiazepines later in this chapter.)

Treatment of Insomnia. Benzodiazepines' sedating effects can make them useful for the treatment of insomnia; in addition, they are inexpensive and readily available. Agents with a rapid onset, a 2- to 3-hour half-life, and no active metabolites may be preferred to minimize daytime sedation; however, few benzodiazepines fit this profile—as shown in Table 3.1, most have half-lives of 8 hours or longer. Another potential advantage of benzodiazepines in treating insomnia is that they may be useful in patients with comorbid anxiety disorders.

Five benzodiazepines have been specifically approved by the FDA for the treatment of insomnia: estazolam, flurazepam, quazepam, temazepam, and triazolam, although others are widely used and similarly effective for this purpose (e.g., alprazolam). Of the five FDA-approved drugs, triazolam has the shortest half-life and is associated with the least daytime sedation; however, it may not provide adequate sedation through the night. Conversely, the other four drugs have longer half-lives and maintain sleep longer but may also have adverse cognitive consequences the next day. (Pharmacological characteristics of these five drugs are shown in Table 13.2, in the section on drugs primarily indicated for the treatment of insomnia, later in this chapter.)

The use of benzodiazepines in treating insomnia is also limited by the development of tolerance and dependence, with rebound increases in insomnia if the drug is discontinued. In addition, if a benzodiazepine with a longer half-life is used, some of it will still be present in the body at the time of administration every evening. This constant presence of the drug in the body means that adverse side effects such as cognitive impairment may also be constantly present until the drug is stopped. (For an extensive review covering the efficacy and safety of benzodiazepines and other hypnotics in the treatment of insomnia, see De Crescenzo et al., 2022.)

TABLE 13.2 Drugs for the Treatment of Insomnia

Drug	Dosage (mg)	Elimination Half-Life (hours)	T_{max} (hours)[a]	Used For[b]
BENZODIAZEPINES				
Estazolam	1, 2	10–24	1.5–2	SOI, SMI
Flurazepam	15, 30	48–120	1.5–4.5	SOI, SMI
Quazepam	7.5, 15	48–120	2–3	SOI, SMI
Temazepam	7.5, 15	8–22	1–2	SOI, SMI
Triazolam	0.125, 0.25	2–4	2–6	SOI
NONBENZODIAZEPINE AGONISTS AT BENZODIAZEPINE RECEPTORS				
Zaleplon	5, 10, 20	1	1	SOI
Zolpidem	5, 10	2.5	1.6	SOI
Zolpidem CR (controlled release)	6.25, 12.5	2.8	1.5	SOI, SMI
Eszopiclone	1, 2, 3	6	1	SOI, SMI
MELATONIN RECEPTOR AGONISTS				
Ramelteon	8	1–2.6	0.75	SOI
Circadin[c]	2	3.5-4.0	1–2	SMI
Tasimelteon	20	1.4	0.5–2.0	N24[d]
OREXIN RECEPTOR ANTAGONISTS				
Suvorexant	5–20	12	2	SOI, SMI
Lemborexant	5	17–19	1–3	SOI, SMI
Daridorexant	25, 50	8	1–2	SOI, SMI
HISTAMINE RECEPTOR ANTAGONIST				
Doxepin	3, 6	15.3	3.5	SMI

[a]T_{max} = time to maximum concentration in blood.
[b]SOI = sleep onset insomnia; SMI = sleep maintenance insomnia.
[c]Not available in the United States; approved for use by prescription in other countries.
[d]Non-24-hour sleep–wake disorder.
[Data from Asnis et al., 2016.]

Use as Anticonvulsants. All benzodiazepines have anticonvulsant effects because they raise the threshold for generating seizures. In general, however, benzodiazepines are used as secondary drugs or as adjuvants to other, more specific anticonvulsants. The benzodiazepines have also been used as muscle relaxants; although they do not directly relax muscles, they reduce the psychological distress that can predispose people to muscle tension (much as alcohol does). However, diazepam is the only benzodiazepine that has been approved by the FDA for treating spasticity and muscle spasms (Fudin and Raouf, 2016).

Use as Amnestics. Benzodiazepines are exceedingly effective in producing anterograde amnesia, called *conscious sedation* in the context of medical procedures in which the patient has to be kept awake and cooperative yet not later able to remember the procedure (for discussion of anterograde amnesia, see the section on blackouts earlier in this chapter). For use in inducing conscious sedation, two injectable benzodiazepines are available: lorazepam for a longer-lasting amnesia and midazolam for a shorter-lasting amnesia.

Use in Older Adults. In general, older adults have a reduced ability to metabolize long-acting benzodiazepines and their active metabolites—for example, the half-life of diazepam and its active metabolite nordiazepam averages about seven to ten days among older adults, versus less than three days in younger people (see Table 3.1). Thus, given that it takes about six half-lives to rid the body completely of a drug, older adults may need six to ten weeks to become drug-free after stopping the drug. With short-acting benzodiazepines, such as midazolam, the pharmacokinetics are not so drastically altered in older adults, but the dose necessary to achieve the desired therapeutic effect is reduced by about half.

In general, clinicians should probably avoid prescribing benzodiazepines for older adults, not just because of these pharmacokinetic issues, but also because benzodiazepines are associated with other increased risks in this population:

- Older adults who suffer from chronic obstructive pulmonary disease are at increased risk of untoward respiratory effects from benzodiazepine use (Baillargeon et al., 2019).
- Increases in the incidence of falls and bone fractures are a significant problem associated with benzodiazepine use in older adults (Amari et al., 2022).
- Older adults can experience cognitive dysfunction as a result of benzodiazepine use, including becoming clinically demented. A study that followed more than 130 benzodiazepine-using older adults for up to four years found that even intermittent use was associated with prolonged decreases in cognitive performance, compared with older adults who did not use benzodiazepines (Paterniti et al., 2002). Here is an older anecdote that vividly illustrates these cognitive risks:

> At the age of 91, the grandmother of one of the authors was growing increasingly forgetful . . . having been taking nitrazepam for insomnia regularly for years. To the author's lasting shame, it took a canny general practitioner to diagnose the problem. Cancellation of the nitrazepam prescription produced a dramatic improvement. (Rang and Dale, 1991)

Use in Pregnancy. Benzodiazepine use is fairly common among women of reproductive age, including among pregnant women—for example, anxiety disorders occur in up to 15% of pregnant women, and 10–26% of pregnant women with anxiety disorders are prescribed benzodiazepines (Najam et al., 2022). Although current recommendations are that short-term use of benzodiazepines can be considered for pregnant women with severe, disabling anxiety or sleep disorders after an individual risk-benefit analysis, the question arises over whether benzodiazepines adversely affect the developing fetus, given that all benzodiazepines freely cross the placenta and accumulate in the fetal circulation. One study aimed at addressing this question found that benzodiazepines administered during pregnancy do not seem to be associated with an increased risk of congenital malformations (Shyken et al., 2019); however, another study found that benzodiazepine use during pregnancy is associated with a slightly increased risk of preterm birth and lower birth weight (Huitfeldt et al., 2020).

Another risk arises if a pregnant woman is taking high doses of benzodiazepines near the time of delivery: the fetus can develop benzodiazepine dependence (even including "floppy-infant syndrome") followed after delivery by signs of withdrawal. After delivery, taking benzodiazepines while breast-feeding is not recommended, because benzodiazepines are excreted in breast milk and so can accumulate in the nursing infant.

General Limitations on Clinical Use. For longer-term treatment of such disorders as insomnia, generalized anxiety, phobias, and panic disorder, a combination of cognitive-behavioral therapies (CBTs) with antidepressant drugs is now preferred over a combination with benzodiazepines, because benzodiazepines have the potential to interfere with CBTs, perhaps significantly reducing the efficacy of the combined treatment (Bandelow, 2017). This is hardly surprising, as cognitive inhibitors such as benzodiazepines could certainly be predicted to have a negative effect on cognitive therapies.

Benzodiazepines should also be avoided in patients who need to maintain fine motor skills or high levels of mental alertness and in patients who habitually drink alcohol or use CNS depressants. As noted above, benzodiazepines should be used only with great caution in older adults, and the same caution should be used in prescribing them for children, adolescents, and anyone with a history of drug abuse. In addition, benzodiazepines should not be used as antidepressants; indeed, they intensify depression in much the same way that alcohol does.

Prescription of benzodiazepines for use before or after common surgical procedures also presents risks, in particular, the risk of persistent use after the procedure. For example, a recent study of about 2.5 million patients who underwent such procedures included about 64,000 who were prescribed benzodiazepines, and 19.5% of those developed persistent use, an unacceptably high rate (Wright et al., 2021).

Finally, the long half-life of many benzodiazepines means that evening use carries the risk that the person will not be free of the drug's effects the next day. The clear conclusion to be drawn from all these risks (including the risks of the types of adverse effects discussed next), is that, as with any type of drug, physicians who are considering prescribing benzodiazepines must find a balance between the risks and the potential benefits for the specific patient (Hirschtritt et al., 2021).

Adverse Effects

Common acute side effects associated with benzodiazepine therapy are usually dose-related extensions of the intended actions, including sedation, drowsiness, ataxia, lethargy, confusion, psychomotor impairments (particularly in older adults), disorientation, slurred speech, amnesia, and induction or extension of the symptoms of dementia. At higher doses, mental and psychomotor dysfunctions progress to hypnosis

DR. J'S MUSINGS 13.2

Benzodiazepines and Impairment

Benzodiazepines prescribed for the symptomatic relief of debilitating anxiety are intended to be used for only a few weeks. Unfortunately, many users continue to take the drugs for much longer periods, even years. Such long-term use results not only in dependence but also in persistent psychomotor impairments. My forensic consulting practice has shown me that benzodiazepines are not infrequently involved in arrests for impaired driving, even when blood concentrations at the time of arrest are within the therapeutic range. In such cases, drivers typically are not aware of their own impairment. It is indeed unfortunate that taking a prescribed medication can lead to such drastic consequences!

(sleep). As noted earlier, chronic use can lead to tolerance, dependence, and withdrawal symptoms; however, these risks can be mitigated with lower doses, treatment with limited duration (ideally, four weeks maximum), and the careful selection of patients (but keeping in mind that some patients do warrant long-term administration).

Impairment of motor abilities—especially a person's ability to drive an automobile—is common, as all benzodiazepines are capable of impairing driving, even at therapeutic concentrations[5] (Papoutsis et al., 2016). This also applies to new "designer benzodiazepines" that have been appearing on the illicit drug scene, including etizolam, flualprazolam, flubromazolam, and phenazepam (Moustafa et al., 2021; Orsolini et al., 2020b). The pharmacology of these drugs has not been worked out but is probably similar to the pharmacology of the prescription benzodiazepines, including an association with driving impairments (Rohrig et al., 2021).

When used for the treatment of insomnia, benzodiazepines usually cause the expected sedation but may instead induce paradoxical agitation as a result of mental confusion and disorientation, with symptoms such as anxiety, aggression, hostility, and behavioral disinhibition. In addition, cessation of use results in rebound increases in insomnia and anxiety. (For a discussion of the complex effects associated with persistent benzodiazepine dependence, see Peng et al., 2022.)

By far, the most contentious issues involving the adverse effects of benzodiazepines concern their effects on mortality and dementia. One study found that regardless of age, patients with delirium who were treated with benzodiazepines had a greater mortality than those who were not given benzodiazepines (Serna et al., 2015). With regard to dementia, a study reported that taking benzodiazepines for three months or more

---

[5]For a review of the literature on specific drugs and their side effects, including references for blood concentrations associated with driving impairments, see Baselt, 2020. Impairment was measured by the standard deviation of lateral position (i.e., tracking the vehicle while it was being driven on a city street).

increased the risk of Alzheimer's disease by as much as 51% and that longer exposure and the use of long-acting agents were more likely to increase the risk (Yaffe and Boustani, 2014; for a review of benzodiazepines as a risk factor for Alzheimer's disease dementia, see Ettcheto et al., 2020). In the American Geriatrics Society's 2019 update of its Beers criteria of inappropriate drugs for older adults, benzodiazepines were included because of the risk of cognitive impairment; however, an earlier analysis concluded that there is no "causal association between benzodiazepine use and dementia" (Gray et al., 2016), while a subsequent review noted conflicting results (Lucchetta et al., 2018).

Tolerance, Dependence, and Withdrawal

We have already noted that tolerance and dependence can develop when benzodiazepines are taken for prolonged periods of time, but an unusual aspect of these drugs is that dependence can develop without being preceded by tolerance (Soyka, 2017). After dependence develops, if the drug is stopped, early withdrawal signs include a return and possible intensification of the anxiety and/or other symptoms for which the drug was originally given. Rebound increases in insomnia, restlessness, agitation, irritability, and unpleasant dreams gradually appear. In rare instances, hallucinations, psychoses, and seizures may occur. Most of these withdrawal symptoms subside within one to four weeks. In cases where the person has developed dependence on a short-acting benzodiazepine, there are effective methods for avoiding withdrawal symptoms by switching to a long-acting benzodiazepine and then slowly tapering the latter drug (Soyka, 2017). It is generally agreed that discontinuation of benzodiazepines should occur gradually over several weeks, with dose reductions ranging from around 50% weekly (or, in severe cases of dependence, every two weeks) to 10–25% every two weeks.

Misuse: Overdose and Abuse

Benzodiazepines are often misused in combination with other drugs: opioid-dependent people undergoing withdrawal may self-medicate with benzodiazepines in order to ameliorate withdrawal symptoms and reduce anxiety; people using methadone may take benzodiazepines in order to intensify the effects of methadone by reducing its metabolism; and people using cocaine or methamphetamine may take benzodiazepines in order to ameliorate the adverse effects of those drugs.

Some of this misuse undoubtedly arises from the prescription of benzodiazepines to people already taking opioids. A federal report in 2022 notes that 16% of overdose deaths involving opioids also involved benzodiazepines (National Institute on Drug Abuse, 2022). (See the discussion of the opioids epidemic in Chapter 10.) A study of U.S. veterans found that about 50% of overdose deaths occurred among those who had received prescriptions for both benzodiazepines and opioids (Park et al., 2015), and these data are all the more sobering in light of the fact that benzodiazepines do not adequately treat patients with either posttraumatic stress disorder (PTSD) or chronic pain, conditions that are especially common among veterans. A more recent and comprehensive study revealed a number of alarming statistics (Liu et al., 2021):

- In 2018, an estimated 10,724 people in the United States died as the result of an overdose involving benzodiazepines, many of these involving combinations with alcohol or opioids.

DR. J'S MUSINGS 13.3

Benzodiazepines and Alcohol

As noted in this chapter, benzodiazepines by themselves are rarely associated with fatal overdoses, but overdose deaths are much more common when benzodiazepines are mixed with alcohol. The most common and perhaps most fatal interaction involves taking benzodiazepines in combination with binge drinking of alcohol. The two drugs "act as one"—that is, their effects are additive—and the resulting impairment can be serious, even leading to death. Basically, alcohol can turn benzodiazepines into potentially fatal drugs.

However, benzodiazepines such as lorazepam and chlordiazepoxide are very effective in treating acute symptoms of alcohol withdrawal. There is also the question of whether benzodiazepines should be prescribed to an alcohol-dependent patient if the patient has a condition that is typically treated with benzodiazepines (e.g., debilitating anxiety). Likely not. Although I am sure exceptions can be made, serious potential problems must be considered, including dual dependence, additive intoxication, and other difficulties. Also, even when just short-term use of benzodiazepines is intended, persistent use can result in about 20% of patients (Wright et al., 2021).

- In 2019, an estimated 92 million benzodiazepine prescriptions were dispensed from U.S. outpatient pharmacies, the most common being alprazolam (38%), clonazepam (24%), and lorazepam (20%).
- From April–June 2019 to April–June 2020, overdose deaths involving prescription and illicit benzodiazepines increased 21.8% and 519.6%, respectively.
- In the period January–June 2020, 92.7% of benzodiazepine-involved deaths also involved opioids, with 66.7% involving illicitly manufactured fentanyls.

There are also misuses related to the amnestic effects of benzodiazepines, particularly with regard to their use as date rape drugs, as described earlier in this chapter. For example, concern has been expressed about flunitrazepam (Rohypnol), a benzodiazepine that is legally prescribed outside the United States but has been illegally imported. When an unknowing person ingests the drug in combination with alcohol, the effect closely resembles the effect of a Mickey Finn (chloral hydrate plus alcohol) in that amnesia is achieved without loss of consciousness.[6]

[6]Flunitrazepam is very similar to triazolam; it produces anxiolysis, sedation, and amnesia, especially when taken with alcohol. When flunitrazepam is taken alone, intoxication and the amnesia it causes can begin within about 30 minutes, peak within 2 hours, and persist for up to 8 hours. When the drug is combined with alcohol, the amnestic and other intoxicating effects can last 8–18 hours. Disinhibition is also a widely reported effect of the drug when it is ingested either alone or in combination with alcohol.

When benzodiazepine overdose is suspected, the drug **flumazenil** (Romazicon) can be used as an antidote, administered by intravenous injection. Flumazenil is itself a benzodiazepine that binds with high affinity to $GABA_A$ benzodiazepine receptors; however, after binding, it exhibits no intrinsic activity. Thus, it competitively blocks the access of pharmacologically active benzodiazepines to the receptors, effectively reversing the antianxiety and sedative effects of any benzodiazepines administered before flumazenil (Gallo and Hulse, 2021; Sivilotti, 2016). Unfortunately, flumazenil is metabolized quite rapidly in the liver and has a short half-life of about 1 hour, much shorter than that of most benzodiazepines. This means that the effects of previously administered benzodiazepines may reappear as flumazenil is eliminated, thus necessitating reinjection of flumazenil. The use of flumazenil as an antidote to benzodiazepine overdose risks precipitating withdrawal seizures, making such use fairly rare.

ALTERNATIVES TO BENZODIAZEPINES FOR THE TREATMENT OF ANXIETY

Given the prevalence of anxiety disorders, and the adverse side effects or modest efficacy of benzodiazepines, there is significant interest in finding better alternatives. As we will see in this section, alternatives to benzodiazepines that have shown promise for the treatment of anxiety disorders include not only various antidepressants and anticonvulsants, but also two noradrenaline receptor antagonists and a melatonin receptor agonist. In addition, many over-the-counter herbal medications are sold for the treatment of anxiety. Finally, cannabidiol has been used as an anxiolytic (and antidepressant), supposedly with good efficacy (Melas et al., 2021).

Antidepressants

Antidepressant alternatives to benzodiazepines for the treatment of anxiety disorders include serotonin-type antidepressants and dual-action antidepressants such as venlafaxine. For example, treatment of panic attacks and phobias with benzodiazepines such as alprazolam may be less efficacious than treatment with serotonin-type antidepressants. Also, unlike the benzodiazepines, serotonin-type antidepressants do not cause impairments in psychomotor performance, do not impair learning and cognition, do not reduce alertness, and have little or no potential for dependence and abuse. However, with regard to treatment of panic disorder, it is worth noting that treatment can be effective with either a benzodiazepine or a selective serotonin reuptake inhibitor (SSRI) (or both), but the majority of patients may relapse, even after long-term therapy (Quagliato et al., 2018). Nevertheless, resumption of therapy with either type of drug (or with a different medication) can be successful in preventing or reducing the incidence of additional attacks in nearly all patients.

Serotonin-type antidepressants may also have efficacy in treating PTSD, reducing such symptoms as reexperiencing, avoidance, numbing, and hyperarousal, while also improving quality of life (Lancaster et al., 2016). The antidepressants sertraline and paroxetine have been approved by the FDA for use in PTSD, while fluvoxamine and citalopram have also been found effective, as has vilazodone (Ramaswamy et al., 2017).

Anticonvulsants

The gabapentinoid anticonvulsants gabapentin and pregabalin (discussed below in the section on anticonvulsant drugs for the treatment of epilepsy) exert sedative, analgesic, and anxiolytic effects in a variety of clinical situations and thus can sometimes be considered as viable alternatives to benzodiazepines. For example, the mood-stabilizing anticonvulsant pregabalin has been used in the treatment of generalized anxiety disorder and panic disorder (Rickels et al., 2012). Anticonvulsants usually show clinical efficacy within only a few days, and clinical improvements are maintained long term with continued use. Pregabalin can be effective in the treatment of several other anxiety disorders, as well as in the treatment of older adults, patients with severe anxiety, and patients with resistant depression (as an adjunct to standard antidepressants).

Noradrenaline Receptor Antagonists

The beta-blocker **propranolol** (an antagonist at noradrenaline beta receptors) has been effective against a variety of anxiety disorders, particularly phobias. Propranolol is widely used to treat various heart conditions by reducing blood pressure and cardiac arrhythmias (especially rapid heart rates) through its action at peripheral noradrenaline receptors. These beneficial effects can also mitigate performance anxiety ("stage fright"), test anxiety, and similar conditions. Propranolol seems to reduce the emotional reaction when a "fear memory" is reactivated, and this suggests that it might be useful in treating anxiety disorders based on disturbing memories, such as PTSD. However, a study concluded that there is insufficient evidence of efficacy to justify using propranolol for treating PTSD or, indeed, for any of the anxiety disorders (Steenen et al., 2016). Interestingly, this very guarded conclusion is contradicted by a study in which propranolol appeared to reduce fear in otherwise healthy persons with arachnophobia (fear of spiders) (Soeter and Kindt, 2015).

In clinical trials, **prazosin** (Minipress), a drug that is somewhat related to propranolol (it is an antagonist at noradrenaline alpha receptors) has shown efficacy in the treatment of PTSD-related symptoms including sleep disruptions, nightmares, and global functioning (Singh et al., 2016).

Melatonin Receptor Agonist

An analysis of data from 45 clinical centers worldwide found that the melatonin receptor agonist agomelatine was modestly effective in the treatment of patients with PTSD (Stein et al., 2014). Patients receiving 25–50 milligrams per day of the drug had lower mean total scores on the Hamilton Anxiety Rating Scale and experienced fewer adverse effects than patients receiving the SSRI antidepressant escitalopram (Lexapro).

However, agomelatine was never marketed in the United States because it can have adverse effects on the liver.

DRUGS PRIMARILY INDICATED FOR THE TREATMENT OF INSOMNIA

About 10% of people experience chronic insomnia, which can manifest itself as difficulty falling asleep, difficulty staying asleep, waking up too early, or waking in the morning without feeling refreshed. And roughly 50% of people with other medical or psychological conditions also complain of insomnia. Consequences of insomnia include daytime fatigue, lack of energy, poor concentration and memory, moodiness and irritability, and difficulty completing tasks.

Treatments for insomnia can be either psychological or pharmacological (or both). Of the psychological treatments, CBTs have been found very effective (Trauer et al., 2015). Advantages of CBTs include lack of drug side effects, no dependence or withdrawal issues, and safety for use with pregnant women. However, CBTs can be expensive, have a delayed onset of effect, and may not be readily available. Pharmacological treatments include the following drugs (pharmacological characteristics of these drugs are shown in Table 13.2, and their potential adverse effects are shown in Table 13.3;

TABLE 13.3 Adverse Effects of Drugs for the Treatment of Insomnia

	Drug Class[a]				
Adverse Effects[b]	BZDs	NBZDs	MRAs	ORAs	HRAs
Morning sedation	+	+	–	+	+
Unsteady gait, falls	++	+	–	+/–	–
Confusion	++	+	–	–	–
Amnesia	+	+	–	–	–
Dependency and abuse	+	+/–	–	–	–
Rebound insomnia	+	+	–	–	–
Respiratory depression	+	+/–	–	–	–
Anticholinergic effects	–	–	++/+	+	–
Orthostasis	–	–	+	+	–
Hypnagogic hallucinations, sleep paralysis	–	–	–	+	–

[a]BZDs = benzodiazepines (e.g., estazolam); NBZDs = nonbenzodiazepine agonists at benzodiazepine receptors (e.g., zaleplon); MRAs = melatonin receptor agonists (e.g., ramelteon); ORAs = orexin receptor antagonists (e.g., suvorexant); HRAs = histamine receptor antagonists (e.g., doxepin).
[b]Some effects (e.g., morning sedation) may depend on the particular compound's pharmacokinetics.
+ and – indicate the frequency of the effect: ++ = common; + = occasional; – = rare.
[Data from Scammell and Winrow, 2011.]

all but Circadin have been approved by the FDA for treatment of insomnia; see De Crescenzo et al., 2022, for a review of the safety and efficacy of all these drugs):

- The benzodiazepines estazolam, flurazepam, quazepam, temazepam, and triazolam. (For discussion, see the section above on treatment of insomnia with benzodiazepines.)
- Three nonbenzodiazepine agonists at benzodiazepine receptors—zaleplon, zolpidem, and eszopiclone.
- Three agonists at melatonin receptors—ramelteon, Circadin, and tasimelteon.
- Three antagonists at orexin receptors—suvorexant, lemborexant, and daridorexant.
- An antagonist at histamine receptors—doxepin.

For many years, attempts have been made to identify *partial* agonists at $GABA_A$ benzodiazepine receptors that, unlike the benzodiazepines and the nonbenzodiazepine receptor agonists listed above, which are all *full* agonists at those receptors, would be clinically effective anxiolytics with fewer, less frequent, or less severe adverse effects. To date, several such drugs have been studied, but none are clinically available. Extracts of valerian are partial $GABA_A$ and serotonin 5-$HT5_A$ receptor agonists (Dietz et al., 2005) and are useful in treating insomnia as over-the-counter products.

Nonbenzodiazepine Agonists at Benzodiazepine Receptors

The drugs discussed in this section were developed in an effort to improve upon the safety and side effect profiles of the benzodiazepines by designing nonbenzodiazepines that would also be agonists at benzodiazepine binding sites on $GABA_A$ receptors but would bind to those sites more selectively. The benzodiazepines bind nonselectively to multiple subtypes of the alpha subunit of the $GABA_A$ receptor, whereas these nonbenzodiazepines were designed to bind selectively to just one or two of the subtypes. Of the three nonbenzodiazepines discussed here, the first and second to be approved by the FDA (zolpidem in 1993 and zaleplon in 1999) selectively bind to only the $\alpha1$ subtype, while the third (eszopiclone, FDA approved in 2004) is predominantly selective for the $\alpha2$ and $\alpha3$ subtypes. Currently, these are the only FDA-approved nonbenzodiazepines for the treatment of insomnia.

The pharmacological significance of the modest variations in action of these three drugs is unknown (their chemical structures are shown in Figure 13.7). Their receptor selectivity and their relatively short half-lives (see Table 13.2) are presumed to result in less motor and neuropsychological impairment and in less frequent dependence, withdrawal, and abuse, relative to the benzodiazepines. However, these presumptions are still being debated, with results of one study indicating that the adverse reactions to these drugs may be as common and serious as those to the benzodiazepines (Cimolai, 2017).

Zolpidem

Presumably, because of its more selective binding to the $\alpha1$ subtype of the $GABA_A$ receptor, **zolpidem** (Ambien) is primarily a hypnotic rather than an anxiolytic. Zolpidem is often compared to triazolam, a benzodiazepine with a similar half-life of about

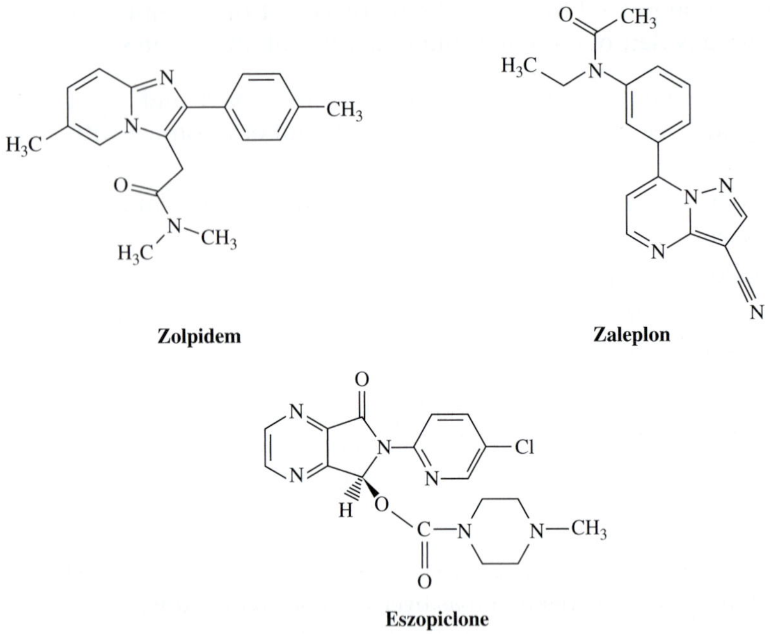

FIGURE 13.7 Chemical Structures of Zolpidem, Zaleplon, and Eszopiclone. Note the similarity of the three-ring structures of these drugs to the benzodiazepine nucleus (see Figure 13.5). The pharmacology of these drugs is also similar to that of the benzodiazepines. Nevertheless, they are not benzodiazepines.

2.5 hours. A controlled-release formulation of zolpidem is available as a tablet to be swallowed (Ambien CR) and as a sublingual tablet (Edluar). Also available is a low-dose formulation of zolpidem (Intermezzo), with recommended doses of 1.75 milligrams for women and 3.5 milligrams for men, intended to be taken when the person wakens in the middle of the night and cannot get back to sleep (but only if there are still at least 4 hours of bedtime left).

At doses of 5–10 milligrams, zolpidem produces sedation and promotes sleep, without anxiolytic, anticonvulsant, or muscle relaxant effects. However, memory is as adversely affected as it is by benzodiazepines, and drug-induced blackouts and complex sleep-related behaviors are common (see the earlier discussion of these types of effects).

Dose-related adverse effects of zolpidem include drowsiness, dizziness, and nausea. At doses of 5 milligrams, zolpidem has minimal next-day effects on memory and on the performance of psychomotor tasks such as driving; however, at doses of 10–20 milligrams, memory and psychomotor performance are significantly impaired, even 4 hours after awakening. In January 2013, the FDA informed zolpidem manufacturers that the recommended dosages for women should be lowered from 10 milligrams to 5 milligrams for immediate-release products and from 12.5 to 6.25 milligrams for extended-release products; for men, the new FDA-recommended dosages were either 6.25 or 12.5 milligrams for both immediate-release and extended-release products.

Further, the FDA told the manufacturers that the labeling should recommend that health care professionals prescribe the lowest effective dose.

A Substance Abuse and Mental Health Services Administration (SAMHSA) report found that, in 2010, women accounted for two-thirds of emergency room visits involving zolpidem overmedication (Substance Abuse and Mental Health Services Administration, 2014). Counting both men and women, the largest age bracket involved in such visits was ages 45–54 years. Huge overdoses have not been fatal, but in older adults, confusion, falls, memory loss, and psychotic reactions have been reported—for example, one study found that older adults taking zolpidem had about double the hip fracture rate of those not taking an insomnia drug and that rates were 21 times higher in older users (ages ≥65 years) than in younger users (ages 18–44 years) (Lin et al., 2014).

Finally, zolpidem is the insomnia drug most associated with parasomnias (complex sleep-related behaviors, such as sleep driving), resulting in thousands of legal cases; a study concluded that there is "a significant association between zolpidem and the induction of these bizarre sleep-related behaviors" (Wong et al., 2017).

Zaleplon

As noted above, **zaleplon** (Sonata) also binds selectively to the $\alpha 1$ subtype of the $GABA_A$ receptor, and in general, its actions are similar in kind to those of zolpidem but different in degree because of pharmacokinetic differences between the two drugs. The half-life of zaleplon is very short (about 1 hour), and only about 30% of the dose reaches the bloodstream because most undergoes first-pass metabolism in the liver. Zaleplon's short half-life and poor absorption mean that it can be taken as needed, if the person is unable to fall asleep or stay asleep, without fear of detrimental effects the next morning. In contrast, people taking a longer-acting and more thoroughly absorbed drug like zolpidem must predict when they will experience insomnia and take the drug before bedtime in order to minimize next-day effects.

At doses of 5–10 milligrams, zaleplon induces sleep quite rapidly, with improved sleep quality and without rebound insomnia. Zaleplon also appears to have few adverse effects on psychomotor function the morning following use, including on driving ability, presuming at least 4 hours from drug intake to driving (at 4 hours after oral administration, most of the drug has been eliminated from the body). Dependence is unlikely to develop because of the short half-life—that is, by morning, the drug has been virtually completely metabolized, which means that the drug does not persist in the body; in essence, a person taking the drug withdraws daily.

Eszopiclone

Eszopiclone (Lunesta) is the active isomer of zopiclone (Imovane), which has been used outside the United States for many years. Although eszopiclone differs from zolpidem and zaleplon in that it preferentially binds to the $\alpha 2$ and $\alpha 3$ subtypes (as opposed to the $\alpha 1$ subtype), its effects are similar to theirs and to the effects of the benzodiazepines. Its half-life of about 6 hours gives it the most prolonged action of the three nonbenzodiazepines, perhaps making it preferable to the others for improving sleep maintenance, and its rapid onset might also result in improved sleep latency (the time it takes to fall asleep after taking the drug). But the benefit of improved sleep maintenance is offset by an increased risk of next-day sedation and, at its highest dose level of 3 milligrams, an increased risk of next-day memory impairments and poor psychomotor performance (Boyle et al., 2008).

In April 2014, the FDA approved the generic formulation of eszopiclone. Then, in May 2014, the FDA recommended that the starting dose be lowered from 2 milligrams to 1 milligram due to an increased risk for psychomotor and memory impairments the next morning. The agency noted that the dose can be increased to 2 or 3 milligrams as needed but that people who take 3 milligrams should avoid driving or engaging in other activities that require their full attention the next day.

Melatonin Receptor Agonists

Melatonin (5-methoxy-N-acetyltryptamine) is a hormone secreted by the pineal gland in a circadian rhythm—that is, in response to the environmental light–dark cycle. When light activates receptors in the retina that project to the pineal gland, norepinephrine is released in the pineal gland, which inhibits the production of melatonin in the pineal gland. In the dark (e.g., at bedtime), norepinephrine production in the pineal gland decreases and melatonin production increases; then, when sleep ends in the morning, melatonin production begins returning to daytime levels (nocturnal plasma melatonin concentrations can be as much as tenfold higher than daytime concentrations). Melatonin has many functions in the body, including sleep promotion via actions in the anterior hypothalamus where there is a high concentration of neurons with two types of high-affinity G-protein-coupled receptors, melatonin-1 and melatonin-2.

Melatonin itself is available as an over-the-counter compound for the treatment of insomnia, but it has a short half-life and limited efficacy, except perhaps in people with disrupted sleep–wake cycles, such as shift workers and people with jet lag (Sadeghniiat-Haghighi et al., 2016); and prolonged-release melatonin may have clinically meaningful efficacy in persons aged 55 years and older (Wade et al., 2007). However, in a review discussing the increase in melatonin use over the past decade, researchers noted the potential dangers of exceeding the recommended 5 mg/day maximum dosage (some over-the-counter products exceed that recommendation by as much as 478%) (Li et al., 2022).

As we will see in the following sections, melatonin receptor agonists may have greater clinical efficacy than melatonin itself in treating insomnia and sleep–wake disorders, but their use comes with greater risk of adverse effects (see Table 13.3).

Ramelteon

Ramelteon (Rozerem), FDA approved in 2005 for the treatment of insomnia characterized by difficulty with sleep onset, was the first commercially available agonist at both types of melatonin receptors. It promotes drowsiness via melatonin-1 receptor stimulation, and it promotes synchronization of the circadian clock via melatonin-2 receptor stimulation. It has a half-life of about 1–3 hours, and if taken in the available 8-milligram dose 30 minutes before going to bed, it is thought to leave little morning drowsiness, although next-morning driving performance can be impaired. In controlled trials, however, its efficacy was quite modest, with sleep onset occurring only about 10 or 15 minutes earlier than after taking a placebo and with little increase in total sleep time (Liu and Wang, 2012). Another study reported some improvement in sleep parameters with short-term use but overall modest clinical impact (Kuriyama et al., 2014). A study of five alcohol-dependent patients noted improvements in insomnia scores, including a shorter time to fall asleep and greater total sleep time (Brower et al., 2011), and a study of older adults found that ramelteon, like melatonin, reduces the risk of delirium (Hatta et al., 2014). The drug is thought to be devoid of abuse potential, and there have not been reports of rebound insomnia following a period of nightly use.

Circadin

Circadin is a prolonged-release melatonin formulation that, like the hormone itself, is an agonist at both types of melatonin receptors. It is designed to match the profile of physiological melatonin secretion (Liu et al., 2016). Not available over the counter in the United States, it has clinically relevant antidepressant properties and sleep-promoting properties and has been approved for use by prescription in other countries. It is reported to improve sleep in older adults with insomnia, including improvements in sleep latency, overall sleep quality, and next-day function; also, the clinical use of Circadin does not impair memory or decrease vigilance, and it is said to have no significant withdrawal symptoms (Quera-Salva and Claustrat, 2018). A British study is underway to investigate whether Circadin might have analgesic and sleep-promoting effects in adults with severe nonmalignant pain of at least three months' duration (Adam et al., 2020).

Tasimelteon

In 2014, **tasimelteon** was approved by the FDA for treatment of non-24-hour sleep–wake disorder, a circadian rhythm disorder in which the person's biological clock fails to synchronize to a 24-hour day. People with this condition typically find themselves going to sleep at later and later times, day after day, and trying to sleep on a normal schedule usually results in severe sleep deprivation. The condition occurs in many, perhaps most, people who are totally blind and cannot perceive enough light for their brain to establish a normal sleep schedule (Nishimon et al., 2021). The FDA estimates that as many as 100,000 people in the United States have this disorder, and there is currently no other treatment for it. Tasimelteon is an agonist at both melatonin-1 and melatonin-2 receptors, with greater affinity at the melatonin-2 receptor. Adverse effects of tasimelteon include potentially significant interactions with other drugs, such as a nearly sevenfold increase in the blood concentration of tasimelteon in patients also taking the SSRI fluvoxamine (Ogilvie et al., 2015).

Orexin Receptor Antagonists

As we have seen, the activation of $GABA_A$ and melatonin receptors has inhibitory effects, among which is sleep promotion, and insomnia drugs that act by binding to those receptors are agonists. A different approach for promoting sleep is to use antagonists that block the activation of receptors involved in promoting wakefulness, including orexin receptors (discussed in this section) and histamine receptors (discussed in the next section).

Orexin is a neuropeptide neurotransmitter that has two forms, orexin-A and orexin-B, both of which bind with somewhat differing affinities to two types of orexin receptors, OX1 and OX2 (both are G-protein-coupled receptors). The orexin system, first described in 1998, was originally thought to be principally involved in promoting feeding behaviors (*orexis* in Greek means "appetite") but is now known to have much more profound effects on arousal, with a key role in supporting and maintaining wakefulness and with less pronounced effects on feeding than originally thought. The regulation of sleep and wakefulness is mediated by the interaction of multiple nuclei within the hypothalamus. Orexin seems to be involved in aiding the transition from sleep to wakefulness by activating neural pathways of the ascending arousal system (Kumar et al., 2016). Orexin-releasing neurons in the lateral hypothalamus project broadly in the CNS, with especially dense connections to other neural systems involved in promoting wakefulness.

Three orexin receptor antagonists—suvorexant, lemborexant, and daridorexant, all of which bind to both types of orexin receptors—have been approved by the FDA for the treatment of insomnia characterized by difficulties with sleep onset or sleep maintenance (see Table 13.2; as of late 2022, no comparative studies of these three drugs had been reported).

Suvorexant

In 2014, **suvorexant** (Belsomra) became the first orexin receptor antagonist to be approved by the FDA for the treatment of insomnia. A dose of is 5–20 milligrams is taken once per night, within 30 minutes of retiring, with at least 7 hours available before the expected wake-up time. The drug has a half-life of 12 hours, and there are no active metabolites.

The efficacy of suvorexant appears good (Herring et al., 2016; Norman and Anderson, 2016). In a three-week study with shift workers, suvorexant (compared with placebo) resulted in improved sleep, with 2 extra hours of total sleep time (Zeitzer et al., 2020). However, it is too soon to know whether suvorexant will be sufficiently effective and safe in the real world to be a first-line insomnia treatment or whether it will be reserved only for those who have not had good results with other treatments.

Suvorexant is well tolerated, with the most common adverse event, somnolence, reported in only a few patients (Berger et al., 2022), but like other insomnia drugs, it carries the risk of complex sleep-related behaviors, including driving while not fully awake (see Table 13.3). In trials of up to one year in duration, no withdrawal or rebound effects were seen after the drug was stopped (Asnis et al., 2016).

Lemborexant

Lemborexant (Dayvigo) was FDA approved in December 2019 to help adults with insomnia fall asleep and stay asleep (Scott, 2020). The drug is taken at a dose of 5 milligrams nightly and has a half-life of 17–19 hours, but with few next-day residual effects (Landry et al., 2020). Studies in adults over 55 years of age found that lemborexant compared favorably with zolpidem (Murphy et al., 2020; Rosenberg et al., 2019). Other studies suggest that lemborexant may have a place in treating insomnia in older adults (Abad and Guilleminault, 2018), maybe particularly in those with Alzheimer's disease (Muehlan et al., 2020). No head-to-head comparisons between suvorexant and lemborexant have been reported; however, review studies indicate that lemborexant is superior to suvorexant in initiating sleep, with this superiority being attributed to its faster binding to orexin receptors and its shorter time to reach maximal concentration in blood (Kishi et al., 2020, 2021).

Daridorexant

In 2022, daridorexant (Quviviq) became the third dual orexin antagonist to be approved by the FDA for the treatment of insomnia in adults. Approval was based on two Phase 3 double-blind trials of the drug versus placebo for a period of three months, which found that doses of 25 and 50 milligrams nightly were consistently superior to placebo, with a very favorable profile of side effects, and that patients receiving the 50-milligram dose nightly also exhibited improved daytime functioning (Mignot et al., 2022).

Histamine Receptor Antagonist

In 2010, the antihistamine and tricyclic antidepressant **doxepin** (Silenor) was approved by the FDA for the treatment of sleep maintenance insomnia. Its observed ineffectiveness for sleep-onset problems is probably related to the fact that it takes about 3.5 hours to reach maximum concentration in blood. At low doses of 3 or 6 milligrams daily, doxepin preferentially blocks histamine H1 receptors, and this action is thought to mediate its effect on insomnia (the antidepressant dose is 150–300 milligrams per day). Doxepin is effective in both younger and older populations for up to three to six months, with minimal side effects.

OFF-LABEL AND ALTERNATIVE TREATMENTS FOR INSOMNIA

Several sedating medications are widely used off-label for the treatment of insomnia, including the antidepressants trazodone (Desyrel) and amitriptyline (Elavil), the antipsychotic quetiapine (Seroquel),[7] the antihistamine diphenhydramine (Benadryl),[8] and the anticonvulsant gabapentin (Neurontin) (see Table 13.4).

Alternative treatments that have been tried as therapy for insomnia include acupuncture, Chinese herbal medicine, and medicinal plants such as valerian and passion flower (Borras et al., 2021).

[7]However, new recommendations issued by leading psychiatric organizations warn against the routine use of antipsychotics to treat primary insomnia.

[8]The "Benadryl challenge" on the social media site TikTok, encouraging viewers to take large doses of Benadryl in order to induce hallucinations, has led to Benadryl abuse by young people. Overdoses (10–12 tablets) have resulted in numerous emergency room visits and a few deaths.

TABLE 13.4 Sedating Drugs Used Off-Label for the Treatment of Insomnia

Drug	Dosage (mg)	Mean Elimination Half-Life in Hours (range)	T_{max} (hours)
ANTIDEPRESSANTS			
Trazodone	25–150	9 (7–15)	1–2
Amitriptyline	10–100	30 (5–45)	2–5
ANTIPSYCHOTIC			
Quetiapine	25–100	6	1–2
ANTIHISTAMINE			
Diphenhydramine	25–50	4–8	1–4
ANTICONVULSANT			
Gabapentin	100–900	5–9	1.6–3

[Data from Asnis et al., 2016.]

ANTICONVULSANT DRUGS

Epilepsy affects about 65 million people worldwide and about 1% of the U.S. population. The primary goal of the pharmacological treatment of epilepsy is to eliminate seizures while minimizing the adverse side effects of antiseizure drugs (for reviews of the efficacy and safety of such drugs, see Kanner and Bicchi, 2022, and Loscher and Klein, 2021). The number of commercially available anticonvulsant drugs has more than doubled during the past 15–20 years. Currently, 28 are available, and of these, 10 have become available since 2009 (see Table 13.5). The chemical structures of some of the older and newer anticonvulsants are shown in Figure 13.8.

In recent years, the uses of anticonvulsant drugs have been expanded beyond just the treatment of seizure disorders (epilepsy): some of these drugs are now used in the treatment of bipolar disorder;[9] treatment of aggressive and explosive behavioral disorders in children, adolescents, and adults; management of alcohol withdrawal and cravings; treatment of chronic pain; and management of certain anxiety disorders, such as PTSD, generalized anxiety disorder, and even certain components of borderline personality disorder. Similarly, older drugs no longer used as anticonvulsants may be repurposed for use in other conditions. For example, fenfluramine, an anticonvulsant that was withdrawn from the market in 1997 due its association with cardiac valve abnormalities, was reintroduced in 2020 (and FDA approved under the trade name Fintepla) for the treatment of two seizure disorders in children—Dravet syndrome and Lennox-Gastaut syndrome (Balagura et al., 2020).[10] In this section, however, we confine

[9]Anticonvulsants not specifically discussed in this section that have found use in the treatment of bipolar disorder include topiramate (discussed in Chapter 5 as a treatment for alcoholism) and zonisamide (also used as an antiobesity drug and in treating binge-eating disorder).

[10]Cannabidiol has also proven effective (and is FDA approved) in the treatment of Lennox-Gastaut syndrome and Dravet syndrome (Devinsky et al., 2018; Lattanzi et al., 2018).

TABLE 13.5 Antiepileptic Drugs Approved by the FDA

Approved Before 1993	Approved 1993–2005	Approved 2006–2019
Carbamazepine	Felbamate	Brivaracetam
Clonazepam	Gabapentin	Cenobamate
Diazepam	Lamotrigine	Clobazam
Ethosuximide	Levetiracetam	Eslicarbazepine
Lorazepam	Oxcarbazepine	Ezogabine
Phenobarbital	Pregabalin	Lacosamide
Phenytoin	Tiagabine	Perampanel
Primidone	Topiramate	Rufinamide
Valproic acid	Zonisamide	Stiripentol
		Vigabatrin

[Data from Abou-Khalil, 2022.]

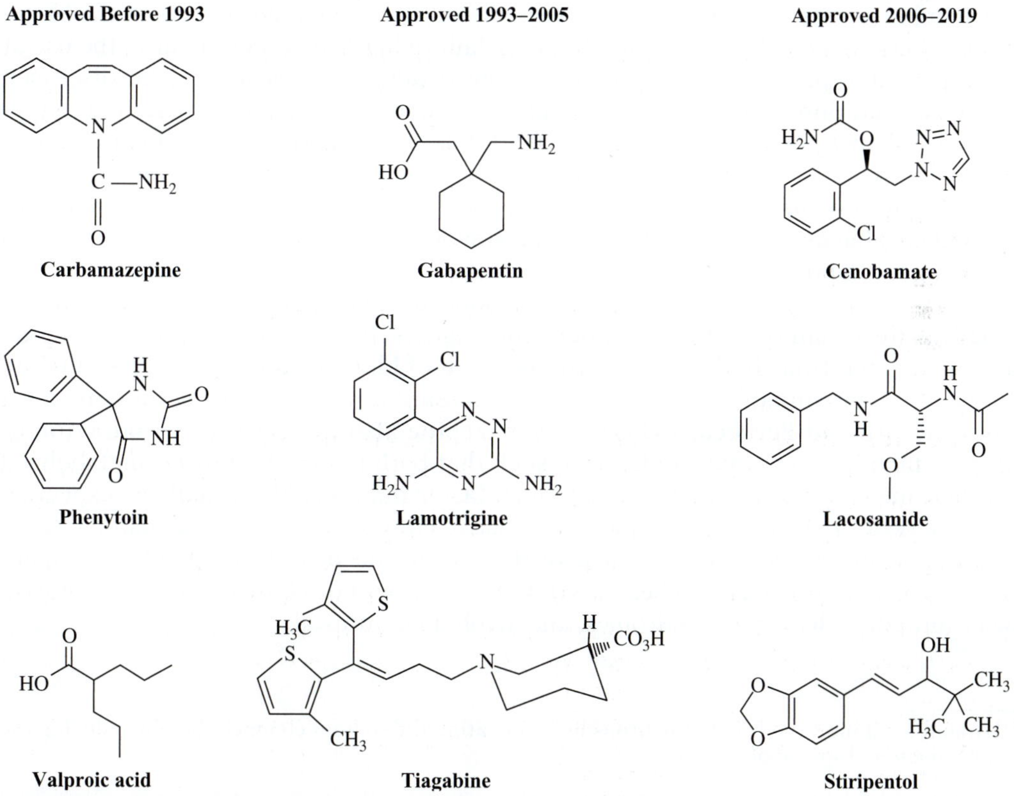

FIGURE 13.8 Chemical Structures of Anticonvulsant Drugs.

our discussion to the uses of anticonvulsants that are currently approved for the treatment of epilepsy.

Drugs Approved Before 1993

The barbiturate phenobarbital (see Figure 13.2) was the first widely effective antiepileptic drug. However, it and other barbiturates are rarely used today, not only because of their sedative and adverse cognitive depressant effects, but also because equally effective, more specific, and less sedating antiepileptics are now available.

Phenytoin (Dilantin), introduced into medicine in 1938, remains a commonly used hydantoin[11] anticonvulsant, producing less sedation than do the barbiturates. It has a half-life of about 24 hours, which means that daytime sedation can be minimized by taking the full daily dose at bedtime. However, its many other bothersome side effects limit its use in favor of newer, less toxic agents. Other currently available anticonvulsants that came into early use include primidone and ethosuximide, both introduced in the late 1950s.

Valproic acid (Divalproex, Depakene, Depakote), introduced in 1974, is effective in treating petit mal seizure disorders in children by augmenting the postsynaptic action of GABA. Valproic acid has a short half-life of about 6 to 12 hours and must therefore be administered two or three times a day. Common side effects include sedation and cognitive impairments, though to a lesser degree than the similar side effects of the barbiturates. Serious side effects are rare, but liver failure has been reported; also, the use of valproic acid by pregnant females can have severe adverse consequences (as discussed below). In addition, valproic acid has been associated with the highest risk of developing type 2 diabetes in adults (Sun et al., 2022). Like many of the newer anticonvulsants, valproic acid is effective in the treatment of other disorders, including bipolar disorder, PTSD, borderline personality disorder, aggressive behaviors, schizophrenia, and alcohol and cocaine dependence. A long-acting, slow-release formulation (Depakote-ER) is approved for the treatment of migraine headache.

Carbamazepine (Tegretol, Equetro), introduced in 1963, perhaps has a less intense sedative effect than that of other antiepileptic agents, but its use is limited by the risk of serious alterations in the cellular composition of blood (reduced numbers of white blood cells), presumably secondary to a depressant effect of the drug on bone marrow (Zaccara and Perucca, 2014). Carbamazepine also increases the production of drug-metabolizing enzymes in the liver, such that both it and other drugs metabolized by the same enzymes are metabolized much faster than would normally be expected, with the result that they all become less effective clinically due to lower-than-expected blood concentrations. Often, the dose of these drugs needs to be doubled to compensate. Carbamazepine has also been used in the treatment of bipolar disorder, explosive behavioral disorders, pain syndromes, and alcohol withdrawal.

---

[11]Hydantoins inhibit the firing of neurons by inactivating the sodium channel, thereby reducing the development and spread of seizures.

Drugs Approved 1993–2005

Gabapentin (Neurontin), introduced in 1993, is a structural analogue of GABA (GABA lacks gabapentin's ring structure, shown in Figure 13.8) that was synthesized with the aim of developing a specifically GABA-mimetic antiepileptic drug. Gabapentin is also effective in treating both an anxiety disorder (phobia) and a pain disorder (reflex sympathetic dystrophy) and has been used in treating a wide variety of other chronic pain states, as well as in treating alcohol withdrawal and preventing relapse to alcohol use (Anton et al., 2020). A related drug, **pregabalin** (Lyrica), also used in treating anxiety disorders (see the discussion earlier in this chapter), was introduced as an anticonvulsant in 2004 for adult patients with partial-onset seizures (i.e., seizures that do not encompass the whole brain, the most common form of epilepsy). Like gabapentin, pregabalin is used to treat several pain disorders, including diabetic peripheral neuropathy, fibromyalgia, postherpetic neuralgia, and neuropathic pain from spinal cord injury. There appear to be significant risks associated with coprescribing gabapentin or pregabalin with opioids or other CNS depressants such as benzodiazepines (Torrance et al., 2020); in late 2019, the FDA issued a warning against such combinations of drugs due to the risk of respiratory depression. Also, the growing off-label use of gabapentin for nonseizure disorders has been associated with an increasing number of overdose deaths, with 90% of the deaths involving combination with opioids, primarily illicitly manufactured fentanyl, and with 83% of those deaths occurring in white males aged 35–54 years (Kuehn, 2022).

Lamotrigine (Lamictal), introduced into medicine in 1995, acts by inhibiting ion fluxes through sodium channels, stabilizing neuronal membranes, and inhibiting the presynaptic release of neurotransmitters, principally glutamate (Pawlik et al., 2021; Sills and Rogawski, 2020). In some epilepsy patients, it also has beneficial effects on mood, mental alertness, and social interactions, and it has the unusual and significant advantage of improving cognitive functioning and exerting antidepressant actions (e.g., it has been used for the treatment of resistant depression as well as the depressive phase in bipolar disorder) (Peters et al., 2021).

Oxcarbazepine (Trileptal) is a structural derivative of carbamazepine that differs from carbamazepine in two ways: it is not itself pharmacologically active but is rapidly metabolized to an active molecule, and it has not been associated with the white blood cell toxicity associated with carbamazepine. Oxcarbazepine is being increasingly used to treat bipolar illness and other disorders for which carbamazepine is also effective.

Tiagabine (Gabitril), introduced into medicine in 1998, acts by inhibiting GABA reuptake transporters located on the presynaptic nerve terminals of GABA-releasing neurons, which serves to prolong GABA's synaptic action. Tiagabine appears to be less useful in the treatment of bipolar disorder than other antiepileptic drugs, but it has shown modest efficacy in the treatment of generalized anxiety disorder.

Levetiracetam (Keppra) is effective in treating partial-onset seizures. It has a unique mechanism of action (Yan et al., 2013) that makes it suitable for add-on therapy with other antiepileptic drugs in both adults and children with refractory seizures. It also has found use in the treatment of bipolar disorder.

Drugs Approved 2006–2019

Lacosamide (Vimpat), introduced in 2008, appears to act differently from traditional anticonvulsants that act by inhibiting the generation of fast action potentials. In contrast, lacosamide modulates sodium channels without affecting fast action potentials. This "novel sodium channel modulator" is useful in the treatment of partial-onset seizures (McGinnis and Kessler, 2016; Vossler et al., 2016) and may have fewer cognition-depressing side effects than other anticonvulsants (Lancman et al., 2016).

Vigabatrin (Sabril), long available in Europe, was introduced into the United States in 2010. Despite serious side effects, it is indicated for treating two forms of severe epilepsy: infantile spasms and refractory partial epilepsy (as an adjunctive therapy for adults who have not responded to other agents). Side effects including loss of peripheral vision and even permanent complete loss of vision mean that it is available only through a single national pharmacy and requires formal ophthalmologic evaluation with continuing follow-up.

Rufinamide (Banzel), FDA approved in 2008 for the treatment of Lennox-Gastaut syndrome in both children and adults (for its use in adults, see McMurray and Striano, 2016), is structurally different from other anticonvulsants. It is also effective in the treatment of refractory partial seizures, and it seems to have no adverse effects on cognitive functioning.

Clobazam (Onfi), approved in the United States in 2011 for the treatment of seizures associated with Lennox-Gastaut syndrome, is a benzodiazepine that is also used for the treatment of refractory epilepsy and for short-term treatment of the severe anxiety and agitation seen in psychotic disorders. Like all benzodiazepines, clobazam has side effects that include adverse sedation and cognitive impairments. Interestingly, the active metabolite of clobazam, N-desmethylclobazam, has some preferential binding to the $\alpha2$ subtype of the alpha subunit of the $GABA_A$ receptor and as a result may have some analgesic activity, in contrast to other benzodiazepines (Raivenius et al., 2016).

Ezogabine (Potiga), FDA approved in 2011 as an adjunctive treatment for adults with partial-onset seizures, appears to act by opening potassium channels in the brain (a unique action among anticonvulsants). Reported side effects include dizziness, somnolence, fatigue, and confusion.

Perampanel (Fycompa), approved by the FDA in 2012, is unique as a blocker of the AMPA subtype of glutamate receptors, giving it a wide spectrum of useful anticonvulsant effects. However, the labeling includes an FDA black box warning of adverse effects, including "aggression, hostility, irritability, anger, and homicidal ideation." Other reported adverse effects include suicidal thoughts and behavior, dizziness, gait disturbances, somnolence, and fatigue.

Eslicarbazepine (Aptiom), FDA approved in 2013 as an ancillary medication to treat partial seizures, is a prodrug to oxcarbazepine, which means it has the same actions as oxcarbazepine. Thus, it has the potential to treat not only epilepsy but also bipolar disorder and certain pain syndromes (Johannessen et al., 2016). Eslicarbazepine is also claimed to be effective in drug-resistant patients and to have fewer side effects, fewer interactions with other drugs, and beneficial effects on quality of life and alertness (Schmid et al., 2016).

Brivaracetam (Briviact) was FDA approved in 2016 for the treatment of both partial and major motor seizures. Its efficacy has been demonstrated (Ben-Menachem et al., 2016; Moseley et al., 2016), but its efficacy does not seem to surpass that of levetiracetam (Zhang et al., 2016).

Stiripentol (Diacomit), was FDA approved in 2018 for the treatment of seizures associated with Dravet syndrome in patients 2 years of age and older taking clobazam. It acts by increasing GABA transmission and by limiting GABA synaptic uptake, which prolongs GABA activity. It strongly inhibits the metabolism of other drugs, making other drugs both more effective—but possibly toxic, too, meaning that dose reductions of other drugs are usually required.

Cenobamate (Xcopri), FDA-approved in 2019, is indicated for the treatment of partial seizures in adults (Loscher and Klein, 2021; Specchio et al., 2021; Steinhoff, 2021). It is a sodium channel blocker (Roberti et al., 2021) that is also thought to enhance presynaptic GABA release, thereby increasing GABA's inhibitory effects (Latimer et al., 2021). In addition, researchers have postulated that cenobamate may have important neuroprotective properties following head trauma (Wicinski et al., 2021).

Effects in Pregnancy

Approximately 1 million women with epilepsy in the United States are in their active reproductive years. Most require anticonvulsant medication during pregnancy, and many anticonvulsants carry a risk of adverse effects on the fetus. In addition, as we have discussed above, anticonvulsants are also used to treat an expanding range of nonepileptic medical conditions, including bipolar disorder, migraine headache, and chronic pain syndromes, and these uses carry the same risk of adverse fetal effects as does use for the treatment of epilepsy (Kaplan and Demir, 2021; Knight et al., 2021). However, most women taking anticonvulsants have a typical pregnancy and give birth to an infant without congenital malformations. Also, women who took an anticonvulsant during a prior pregnancy and delivered an infant without any congenital malformation are not at increased risk during a subsequent pregnancy of delivering an infant with a congenital malformation. In the words of one group of researchers, "The large majority of pregnancies in women with epilepsy do not have significant adverse fetal outcomes" (Meador et al., 2020).

However, if a prior pregnancy resulted in an infant with a malformation, the risk of a malformation in the next pregnancy was two or three times greater (Vajda et al., 2017). The use of multiple anticonvulsants during pregnancy also triples the risk of adverse fetal effects, especially when valproic acid is included (Daugaard et al., 2020). Even alone, without other anticonvulsants, valproic acid use during pregnancy is especially problematic, carrying a significantly increased risk of cognitive impairments in offspring[12] (Bromley et al., 2019). In sum, extreme care and counseling are important when contemplating the use of anticonvulsants during pregnancy.

---

[12]In 2011, the FDA issued a safety announcement on the adverse impact of valproic acid on cognitive impairments in offspring of mothers who took valproic acid during pregnancy.

Risk of Suicidality

In December 2008, the FDA issued a warning that the use of antiepileptic drugs as a class may increase the risk of suicidal thoughts and behaviors, or **suicidality**. The medical community received this warning with skepticism, stemming from the understanding that multiple other factors may be involved in the increased rate of suicidality in patients taking anticonvulsants, whether for epilepsy, for surgery, or for conditions such as depression, bipolar disorder, substance abuse disorders, and anxiety disorders. A study of patients later diagnosed with epilepsy found that they had a prediagnosis and pretreatment incidence of at least one suicide attempt that was about two or three times greater than the incidence in a control group (Hesdorffer et al., 2016); given that anticonvulsant medications had not yet been prescribed, this increase was clearly not due to taking such medications. Probably, the increase was due to a comorbid disorder, such as depression or bipolar disorder (Ferrer et al., 2014). Nevertheless, patients taking anticonvulsants should be carefully monitored for behavioral changes that could be precursors to emerging suicidality, including drug-induced anxiety, agitation, hostility, and mania or hypomania (Mula and Sander, 2015). This applies regardless of whether the anticonvulsants are being used to treat seizures, psychiatric disorders, pain, migraine headaches, or other conditions. Interestingly, as illustrated in Figure 13.9, studies of risk factors for suicidality that included anticonvulsants indicate that anticonvulsants alone are not associated with suicidality (Klein et al., 2021; Roberson et al., 2019).

Therapeutic Drug Monitoring with Anticonvulsants

The widespread use of the many anticonvulsant drugs currently available in the United States (see Table 13.5) has highlighted the importance of therapeutic drug monitoring (TDM) with these medicines (Landmark et al., 2020; Patsalos et al., 2018).

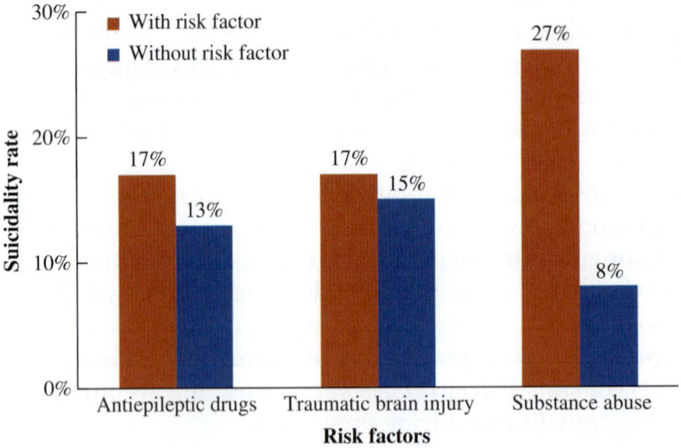

FIGURE 13.9 Suicidality Rate. A study of patients with seizures at a Veterans Administration hospital revealed a significant association between substance abuse and the risk of suicidality, but no significant association between suicidality risk and the use of antiepileptic drugs or the presence of traumatic brain injury. [Data from Roberson et al., 2019.]

(As discussed in Chapter 1, TDM is the process of correlating the plasma level of a drug with its therapeutic response.) TDM is especially important as a clinical guide during pregnancy in women taking anticonvulsants (Arfman et al., 2020). The marked pharmacokinetic variability of anticonvulsants, as well as their multiple drug interactions, can make TDM the basis for a more scientific approach to the optimal clinical care (and safety) of patients taking anticonvulsants, by allowing dose adjustments based on measured plasma concentrations. Essentially, an ED_{50} (see Chapter 3) is determined based on animal studies and clinical trials, and this value often points to reliable clinical dosage and blood concentrations for both established and experimental anticonvulsants (Apraku and Okoro, 2019).

GENERAL ANESTHETICS

All of the sedative-hypnotic drugs in sufficient doses can produce amnesia and loss of consciousness. **General anesthetics** are drugs used to produce these effects during surgery. The two types of general anesthetics are those administered by inhalation through the lungs and those administered by injection into a vein. Inhalation anesthetics in current use include one gas, nitrous oxide (with low anesthetic potency), and five volatile liquids: isoflurane, halothane, desflurane, enflurane, and sevoflurane. These drugs produce a dose-related depression of all functions of the CNS—an initial period of sedation followed by the onset of sleep. As anesthesia deepens, both amnesia and unconsciousness are induced. Adding an opioid narcotic such as morphine to a volatile anesthetic adds analgesic action to this state of unconsciousness.

The inhaled anesthetics are subject to misuse. Nitrous oxide, for example, which induces behavioral disinhibition, analgesia, and mild euphoria, is used as a carrier gas in whipped cream charger cans and abused by people who break open the cans and inhale the gas (referred to as "whippets"). Whether used clinically or abused recreationally, the inhalation of nitrous oxide dilutes the air that a person is breathing, so extreme caution is needed to prevent hypoxia, which could produce irreversible brain damage. (Other forms of inhalant abuse are discussed in Chapter 5; the use of nitrous oxide as an antidepressant is discussed in Chapter 12.)

Injectable anesthetics in current use include thiopental, methohexital, propofol, fospropofol, etomidate, and dexmedetomidine. Thiopental (Pentothal) and methohexital (Brevital) are ultrashort-acting barbiturates. Propofol (Diprivan) and etomidate (Amidate) are structurally unique (propofol structurally resembles the neurotransmitter GABA). After propofol and etomidate became generically available, more expensive preparations were marketed: fospropofol (Lusedra), a prodrug that is rapidly converted to propofol (Bengalorkar et al., 2011), and dexmedetomidine (Precedex), which is structurally related to etomidate and likely works with identical efficacy (Mizrak et al., 2010).

Recently, the veterinary anesthetic xylazine (Rompun, Sedazine, "tranq") has been found as an additive to fentanyl pills. Xylazine is a potent sedative and amnestic; it potentiates the effects of fentanyl, increasing its lethal toxicity (Ball et al., 2022). The effects of xylazine are not reversible by naloxone, and the drug has become increasingly responsible for fatal overdoses (Chhabra et al., 2022).

CHAPTER REVIEW

1. In the term *sedative-hypnotic drugs*, what do the words *sedative* and *hypnotic* refer to?
2. Starting in the 1960s, which class of sedative-hypnotic drugs replaced the barbiturates in many of their uses?
3. Describe these three types of brain dysfunctions associated with the use of sedative-hypnotic drugs; blackouts, dysfunction associated with loss off nerve cell function, and complex sleep-related behaviors.
4. Describe an important difference between barbiturates and benzodiazepines in how they interact with $GABA_A$ receptors.
5. Why has the clinical use of barbiturates declined? What are some of their current clinical uses?
6. What is a Mickey Finn?
7. Why are nonbarbiturate sedative-hypnotics such as meprobamate, methaqualone, and gamma hydroxybutyrate now considered obsolete for use in medicine but still sometimes encountered as drugs of abuse?
8. What is the most important pharmacokinetic difference among the benzodiazepines?
9. Discuss the pros and cons of the clinical use of benzodiazepines in the treatment of anxiety and insomnia and as anticonvulsants and amnestics. What are the risks associated with the clinical use of benzodiazepines in older adults and in pregnant women?
10. What are the main reasons for the large numbers of benzodiazepine overdoses? How does flumazenil work as antidote to such overdoses, and why is it rarely used?
11. What are the four main classes of drugs used as alternatives to benzodiazepines for the treatment of anxiety?
12. Match each numbered drug used in the treatment of insomnia with the lettered drug class to which it belongs.
    1. zolpidem; 2. ramelteon; 3. suvorexant; 4. Doxepin
    A. melatonin receptor agonist; B. histamine receptor antagonist; C. nonbenzodiazepine agonist at benzodiazepine receptors; D. orexin receptor antagonist
13. True or false: Anticonvulsant drugs are used in the treatment of a wide variety of disorders in addition to epilepsy.
14. Which anticonvulsant drug is especially risky to use during pregnancy?
15. True or false: Studies indicate that the use of anticonvulsant drugs significantly increases the risk of suicidal thoughts and behaviors.
16. What are the desired effects of sedative-hypnotic drugs used as general anesthetics?

KEY TERMS

anticonvulsant drugs
anxiolytic drugs
barbiturates
benzodiazepines
brivaracetam
carbamazepine
carisoprodol
cenobamate
chloral hydrate
Circadin
clobazam
complex sleep-related behaviors
doxepin
eslicarbazepine
eszopiclone
ezogabine
flumazenil
gabapentin
gamma hydroxybutyrate (GHB)
general anesthetics
lacosamide
lamotrigine
lemborexant
levetiracetam
melatonin
meprobamate
methaqualone
orexin
oxcarbazepine
paraldehyde
perampanel
phenobarbital
phenytoin
prazosin
pregabalin
propranolol
ramelteon
rufinamide
sedative-hypnotic drugs
stiripentol
suicidality
suvorexant
tasimelteon
tiagabine
valproic acid
vigabatrin
zaleplon
zolpidem

CHAPTER 14

Drugs Used to Treat Bipolar Disorder

CHAPTER OUTLINE

Bipolar disorder, also known as *manic-depressive disorder*, is one of the ten most disabling mental health disorders, with a lifetime prevalence of about 2% across all populations, regardless of nationality, race, or socioeconomic status (Carvalho et al., 2020). It "is a mental health disorder characterized by extreme shifts in mood, high suicide rate, sleep problems, and dysfunctions of psychological traits like self-esteem (feeling inferior when depressed and superior when manic)" (Rantala et al., 2021). Persons who have bipolar disorder lose many years of healthy functioning, and their livelihood, marriage, schooling, social relationships, and even lives may be destroyed. The illness is episodic, with alternating periods of mania or depression nearly a third of the time and intervening periods of at least some degree of recovery and sometimes remission (Figure 14.1).

Clinical onset averages about 20–25 years of age, with various subgroups showing even earlier onset, averaging about 14 years (+/– 5 years). The younger the onset, often the longer the delay to treatment, the greater the depressive symptomatology, and the higher the levels of comorbid anxiety and substance abuse (Yatham et al., 2018). There is typically a significant delay between the appearance of symptoms and a correct diagnosis and treatment. In fact, estimates of the delay between onset of symptoms and correct diagnosis and appropriate treatment range from six to ten years (Dagani et al., 2016). The most common initial misdiagnosis is unipolar depression (a topic we'll discuss in the next section).

There are several subtypes of the disorder. **Bipolar I disorder** includes at least one episode of full-blown mania with or without an episode of major depression. In **bipolar II disorder** the manic episode is less severe, or hypomanic, and episodes of major depression are more frequent. A patient is said to be a **rapid cycler** if at least four episodes occur in a 12-month period. Several other bipolar subtypes have been described, exhibiting varying degrees of severity in recurrent mood swings.

Despite intensive care and treatment, outpatients with bipolar disorder have a considerable degree of illness-related morbidity and variability in illness cycles, including a three- to sixfold greater amount of time spent depressed than time spent manic (Figure 14.1). Moreover, as noted, there is a high rate of mortality, with 25–50% of bipolar patients attempting suicide at least once over their lifetime, and 8–19% completing suicide (Latalova et al., 2014). To be clear, bipolar disorder has the highest rate of suicide of all psychiatric conditions, approximately 20–30 times that of the general population

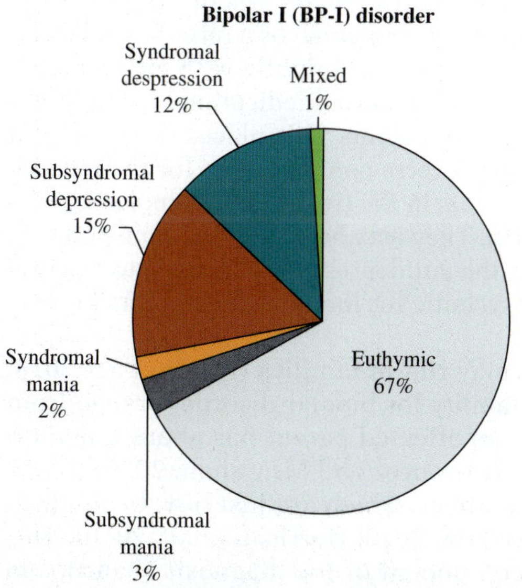

FIGURE 14.1 Bipolar I (BP-1) Disorder. Percentage of time spent in each mood state for individuals who have bipolar I disorder. Two-thirds of the time they have no symptoms, and they are depressed (subsyndromal or syndromal) more than three times more frequently than they are manic (subsyndromal and syndromal mania) during the course of the disorder. [Data from Parikh et al., 2015.]

(Miller and Black, 2020). Other predictors of mortality in bipolar patients include being male, having a history of alcoholism, and poor occupational status before the index episode, as well as a history of previous episodes, psychotic features, mixed episodes, and residual affective symptoms between episodes. This speaks to the need for aggressive treatment of bipolar disorder with a goal of reaching full remission from each episode, if possible.

DIAGNOSTIC AND TREATMENT ISSUES

Similar to unipolar depression, the symptoms of bipolar depression include, in decreasing order of prevalence, sadness, insomnia, feelings of worthlessness, loss of energy and ability to concentrate, inability to enjoy everyday activities, thoughts of death and suicide, and an inability to function. Manic symptoms include various aspects of behavioral and physiological hyperactivity, such as erratic sleep, increased sexual interest, emotional elation, racing thoughts, increased physical activity, impulsiveness, poor judgment, and reckless and aggressive behavior; in other words, extreme disinhibition, irritability, overconfidence, and highly elevated mood (Carvalho et al., 2020). Up to 75% of individuals presenting with mania will have psychotic symptoms, such as delusions of grandeur and hallucinations.

Comorbid substance abuse affects up to 70% of bipolar I and 50% of bipolar II patients (Grunze et al., 2021), with reported rates for alcohol (82%), cocaine (30%), marijuana (29%), sedatives or amphetamines (21%), and opioids (13%). It may, at least initially, represent an attempt at self-medication for the symptoms accompanying the affective disorder. Unfortunately, substance abuse is associated with a greater risk of "switching" or "flipping" from a depressive episode to one of mania, hypomania, or a mixed mood state.

Although a patient with bipolar disorder may present initially with either mania or depression, most patients seek treatment for and receive medications for unipolar depression, as noted, typically with antidepressants alone. This places the patient at risk for a manic flip, which can result in serious adverse consequences for the individual (Gitlin, 2018). Indeed, the use of antidepressants in the treatment of bipolar depression is controversial (Cheniaux and Nardi, 2019). They may be useful for some patients, but they may be harmful for others. If chosen, the antidepressant may need to be combined with a mood stabilizer or atypical antipsychotic for longer-term stability (a topic discussed in more detail later).

Bipolar disorder is highly heritable and may run in families (Hibar et al., 2018; Sandstrom et al., 2019). Estimates of inheritability for bipolar disorders range from 70 to 90% (Carvalho et al., 2020). A child of an affected parent has about a tenfold increased risk of developing bipolar disorder (Gordovez and McMahon, 2020). There are multiple susceptibility loci, each of small effect, which are just now being identified (Ching et al., 2022; Gordovez and McMahon, 2020; Harrison et al., 2018). This makes a thorough family history a crucial component of the diagnosis (Sandstrom et al., 2019). Similarly, a personal history of disruptive behavioral patterns or evidence of mania, hypomania, increased energy, or decreased need for sleep may suggest a bipolar diagnosis, as would treatment-emergent mania or hypomania during antidepressant monotherapy. Early interventions are necessary for persons at risk for developing bipolar disorder. This may include pharmacotherapy.

Overview of Pharmacotherapy

Pharmacotherapy forms the foundation for the successful treatment of bipolar disorder (Fountoulakis et al., 2020) and addresses three phases of bipolar illness: mania, depression, and long-term recurrences (Baldessarini et al., 2019). Table 14.1 summarizes the relative effectiveness of the available agents for each phase. We will discuss specific drugs associated with each of these phases later in the chapter, but following is a quick overview.

TABLE 14.1 Comparison of the Efficacy of Drugs for the Treatment of Bipolar I Disorder[a]

Drug	Acute mania/mixed	Acute bipolar depression	Mood stabilizer prophylaxis
Lithium	++++	++	+++
Valproic acid	+++	++	+
Carbamazepine	+++	++	+
Oxcarbazepine	+++	+	+
Lamotrigine	0	+++	+++
Gabapentin	0	0	0
Topiramate	0	0	0/+
Aripiprazole	+++	0	0
Haloperidol	+++	0	0
Olanzapine	+++	++	+++
Risperidone	+++	0	+++
Paliperidone	++	?	++
Quetiapine	+++	+++	+++
Ziprasidone	+++	0	0
Asenapine	+++	0	?
Lurasidone	+	+++	?
Cariprazine	+++	++	?

[a]Key
++++ = Highly effective
+++ = Substantially effective
++ = Effective
+ = Possibly effective
0 = Not effective
? = Not enough information
Note: It should be noted that most antipsychotic medications can be used to treat acute mania in bipolar disorders either alone or in combination with a mood stabilizer. Antipsychotic medications can also be used as adjunctive treatment with mood stabilizers to treat bipolar depression and combined with mood stabilizers for ongoing maintenance treatment of bipolar disorder. The combination drug olanzapine–fluoxetine is indicated for and is effective for the treatment of acute bipolar depression and for maintenance therapy.
[Data from author's review of the literature.]

For over 70 years lithium has remained the "gold standard" for the treatment of bipolar 1 disorder (Hafeman et al., 2020; Volkmann et al., 2020). Although lithium may effectively control manic symptoms and reduce the recurrence of both manic and depressive episodes, its bothersome and potentially serious side effects have necessitated a search for equally effective, safer, and more tolerable agents. (Again, we will discuss lithium in more detail later in the chapter.)

Acute Mania and Agitation

Until lately, lithium, valproic acid, and antipsychotic drugs were first-line treatments for acute mania and severe bipolar agitation (Fountoulakis et al., 2020; Kishi et al., 2022; Malhi et al., 2020; Verdolini et al., 2021). Bipolar agitation may affect up to a quarter of the estimated 7 million people in the United States who are diagnosed with schizophrenia or bipolar disorders, with episodes that can occur 10–17 times a year. Symptoms of bipolar agitation can range from mild (uneasiness, restlessness) to severe (aggression, violence), and escalation can occur quickly. In general, early identification and intervention are necessary. For the past three quarters of a century, treatment has largely involved behavioral calming, physical restraint, and seclusion combined with various antipsychotic agents, benzodiazepines, or ketamine.

In 2022, a new medication, dexmedetomidine (Igalmi), was approved by the FDA for the acute treatment of agitation associated with either schizophrenia or bipolar disorder in adults. Available in a sublingual film, this sedative agent can ameliorate acute episodes of agitation and make the acute patient more susceptible to treatment.

Bipolar Depression

Bipolar depression remains a major clinical and medical challenge (Baldessarini et al., 2020). First-line treatment of acute bipolar depression is monotherapy, often with lamotrigine or aripiprazole, adding either lithium or an antipsychotic if there is a history of mania. Other antiepileptic drugs found useful for the treatment of bipolar depression include carbamazepine, oxcarbazepine, and valproic acid. Many second-generation antipsychotics and some anticonvulsant drugs have been found to be useful for the treatment of bipolar depression, although treatment remains a challenge (Bahji et al., 2020; Cohen, 2019; Earley et al., 2019).

Mixed States

Mixed episodes, presenting with both depressive and manic symptoms, are relatively frequent in bipolar disorder (Stahl et al., 2017). As many as 40% of cases show this combination of symptoms, and individuals who present with mixed features may have more severe pathology, higher frequency of comorbidities, higher rates of suicide, and poorer outcomes. Treatment for individuals with mixed features can include atypical antipsychotics, particularly lurasidone, asenapine, pramipexole, or (again) an anticonvulsant such as valproic acid or lamotrigine (Chakrabarty et al., 2020; Marazziti et al., 2019). For individuals who have a pattern of rapid cycling, lithium and the anticonvulsants have relatively low efficacy, and these patients have an even higher risk for suicide and comorbidity with substance use and anxiety disorders.

Relapse Prevention

For maintenance treatment, regardless of whether the most recent episode was manic, depressed, or mixed, it is acceptable to stay on the acute-phase medication if it is well tolerated. If the most recent or predominant phase is manic, the medications with the most research support for maintenance treatment include lithium, valproic acid, and antipsychotics (Verdolini et al., 2021), or olanzapine, quetiapine, ziprasidone, aripiprazole, asenapine, clozapine, paliperidone long-acting injectable, and risperidone long-acting injectable. Of note, researchers reviewed the efficacy of long-acting injectable antipsychotics in bipolar disorder, concluding that they show efficacy in reducing manic symptomatology, but they may worsen depressive symptoms (Pacchiarotti et al., 2019). If the most recent or predominant phase is depressed, the medications with the most research support include lithium, lamotrigine, valproic acid, olanzapine, quetiapine, and aripiprazole (Grande et al., 2016; Shah et al., 2017). In many cases, some combination of the aforementioned drugs may be necessary to achieve long-term stability (Verdolini et al., 2021). Long-term relapse prevention in bipolar disorder is challenging, with a significant number of patients relapsing following the initial stabilization of mood (Joshi et al., 2019).

Pathophysiology and Mechanisms of Drug Action

Neither the pathophysiology underlying bipolar illness nor the mechanisms through which medications used in its treatment act are known. Indeed, it is difficult to conceive how any single drug class can reduce symptoms of both mania and depression. Furthermore, it has proven difficult to find a mechanism among the relevant drug classes that would account for this dual therapeutic efficacy.

Like antidepressants, mood-stabilizing anticonvulsants may reverse some of the impairments in brain structure and levels of brain-derived neurotrophic factor (BDNF), reversals that could be relevant to the therapeutic benefit of mood stabilizers in bipolar disorder (Haupt et al., 2021). Lithium protects neurons against a variety of toxic agents and promotes the growth of neuronal processes; in the human brain, lithium increases levels of N-acetyl-aspartate and gray matter volume. But in spite of their common neuroprotective effects, no universal mechanism has yet been identified to account for the therapeutic and neurobiological similarities between antidepressants and mood stabilizers. While antidepressants and antipsychotics have some common effects on neurotransmitter receptors in the brain, which could be relevant to their common antidepressant efficacy, neither lithium nor the anticonvulsants share these mechanisms of action. That is, unlike antidepressants and antipsychotics, lithium and many of the anticonvulsants do not exert their primary effect at neuronal synapses. Instead, anticonvulsants seem to act intracellularly to produce changes that stabilize neuronal membranes (hence the term mood stabilizer).

Currently, the most extensively studied putative mechanisms of mood stabilizers are the second- and third-messenger systems, that is, the intracellular biochemical processes produced by activation of G-protein-coupled receptors. It has already been established that lithium, valproic acid, and carbamazepine interact with various enzymes involved in these intracellular signaling pathways, especially involving glutamate neural transmission in the hippocampus (Kato, 2019).

Although individual drugs may interact at different sites, they may all ultimately produce a yet unknown final common effect that is responsible for their clinical efficacy in bipolar disorder (Rapoport et al., 2009).[1] The target sites of the hippocampus and its connections with the prefrontal cortex and amygdala make these actions relevant. Finally, there is increasing evidence of the impact of circulating glucocorticoids on mood disorders (Podgorny and Gulyaeva, 2021). Hypercortisolemia can produce mood changes, may occur in patients with bipolar disorder, and has deleterious effects on the brain. Cortisol elevation can be reversed by chronic treatment with lithium and valproic acid, suggesting new targets for drug development.

Other mechanisms postulated to be involved in the etiology of bipolar disorder include circadian dysregulation; genetic mutations; immunological, endocrine, and neurophysiological alterations; neuroinflammation; oxidative stress; and changes in calcium signaling and membrane and vesicular transport (Ashok et al., 2017a; Buoli et al., 2016; Özerdem et al., 2016). The drugs used to treat bipolar disorder have been theorized to affect a wide range of receptors, proteins, transporters, and intracellular transcription processes. The research challenge continues, partly because we have no laboratory models of human bipolar illness and partly because of the complexity of the illness. (The Did You Know? box later in the chapter discusses mechanisms in a bit more depth.)

STEP-BD Study

To provide therapeutic guidelines for practitioners, a large-scale, federally funded trial, the **STEP-BD study**, compared pharmacological treatments for bipolar disorder in a semicontrolled, real-world environment. STEP-BD stands for Systematic Treatment Enhancement Program for Bipolar Disorder and was one of several studies funded by the National Institute of Mental Health designed to determine the real-world effectiveness of the major psychiatric drug classes. Like its companion studies for depression (the STAR*D trial; Chapter 12) and schizophrenia (the CATIE trial; Chapter 11), STEP-BD involved large numbers of typical patients and used few exclusion criteria in an effort to make the results more generalizable for treatment in standard clinical practice.

The nature, scope, and overall design of the STEP-BD study were initially described in Sachs and coworkers (2003), and a summary of the initial results is described in Bowden and colleagues (2012). The data from STEP-BD continue to be analyzed, and multiple studies are published yearly based on these subsequent analyses (Ballard et al., 2020; Costa et al., 2020). One research group found that only 58.4% (858 patients)

[1]One possibility is suggested by the fact that lithium and valproic acid, like antidepressants, increase the levels of proteins, such as the *cAMP response-element binding protein* (CREB), that activate genes that produce additional proteins (bcl-2) and a neurotrophic factor (BDNF), which is known to protect neurons from the toxic effects of injury or trauma. Because of this, the two drugs are sometimes referred to as neuroprotective agents.

of a subset of 1469 patients who participated for at least two years achieved recovery, defined as having only two symptoms of the disorder for at least eight weeks; almost half of this group, 48.5%, or 416 patients, had a recurrence at some point, most commonly to a depressive episode (72%) (Perlis et al., 2006).

Other researchers noted five main lessons from the STEP-BD study that could inform clinical practice (Peters et al., 2011):

1. Antidepressants added to mood stabilizers are no more effective than placebo for treatment of bipolar depression.
2. Antidepressants did not induce mania more frequently than placebo in bipolar depressed patients receiving mood stabilizers who had no history of antidepressant-induced mania.
3. Patients with an acute depressive episode who also had subsyndromal manic symptoms did not recover any faster with the addition of antidepressants to their mood stabilizers compared to similar patients who did not receive add-on antidepressants. If anything, those who received the antidepressants were more likely to relapse or have an exacerbation of their manic symptoms, as mentioned earlier.
4. The anticonvulsant lamotrigine (Lamictal) showed benefit for treatment-resistant bipolar depression, as noted.
5. Intensive psychosocial treatments provided more rapid recovery, improved social functioning, and greater life satisfaction compared to simple collaborative care (a topic we will discuss at the end of the chapter).

More recent examination of the data from the STEP-BD study identified several interesting aspects of bipolar disorder and use of certain medications for treatment. A group of researchers determined that use of antidepressants to treat bipolar disorder, even with mood stabilizers on board, tended to increase the rate of rapid cycling in patients who were identified as rapid cyclers (El-Mallakh et al., 2015). The authors noted that the mood stabilizer medications were not protective against the increased rate of depressive episodes and that bupropion was the only antidepressant that did not seem to induce a worsening of rapid cycling. This supports concern for use of antidepressants to treat bipolar depression, even when mood stabilizers are present.

Of all the symptoms of bipolar disorder listed in the DSM-V-TR, researchers found that (1) improvement in rating scale scores for self-esteem and loss of energy within two weeks of starting treatment predicted a more sustained period of recovery; and that (2) improvement in scores measuring psychomotor retardation predicted a potential risk to switch to mania (Mizushima et al., 2017).

In a recent analysis of STEP-BD data, researchers examined suicidal ideation in a subset of STEP-BD participants who attempted suicide during the trial (Ballard et al., 2020). Of the 4100 participants, 245 (5.9%) attempted suicide. The authors focused on suicidal ideation during the 120 days before and 120 days following the suicide attempt. Suicidal ideation worsened in the 120 days pre-attempt, but improved afterward, reaching non-attempt levels by 90 days post-attempt. Other markers followed a similar trajectory: depressed mood, loss of interest, guilt, and self-esteem.

LITHIUM

As mentioned earlier, **lithium** continues to be a prototype for treating bipolar disorder and reducing its rate of relapse.[2] Today, it remains useful for the treatment of acute episodes of bipolar mania, long-term treatment of bipolar disorder, and augmentation of antidepressant drugs in persons with treatment-resistant depression. Unfortunately, its real-world effectiveness is less than that predicted by clinical trials, and relapse often occurs because of patient nonadherence to therapy, as soon discussed.

Lithium (Li^+) is the lightest of the alkali metals and shares some characteristics with sodium (Na^+). In nature, lithium is abundant in some alkaline mineral spring waters. Devoid of psychotropic effects in people who do not experience acute manic or hypomanic episodes, lithium is effective in treating 60–80% of acute manic and hypomanic episodes, although, as mentioned, in the past few years its use has declined because of toxicity, side effects, nonadherence, and resulting relapse as well as the availability of alternatives (we will soon discuss this in more detail).

The history of lithium as a medicine is fascinating (Tondo et al., 2019). In 1948, John Cade, an Australian psychiatrist, discovered the effects of lithium carbonate as a mood stabilizer (Lopez-Munoz et al., 2018) while conducting a study with guinea pigs. Cade noted that when lithium was administered to guinea pigs (lithium was used as a solvent in which to dissolve the injectable drugs he was studying), the animals became lethargic. Taking an intuitive leap, he administered lithium to patients with acute mania and noted remarkable improvement. However, because of earlier problems with lithium as a salt substitute that had resulted in some deaths, the medical community took more than 20 years to accept this agent as an effective treatment for mania. Fortunately, research in the 1970s found lithium to be clearly superior to placebo in the prophylaxis of bipolar disorder; less than a third of lithium-treated patients relapsed, compared with 80% of placebo-treated patients. In 1970, the FDA approved lithium for the treatment of acute mania, and in 1974 lithium became the first FDA-approved treatment for prevention of recurrences in bipolar disorder. At a time when the standard treatments for psychosis were electroconvulsive therapy and surgical lobotomy, lithium had the distinction of being the first effective medication available to treat a mental illness.

Many controlled studies demonstrate lithium's efficacy for acute mania, acute depressive episodes, and maintenance treatment for relapse prevention. One research group recommended lithium as a drug of first choice for both the treatment of acute manic attacks and the long-term management of bipolar disorder (Baldessarini and Tondo, 2000). They concluded that:

> No other proposed mood-stabilizing treatment has such substantial research evidence of long-term efficacy in both type I and type II bipolar disorders, as well as yielding a substantial reduction of mortality risk (p. 190).

---

[2]For a historical overview of lithium therapy and commentaries on lithium, see four related letters in Schou (1997).

Despite being the gold standard of bipolar treatment, real-world experience indicates that lithium is utilized far less often now than are anticonvulsants or antipsychotic medications, with antipsychotics being more commonly prescribed than ever before, supplanting traditional anticonvulsants (Rhee et al., 2020). It has been argued that lithium is less effective than these other agents due to findings indicating that lithium may be most effective for a subpopulation of individuals with bipolar disorder; that requirements for routine periodic blood tests to measure lithium levels may make it inconvenient and costly for some patients; and that its spectrum of side effects may limit its choice for many patients.

Despite these disadvantages, reviews of the historical effectiveness of lithium support its stature as a first-line treatment for individuals with the more classic presentation of bipolar disorder (Table 14.2). When used properly in accurately diagnosed patients, lithium has the greatest efficacy compared to other drugs, reducing suicidal risk and self-harm rates (Hayes et al., 2016; Toffol et al., 2015) (Figure 14.2); however, one group of researchers reported from a large veteran's study that lithium did not reduce the incidence of suicide-related events in veterans with major depression or bipolar disorders and who had experienced a recent suicide event (Katz et al., 2022). Moreover, a recent study suggests that lithium may also reduce the risk of developing dementia in patients with bipolar disorder (Velosa et al., 2020). This is likely the result of a neuroprotective effect of lithium (Rybakowski et al., 2018). Finally, lithium may exert a protective role in lessening the risk of osteoporosis in patients with bipolar disorder (Kohler-Forsberg et al., 2022). Osteoporosis is unfortunately commonly seen in persons with bipolar disorder and may lead to long-term morbidity.

TABLE 14.2 Signature of a Lithium Responder[a]

Essential features
Recurrent mood disorder
Episodic course of illness with distinct mood periods
Remission is complete between episodes
Pattern of mania, then depression sequence
Later age of onset
Indicative features
Absence of rapid-cycling pattern
Family member who is lithium responder
Episodic course in another family member
No significant psychiatric comorbidity

[a]The features tabulated can be broadly regarded as a "signature" of potential lithium response, and although not predictive in an absolute manner, are suggestive of an increased likelihood of a response to treatment with lithium. However, when determining treatment choice, the overall clinical profile of the patient needs to be considered along with tolerability and patient preference.

[Data from Gershon et al., (2009), Grof (2009), and Rybakowski (2014).]

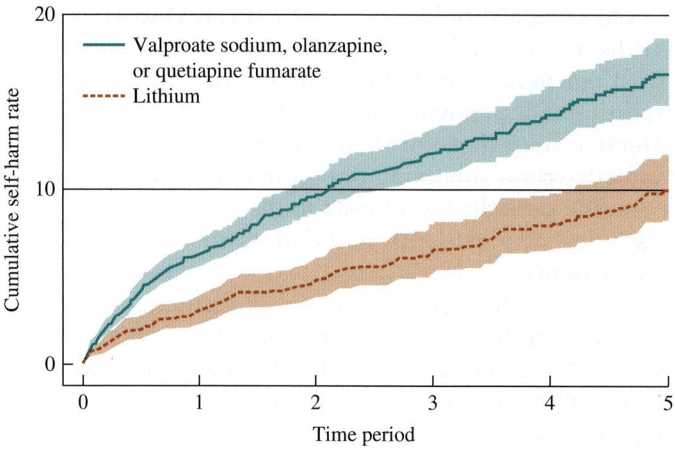

Valproate, olanzapine, or quetiapine	4523	2482	1561	1026	708	493
Lithium	2148	1458	1066	804	649	509

FIGURE 14.2 Self-harm Rates. Cumulative rates of individuals who were seen either in an emergency department or in primary care after attempting to harm themselves intentionally over a five-year period. The top curve represents individuals who had been receiving either valproate, olanzapine, or quetiapine; the lower curve represents individuals who had been receiving lithium. At each time point, individuals receiving lithium had lower rates of self-harm than individuals receiving any of the other drugs listed. The table below the graph indicates the total number of individuals in both groups who were at risk for self-harm at each time point. Total number in the group at time point 0 was 6671 (4523 were receiving valproate, olanzapine, or quetiapine, and 2148 were receiving lithium). [Data from Hayes et al., 2016.]

Pharmacokinetics and Pharmacodynamics

The therapeutic efficacy of lithium is directly correlated with its blood level. Peak blood levels of lithium are reached within 3 hours of oral administration, with complete absorption within 8 hours. The drug crosses the blood-brain barrier slowly and incompletely. Although the clinical significance of this observation is unclear, there can be a twofold variation in the concentration of lithium in the brain compared with its concentration in plasma.

Lithium is not metabolized and is excreted unchanged by the kidneys, with only small amounts excreted through the skin. About half an oral dose is eliminated within 18–24 hours, and the rest, which is taken up by the cells of the body, is excreted over the next one to two weeks. Thus, when therapy is initiated, lithium slowly accumulates over about two weeks until a steady state is reached.

Lithium has a very narrow therapeutic range below which the drug is ineffective and above which side effects and toxicity are prevalent. Practice guidelines recommend a blood level of about 0.8–1.2 milliequivalents per liter (mEq/L) for acute treatment and 0.6–0.8 mEq/L for maintenance. More adverse effects, increasing the likelihood of discontinuation, occur at levels above 1.5 mEq/L, and levels above 2.0 mEq/L are potentially lethal. Because lithium closely resembles table salt, when a patient lowers their normal salt intake or loses excessive amounts of salt via excretion of bodily fluids such as through sweating, lithium blood levels may rise and quickly produce toxicity. Consequently, patients taking lithium should avoid marked changes in sodium intake or excretion and replenish salts after excessive exercise or illness-induced dehydration via decreased fluid intake, vomiting, and diarrhea (Vosahlikova and Svoboda, 2016).

In therapeutic concentrations, lithium has almost no discernible psychotropic effect in normal persons and, unlike many psychoactive drugs, does not produce sedation, depression, or euphoria. Despite clinical utility, the mechanism through which lithium exerts its antimanic effect remains elusive, as noted earlier. Some theories of potential mechanisms are included in the Did You Know? box.

Did You Know?

Mechanism of Action of Lithium

Although the mechanism of action has not been proved, lithium, valproic acid, and lamotrigine are all known to inhibit the intracellular enzyme glycogen synthase kinase-3 (GSK-3). One consequence is an increase in the level of a protein, β-catenin, which promotes cell survival and stimulates axonal growth. Lithium's effect on GSK-3, in animal and tissue models, has been shown to be related to effects on neurotransmitter systems, several signaling pathways, and levels of BDNF, among other physiological effects (Vosahlikova and Svoboda, 2016). Based on the wide array of effects listed earlier, it is difficult to pinpoint exactly how lithium works and through what mechanisms.

Researchers found that lithium and valproic acid protected neurons in the brains of rats (in culture) from damage due to oxidative stress (Vosahlikova and Svoboda, 2016). Oxidative stress occurs when intracellular enzymes cannot sufficiently reduce the levels of toxic substances produced by metabolic activity. In this environment, lithium and valproic acid increased the amount of the antioxidant enzyme glutathione, which plays an important role in reducing oxidative damage. Chronic treatment with lamotrigine and carbamazepine had similar effects. Valproic acid also influences DNA to alter genetic processes in ways that could protect cells from injury or toxic agents. The interaction of valproic acid with DNA is believed to increase levels of cellular protective proteins, such as cAMP response-element binding protein (CREB) and *bcl-2* and other neurotrophic substances, such as BDNF.

Another study found that the volume of gray matter in the brains of patients with bipolar disorder who were taking lithium was as much as 15% larger in areas that are critical for paying attention and controlling emotions, compared to the brain volume of people without the disorder and of patients with bipolar disorder who were not taking lithium (Vosahlikova and Svoboda, 2016).

Side Effects and Toxicity

Because of lithium's extremely narrow therapeutic range, lithium blood levels must be closely monitored. The occurrence and intensity of side effects and toxic reactions are usually related to plasma drug concentrations and involve the nervous system, gastrointestinal (GI) tract, kidneys, thyroid, cardiovascular system, and skin.

DR. J'S MUSINGS 14.1

Lithium

I recall two friends/neighbors with bipolar disorder who experienced lithium side effects that were seriously impacting their lives. One was a 45-year-old male who made his living as a fundraiser for local charities. He had bipolar disorder, inherited from his mother, and was taking lithium. One morning he approached me and said, "Bob, I'm going to lose my job." I asked what was wrong. He replied that he had gained 30 pounds and could not remember names. This was deadly for a person in his business. He told me he was on lithium. I suggested that he talk to his psychiatrist about considering a change to lamotrigine (an anticonvulsant mood stabilizer with antidepressant properties). I saw him a few weeks later, after the switch, and he was doing much better. Now, 25 years later, he remains on lamotrigine and is doing well.

The second person was a 27-year-old female, also with bipolar disorder and on lithium. She would stay on the drug for a while, experience intolerable side effects, quit the drug, become manic, and eventually restart the lithium. The cycle was never-ending. I asked why she would follow this pattern, and she replied, "Every time I went on lithium, I became fat as a house and dumb as a stone." This reflected two of the major side effects of lithium: weight gain and cognitive impairment. Again, I recommended that she consult with her psychiatrist about a switch to lamotrigine. Now 12 years stable, she continues to take lamotrigine.

Early signs of lithium toxicity include ataxia, dysarthria, and impairment in coordination. These effects can be seen at plasma levels below but approaching 1.5 mEq/L. In addition, lithium-induced tremor is very common, and more than 30% of patients report this reaction even at therapeutic blood levels of 0.6–1.2 mEq/L. At plasma levels of 1.5–2.0 mEq/L, patients may experience listlessness, nausea, slurring of speech, diarrhea, nystagmus (uncontrollable, jerky eye movements in any direction), memory impairments, and the appearance of a coarse tremor. Weight gain may be substantial during long-term therapy—up to 30% of patients become obese, a prevalence three times greater than in the general population that can profoundly affect adherence. At plasma levels of 2.0–2.5 mEq/L, patients experience further coarsening of the tremor, confusion, delirium, and pronounced ataxia (Gitlin, 2018; Murru et al., 2015). Lastly, at plasma levels of 2.5 mEq/L and above, patients experience significant alterations of consciousness, hyperextension of the extremities, seizures, and possibly death. Fortunately, the mortality rate of lithium overdose or toxicity is less than 1% (Gitlin, 2018).

In addition to the plasma-level-related side effects noted earlier, lithium may elicit a variety of dermatological reactions. These include rashes, acne, psoriasis, hair and nail disorders, lesions of the mucosal tissue, and like conditions (Gitlin, 2018; Murru et al., 2015). As many as 60% of patients on lithium may experience increased thirst and water intake (polydipsia) and urine output (polyuria) due to an impairment of renal concentrating ability, which can lead to a nephrogenic diabetes insipidus. Kidney function should be assessed periodically to identify those individuals who may be developing kidney dysfunction. Lithium does lead to a small decrease in glomerular filtration rate that is not functionally significant. Permanent kidney damage is rare, occurring in about 1% of patients taking lithium continuously for 15 years (Clos et al., 2015; Shine et al., 2015).

A hypothyroid condition may develop, and enlargement of the gland, such as hypertrophy or goiter, can occur at normal doses along with effects on the parathyroid gland. Adverse effects on memory and cognition are common, and patients often complain of memory problems, as was discussed in Dr. J's Musings 14.1. Consistent with these effects, some researchers found improvements in motor performance, cognition, and creative ability after lithium withdrawal.

Treatment of poisoning or overdose is nonspecific; there is no antidote to lithium. Usually, drug administration is stopped and sodium-containing fluids are infused immediately. If toxic signs are serious, hemodialysis, gastric lavage, diuretic therapy, antiepileptic medication, and other supports may be needed. Complete recovery may be prolonged, with full return of renal and neurological function taking weeks or months. One researcher summarizes how to use lithium most effectively for clinical treatment of bipolar disorder as well as how to reduce the risk of lithium-induced side effects and to manage side effects when they occur (Gitlin, 2016).

Effects in Pregnancy

Lithium can produce adverse effects when taken during pregnancy, particularly in the first trimester, as there is a risk of fetal malformation of the cardiovascular system involving the tricuspid valve; therefore, lithium is generally inappropriate during pregnancy (Fornaro et al., 2020). In addition, valproic acid, typically a good choice for treatment-resistant bipolar disorder, should also be avoided during pregnancy as it can be fetotoxic (Seshachala et al., 2021; Wiggs et al., 2020). As a result, alternative medication is often used, including several antiepileptic drugs (e.g., lamotrigine) or any of several antipsychotic drugs (e.g., quetiapine, olanzapine, or aripiprazole). Because of the risk of recurrence, merely stopping drug therapy during pregnancy is considered unwise. Early switch to lamotrigine seems the most appropriate choice (Kong et al., 2018). Note that the risk of neonatal problems (usually fetal malformations or later neurodevelopmental delays) with lamotrigine or another mood-stabilizing drug must be balanced against the risks of uncontrolled maternal symptoms (Kong et al., 2018).

Breast-feeding is also a consideration during lithium therapy because lithium passes easily into breast milk and the level in breast milk is about 50% of the level in the mother's blood. When considering all the risks and benefits to treatment, most guidelines consider lithium generally a reasonable choice among the class of mood-stabilizing drugs for use in pregnancy. (For a summary of the approaches to treating bipolar disorder before, during, and after pregnancy, see Pacchiarotti et al., 2016; Uguz and Sharma, 2016.)

Nonadherence

Despite demonstrated efficacy in treating bipolar disorder in clinical studies, up to 50% of patients stop taking lithium against medical advice. Nonadherence seems to result primarily from intolerance of side effects, particularly memory impairment, cognitive slowing, weight gain, and the subjective feeling of reduced energy and productivity. Other reasons include missing the manic "highs," belief that the disorder has resolved and the drug is unnecessary, and feelings of stigmatism in having a psychiatric illness. Indeed, management of complications of side effects often becomes a clinician's greatest challenge.

Combination Therapy

Combination therapy—usually lithium plus an antiepileptic or antipsychotic drug—can provide both greater therapeutic efficacy and better protection against relapse than lithium therapy alone. In fact, combination therapy has become the rule rather than the exception (Grande et al., 2016; Shah et al., 2017), with lithium most effective for mania, augmenting antidepressant efficacy in refractory patients, and maintenance. Furthermore, as noted, an anticonvulsant such as lamotrigine is often helpful against bipolar depression (Baldessarini et al., 2020; Jann, 2014).

A federally sponsored six-month study, the **Lithium Treatment Moderate-Dose Use Study (LiTMUS)**, was intended to answer the question of whether combining lithium with other mood stabilizers or second-generation antipsychotics resulted in any greater benefit, relative to the additional side effect risk, than just using the mood stabilizers or antipsychotics alone. Overall, adding an antidepressant to the treatment regimen failed to either lower depressive symptoms or increase manic symptom (Kohler-Forsberg et al., 2021).

Similarly, in another study, the **Bipolar CHOICE (Clinical Health Outcomes Initiative in Comparative Effectiveness)**, either lithium or quetiapine was administered to 480 patients over a six-month trial. Improvements with both drugs were observed, with 20% having a sustained response. Overall, outcomes with both drugs were very similar (Nierenberg et al., 2016).

MOOD STABILIZERS: ANTIEPILEPTIC DRUGS

Only about 60–70% of patients with bipolar disorder can be adequately helped by lithium alone, both for maintenance and for relapse prevention, and lithium is even less effective in controlling episodes of rapid-cycling mania. Therefore, there is a need for alternative agents in patients who are treatment refractory, nonadherent, or intolerant of lithium's side effects (Post et al., 2019). Such alternative or adjuvant drugs include either a second-generation antipsychotic or an anticonvulsant mood stabilizer that is an antiepileptic drug. Here we discuss anticonvulsants, and later we discuss antipsychotics.

Anticonvulsants were originally FDA-approved for the treatment of epilepsy. Today, their uses have expanded to include use in alcohol detoxification and relapse prevention (Chapter 5), treatment of anxiety disorders and the control of emotional outbursts in such disorders as posttraumatic stress disorder (PTSD) (Chapter 13), treating aggressive and explosive behavioral disorders in children and adolescents (Chapter 15), and treatment of certain chronic pain syndromes (Chapter 10).

The older first-generation anticonvulsants (e.g., phenobarbital and phenytoin) are not terribly useful in treating bipolar illness;[3] however, second-generation anticonvulsants (e.g., valproic acid, carbamazepine, and lamotrigine) are widely used in the treatment of bipolar illness. Third-generation anticonvulsants began in 2008 with the approval of lacosamide and include at least nine other drugs, most of which have yet to be extensively studied in the treatment of bipolar illness.[4]

Of particular note is the fact that many of the anticonvulsants can be teratogenic. (This topic is covered at length in Chapter 15.) In addition, the FDA issued a warning in 2008 about increased suicidal behavior related to use of anticonvulsants. The evidence for antisuicidal effects of anticonvulsants is unclear, and monotherapy should likely be avoided in patients at risk of suicidal ideation or attempts (Johnson et al., 2020; Marzani and Neff, 2021).

Carbamazepine

Studies conducted in the early 1990s indicated that carbamazepine (Tegretol, Equetro) might be as effective as lithium in preventing the recurrence of mania (Dea et al., 2016; Muneer et al., 2016; Shah et al., 2017). Equetro is an extended-release form of carbamazepine approved by the FDA in 2005 for the treatment of manic and mixed episodes of bipolar disorder. In bipolar patients not previously treated with mood stabilizers, lithium is superior to carbamazepine in prophylactic efficacy (Grande et al., 2016). Because of the correlation between therapeutic effectiveness and plasma level, one reason patients may fail to respond to carbamazepine is inadequate blood levels. The therapeutic level for epilepsy and for bipolar disorder is estimated to be the same, between 4 and 12 mg/L.

Several possible mechanisms have been proposed to explain carbamazepine's action in treating epilepsy and bipolar disorder. Its anticonvulsant effects may occur because it reduces neuronal excitation by blocking sodium channels and thus the ability of sodium to initiate action potentials. Its benefit for bipolar disorder may be related to the fact

[3]Phenytoin was never widely used as a mood stabilizer, although there are some positive reports relevant to phenytoin as an antimanic drug.

[4]Third-generation anticonvulsants include lamotrigine, lacosamide, eslicarbazepine, rufinamide, brivaracetam, perampanel, vigabatrin, clobazam, and ezogabine.

that carbamazepine, like lithium, inhibits enzyme activity in intracellular second-messenger systems. In the treatment of bipolar disorder, carbamazepine is useful as a prophylaxis for reducing the frequency of episodes, and it may be the better choice for episodes of mixed mania and rapid cycling.

Adverse effects of carbamazepine include GI upset, sedation, ataxia, tremors, visual disturbances, and rare but life-threatening dermatological reactions, namely, Stevens-Johnson syndrome. While the risk of the skin reactions is generally low, the risk is estimated to be about ten times higher for people of Asian ancestry. Therefore, an FDA requirement stipulates that manufacturers add a recommendation to the labeling of this drug that patients of Asian ancestry get a genetic blood test that would indicate whether they were in the population at risk (Thong et al., 2020). Other serious reactions involve the blood and range from a relatively benign reduction in white blood cell count (leucopenia) to, on rare occasions, a severe reduction in white blood cell count (agranulocytosis). For this reason, carbamazepine has an FDA black box warning and a recommendation for periodic blood tests.

Drug interactions involving carbamazepine are common and result from drug-induced stimulation of drug-metabolizing enzymes, especially CYP-3A4 in the liver. As a result, acute blood levels may decrease, which may require increasing the dose by up to 100% to maintain a therapeutic blood level. This effect also extends to other drugs metabolized by the same enzyme family when combined with carbamazepine. For example, aripiprazole and valproic acid blood levels are reduced when combined with carbamazepine such that it may be necessary to increase the dose of these drugs to compensate if carbamazepine is added. With all this, today carbamazepine is considered a second- or even third-line drug for the treatment of bipolar disorder.

Oxcarbazepine

Oxcarbazepine (Trileptal) can be considered a safer carbamazepine, capable of replacing carbamazepine for all its uses with comparable efficacy and greatly improved safety. Oxcarbazepine is essentially carbamazepine with an oxygen molecule attached to one of the rings. The liver can thus easily metabolize the drug by a process called hydroxylation. In fact, this process occurs within 5 minutes after drug absorption, and the monohydroxy derivative is the active form of the drug; oxcarbazepine is, therefore, an inactive prodrug. Because of this easy metabolic process, there is no enzyme induction, no alteration in liver enzymes, no white blood cell problems, no required blood monitoring, and few drug interactions.

Oxcarbazepine, approved for use in epilepsy, is used off-label to treat bipolar disorder and other disorders treatable with carbamazepine. It may be superior to placebo in the treatment of acute mania in adults but less effective when compared to lithium, valproic acid, and the antipsychotics.

Side effects of oxcarbazepine include tiredness, headache, dizziness, and some allergic reactions. Teratogenic effects are also possible (Gimenez et al., 2019). Like carbamazepine, prescribers should check the genetic profile of individuals of Asian ancestry to determine if they carry a particular allele that would increase their risk of developing the serious and potentially lethal dermatological skin reactions when treated with oxcarbazepine.

Valproic Acid

Valproic acid (Divalproex, Depakene, Depakote) is the second anticonvulsant that was systematically studied for treatment of bipolar illness (second to carbamazepine) and has been used for this disorder since 1994.

Several actions of valproic acid have been identified (Romoli et al., 2019). First, it binds to and inhibits gamma aminobutyric acid (GABA) transaminase, the enzyme that breaks down GABA. Therefore, the drug's anticonvulsant activity may be related to increased brain concentrations of GABA. Second, valproic acid may increase GABA by blocking its reuptake into glia and nerve endings. Third, valproic acid may also work by suppressing repetitive neuronal firing through inhibition of voltage-sensitive sodium channels.

Clinically, valproic acid is effective in the treatment of acute bipolar mania (Kishi et al., 2022), mixed states, schizoaffective disorder, and rapid-cycling bipolar disorder. It may be more effective than other agents in treating lithium-resistant patients, producing a positive response in up to 71% of patients. One group of researchers noted that valproic acid is the most common alternative to lithium when suicidal behavior is a concern (Song et al., 2017). Recently, the drug has been reported useful for the management of agitation and delirium in both bipolar and nonbipolar patients in intensive care units (Crowley et al., 2020; Quinn et al., 2021).

Valproic acid has traditionally been administered in divided doses through the day. An extended-release preparation allows once-daily dosing, usually at bedtime, to improve adherence and help alleviate daytime sedation and memory impairment. Effective doses are determined by evaluation of blood concentrations (as with lithium), and normal therapeutic blood levels should be between 50 and 150 mg/L.

Side effects associated with valproic acid include GI upset, sedation, lethargy, weight gain, hand tremor, alopecia (hair loss), and some metabolic changes in the liver (Romoli et al., 2019). In females, the drug has been associated with obesity, polycystic ovaries, menstrual disturbances, and increases in testosterone levels. Valproic acid may be slightly more detrimental to cognitive function than carbamazepine. Like lithium and carbamazepine, valproic acid can be teratogenic and should be avoided in pregnancy (Anmella et al., 2019; Seshachala et al., 2021). As stated by one researcher (Andrade, 2018):

> It (valproic acid) is significantly more teratogenic than many other antiepileptic drugs. In observational studies, gestational exposure to valproate is also associated with higher risks of cognitive, language, and psychomotor delay during early childhood and possibly with an increased risk of autism, as well (p. e1).

An analogue of valproic acid, valnoctamide, has long been available as a sedative in Europe. It is antiepileptic, but its utility in treating mania is not robust (Sparacino et al., 2022). The drug is not available in the United States. Valnoctamide does not go through the same metabolic pathway, and its chemical structure is sufficiently different from valproic acid such that it is less teratogenic (Lin et al., 2019).

Lamotrigine

Lamotrigine (Lamictal) is an antiepileptic and antimanic drug that appears unique in that it has antidepressant properties. Indeed, "sound evidence supports lamotrigine for acute bipolar depression and prophylaxis..." (Naguy and Al-Enezi, 2019). Lamotrigine is equal to lithium in preventing relapse to any manic episode and better than lithium in preventing relapse to a depressive episode. As stated by researchers (Parker et al., 2021):

> Lithium and lamotrigine are likely to have equal efficacy as mood stabilizers for those with a bipolar II condition but that, as maintenance treatments, lithium has more distinctive side effects (p. 381).

Similarly, other researchers stated (Hashimoto et al., 2021):

> In the comparison between lamotrigine and lithium, efficacy was similar except for recurrence of mania episode at one year. Recurrence of manic symptoms was higher in the lamotrigine group than that of the lithium group (p. 1).

Lamotrigine's major mechanism of action is the blockade of voltage-dependent sodium channel conductance, which reduces glutamate release, particularly in the cortex and hippocampus (Silva de Miranda et al., 2019). This decrease in neuronal excitability may account for its antiepileptic, mood-stabilizing, and analgesic effects, and it may also have some neuroprotective effects in people with traumatic brain injuries.

After oral administration, lamotrigine is rapidly and completely absorbed, reaching peak plasma concentrations in 1–5 hours. It is metabolized before excretion, with a half-life of 26 hours, which can decrease to about 7.4 hours when used with carbamazepine, requiring increased doses of lamotrigine, or the half-life can increase to 60 hours when used with valproic acid, requiring decreased doses of lamotrigine.

Side effects include dizziness, tremor, blurred vision, somnolence, headache, nausea, constipation, increased liver enzymes, menstrual disturbances, and rash. The most serious side effect is Stevens-Johnson syndrome (Parker, 2018), which can be fatal. Adolescents are believed to be more prone to this reaction, so the drug is not indicated for patients younger than 16. In marked contrast to other antiepileptic agents, lamotrigine can improve cognitive functioning (Moavero et al., 2017).

Of all the antiepileptic drugs, lamotrigine is the safest to use in pregnancy (Tomson et al., 2019). Lastly, lamotrigine is considered relatively safe with careful monitoring when breastfeeding (Yashima et al., 2021).

Gabapentin and Pregabalin

Gabapentin is an anticonvulsant used for the treatment of partial complex seizures. The drug is also used off-label for the treatment of anxiety, chronic neuropathic pain, substance dependency, and behavioral dyscontrol. Mechanistically, it is a GABA analogue, but it has little or no action on the GABA receptor. Although it increases GABA levels, it is not clear how much the increase contributes to its efficacy. A derivative of gabapentin, pregabalin (Lyrica), is available for the treatment of pain states, such as diabetic peripheral neuropathy and postherpetic neuralgia, and as adjunctive therapy in the treatment of partial seizures in adults.

Since both of these drugs have antiepileptic effects, it was thought that like other anticonvulsants they might have usefulness for the treatment of bipolar disorder. Some open-label studies have suggested that these drugs might be useful as adjunctive treatment for individuals who do not derive full benefit from treatment with other mood stabilizers or who may be presenting with anxiety or agitation along with symptoms of bipolar disorder (Muneer, 2016). Gabapentin and pregabalin, however, are not effective as monotherapy for bipolar disorder. As stated (Ng et al., 2021):

> Studies show that gabapentin and its related drug pregabalin do not have significant clinical efficacy as either monotherapy or adjunctive therapy for bipolar disorder. Gabapentin and pregabalin are probably ineffective for acute mania with only small open-label trials to support its potential adjunctive role (p. 834).

Topiramate

Topiramate (Topamax) was discussed in Chapter 5 as an antiepileptic drug used to prevent relapse in people with alcoholism. It is also an effective anticonvulsant and has been shown to be a useful adjunct in the treatment of bipolar disorder, especially in cases where bipolar disorder occurs with comorbid substance abuse, binge-eating disorder, or weight gain from other medications (Duan et al., 2019; Hiluy et al., 2019). Caution must be taken to monitor for precipitation of a manic episode.

Unfortunately, up to 40% of topiramate-treated patients can experience cognitive impairments, including word-finding difficulties, concentration and attention deficits, confusion, and memory problems (Callisto et al., 2020). This appears to be a side effect unique to topiramate among other anticonvulsants. Other side effects of topiramate include tingling in the extremities, irritability, anxiety, somnolence, ataxia, dizziness, impaired or slurred speech, fatigue, and depression. In pregnancy, rates of congenital malformations are lower than with valproic acid but higher than with lamotrigine (Veroniki et al., 2017). As a result, the FDA changed topiramate's pregnancy classification to category D, that is, there is evidence of teratogenicity in humans (Ornoy, 2017).

Topiramate has multiple mechanisms of action. It inhibits sodium conductance, decreasing the duration of spontaneous bursts and the frequency of generated action potentials; it enhances GABA by unknown mechanisms; and it blocks the AMPA subtype glutamate receptor.

ANTIPSYCHOTIC DRUGS FOR BIPOLAR DISORDER

We mentioned earlier the various phases of bipolar disorder and have discussed them throughout the chapter. Following is a more detailed account of the specific antipsychotic agents involved in the treatment of each phase.

Acute Manic Episodes

For decades, predating the use of lithium by 20 years, traditional, first-generation antipsychotic drugs were used to help control the symptoms of acute manic episodes, as noted. The fact that the antimanic potency of the drugs was positively associated with their affinity for D_2 receptors supported a "dopamine blockade" hypothesis of mania and depression. This was consistent with the possibility that schizophrenia and bipolar disorder share some common genetic origin, an idea that continues (Ashok et al., 2017a).

Currently, both the first- and second-generation antipsychotics have efficacy either as monotherapy or as adjunctive agents for the treatment of acute mania. Today, because of less toxicity (Chapter 11), most focus is on the second-generation agents. However, recently, clozapine, a first-generation antipsychotic, was found to be superior to other antipsychotic agents in treatment-resistant bipolar disorder, despite a small risk of agranulocytosis (Delgado et al., 2020). Indeed, clozapine has been regarded as the top treatment when other medication have not been effective.

Among second-generation agents, there is much support for the efficacy of aripiprazole in reducing mood symptoms in people at high risk of developing bipolar disorder (Cuomo et al., 2019; Saraf et al., 2021). As noted earlier, other effective antipsychotic drugs include olanzapine, risperidone, and quetiapine. Even the newest antipsychotics are useful in the treatment of bipolar disorder (discussed below).

Cariprazine (Vraylar) is a newer atypical antipsychotic approved for the treatment of acute mania as well as schizophrenia, mixed mania/depression, and bipolar depression (Patel et al., 2021; Pinto et al., 2020; Saraf et al., 2019; Stahl et al., 2020). The drug may also have efficacy for the treatment of unipolar depressive disorder. Cariprazine is a broad-spectrum dopamine antagonist/partial agonist with dopamine D_3/D_2 (preferring D_3) and serotonin 5-$HT1_A$ receptor partial agonist properties (Tohen, 2021). The drug is generally well tolerated, with extrapyramidal side effects, restlessness and akathisia being the most common (Citrome et al., 2021).

Bipolar Depression

As we've noted, bipolar depression remains one of the more difficult psychiatric conditions to treat (Bahji et al., 2020a). In past years, olanzapine (a second-generation antipsychotic) and fluoxetine (a selective serotonin reuptake inhibitor [SSRI] antidepressant) either alone or in combination (as Symbyax) were reported as effective for bipolar depression. Studies have examined the relative risk of three other antidepressants—sertraline, bupropion, and venlafaxine—for producing a manic switch when used as adjuncts to mood stabilizers. Venlafaxine may be more likely than the other two antidepressants to produce such a switch (Patel et al., 2015).

Several other studies have supported the use of quetiapine, valproic acid, and cariprazine (noted above) in treating bipolar depression (Bahji et al., 2020a). One of the newer antipsychotic agents, asenapine, is effective as short-term treatment for reducing manic symptoms compared to placebo as monotherapy. Furthermore, asenapine was also found to be equal to olanzapine in an extension study at reducing both manic and depressive symptoms and, when added to either lithium or valproic acid, was more effective than placebo at reducing manic symptoms. One set of researchers reviewed the pharmacology of asenapine and its use in bipolar disorder (Vieta and Montes, 2018). Another stated, "Asenapine appears to have a beneficial effect on both depression and anxiety in depressed Bipolar I patients compared to treatment with placebo" (El-Mallakh et al., 2020).

Today, second-generation antipsychotics are widely used in the treatment of acute bipolar depression. These drugs include quetiapine, aripiprazole, and olanzapine. Adverse events like weight gain, akathisia, and sedation produced by the second-generation antipsychotics may reduce overall clinical effectiveness. Significantly, although second-generation agents may be less likely to elicit movement disorders than the older drugs used by patients with schizophrenia, there is evidence that patients with bipolar disorder may be more susceptible to these side effects. Indeed, patients with bipolar disorder are approximately twice as likely as patients with schizophrenia to experience movement disorders, such as extrapyramidal symptoms and akathisia (as noted with cariprazine, above) and may require an increase in the use of anticholinergic drugs to treat these symptoms.

Lurasidone (Latuda) is a new atypical antipsychotic drug approved for the treatment of acute bipolar depression, either as monotherapy or adjunctive to lithium or valproic acid (Tran and Ford, 2020). As stated by researchers (Ali et al., 2020):

> Lurasidone has not been studied in patients with mania or bipolar psychosis. It has been studied, both as a monotherapy and adjunctive treatment to lithium or valproate, in acute depression and in prevention of recurrence *of any mood episode* in patients with bipolar disorder initially treated for bipolar depression (p. 253).

Another new atypical antipsychotic drug FDA-approved for the treatment of bipolar depression is lumateperone (Caplyta) (Blair, 2020; Calabrese et al., 2021; D'Souza et al., 2021), which was originally approved in December 2019 for the treatment of schizophrenia (Kumar et al., 2018). Other potential uses of lumateperone include the treatment of behavioral disorders associated with dementia, insomnia, and major depression (Calsolaro et al., 2019; Corponi et al., 2019). Lumateperone is primarily a potent inhibitor of the $5\text{-HT}2_A$ receptor.

Acute Bipolar Agitation

To date, the only approved medications for acute bipolar agitation have been loxapine (Loxitane) and intramuscular olanzapine. Although considered a first-generation antipsychotic drug, loxapine more closely resembles a second-generation antipsychotic in its activity profile. A new formulation of the drug, Adasuve, has been approved. This formulation of loxapine is a powder that is aerosolized and administered via inhalation. In clinical trials, the drug rapidly reduced psychomotor agitation within 10 minutes[5] (Faden and Citrome, 2019). Due to the risk of causing bronchospasm, the drug should only be used only in facilities that are capable of providing immediate treatment for this reaction.

As discussed, providing an alternative medication approach, researchers studied a sedative medication, dexmedetomidine sublingual, that can rapidly relief agitation and prevent escalation to aggressive behavior (Preskorn et al., 2022). In a Phase 3 study of 362 adults with bipolar I or II disorder, this medication had an onset of sedative effect

[5]Psychomotor agitation is defined as "excessive motor activity associated with a feeling of inner tension." Patients experiencing agitation often manifest behaviors that interfere with their care (e.g., threatening behaviors, escalating or urgently distressing behavior, self-exhausting behavior), leading clinicians to the use of rapidly absorbed antipsychotic medications to achieve rapid control of the agitation.

within 20 minutes and offered reductions in agitation superior to placebo therapy. The FDA formally approved this medication in April 2022, and it is available under the trade name *Igalmi*.

Relapse Prevention

As we've stated, lithium is typically the first choice for long-term maintenance. As alternatives, monotherapy with valproic acid can be considered as a reasonable option. However, in terms of antipsychotics used for relapse prevention, many of the second-generation agents (e.g., aripiprazole) can also be used as monotherapy. If that approach is ineffective, the next step usually involves combining two agents or substituting an antipsychotic (if one was not used as a first-line treatment). Alternatively, lamotrigine can be added to the monotherapy agent if the primary phase of illness is depression (Hashimoto et al., 2021). Table 14.3 summarizes the current treatments approved by the FDA for the various states of bipolar disorder in adults.

Although not an antipsychotic agent, it should be noted that there has been a long and continuing interest in nutraceuticals, such as **omega-3 polyunsaturated fatty acids**, for the treatment of psychiatric disorders, including bipolar disorder (Ashton et al., 2021). In a recent summary, researchers concluded that studies of efficacy

TABLE 14.3 FDA-approved Treatments for Bipolar Disorder in Adults

Generic name	Mania	Depression	Mixed	Maintenance
Lithium	X			X
Carbamazepine[a]	X		X	
Divalproex	X			X
Lamotrigine		X		X
Olanzapine/fluoxetine		X		
Aripiprazole[b]	X		X	
Quetiapine[b]	X	X	X	X
Risperidone[b]	X		X	X[c]
Olanzapine[b]	X		X	X
Ziprasidone[b]	X		X	X
Asenapine[b]	X		X	X
Lurasidone[b]		X	X	X
Cariprazine	X	X	X	X

[a]Equetro XR version.
[b]Monotherapy or as adjunct agent.
[c]As the long-acting injection (LAI) formulation.

against bipolar depression are inconclusive, with strong evidence of research and publication bias (Nasir and Bloch, 2019). Also, evidence of efficacy of omega-3 fatty acids in the treatment of psychosis, PTSD, anxiety, and bipolar mania is minimal. From these studies, there seems to be little harm in using relatively high doses (>2 grams/day) as adjunctive therapy for bipolar depression. In addition, intranasal (S)-ketamine could be a promising treatment in depressed patients with suicidal ideation (Corriger and Pickering, 2019).The drug has also been used in subanesthetic doses successfully in the treatment of bipolar depression (McCloud et al., 2015; Rong et al., 2018). Onset of effect is rapid (within 40 minutes), and the duration of the effect is short (up to three days).

In the Pipeline

The following drugs may soon be used in the future to treat bipolar disorder:

- *Brilaroxazine.* Reviva Pharmaceuticals is testing brilaroxazine, which they refer to as a dopamine-serotonin stabilizer antipsychotic. It is structurally nearly identical to aripiprazole, brexpiprazole, and cariprazine. Brilaroxazine is a potent multimodal dopamine/serotonin modulator. It is a partial agonist of dopamine D_2, D_3, and D_4 receptors, 5-$HT1_A$ and 5-$HT2_A$ and has antagonist activity at 5-$HT2_B$ and 5-HT7 receptors. Brilaroxazine is an atypical antipsychotic agent and has the potential to improve cognitive impairments in neuropsychiatric and neurological diseases in vivo. As of late 2022, brilaroxazine was in Phase 3 clinical trials for the treatment of schizophrenia. Reports of the drug being used in the treatment of bipolar disorder have not been recorded.
- *Cenobamate* (*Xcopri*). SK Biopharmaceuticals has recently marketed cenobamate (Xcopri) for the treatment of focal seizures (Barbieri et al., 2022; Krauss et al., 2020). The drug may have utility in the treatment of bipolar and other CNS disorders, but clinical reports remain unavailable.

PSYCHOTHERAPEUTIC AND PSYCHOSOCIAL TREATMENTS

Due to a variety of factors, including lack of adherence to treatment, high relapse rates, and psychological impact, the social impact of bipolar disorder is high. Patients with bipolar disorder experience the psychosocial consequences of past episodes, the ongoing vulnerability to future episodes, and the burden of adhering to long-term medication treatment plans that may involve some unpleasant side effects. The longitudinal course of bipolar disorder is highly variable, with the highest level of psychosocial disability in persons with chronic mixed and depressive symptoms who show limited improvement despite guideline-based treatment (Mignogna and Goes, 2022). Indeed, psychological therapies seem to have less effect in reducing depressive symptoms in patients with bipolar I or II disorder (Yilmaz et al., 2022).

Successful treatment involves a social network primed to recognize the early symptoms of an episode, to seek help for patients who lack insight into their condition, and to assist with recognition of side effects and toxicities, hopefully improving adherence to the treatment plan.

It is important to ensure that the manic state is not being caused by medications, such as antidepressants, caffeine, herbals containing ephedrine, behavioral stimulants, including illegal drugs such as cocaine, corticosteroids (cortisone), anabolic steroids, antiparkinsonian drugs, over-the-counter cough and cold preparations, and diet aids. Also, a good physical examination is important in order to rule out an underlying medical condition, such as hyperthyroidism, that could trigger or exacerbate a manic episode.

Psychotherapy combined with pharmacotherapy is associated with 30–40% reduction in relapse rates over 12–30 months (Yatham et al., 2018). Evidence-based psychotherapeutic and psychosocial treatments when combined with medication treatment have been shown to produce improved outcomes compared to medication alone. For example, **family-focused therapy** teaches families about the disorder, how to recognize signs of episodes, how to support the individual's efforts to manage the illness through adherence to the treatment plan, how to avoid negative communication styles that exacerbate or trigger episodes, and other skills. Family-focused therapy has been shown to reduce the frequency of relapse and rehospitalization, improve medication adherence, reduce symptom severity, and reduce frequency of depressive episodes (Weintraub et al., 2022).

Interpersonal and social rhythm therapy stresses the importance of establishing and maintaining a regular life schedule and teaching the individual and their family problem-solving skills that will improve the individual's satisfaction within social situations. This therapy may reduce illness recurrence. Dou and coworkers (2022) emphasize that enhanced social support and resilience support are important, while paying particular attention to suicidal ideation. Brickman and Fristad (2022) critically review prevention interactions for bipolar disorder in children and adolescents.

Cognitive-behavioral therapy teaches the individual about their illness, how to recognize signs and symptoms of episodes, and cognitive coping strategies. Cognitive-behavioral therapy has been shown to reduce the rate of rehospitalization, improve social functioning, and reduce severity of symptoms within episodes. Psychoeducational interventions have been shown to decrease recurrence rates and improve functional outcomes, including suicidal ideation, which can occur in up to 39% of youth with bipolar disorder (Weinstein et al., 2018).

CHAPTER REVIEW

1. Discuss the symptomatology of bipolar disorder, including the subtypes. Why is it important to try to differentiate them?
2. What are the phases of bipolar disorder and the major pharmacological drug categories useful in its treatment? Explain the mechanism of action for each of the drugs in these categories.
3. Why is lithium considered the gold standard in drug treatment for bipolar disorder? What are some of its side effects and toxicity as well as the effects on pregnancy?
4. Compare and contrast the anticonvulsants that have some efficacy in treating bipolar disorder. Be sure to note major side effects associated with these drugs.

5. Which antipsychotics have been found useful for treatment of bipolar disorder?
6. What are the most effective psychotherapeutic interventions for the treatment of bipolar disorder and how do they improve treatment outcomes?

KEY TERMS

Bipolar CHOICE (Clinical Health Outcomes Initiative in Comparative Effectiveness)
bipolar disorder (manic-depressive disorder)
bipolar I disorder
bipolar II disorder
cognitive-behavioral therapy
family-focused therapy
interpersonal and social rhythm therapy
lithium
Lithium Treatment Moderate-Dose Use Study (LiTMUS)
omega-3 polyunsaturated fatty acids
rapid cycler
STEP-BD study
topiramate

PART 4

Special Populations

Part 4 of this text focuses on the uses and misuses of psychoactive drugs in three special populations—pregnant women (Chapter 15), children and adolescents (Chapter 16), and older adults (Chapter 17)—and on psychopharmacological issues that have become apparent during the COVID-19 pandemic, as well as the implications of those issues going forward (Chapter 18).

Chapter 15 covers the effects of psychoactive drugs on pregnant women, the fetus, and the newborn, while also looking at effects that carry forward into childhood. The chapter begins with discussions of substance abuse during pregnancy and then examines the use of psychotherapeutic drugs to treat mental disorders during and after pregnancy, including postpartum depression.

Chapter 16 starts out by discussing substance abuse in children and adolescents. It then moves to an examination of the use of psychoactive medications to treat a variety of disorders in youngsters from preschool age through adolescence, including substance abuse, anxiety disorders, depression, bipolar disorder, autism spectrum disorders, attention deficit/hyperactivity disorder (ADHD), and behavioral disorders marked by aggression, as well as the treatment of disorders with antipsychotic medications and analgesics. The chapter concludes with a detailed discussion of treatments for ADHD.

Chapter 17 shifts to the other end of the life span, focusing on geriatric psychopharmacology—the use of psychoactive medications in older adults. The chapter begins with a discussion of inappropriate drug use in that population and then discusses the treatment of agitation, aggression, and psychosis. This is followed by a look at the treatment of depression and then a detailed look at Parkinson's disease, including discussions of treatment issues and of apathy associated with that condition. The chapter concludes with an equally detailed discussion of Alzheimer's disease and its treatment.

The first part of Chapter 18 discusses the effects of the COVID-19 pandemic on the use of psychoactive medications, focusing successively on health care workers; children, adolescents, and adults; COVID-19 long haulers; and inequities in health care. The second part of the chapter discusses how pharmacological issues and the limitations of pharmacological therapies relate to mental health support.

CHAPTER 15

Pregnancy and Psychoactive Drugs

CHAPTER OUTLINE

In previous chapters, we often focused on how various drugs affect pregnant females and their developing fetuses. Now, in this chapter, we will review much of that information and add to it as we examine the subject from two broad perspectives, looking first at the effects of various types of abused substances and then at the effects of psychotherapeutic drugs.

In the United States, approximately 3% of all pregnancies involve fetuses with congenital malformations, or birth defects (Centers for Disease Control and Prevention, 2020b). In most cases, the causes of the malformation are unknown. In 1979, the U.S. Food and Drug Administration (FDA) established five risk categories—A, B, C, D, and X—for classifying drugs according to their risk for producing malformations if taken during pregnancy (however, the risks associated with the passage of drugs and their metabolites into breast milk were not considered). In 2015, these letter categories were replaced with narrative sections for specific medications (including a lactation subsection for each medication with information about using the drug while breast-feeding) and with a pregnancy drug exposure registry to track pregnancy outcomes in women taking the medications.

The FDA's Pregnancy and Lactation Labeling Final Rule went into effect in 2015, requiring for each drug more detailed information based on specific research regarding the risk of taking the drug during pregnancy, labor, and delivery and the risk of using the drug during lactation and breast-feeding; in addition, the rule included an entirely new requirement for providing information about the drug in regard to pregnancy testing, contraception, and infertility effects, for both females and males. However, the implementation schedule for including the required information in drugs' package inserts varies.

Although an improvement over the previous version, the new labeling rule still does not guarantee a definitive answer to the question of whether a drug is safe for a specific patient during pregnancy and breast-feeding. In addition, according to a recent report, more than one-third of drug labels have remained out of compliance, and data on pregnancy and lactation are included in fewer than 20% of new product labeling (Byrne et al., 2020). The FDA's work in this area continues (Baisden and Dinatale, 2019).

According to the FDA, several developments prompted the 2015 reassessment of its labeling rules. First, most women take at least one prescribed medication during pregnancy, while the proportion of women using four or more medications during pregnancy has more than doubled over the last 30 years. Second, many women have chronic conditions, such as asthma, high blood pressure, depression, and diabetes, requiring them to continue taking medications after they become pregnant. Third, women who abuse substances before becoming pregnant tend to continue doing so during pregnancy, and commonly abused substances such as nicotine, alcohol, cannabis, stimulants, and opioids present significant risks to the unborn. Lastly, a woman's body changes throughout her pregnancy, which may affect the medications she needs.

The FDA's new rules are intended to address the risks to women, fetuses, and newborns associated with taking psychoactive drugs while pregnant or while breast-feeding. For each drug, the questions are whether the drug has a potential to cause a malformation in the fetus and whether it has a potential to cause later developmental problems. Conversely, when pregnant women with mental health disorders do *not* take psychoactive medications to treat their disorders, there is a risk that the symptoms and effects of the untreated disorder in the woman will cause fetal or later developmental problems (Chan et al., 2014).

As a general rule, when a pregnant woman takes a psychoactive drug, the blood level of the drug in the fetus will reach about the same level as in the woman because the placental barrier is easily crossed, and of course, by definition, psychoactive medications also cross the blood-brain barrier and reach the fetal brain (these physiological barriers to drug distribution are discussed in Chapter 1). This means that the use of psychoactive drugs during pregnancy risks causing teratogenic effects on the fetus (see Table 15.1), perinatal syndromes (i.e., within several weeks immediately before or after birth), postnatal behavioral abnormalities, and toxicity in the child if the mother continues taking medications while breast-feeding. In contrast, the risks associated with untreated mental health disorders in pregnant women include poor compliance with prenatal care; inadequate nutrition; exposure to dangerous drugs, including increased use of alcohol, caffeine, and nicotine; deficits in mother-infant bonding; neglect of proper postnatal infant care; and disruption of the family environment.

TABLE 15.1 Teratogenic Effects of Selected Psychoactive Drugs

Drug	Trimester	Effect
Amphetamines	All	Suspected abnormal developmental patterns, impaired school performance
Antidepressants, tricyclic	Third	Neonatal withdrawal symptoms in a few cases with clomipramine, desipramine, and imipramine
Barbiturates	All	Neonatal dependence with chronic use
Carbamazepine	First	Neural tube defects
Clomipramine	All	Prolonged symptomatic neonatal hypoglycemia
Cocaine	All	Increased risk of spontaneous abruption of placenta and premature labor, neonatal cerebral infarction, abnormal development, and decreased school performance
Diazepam	All	Neonatal dependence with chronic use
Alcohol	All	Risk of fetal alcohol syndrome and alcohol-related neurodevelopmental defects
Heroin	All	Neonatal dependence with chronic use
Lithium	First and third	Ebstein's anomaly (cardiac malformation), neonatal toxicity after third trimester
Methadone	All	Neonatal abstinence syndrome after chronic use

Information from G. Koren (2018). "Special Aspects of Perinatal and Pediatric Pharmacology," Chapter 59 in B. G. Katzung, *Basic and Clinical Pharmacology*, 14th ed. (McGraw-Hill Education).

SUBSTANCE ABUSE AND PREGNANCY

Substance abuse among pregnant women in the United States is a major public health concern, especially among adolescents. In one study, 59% of pregnant teenagers reported having used one or more commonly abused substances in the previous 12 months, a rate that is nearly two times as great as that of nonpregnant teenagers (35%) (Salas-Wright et al., 2015). The most commonly used substance was alcohol (16%). Another study found that, among adolescents, 75–82% of pregnancies are unintended (Ranganathan and Gupta, 2020), increasing these young women's risk of substance abuse and the risk that their fetuses will be exposed to drugs of abuse. The authors of a recent study note that polysubstance abuse among pregnant women increases the likelihood of a future diagnosis of ADHD in offspring (Garrison-Desany et al., 2022).

Nicotine

Tobacco smoking during pregnancy is linked to multiple problems, including miscarriage, preterm delivery, low birth weight, fetal growth restriction, and SIDS (sudden infant death syndrome) (Gould et al., 2020; Sealock and Sharma, 2020). Unfortunately, some women who smoke during pregnancy may not acknowledge the extent of their habit, which means that the degree of fetal exposure to nicotine from pregnant smokers is not easily determined; nor is it easy to determine the degree of fetal exposure to secondhand smoke. "Heavy" maternal nicotine use is associated with higher rates of movement, eating, and developmental disorders in offspring, as well as with higher rates of ADHD and neurological-related hospitalizations (Gutvirtz et al., 2019). A recent neuroimaging study of 2700 children 9–11 years of age whose mothers had smoked during their pregnancy found that "continued maternal tobacco use during pregnancy was associated with lower brain volumes and suboptimal cortical traits of offspring in preadolescents" (Zou et al., 2022). However, children exposed to maternal smoking in only the first trimester of pregnancy showed no difference in brain morphology compared with nonexposed children.

Pregnant females should be helped to quit smoking before, during, and following pregnancy, using both nonpharmacological interventions (Grange et al., 2020) and nicotine replacement therapies (Claire et al., 2020). As stated by one team of researchers:

> [C]igarette consumption during either the first or second trimester of pregnancy, even as low as 1–2 cigarettes per day, was associated with an increased risk of preterm birth. These findings suggest that there is no safe level or safe trimester for maternal smoking during pregnancy. (Liu et al., 2020, p. 2)

Alcohol

The damaging effects of heavy drinking on the fetus have been well established, but there is still no consensus on the impact of low to moderate amounts of alcohol. In a study aimed at addressing this deficiency (Lees et al., 2020), 10,000 youths 9–11 years of age from the Adolescent Brain Cognitive Study (Lisdahl et al., 2018) were surveyed to establish whether participants had been exposed to alcohol in utero and whether such exposure was associated with adverse outcomes. The 2020 study revealed that 26% of the participants had been exposed and that "exposure of any severity was associated with greater psychopathology, attention deficits, and impulsiveness, with some effects showing a dose-dependent response." The researchers concluded as follows:

> Any alcohol use during pregnancy is associated with subtle yet significant psychological and behavioral effects in children. Women should continue to be advised to abstain from alcohol consumption from conception throughout their pregnancy. (Lees et al., 2020, p. 1060)

In the United States, the surgeon general has advised women against drinking alcohol during pregnancy. Nevertheless, according to a federal government survey, 10% of pregnant women in the United States do drink alcohol, and about 3.3% binge drink (Tan et al., 2015). The survey also found that unmarried pregnant women were nearly five times more likely to binge drink than were married pregnant women. Unfortunately, as many as 6% of pregnant women binge drank during their pregnancy (Howard et al., 2022). Binge drinking was defined as consuming four or more drinks during a single occasion.

Alcohol use during pregnancy is common in many other countries as well, and fetal alcohol syndrome (FAS) is a relatively prevalent alcohol-related birth defect (see the discussion of FAS in Chapter 5). The global prevalence of alcohol use during pregnancy was recently estimated to be 9.8%, and the estimated prevalence of FAS in the general population might be as high as 1–5 per 100 school children, or 1–5% of the school-age population (Centers for Disease Control and Prevention, 2022c). A study of the populations of Canada and the United States concluded that 1 in every 67 women who consume alcohol during pregnancy would deliver a child with FAS, which translates to about 119,000 children born with FAS every year (Popova et al., 2017).

Cannabis

Several surveys of the U.S. general population in since 2010 have shown an increase in cannabis use during pregnancy, from 1.95% at the beginning of that decade to 7% at the end, with 0.5% using the drug for medical purposes only (Giacomo et al., 2021). The widespread legalization of cannabis use means we need to understand its impact on human health and behavior, especially among sensitive subgroups such as pregnant women (Grant et al., 2018). In 2017, the American College of Obstetricians and Gynecologists updated its position on the use of cannabis during pregnancy and breast-feeding, essentially recommending that such use, even for medical purposes, should be discouraged (American College of Obstetricians and Gynecologists Committee on Obstetric Practice, 2017). Specifically with regard to breast-feeding, a recent review found the following:

> Cannabinoid receptors are present in the placenta and they appear in the fetal brain at 14 weeks after conception and increase in density throughout the third trimester. Given its lipophilic nature, one third of the THC in the maternal plasma crosses the placenta and it can be excreted into breast milk. (Roncero et al., 2020, p. 4)

A systematic review of research reported a potential for adverse maternal, fetal, and neonatal outcomes up to six weeks postpartum after maternal cannabis use (Marchand et al., 2022; Metz and Borgelt, 2018). Fetuses exposed to cannabis in utero may exhibit growth restriction and preterm birth (Klebanoff et al., 2021; Nguyen and Harley, 2022; Paul et al., 2021). The authors of another study came to this conclusion:

> The neurodevelopmental data . . . suggest that prenatal exposure to THC may lead to subtle, persistent changes in targeted aspects of higher-level cognition and psychological well-being. . . . Until more information is available, pregnant women should not assume that using cannabis during pregnancy is safe. (Grant et al., 2018, p. 133)

Long-term outcomes of persons born to mothers who used cannabis during pregnancy are consistent with the idea that the drug has an adverse effect on "externalizing behaviors such as delinquency and substance use, which persists into adulthood" (De Genna et al., 2022). However, adverse cognitive effects have not been reported (Torres et al., 2021).

Stimulants

A recent review noted that stimulants—including prescription medications as well as illicit drugs such as cocaine, MDMA (ecstasy), and methamphetamines—are the second most widely used and abused substances in the United States, after cannabis (the lifetime prevalence among adults for stimulant use was found to be 29.2%, second to cannabis at 46.9%) (Smid et al., 2019). The same review noted that, in 2015, 1.38 million women of reproductive age (15–44 years old) reported having used a stimulant in the past month (misuse of stimulant prescriptions was reported by 1.0% of those 1.38 million women, cocaine by 0.7%, methamphetamine by 0.7%, and MDMA by 0.3%). After observing that stimulant use among pregnant women in the United States has increased at a rate consistent with the overall nationwide rise in rates of stimulant use, the authors of the review noted the growing public health concerns over the adverse effects associated with such use during pregnancy, "including psychiatric co-morbidities, poverty and social isolation, history of trauma and domestic violence, all of which impact maternal and child health outcomes."

As a general rule, stimulants are not teratogenic, but their use, both licit and illicit, can be associated with adverse neurodevelopmental outcomes in newborns exposed to them in utero. Pregnant females' use of stimulants such as cocaine, methamphetamine, and MDMA is associated with preterm delivery, low birth weight, and infants who are small for gestational age, as well as with reduced birth rates (Smid et al., 2019). Long-term neurotoxicities can follow from the effects of these drugs on the permeability of the blood-brain barrier, an effect that presumably can also occur in utero. Specifically with regard to methamphetamine:

> [P]renatal methamphetamine exposure has transient effects on gross motor development, no effect on language and cognition, and modest effects on behavior and executive functioning with poor inhibitory control. (Sankaran et al., 2022, p. 293)

Drug discontinuation and abstinence should be the goals of treatment for pregnant females addicted to methamphetamine (Charlotte et al., 2019). However, immediate discontinuation can cause withdrawal symptoms such as depression, fatigue, and psychosis, as well as have adverse effects on the fetus. Therapy should be individualized and should include prenatal care, cognitive-behavioral therapy, parenting support, a 12-step program, and regular urine testing. Pharmacological therapies are not generally recommended.

Opioids

Opioid use by pregnant women represents a significant public health concern given the association of opioid exposure with adverse maternal and neonatal outcomes, including preterm labor, stillbirth, **neonatal abstinence syndrome**, and maternal mortality (Haight et al., 2018). Nationally, the prevalence of opioid use disorder in pregnant females more than quadrupled during the period 1999–2014, from 1.5 to 6.5 cases per 1000 delivery hospitalizations (see Figure 15.1). Continued efforts are needed to prevent, monitor, and treat opioid use disorder among pregnant women and all other women of reproductive age, including improved access to substance abuse screening,

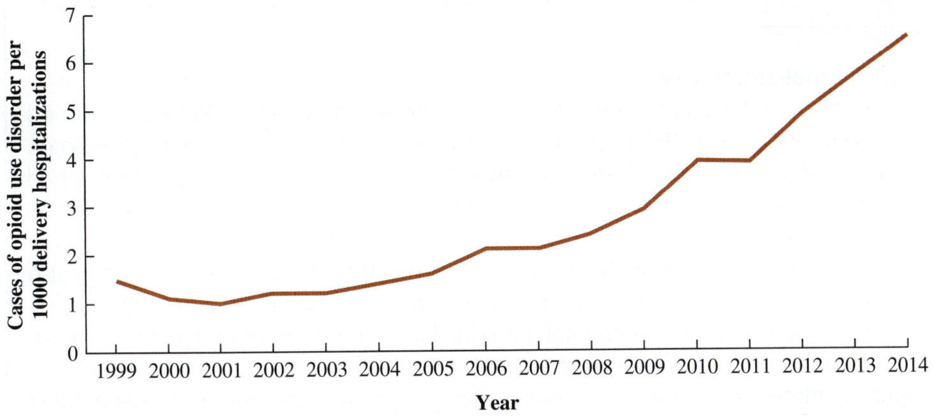

FIGURE 15.1 Prevalence of Opioid Use Disorder in Pregnant Women in the United States, 1999–2014. [Data from Haight et al., 2018.]

use of medication-assisted therapy, and substance abuse treatment referrals. A study of women with a history of prenatal opioid use found that the women could be separated into five categories reflecting their relative risk of overdose and death within one year postpartum, with the highest risk occurring in women with a history of mixed opioid use plus high levels of need for social and medical support (Camden et al., 2022).

The American College of Obstetricians and Gynecologists recommends universal substance use screening at the first prenatal visit. Patients who are diagnosed with opioid use disorder should be prescribed medication-assisted therapy when possible and appropriate. Concerning medications, buprenorphine seems to have advantages over methadone (Rausgaard et al., 2020). Those with opioid use disorder involving heroin might require referral to harm reduction services (e.g., comprehensive syringe services). Arrangements can be made for pregnant patients with opioid use disorder to deliver at facilities prepared to monitor and care for their infants, including watching the infants for withdrawal signs and symptoms indicating neonatal abstinence syndrome (such infants may need treatment to help them sleep and eat). After delivery, women with opioid use disorder might need referrals to postpartum psychosocial support services, substance use treatment, and relapse prevention programs. The following general guidelines for management of opioid use disorder in the pregnant female are based on recommendations from both the Centers for Disease Control and the American College of Obstetricians and Gynecologists:

1. Patients should avoid hiding their opioid use disorder or their pregnancy from clinicians. They should not let fear or embarrassment keep them from getting the help they need.
2. Patients and clinicians should keep in mind that opioid use disorder is a treatable illness, like diabetes or high blood pressure. Clinicians should discuss treatment plans with patients.
3. Patients should make sure to arrange for good prenatal care throughout their pregnancy.

Did You Know?

Pregnancy Criminalization Laws

In 2017, an Amnesty International report described the effects of what the report termed "pregnancy criminalization laws" in the United States—that is, laws that punish women for engaging in behaviors that could damage their fetus. As of 2021, some U.S. states had expanded such laws to include prenatal substance use, with provisions whereby parental rights can be terminated because of drug abuse. Currently, 24 states and the District of Columbia consider substance use during pregnancy to be child abuse, and an additional three states also consider substance abuse as grounds for civil commitment (Guttmacher Institute, 2022). These pregnancy-related laws stem from state fetal homicide laws, which aim to protect fetuses from harm. While 38 states have general fetal homicide laws, 29 states specify that fetal age is irrelevant in applying these laws—that is, the laws would apply at any time after conception. Most of the time, pregnancy criminalization laws are applied to women who have abused drugs during their pregnancy, but their reach may be much broader. Punishments have been meted out to women for falling down stairs, not putting on seat belts when riding in cars, attempting suicide, and declining medical treatment. Consequently, women may seek abortions or may even abandon their newborns in order to avoid potential criminal punishment. Moreover, pregnant women struggling with substance abuse or mental health problems may not seek help because they fear prosecution. The Amnesty International report argues for more support, assistance, and access to treatment services, rather than criminalization and incarceration.

4. Patients should not try to stop opioid use on their own, as suddenly stopping the use of opioids can lead to withdrawal for both the patient and the fetus. Patients experiencing withdrawal are at increased risk of starting to use drugs again and even overdosing.
5. Opioid use disorder in pregnant women is best treated with methadone or buprenorphine, along with counseling and recovery support services. Both of those medications stop and prevent withdrawal symptoms and reduce opioid cravings, allowing patients to focus on recovery and infant care.
6. Keep in mind that tobacco, alcohol, and benzodiazepines may harm the fetus, so treatment should include efforts to stop using these substances.
7. Depression and anxiety are common in women with opioid use disorder, and new mothers may also experience depression and anxiety after giving birth. Clinicians should check for these conditions regularly and help patients get treatment for them.
8. Women with opioid use disorder are at risk for hepatitis and HIV infection, which can be transmitted to a fetus or newborn. Clinicians should do regular lab tests to detect any infections and provide treatment.

In addition, women without opioid use disorder but taking prescription opioids during pregnancy should probably try to reduce their use, especially given that some minor congenital malformations have been reported for women taking hydrocodone in the second trimester and similar malformations reported with oxycodone taken during the third trimester, although the cause of the malformations could not be determined (Wen et al., 2021).

More generally, the Centers for Disease Control and the American College of Obstetricians and Gynecologists recommend that before prescribing opioids for chronic pain, clinicians should ensure that they are appropriate and that the expected benefits are anticipated to outweigh the risks, as well as review the prescription drug monitoring program, provide contraception counseling, and discuss the risks of opioid use in pregnancy.

PSYCHOTHERAPEUTIC DRUGS AND PREGNANCY

Pregnant females are at least as likely as nonpregnant females to experience psychiatric disorders and thus to become candidates for pharmacotherapy with one or more psychotherapeutic drugs. In this section, we will examine the effects of different types of such drugs on the mothers and their fetuses, as well as on offspring after birth.

Antidepressants

About 9–16% of pregnant women have depressive disorders, with some estimates of up to 20%; and about 2.4% of pregnant women take antidepressants during their pregnancy (Sun et al., 2019). As stated by one team of researchers:

> Affective disorders are among the most commonly diagnosed mental diseases. In pregnancy, they can occur as pre-delivery depression, recurrent depressive disorder, or postnatal depression. (Dubovicky et al., 2017, p. 30)

Treatment of depression during pregnancy and breast-feeding is a complicated and controversial issue, as antidepressants administered during pregnancy are associated with a variety of adverse effects on the developing fetus, including intrauterine growth retardation, premature birth, low birth weight, and pulmonary hypertension. However, untreated maternal depression can adversely affect maternal health and increase the risk of preeclampsia and eclampsia, as well as the risk of subsequent postpartum depression, which can lead to disruption of the mother-child relationship. Other problems related to untreated maternal depression during pregnancy include drug abuse, malnutrition, suicidal ideation, and premature birth. Thus, the basic question is whether to treat depression with medications during pregnancy and lactation.

Some data suggest that the anti-irritability and antianxiety effects of several SSRIs (selective serotonin reuptake inhibitors) may help mothers improve their capacity to listen and respond to their children and that the children are likely to respond positively (Weissman et al., 2015) (see Chapter 12 for a detailed discussion of SSRIs). How safe are these and other antidepressants taken during pregnancy? Although some antidepressants are associated with a higher risk of birth defects than are others, the overall risk for babies of mothers who take antidepressants during pregnancy is very low. Nevertheless, treatment decisions require discussions between the patient and the clinician who would be prescribing any antidepressants. Certainly, one goal would be to minimize fetal exposure to the medication, and this goal can be achieved by prescribing a single medication (monotherapy) at the lowest effective dose, particularly during the first trimester. Patients and clinicians should always keep in mind that psychotherapy is an effective treatment for mild to moderate depression and should be instituted before and during any medication treatments. In any case, counseling should accompany any decision to use an antidepressant during pregnancy, and the decision should be based on balancing the risks to the developing fetus and the benefits of the medication to the mother.

Regarding drug choice, SSRIs are generally considered the first option during pregnancy, including citalopram and sertraline. Potential complications include maternal weight changes and premature birth, but most studies show that SSRIs are not associated with birth defects. However, paroxetine might be associated with a small increased risk of a fetal heart defect and is generally discouraged during pregnancy (Gao et al., 2018). Should SSRIs be ineffective, SNRIs (serotonin-norepinephrine reuptake inhibitors) such as duloxetine and venlafaxine are considered as alternatives (see Chapter 12 for discussion of SNRIs). Of note, for up to a month after birth, infants of mothers taking antidepressants might show signs and symptoms of discontinuation, such as jitters, irritability, poor feeding, and respiratory distress.

Recent research has repeatedly indicated that there is no long-term neurodevelopmental impairment of children exposed to antidepressants in utero, even if some short-term deficits occur (Rommel et al., 2020). However, substantial attention has been given to concern about the risk of autism in the offspring of mothers who took antidepressants during pregnancy. Although early evidence supported a relation, the preponderance of newer data does not indicate that antidepressants taken during pregnancy carry a significant risk of later development of autism in offspring (Vega et al., 2020).

In July 2022, the Canadian Task Force on Preventive Health Care recommended against instrument-based screening for depression during pregnancy and lactation, stressing that clinicians currently give adequate attention to mental health and well-being and that arbitrary scores on screening tests do not appear to add further benefit (Lang et al., 2022).

Women who did not experience depression before or during their pregnancy may develop postpartum depression after giving birth. In 2020, a new medication, brexanolone, became the first drug to receive FDA approval for the treatment of postpartum depression. Administered by intravenous infusion, the drug has been shown to rapidly decrease depressive symptoms. In addition, an even newer antidepressant, zuranolone, has been shown to be useful in treating not only depression in general but also postpartum depression (Althaus et al., 2020; Deligiannidis et al., 2021), and zuranolone has the advantage over brexanolone of being administered orally instead of by infusion. Both brexanolone and zuranolone activate $GABA_A$ receptors and are referred to as allopregnanolone agonists because they increase the amount of allopregnanolone in the CNS, resulting in reduced GABA and glutamate neurotransmission (Walkery et al., 2021). Certainly, these two allopregnanolone agonists offer new opportunities for the treatment of postpartum depression. (See Chapter 12 for further discussion of postpartum depression and its treatment.)

Antipsychotics

The increased use of antipsychotic drugs by pregnant women during the last 15 years is largely due to the overall greater use of more tolerable atypical antipsychotics in treating bipolar disorder and major depression as well as in treating schizophrenia. Atypical antipsychotic drugs (discussed in detail in Chapter 11) may also be prescribed for other mental health disorders, many of which occur in women of childbearing age.

The safety of pharmacotherapy with atypical antipsychotics during pregnancy and lactation remains a subject of debate and uncertainty (Tomson and Battino, 2009). However, one team of researchers concluded, "The antipsychotic drugs are safe for the developing fetus and do not seem to induce developmental delay" (Ornoy et al., 2017). Currently, most second-generation antipsychotics are considered relatively safe, apart from possible extrapyramidal and other motor signs of withdrawal after delivery (Albertini et al., 2019). The results of an earlier study support a similar conclusion, that antipsychotic medications used during pregnancy are associated with only a modest risk of adverse outcomes (Petersen et al., 2016). Monotherapy with antipsychotics is considered safer than polypharmacy, with doses kept as low as possible (Breadon and Kulkarni, 2019). Other studies demonstrated only a very modest risk of congenital malformations, which, if it exists, might be due to other factors, particularly polypharmacy (Betcher et al., 2019; Cohen et al., 2016; Straub et al., 2022).

In general, current evidence suggests that patients with major psychiatric disorders responding well to atypical antipsychotics are best served by continuing their medications during pregnancy. Of course, psychological interventions are essential to optimize symptom control and to minimize the need for pharmacotherapy. No specific atypical antipsychotic has emerged as clearly having fewer or less severe adverse reproductive effects than any other. Certainly, neonates exposed to antipsychotic medications during the third trimester of pregnancy are at risk for extrapyramidal and/or withdrawal symptoms following delivery, including agitation, hypertonia, hypotonia, tremor, somnolence, respiratory distress, and feeding disorder (Convertino et al., 2016).

Stimulants

Pregnant women who take a stimulant medication to treat their own ADHD (usually methylphenidate) expose their fetus to the drug. In addition, given that many stimulants are excreted in breast milk, the breast-feeding infant may be further exposed (Ornoy, 2018). However, research to date does not link stimulant medications to major congenital malformations; in particular, use of ADHD medications during pregnancy has not been associated with an increased risk of ADHD in children (Lemelin et al., 2021). Thus, women who continue their prescription stimulants during pregnancy do not appear to be at increased risk of adverse fetal or postnatal outcomes, but caution is warranted:

> [M]ethylphenidate might slightly increase the rate of cardiac malformations and of spontaneous abortions, while amphetamines slightly increase the risk for premature birth [and] low birth weight . . . . (Ornoy and Koren, 2021, p. 1794)

Lithium and Anticonvulsants

Untreated bipolar disorder in the pregnant female is associated with relapse to drug and alcohol abuse, manic episodes (including early postpartum mania), disrupted interpersonal relations, depression, and psychosis. Research indicates that medication-free patients with bipolar disorder are at much greater relapse risk than those receiving medication during pregnancy (66% versus 23%) and in the postpartum period (65% versus 29%) (Wesseloo et al., 2016). The symptoms of pregnant women with bipolar disorder tend to be much more severe than those of women seeking care for other psychiatric conditions including symptoms such as suicidal behavior, substance abuse, and difficulties during childbirth and while breast-feeding (Battle et al., 2014). Regarding breast-feeding, blood concentrations of anticonvulsants in infants breast-fed by mothers with epilepsy taking these drugs tend to be low compared with the mother's blood concentrations (Birnbaum et al., 2020).

When choosing among the mood stabilizers and anticonvulsants discussed in the sections below (and in more detail in Chapters 13 and 14), experts tend to avoid both valproic acid and carbamazepine and to consider lamotrigine relatively benign, while lithium generates strong opinions both for and against (Albertini et al., 2019). As summarized by one group of researchers:

> [L]ithium, and several antiepileptic drugs may adversely affect the developing embryo and fetus. While valproic acid, carbamazepine and topiramate are teratogenic and may also affect postnatal development, the newer [drugs], lamotrigine and levetiracetam, seem to be safe in pregnancy and apparently have no long-term neurodevelopmental damage. (Ornoy et al., 2017, p. 933)

Lithium

Lithium is widely considered to be the gold-standard mood stabilizer for the treatment and prevention of relapses in bipolar disorder, particularly relapses into manic episodes. During pregnancy and the postpartum period, however, its use is limited by concerns about teratogenicity and perinatal complications, including congenital cardiac anomalies (Munk-Olsen et al., 2018). A large study comparing pregnant women who were treated with lithium to those who were not found that the lithium-treated group had more miscarriages, terminations, and preterm births than the nonlithium group and that lithium use was associated with increased cardiovascular risk to the fetus, even after accounting for confounding variables such as smoking, birth order, and bipolar disorder (Diav-Citrin et al., 2014). Another study, however, did not find worse obstetric outcomes in women with bipolar disorder taking lithium during pregnancy (Sague-Vilavelia et al., 2022).

If lithium is absolutely necessary during pregnancy, doses should be minimized, and the fetus should be closely monitored. At any given dose, the serum concentration of maternal lithium declines during pregnancy, which may require dose increases of as much as 50% during the third trimester (Clark et al., 2022). During periods of breast-feeding, small amounts of lithium are transferred to the infant but with no apparent adverse effects (Imaz et al., 2021).

Valproic Acid

Among all the drugs used in the treatment of bipolar disorder, valproic acid is associated with the highest rate of major congenital malformations, with a relative risk estimated to be up to 16% compared to about 2.9% in nonmedicated females (Tomson and Battino, 2009). In addition, use of valproic acid during pregnancy has been associated with impaired cognitive functioning and intellectual disability in offspring, including

IQ scores 9 points lower than in those exposed to lamotrigine, 7 points lower than those exposed to phenytoin, and 6 points lower than those exposed to carbamazepine (Daugaard et al., 2020; Meador et al., 2013). Finally, there is evidence that fetal exposure to valproic acid is associated with an increased risk for autism spectrum disorders, with incidence rates ranging from less than 1% in control children to 2% in children with fetal exposure to lamotrigine monotherapy to 6% with exposure to valproic acid monotherapy (Chaliha et al., 2020). The FDA has concluded that women of childbearing potential should use valproic acid only if it is essential to manage their medical condition and only if they have been adequately warned of its potential for causing harm.

Carbamazepine

A review of the effects of carbamazepine and several other antiepileptic drugs taken during pregnancy and during periods of breast-feeding indicated that carbamazepine is slightly teratogenic, increasing the incidence of adverse effects on the fetus and offspring by about 3% over the incidence with unmedicated females (Kaplan and Demir, 2021). Interestingly, abnormal effects on postnatal growth and development have not been reported for the drug's close structural derivative, oxcarbazepine.

Lamotrigine

Lamotrigine is not considered to be a major teratogen, although a slightly increased incidence of cleft lips and cleft palates has been reported (Kaplan and Demir, 2021). Given reassuring safety data, including an extremely low incidence of congenital malformations when used by pregnant females, clinicians often favor it for treatment of bipolar disorder in women of reproductive age. Data also suggest that there is no significant impact on long-term neurodevelopment in children exposed to lamotrigine in utero (Knight et al., 2021).

Topiramate

Topiramate has been associated with an increase in congenital malformations, although the numbers of pregnancies studied were small—in one study, for example, the risk of oral clefts at birth was found to be 4.1 per 1000 in the 2425 infants born to women exposed to topiramate compared with 1.1 per 1000 in the unexposed group (Hernandez-Diaz et al., 2018). Monotherapy with topiramate does seem to correlate with a modestly increased risk of postnatal intellectual disability (Bjork et al., 2022).

Benzodiazepines

Benzodiazepine use and dependence are on the rise, as are as the number of deaths attributable to the combination of opioids and benzodiazepines (Shyken et al., 2019). Benzodiazepines are frequently prescribed for the treatment of anxiety, and such prescriptions have increasingly coincided with pregnancy. Unfortunately, both benzodiazepine use and untreated anxiety in pregnancy are associated with preterm delivery and low birth weight. Short-term neonatal effects of benzodiazepines taken near the time of delivery include floppy infant syndrome and neonatal withdrawal syndrome. Long-term effects, if any, are poorly understood. Patients and clinicians should keep in mind that benzodiazepine use is associated with physical dependence and potentially serious withdrawal symptoms; to avoid withdrawal, tapering off these medications is recommended (Bais et al., 2020).

SUMMARY AND CONCLUSION

Overall, infants exposed to psychoactive drugs (either prescribed or illicit) during pregnancy are at risk of adverse drug-induced outcomes and should be considered a high-risk population (Kaplan and Demir, 2021). Health care workers should help patients withdraw from illicit drug use and begin aggressive counseling as a replacement. For women who require medication for their psychiatric disorder, psychological and psychosocial interventions should always accompany carefully chosen medication therapy to maximize benefits while minimizing drug exposure. Monotherapy with the lowest possible doses consistent with good control of symptoms is a reasonable therapeutic goal.

CHAPTER REVIEW

1. How did the FDA's 2015 Pregnancy and Lactation Labeling Final Rule change the requirements for drug labeling?
2. What risks are associated generally with psychoactive drug use by females during pregnancy and when breast-feeding?
3. Summarize the specific risks associated with pregnant or breast-feeding females' abuse of each of these specific types of drugs: nicotine, alcohol, cannabis, stimulants, and opioids.
4. Summarize the specific risks associated with pregnant or breast-feeding females' use of each of these specific types of prescription psychotherapeutic drugs: antidepressants, antipsychotics, stimulants, lithium, and anticonvulsants.
5. What are the risks of not using psychotherapeutic drugs to treat pregnant or breast-feeding females with psychiatric disorders?
6. What should be the main goals and considerations when deciding whether to use psychotherapeutic drugs to treat pregnant or breast-feeding females with psychiatric disorders?

KEY TERM

neonatal abstinence syndrome

CHAPTER 16

Child and Adolescent Psychopharmacology

CHAPTER OUTLINE

In 2020 the London-based Wellcome Trust, a foundation that focuses on health research, initiated a new strategy committing $258 million over five years in support of mental health research, primarily addressing depression and anxiety in youth. Because of inadequate treatment regimes, the mission was to find the next generation of approaches to prevent, intervene, manage, and minimize relapse of anxiety and depression in young people. The Trust stated: “Mental health is not just a pressing public health problem, it’s a huge productivity and economic issue.”

Therefore, this chapter offers an introduction to the pharmacology of drugs to treat disorders of children and adolescents. This is done not only to present the treatment of important mental health problems in children and adolescents, but also in the hope of preventing their progression and worsening as these children develop into young adulthood.

Childhood and adolescence are crucial times of biopsychosocial and brain development. Many, if not most, severe mental disorders have their onset prior to age 18 (Solmi et al., 2020). Based on this, early intervention is a cornerstone of modern psychiatry. In addition to psychological interventions, psychotropic medications are often necessary to assist in the alleviation of distress and dysfunction in youth. Many of the medications discussed in this book have received U.S. Food and Drug Administration (FDA) approval for use in children and adolescents for specific indications; many are also used off-label in this same population for other purposes; and many of these drugs and others are subject to compulsive use and abuse by children and adolescents, an important topic we address first.

SUBSTANCE ABUSE IN CHILDREN AND ADOLESCENTS

Substance abuse is a significant contributor to three of the leading causes of death among adolescents—vehicular accidents, homicide, and suicide—and increases risk-taking behaviors while the youths are under the influence, including driving while impaired, unsafe sexual activity, and violence. It is also associated with low educational achievement.

According to research:

> Unhealthy drug use is more commonly reported by young adults ages 18–25 years (24%) than by older adults (10%) or adolescents ages 12 to 17 years (8%). (U.S. Preventive Services Task Force, 2020a, 2301)

In addition, it's been stated that:

> In 2017 . . . an estimated 50% of adolescents in the U.S. had used an illicit drug by the time they graduated from high school. . . . Similar to adolescents, the illicit drugs most commonly used by young adults are marijuana (20.8%) and prescription psychotherapeutics (4.6%). (U.S. Preventive Services Task Force, 2020b, 2060)

Common Addictive Substances

The following are some of the most common addictive substances used by children and adolescents.

Nicotine

Tobacco use is the leading cause of preventable death, with "more than 480,000 adults in the United States dying annually from the effects of cigarette smoking and approximately 16 million having a smoking-related illness" (Selby and Zawertailo, 2022). Regarding youth:

> It is estimated that every day about 1600 youth aged 12 to 17 years smoke their first cigarette and that about 5.6 million adolescents alive today will die prematurely from a smoking-related illness. (U.S. Preventive Services Task Force, 2020c, 1590)

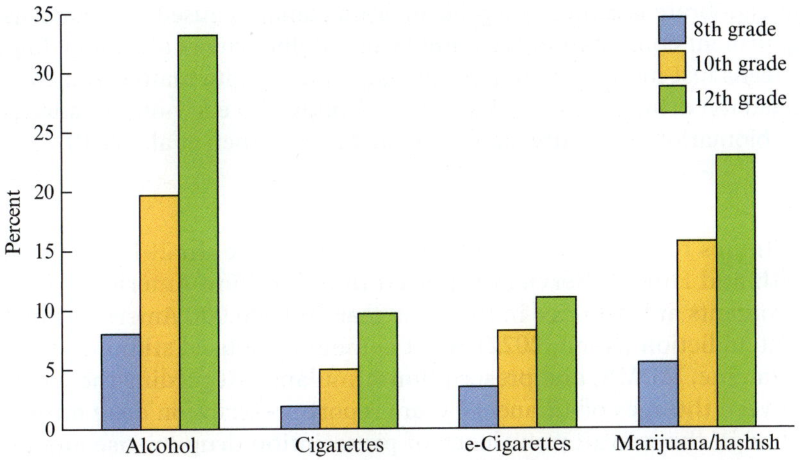

FIGURE 16.1 Prevalence of E-cigarettes. Percent of 8th, 10th, and 12th grade students who used alcohol, cigarettes, e-cigarettes, or marijuana/hashish in the past month. [Data from Johnston et al., 2018.]

While smoking traditional cigarettes has declined gradually, tobacco use via electronic cigarettes is quickly rising and is now more common among youth than cigarette smoking (Figure 16.1). However, compared with nonusers, teenage e-cigarette users were more than four times as likely to use cigarettes or other smokable tobacco products, with a corresponding increase in adverse cardiopulmonary complications (Ruder, 2022).

Most e-cigarettes contain nicotine; nicotine use during adolescence can harm the developing brain and may affect brain function and cognition, attention, and mood (U.S. Preventive Services Task Force, 2020c). Therefore, there is an urgent need for targeted youth tobacco prevention efforts (U.S. Food and Drug Administration, 2022). As of December 2019, persons under 21 years of age can no longer legally purchase cigarette products in the United States (U.S. Food and Drug Administration, June 29, 2022).

Alcohol

Adolescents use alcohol more than any other drug, including tobacco and marijuana. Researchers cited results indicating that children start to think positively about alcohol between ages 9 and 13; that 4.5% of 14- and 15-year-olds reported binge drinking, that is, depending on age and sex, three or more to five or more drinks on one occasion; and nearly two-thirds of high school students reported binge drinking on more than one occasion in the past 30 days (Squeglia et al., 2015). Australian researchers noted that 50% of adolescents report using alcohol and 36% report binge drinking; in addition, parental supplying of alcohol was associated with increased odds of binge drinking and alcohol-related harms (Aiken et al., 2018, 2020). Similarly, other researchers concluded:

> Providing alcohol to children is associated with alcohol-related harms. There is no evidence to support the view that parental supply protects from adverse drinking outcomes by providing alcohol to their child. (Mattick et al., 2018, e64)

The developing adolescent brain is more vulnerable to brain damage caused by alcohol as well as cognitive impairment compared to the adult brain (Melbourne et al., 2021). Further, heavy-drinking teens lost more gray matter and gained less white matter over time than their peers who did not drink (Squeglia et al., 2015). Youth with early-onset patterns of heavy drinking is a biomarker for future alcohol-related harm (Yuen et al., 2020).

Stimulants

Stimulant abuse continues to be a widespread public health issue. In 2018, the U.S. Department of Health and Human Services reported that 5 million Americans misused prescription stimulants at least once in the prior year and 400,000 Americans had prescription stimulant addiction (Nenn, 2022). Most commonly abused stimulants are cocaine, methamphetamine, MDMA, and prescription stimulants. Regarding the latter, over 4% of youth between the ages of 12 and 17 years report prescription drug misuse in the past year. Although the overall prevalence of prescription drug misuse among youth and young adults has declined in recent years, the rates of prescription stimulant misuse are higher than the rates of misuse for other categories of prescription medications (Substance Abuse and Mental Health Services Administration, 2021a).

Adolescents in treatment for methamphetamine (MA) abuse are more likely to be female and have a greater likelihood of past psychiatric treatment, a family history of substance abuse, higher depression rates, and more suicidal ideation relative to adolescents being treated for addiction to other drugs of abuse. Adolescents who use MA are more likely to engage in risky sexual activity, become pregnant, and exhibit greater antisocial behavior. Even after MA use stops, among former MA users there is more depression, anxiety, increased cortisol secretion in response to a social stressor, and more executive function impairments relative to non-MA users for up to 11 months (Buck and Siegel, 2015). Compared with adult MA users, adolescent users had greater decreases in cortical thickness in several brain areas and white matter tracts. MA abuse with cannabis abuse is associated with significantly more neurocognitive impairment than MA abuse alone, and such deficits may be enduring. In a study of Brazilian adolescents, the mean age at which they had started using cocaine was between 13 and 14 years, usually after two and a quarter years of using tobacco, alcohol, or cannabis. Comorbid conduct disorder, oppositional defiant disorder, and attention deficit/hyperactivity disorder (ADHD) were diagnosed significantly more in users than in nonusers (Pianca et al., 2016).

Cannabis

As of June 2022, 37 states, three territories, and the District of Columbia had laws legalizing marijuana for medicinal purposes. As of May 2022, 19 states, two territories, and the District of Columbia had enacted measures to regulate cannabis for adult nonmedical use. In 2015, the American Academy of Pediatrics opposed outright marijuana legalization but supported decriminalization for those 21 and younger (Ammerman et al., 2015). It's clear from all this that marijuana is widely available to children and adolescents. Indeed, marijuana is the exception among drugs as being the only substance whose use is known to be increasing. Much of this increase is due to widespread vaping of flavored marijuana products (Cullen et al., 2019). The terminology regarding e-cigarettes and vaping is confusing: "e-cigarettes," "vapes," "vape pens," "Juul," etc. all refer to the same class of products, with e-cigarette being the product itself and vaping referring to use of the product, either nicotine or marijuana. There are three formats of cannabis vaping: herb vaporizers, oil pens, and wax pens.

Both smoking and vaporizing cannabis are associated with severe and potentially life-threatening conditions, especially damage to the lungs. In adolescents it is associated with an increased risk of developing affective and psychotic disorders, including schizophrenia. The association is strongest in vulnerable youth, such as those who have suffered child abuse or have a family history of schizophrenia and may not be a concern in less susceptible populations. In addition, early and heavy use of cannabis has been associated with deficiencies in brain structure, including cerebral cortical maturation and thickness, dopaminergic alterations, and alterations in thalamic connectivity. Long-term daily marijuana use in young adults has been associated with an abnormally shaped hippocampus and deficits on long-term memory tests relative to their nonusing peers (Smith et al., 2015). Other functional impairments include amygdalar hypersensitivity to threat, impaired decision-making capabilities, poor intelligence test performance, and poorer academic performance.

All these complications imply long-term problems with societal achievement. In analyses that controlled for key social confounding factors, including parental and peer variables, a dose-response relationship was found between use frequency and dropping out of high school, failure to get a college degree, marijuana dependence, use of illicit drugs, and suicide attempts (Silins et al., 2014). A study that followed nearly 950 people from birth through midlife found a link between regular marijuana use and negative job prospects as adults. As compared to their parents, those involved in the study were more likely to face financial difficulties, including food insecurity and debt, if they were heavy marijuana users (Cerdá et al., 2016). Researchers document that cannabis abuse is a common comorbidity and risk marker for self-harm, all-cause mortality, and death by overdose (of other drugs) and homicide among youths with mood disorders (the most prevalent of which was depression) (Fontanella et al., 2021).

The use of synthetic cannabinoids is of equal or greater concern than plant-derived cannabis products. In the first prospective study of synthetics, researchers have found that symptoms of depression, drinking alcohol, and using marijuana were linked to an increased risk of synthetic cannabinoid use one year later (Ninnemann et al., 2017). Depressive symptoms, but not anxiety or impulsivity, were predictive of later synthetics use. One group of researchers reported that when compared to students who used marijuana only, students who used synthetic cannabinoids were more likely to engage in substance use and sexually risky behavior and to engage in more aggressive behaviors if they (1) used the drug before the age of 13 years or (2) used the drug more than 20 times in the last 30 days (Clayton et al., 2017).

Guidelines for Prevention, Diagnosis and Treatment of Substance Abuse in Children and Adolescents

As noted earlier in this section, more adolescents use illicit drugs or intentionally misuse prescription drugs than use tobacco (see Figures 16.2 and 16.3). Previously, the American Academy of Pediatrics recommended that clinicians screen all adolescents for alcohol or drug use and, based on those results, provide guidance, appropriate counseling interventions, and, if necessary, referrals for treatment (Levy et al., 2016).

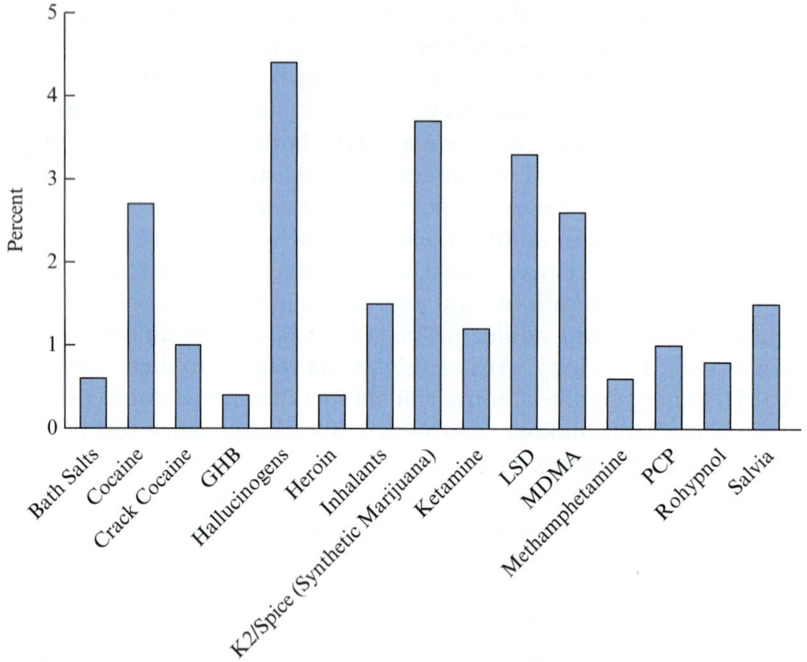

FIGURE 16.2 Illegal Drug Use in the Past Year Among 12th Graders.
[Data from Johnston et al., 2018.]

However, more recently, the **U.S. Preventive Services Task Force (USPSTF)**, an independent agency that reviews medical evidence and makes recommendations about specific preventive care services, advocated that clinicians screen for unhealthy drug use in adults age 18 years and older, stating that evidence was insufficient to recommend such screening in children, adolescents, and young adults. The federal government is actively involved in efforts to prevent and treat substance use in children and adolescents and has published important guidelines on the prevention of substance abuse (National Institute on Drug Abuse, 2011; Substance Abuse and Mental Health and Mental Disorders, 2022), suicide (Wasserman et al., 2021), and mental health disorders, including anxiety and depression (Center for Disease Control and Prevention, 2022).

Chapter 6 described medications that can be used to treat nicotine dependence. Of these, Chantix is not approved for persons under 18 years, and nicotine replacement products and over-the-counter nicotine replacement therapies are available only by prescription for those under 18. They are not approved for persons under 18; prescriptions need to be written for off-label use. This is a major medical/cultural dilemma that has not yet been addressed.

The treatment of substance use co-occurring with other, severe mental health disorders (such as depression) is a special concern, given the enormous burden that they pose (Murthy et al., 2019). Researchers noted less than 12% of adolescents with major depression and a substance use disorder received treatment for both conditions (Lu et al., 2021). To that end, we now turn to a more in depth look at child and adolescent mental health disorders.

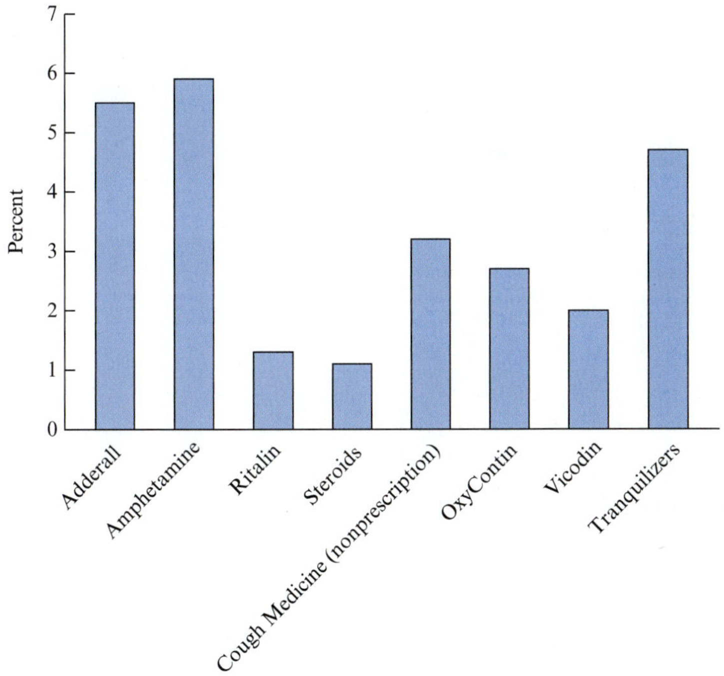

FIGURE 16.3 Illicit Use of Prescription and Over-the-Counter Drugs in the Past Year Among 12th Graders. [Data from Johnston et al., 2018.]

MENTAL HEALTH DISORDERS IN CHILDREN AND ADOLESCENTS

Researchers studied a large community sample of adolescents at several time points over a 14-year period from mid-adolescence into their late 20s. Depression and anxiety were common during adolescence, with anxiety affecting about 9% of children and depression affecting 4–5% of children (Lebrun-Harris et al., 2022; Selph and McDonagh, 2019). By their late 20s, however, the prevalence of disorder had decreased, and many of the participants who had an adolescent episode did not have another episode as a young adult. Several characteristics predicted ongoing disorder into adulthood, namely, longer duration of adolescent disorder, parental separation or divorce, and being female. Because the risk for persistence into adulthood is greater for adolescents with more than one episode, prompt recognition and treatment of the first episode might lead to fewer cases after age 21. While these results are encouraging, the consequences of childhood psychiatric disorders are still severe. Researchers found that such adults who had a childhood psychiatric disorder were more than three times as likely to have health, legal, financial, and social problems as adults, even if they had never received a formal psychiatric diagnosis (Copeland et al., 2015).

In a 13-year-long analysis of mental health care for adolescents in the United States, researchers reported that a total of 47,090 (19.7%) of 230,070 between 2005 and 2018 received mental health care. Of these, 57.5% were female; 31% were ages 12–13 years;

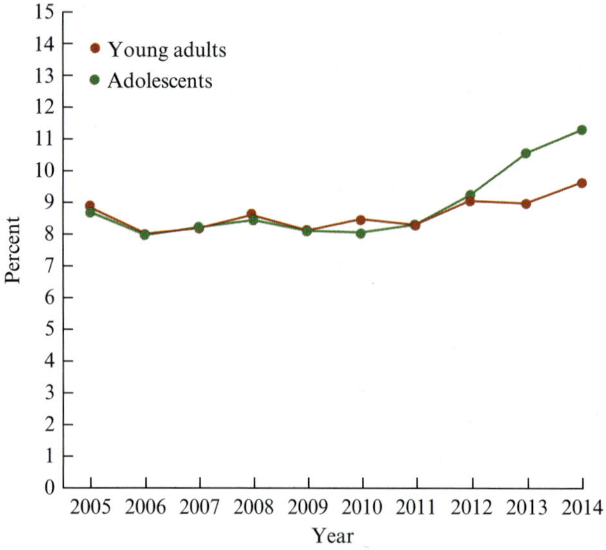

FIGURE 16.4 Major Depressive Episodes. Prevalence of 12-month major depressive episodes in (A) adolescents ages 12–17 years and (B) young adults ages 18–25 years in the United States. [Data from Mojtabai et al., 2016.]

35% were 14–15 years; and 32% were 16–17 years. "Internalizing" diagnoses, including suicidal ideation, anxiety disorders and depressive symptoms, while "externalizing" problems, including substance abuse decreased. Referring only to major depression, the 12-month prevalence increased from 8.7% in 2005 to 11.3% in 2014 in adolescents (ages 12–17 years) and from 8.8.% to 9.6% in young adults (ages 18–25 years) (Mojtabai and Olfson, 2020) (see Figure 16.4). Reductions in school-based counseling decreased, while outpatient mental health counseling increased. With almost one in five adolescents receiving mental health services yearly, discussion regarding treatment approaches, including use of pharmacological agents as a part of treatment, is necessary.

TREATMENT OF ANXIETY DISORDERS

As stated by researchers:

> More than 30% of youths experience an anxiety disorder by age 18, with impairment across family, social, and academic domains. Youth with anxiety are significantly more likely than counterparts without anxiety to go on to develop mood and substance use disorders, drop out of school early, and die by suicide. (Allen et al., 2020, 887)

It is now generally agreed that psychotherapy and pharmacotherapy are effective in treating anxiety disorders and maintaining improvements. Selective serotonin reuptake inhibitors (SSRIs) usually combined with cognitive-behavioral therapy (CBT) are evidence-based treatments and have resulted in the recent publication of a clinical practice guideline for the treatment of anxiety disorders in children and adolescents (Walter et al., 2020). Continuation treatment is recommended for about one year following remission in symptoms, as some symptoms of anxiety persist, even among those children showing improvement after 12 weeks of treatment. If symptoms return, medication reinitiation should be seriously considered.

The largest randomized, controlled treatment study of anxiety in children and youth, the Child/Adolescent Anxiety Multimodal Study, included 488 patients (74% less than 12 years old) with disorders of separation anxiety, generalized anxiety, or social phobia. After 12 weeks, a combination therapy of sertraline (Zoloft) and CBT was associated with a significantly higher response rate (81%) than CBT alone (60%), sertraline alone (55%), or placebo (28%), based on a standardized clinician rating of severity of illness (Gibby et al., 2017; Walkup et al., 2008). During maintenance treatment, 412 responders in the three active treatment groups continued their assigned treatments for an additional six months; 325 completed the extended treatment study. Overall, more than 80% of acute (within 12 weeks) responders maintained positive outcomes at 24 and 36 weeks. Recently the U.S. Preventive Services Task Force (2022a) recommended screening for anxiety disorders in children and adolescents aged 8 to 18 years. Data was insufficient to assess the balance of benefits and harms of screening for anxiety disorders in children 7 years of age or younger. These recommendations were for asymptomatic children and adolescents and do not apply to children and adolescents with a diagnosed anxiety disorder or who show signs or symptoms of anxiety.

Obsessive-Compulsive Disorder

There is little research on obsessive-compulsive disorder (OCD) in preschoolers. However, OCD may emerge in preschool children as early as 2 years of age, being more common in males (Coskun et al., 2012). As stated in the classic Pediatric OCD Treatment Study (POTS), partial response to SSRIs is the norm, and augmentation with short-term OCD-specific CBT provides additional benefit (Franklin et al., 2011, p. 1224). Study results revealed that 68% of OCD youths receiving medication management plus CBT strategy were considered responders, which was superior to 34% in the CBT group and 30% in the medication-only group.

Even so, nearly 30% of all young people diagnosed with OCD are resistant to SSRI plus CBT. Augmentation strategies include addition of an atypical antipsychotic (discussed later in the chapter). For example, in one study 39 adolescents (mean age 12 years) were titrated to a final dose of 12 milligrams of aripiprazole per day, and the drug was effective in more than 50% of patients resistant to continuing SSRI therapy (Masi et al., 2010). (See Aspvall et al., 2021, for a discussion on CBT treatments for OCD.)

Posttraumatic Stress Disorder

If a child is feeling severe anxiety, fear, and hopelessness as a result of PTSD, medication can be a useful addition to psychotherapy. Antidepressants can help the child feel calmer, more in control, and ready to apply the coping strategies they are learning in therapy. Medication, however, is not a "stand-alone" treatment; as noted, psychotherapy is a necessary component.

In a meta-analysis of published literature, researchers noted that the data do not support the use of SSRIs as first-line treatments for PTSD in children and adolescents (Strawn et al., 2010). For example, sertraline was ineffective in a placebo-controlled study in 131 youths (6–17 years) with PTSD (Robb et al., 2010). Limited evidence notes that atypical antipsychotics and several mood stabilizers may attenuate some symptoms, such as intrusive thoughts. Antiadrenergic agents, such as clonidine, guanfacine, and prazosin (Akinsanya et al., 2017), can reduce symptoms such as hyperarousal, intrusive thoughts, nightmares, and impulsivity. (We will discuss clonidine and guanfacine later in the chapter.) Other medications may be needed to target various associated PTSD symptoms such as depression, affect instability, disruptive behavior, and dysregulated attachment.

Cognitive inhibitors (e.g., benzodiazepines, tricyclic antidepressants) are not indicated for use in children and adolescents. Currently, it is thought that prolonged exposure therapy and CBT are more effective in treating PTSD than is medication.

Social Anxiety Disorder

Social anxiety disorder is prevalent in childhood and is associated with lifelong impairment and high societal costs. CBT is effective in children and adolescents with social anxiety disorder and is considered first-line treatment. Researchers recently reported that Internet-delivered CBT was an efficacious and cost-effective treatment for social anxiety disorder (Nordh et al., 2021).

TREATMENT OF DEPRESSION

One of the major controversies in child and adolescent psychopharmacology is the use of antidepressant medication to treat major depressive disorders in children and adolescents. With confirmation of diagnosis, treatment should be initiated for persistent, moderate, and severe depression (Selph and McDonagh, 2019). Do these medications work? Do they increase the risk of suicide? Is their cost-benefit ratio worth the risks involved? These and other questions plague prescribers, parents, and patients. In essence, controversy surrounds the balance between expected benefits and effectiveness in relieving depression versus potential risks, especially the risk of suicide. Research conducted in the late 1990s and early 2000s demonstrated several important points:

- There was a high prevalence of suicidal ideation and completed suicides among untreated children and adolescents with depressive disorders.
- Sixty-two percent of children with depression had experienced childhood adversity, with traumatic events (35%) and bullying victimization (29%) most commonly reported.
- Not only does depression exist in adolescence, but adolescence is the period of highest risk for onset of depression.

- Adolescent depression has a protracted, longitudinal course with persistence into adult life (adolescents do not "grow out of it"), which results in ongoing disruption of interpersonal relationships, risk for substance abuse, early pregnancy, low educational achievement, poor occupational functioning, unemployment, and continued risk of suicide.
- Untreated childhood and adolescent depression is associated with later development of serious personality disorders in early adulthood; dependent, antisocial, passive-aggressive, and histrionic personality disorders; as well as high rates of substance abuse.

Antidepressant Medication

About 25 years ago, researchers demonstrated that fluoxetine (Prozac) was superior to placebo treatment in lowering scores on the Children's Depression Rating Scale (Emslie et al., 1997). This led to widespread off-label use of fluoxetine for child and adolescent depression, culminating in the NIMH-funded Treatment for Adolescents with Depression Study (TADS), the first phase of which was published in 2004 (Treatment for Adolescents with Depression Study [TADS] Team, 2004). The 12-week TADS study compared usual clinical management with fluoxetine (10–40 milligrams per day) alone, CBT alone, or the combination of CBT and fluoxetine. Response to combination treatment (71%) was significantly greater than to fluoxetine alone (61%), CBT alone (43%), and placebo (usual clinical management, 35%). Fluoxetine monotherapy was superior to placebo and to CBT alone. This study set the standard that the best treatment of child and adolescent depression is a combination of fluoxetine and CBT.

Today fluoxetine is one of two SSRIs (the other being escitalopram [Lexapro]) FDA-approved for treating depression in children and adolescents; fluoxetine is approved for use in patients older than 8 years, and escitalopram is approved for use in patients 12 years and older. Medication should likely only be used concomitant with CBT, and decision to modify treatment should be made after about four to eight weeks (Selph and McDonagh, 2019). (See Miller and Campo, 2021, and Cheung and coworkers, 2018, to review the treatment of adolescent depression.)

Results of the landmark **Treatment of Resistant Depression in Adolescents (TORDIA) study** have supported the conclusions previously mentioned. The TORDIA study showed very clearly that combining pharmacological and psychological treatments is more effective than using medication alone. Published in 2008, the study remains a key piece of clinical evidence for helping young people with treatment-resistant depression (Brent et al., 2008). It included about 300 teens who were unresponsive to their initial eight-week SSRI therapy. They were then randomized to 12 weeks of switching to a different SSRI alone; or switching to venlafaxine alone; or switching to either of the drugs plus CBT. Adding CBT to either medication showed a higher response rate (55%) than did the medication alone (40%). The new drugs alone were equally effective (new SSRI, 47%; venlafaxine, 48%). Other researchers confirmed that adding six months of CBT to the medication management of children and adolescents with major depressive disorder reduced the likelihood of depression relapse (Kennard et al., 2014). During the six months studied, participants who received medication management plus CBT had a 9% relapse rate compared to a 26.5% relapse rate for participants who received medication alone. In addition, the superiority of fluoxetine is supported by the results of researchers (Le Noury et al., 2015), who showed that neither paroxetine nor high-dose imipramine showed efficacy for major depression in adolescents, and that there was an increase in harms with both drugs. (Paroxetine may actually be associated with a higher risk of serious adverse effects, including suicidal ideation or behaviors among adolescents [Viswanathan et al., 2020].) A review of 34 trials including 5260 participants and 14 antidepressant treatments (Cipriani et al., 2016) also found that only fluoxetine was statistically significantly more effective than placebo. Of note, psychotherapy trials are not associated with harm (NICE Guideline Updates, 2019; Viswanathan et al., 2020).

In another study, researchers reviewed 80 medications used in the treatment of child and adolescent disorders (Solmi et al., 2020). The safety/coverage ratio was best for escitalopram and fluoxetine, progressively decreasing through vilazodone, paroxetine, sertraline, and venlafaxine, which had the worst safety/coverage ratio.

Antidepressants and Suicidality

> Suicide is the second leading cause of death in the United States among individuals ages 10-24 years, and severe youth depression is often refractory to the current standards of care. (Kim et al., 2021, 1485)

The majority of children and adolescents who attempt suicide have significant mental health disorders, often depression. Among younger children, suicide attempts may be associated with feelings of sadness, confusion, anger, or problems with attention and hyperactivity. Among teenagers, suicide attempts may be associated with feelings of stress, self-doubt, pressure to succeed, financial uncertainty, disappointment, and loss.

Depression and suicidal feelings are treatable mental disorders. The child or adolescent needs to have his or her illness recognized and diagnosed, and appropriately treated with a comprehensive treatment plan. The major question arises as to whether antidepressant medication contributes to suicidality, prevents suicides, or both, depending on the individual. For years, the FDA has required a black box warning for children and for young adults (18–24 years) taking antidepressant medication, who may be at greater risk for suicidal ideation. There is no evidence of increased risk for persons ages 24 years and older.

Within two years after the FDA advisory was issued, antidepressant use plunged 31% among adolescents and 24% among young adults. Unexpectedly, the reduction in antidepressant use due to FDA warnings resulted not only in reduced SSRI prescriptions, but also in an increase in suicides (Lu et al., 2014). This indicated that perhaps SSRI therapy was indeed effective. Researchers argued that the FDA should consider removing the warning, as it may have unintentionally discouraged young persons from seeking treatment and doctors from prescribing antidepressants (Friedman, 2014). Researchers also performed a meta-analysis on the treatment of major depressive disorder from 2007 forward. They noted the superiority of fluoxetine and escitalopram and that there were no increases in treatment-emergent suicidality associated with antidepressant medication in any study (Ignaszewski and Waslick, 2018). More recently, there has been interest in expanding the use of esketamine therapy from adults only to children and adolescents, an approach that might treat both depression and suicidal ideation (Zimmermann et al., 2020).

In addition, the U.S. Preventive Services Task Force (2022b) has recommended screening for major depressive disorder of asymptomatic adolescents aged 12 to 18 years. They concluded that evidence was insufficient to assess the balance of benefits and harms of screening asymptomatic children aged 11 years or younger. They also stated that data was insufficient to assess balances of benefits and risks of screening for suicide risk in asymptomatic children and adolescents.

TREATMENT WITH ANTIPSYCHOTIC MEDICATIONS

Atypical antipsychotics are currently first-line treatments for early-onset psychosis and schizophrenia spectrum disorders. Recently, there has been an increase in the use of antipsychotics in children and adolescents for neurodevelopmental, behavioral, and psychiatric disorders, while, at the same time, the age of persons receiving prescriptions has decreased. According to information from the Citizens Committee on Human Rights International watchdog organization (Eastgate, 2021), nearly 77 million Americans took a psychiatric drug in 2020. More than 11.1 million were taking antipsychotics, of which 829,372 were ages 6–17.

Unfortunately, we do not know much about the safety of these medications in this group of patients. Lurasidone had the best safety/coverage ratio, progressively decreasing through asenapine, quetiapine, ziprasidone, paliperidone, risperidone, aripiprazole, and olanzapine, which had the worst safety/coverage ratio (Solmi et al., 2020). Side effects are the same as in adult patients, namely, extrapyramidal symptoms, tardive dyskinesia, weight gain, metabolic syndrome, and symptoms of hyperprolactinemia. Because the use of second-generation antipsychotics also increases the risk for elevated glucose, insulin resistance, hyperlipidemia, and development of type 2 diabetes, monitoring is recommended but often omitted.

Almost 60% of prescriptions were for off-label use, and antipsychotics were the only psychotropic prescribed in 15–28% of cases (Olfson et al., 2015). In looking at clinical diagnoses, researchers found that ADHD and disruptive behavior disorders were the most common diagnoses among boys ages 1–18 years receiving antipsychotics, suggesting clinicians are prescribing the drugs off-label. Indeed, besides their FDA-approved indications, these agents are also prescribed for a variety of off-label conditions, including depression, anxiety, mood dysregulation, and aggressive behavior, as noted. Researchers reported that there were significant increases in diagnoses of mood disorder among youth treated with antipsychotics due to an increase in those with bipolar spectrum disorders (Cervesi et al., 2017).

Although data are scarce, long-acting injectable (LAI) use in youth appears to be effective, with adverse reactions comparable to those of oral preparations (Lytle et al., 2017). Primary diagnoses included bipolar I disorder, schizophrenia, and bipolar spectrum disorders. The LAIs used were mostly risperidone, paliperidone, fluphenazine, aripiprazole, and olanzapine. These medications are usually well tolerated, with clinical improvement described in most cases.

Researchers summarized the overall clinical outcomes of atypical antipsychotics, that is, second-generation antipsychotics, in children and adolescents relative to placebo (Pillay et al., 2017):

- The second-generation antipsychotics have a slight positive effect in schizophrenia, increasing response rates with clinically insignificant effects for negative and positive symptoms, but an overall functional improvement. The evidence for many drug comparison outcomes was often insufficient.
- In bipolar disorder, the second-generation antipsychotics may reduce manic and depressive symptoms and slightly improve overall functioning. Aripiprazole may improve response and remission rates for manic or mixed states, while quetiapine has no benefit for depression.
- In regard to autism spectrum disorders, second-generation antipsychotics and especially risperidone and aripiprazole may decrease irritability and also reduce lethargy/social withdrawal, stereotypy, and inappropriate speech.
- For ADHD and disruptive, impulse-control, and conduct disorders, second-generation antipsychotics as a group may decrease some behavior problems and aggression. In children who have a diagnosis of conduct disorder or ADHD that does not respond to stimulants, risperidone by itself may reduce hyperactivity.

TREATMENT OF BIPOLAR DISORDER

Over the past decade, bipolar disorder in children and adolescents has been the focus of increasing attention mainly due to controversies surrounding its prevalence, diagnosis, and treatment (Findling et al., 2018). It can easily be misdiagnosed with other disorders such as ADHD, conduct disorder, oppositional defiant disorder, severe mood dysregulation, disruptive mood dysregulation disorder, and temper dysregulation disorder (Cichon et al., 2020). Studies have reported the efficacy of mood stabilizers (lithium and anticonvulsants) as well as second-generation antipsychotics. Here we discuss the mood stabilizers.

Lithium

Lithium is a first-line treatment for bipolar disorder in adults, but few studies document the efficacy or limitations in children or adolescents with the disorder (Pisano et al., 2019). Researchers reported on a double-blind, placebo-controlled eight-week study of lithium in youths (ages 7–17 years) with bipolar disorder (Findling et al., 2015) (Figure 16.5). Authors concluded that lithium was more effective than placebo in reducing manic symptoms and generally well tolerated, and that there was no weight gain with its use. Comparative studies of lithium versus other effective drugs are incomplete. Larger, longer studies are needed to assess the continuing efficacy and the side effects of weight gain and cognitive difficulties; however, researchers reviewed subsequent studies, stating:

> There is evidence that lithium monotherapy is reasonably safe and effective in children and adolescents, especially for acute mania and for prevention of mood episodes. (Amerio et al., 2018, 85)

Others added:

> Studies do not support its [lithium's] use in pediatric bipolar depression and severe mood dysregulation, although it might be effective on aggression in the context of conduct disorder. (Pisano et al., 2019, 318)

This stands in contrast to the opinion of other researchers:

> In recent years, additional clinical trial data have enabled lithium to re-emerge as a valuable and, in many cases, preferred treatment [for child and adolescent bipolar disorder]. (Grant and Salpekar, 2018, 303)

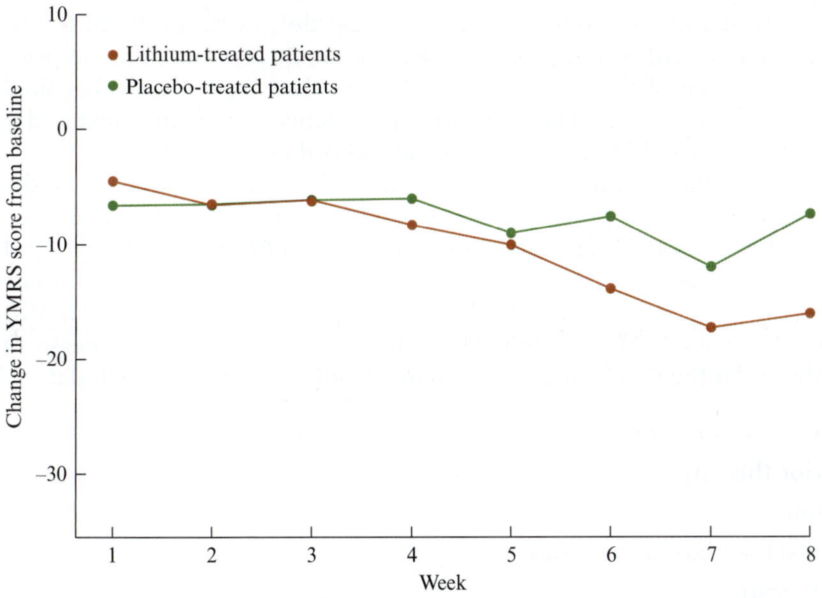

FIGURE 16.5 YMRS Summary Score. Changes in the Young Mania Rating Scale (YMRS) score in either lithium-treated or placebo-treated patients. Baseline was defined as the first visit of the efficacy phase. Data were collected over eight weeks of visits. Scores at weeks 6, 7, and 8 were significantly different from placebo. The median lithium blood concentration averaged 1.4 mEq/l. Body weight was unchanged over the study period. [Data from Findling et al., 2015.]

Anticonvulsants

Researchers reviewed clinical trials of anticonvulsant drugs to treat psychiatric disorders in children and adolescents, particularly bipolar disorder or to manage aggression (Davico et al., 2018). Valproic acid was the most studied drug, with most research showing lack of efficacy in bipolar disorder. The drug was slightly better than placebo in treating recurrent aggression and behavioral dyscontrol. One group of researchers reviewed the literature on valproic acid for acute mania and concluded, "There is no evidence of a difference in efficacy between valproate and placebo for children and adolescents" (Jochim et al., 2019). Other anticonvulsants have not been evaluated for efficacy in child and adolescent bipolar disorder. Researchers discuss the adverse effects of these various medications on youths with bipolar disorder (Sun et al., 2019). Comparing safety versus efficacy of mood stabilizers in children and adolescents, lithium has the best safety/coverage ratio while valproate showed the worst ratio.

TREATMENT OF AUTISM SPECTRUM DISORDERS

Autism is a pervasive developmental disorder characterized by severe impairment in several areas of development, including deficits in social interactions and communication skills and the presence of "repetitive behaviors, highly restricted interests, and/or sensory behaviors" (Lord et al., 2020). Developmental delays range from 0.7 to 20 months when compared with sibling controls (Kuo et al., 2022). Autism must present before age 3; this is true of the many other disorders that are collectively called **autism spectrum disorders (ASDs)**. "The worldwide prevalence of autism is just under 1%, but estimates are higher in high-income countries" (Lord et al., 2020).

Researchers reviewed the etiology of ASDs and noted that genetic factors played a consistently larger role than environmental factors (Taylor et al., 2020). No medication is proven to be effective in treating the core symptoms or the etiology of autism (Goel et al., 2018). Current treatments only target the emotional and behavioral symptoms associated with the disorder. Because there can be overlap in symptoms between ASD and other disorders, such as ADHD, it's important that treatment focus on a person's specific needs, rather than the diagnostic label. Nonmedication treatments include:

- Behavioral management therapy
- Cognitive-behavior therapy
- Early intervention
- Educational and school-based therapies
- Joint attention therapy
- Nutritional therapy
- Occupational therapy
- Parent-mediated therapy
- Physical therapy
- Social skills training
- Speech-language therapy

In terms of medication, the FDA has approved the use of two antipsychotic drugs, risperidone and aripiprazole, for treating irritability associated with ASD in children between certain ages (Alsayouf et al., 2021). Other medications are used to treat other symptoms associated with autism (U.S. Department of Health and Human Services, 2021). For example, in the treatment of hyperactivity, impulsiveness, and attention deficit associated with autism, traditional anti-ADHD medications (discussed later in the chapter), including methylphenidate, atomoxetine, and guanfacine and clonidine, have demonstrated modest efficacy (Goel et al., 2018). Side effects, mostly irritability, often limit therapeutic use. In 1975, bumetanide (Bumex) was introduced into medicine as a diuretic drug. Bumetanide reduces chloride ion levels and seems to restore GABAergic inhibition within the brain (Mollajani et al., 2019). Indeed, in early development of the brain, GABA acts as an excitatory agent that leads to the accumulation of chloride ions within neurons. Researchers reported positive effects of bumetanide in patients with autism (208 total patients, ages 2–18 years). "Behaviors most improved included social communication, interactions, and restricted interest" (James et al., 2019). Other researchers reviewed bumetanide for core symptoms of autism in a carefully controlled trial and reported that the drug was not superior to placebo, casting a negative light on its potential usefulness (Sprenger et al., 2020).

Recently, cannabidiol (CBD) has been suggested as a "candidate for treatment of autism spectrum disorder" (Poleg et al., 2019). Researchers noted that results of cannabidiol in children with autism were "promising," with improvements in problem behaviors, sleep problems, and hyperactivity (Fusar-Poli et al., 2020). Other researchers reported positive effects (30% CBD and 1.5% tetrahydrocannabinol [THC]) in a cohort of children with autism, including improvements in restlessness, rage attacks, anxiety, and agitation, with fewer responses on sleep difficulties and cognitive impairments (Schleider et al., 2019). Two other studies examined the efficacy of cannabidiol-rich marijuana preparations of symptomatology of autism. In both reports, efficacy was quite good with an acceptable incidence of side effects (Aran et al., 2019; Schleider et al., 2019).

Interest has also grown in the possible role of oxytocin in social communication in animals. Researchers have begun exploring whether oxytocin administration in humans might affect social behaviors and attachment in individuals with autism (Baker and Stavropoulos, 2020). Unfortunately, in clinical studies, oxytocin has so far proven to be nonsuperior to placebo (Sikich et al., 2021).

TREATMENT OF BEHAVIORAL DISORDERS MARKED BY AGGRESSION

Severe childhood aggression is one of the most challenging disorders to treat. Preschoolers diagnosed with psychiatric disorders were three times as likely as typical preschoolers to be classified as aggressors, victims, and aggressive victims; children diagnosed with preschool-onset disruptive, depressive, and anxiety disorders were at least six times more likely to become aggressive victims during elementary school.

Behavioral treatments have advantages over medication treatment, but efficacy is variable. Once nonpharmacological approaches have been tried and found inadequate, the second choice is medication. Disruptive behavioral disorders include conduct disorder, oppositional defiant disorder, and disruptive behaviors. Tragically, about 50% of youth with behavioral disruptive disorders progress to antisocial personality disorder as adults, suggesting that their externalizing disruptive symptoms in childhood can be a marker for more pervasive psychopathology as adults.

As stated earlier, mood stabilizers, such as lithium, and anticonvulsants may reduce aggressive behaviors in children with explosive tempers and mood lability. Atypical antipsychotic medications are currently the mainstay in the treatment of aggressive disorders in children and adolescents, with risperidone and aripiprazole both being FDA-approved for such use (Van Schalkwyk et al., 2017). Risperidone is considered to be the most effective drug for aggression (Balia et al., 2018). Other antipsychotics show efficacy, but evidence is less documented.

Polypharmacy, while generally avoided in most treatment situations, may be necessary in some situations involving aggression. Here, risperidone may need to be combined with a stimulant such as methylphenidate or clonidine (Gurnani et al., 2016). Efficacy of anticonvulsants combined with other agents for reducing challenging behavior has been inconclusive.

TREATMENT WITH ANALGESICS

In the pediatric population, pain is frequently underrecognized and inadequately treated. Behavioral research demonstrating long-lasting effects of inadequate pain control during childhood supports the concepts of early and adequate treatment for children suffering from painful conditions in the acute care setting (Gaglani and Gross, 2018; Uspal et al., 2019). Perhaps prompted by the ongoing opioid epidemic, several recent studies have reviewed the epidemiology of pain and surveyed the use of opiate drugs in children and adolescents (Gai et al., 2020; Yaster et al., 2020). Opioid use in children and adolescents involves two patterns: (1) medical prescriptions for postsurgical, acute, and/or chronic pain, and (2) illicitly obtained or diverted opioids intended for other persons.

Regarding the former (prescribed opioids), researchers reported that in children and adolescents, the median prevalence of idiopathic pain is 11–38% (Liossi and Howard, 2016). The highest rates are associated with headaches (23–51%), functional abdominal pain (2–41%), back pain (14–24%), and musculoskeletal pain (4–40%). High rates are also reported in children with organic diseases, such as sickle cell disease, and with persistent postoperative pain after major surgery. Most discomfort can be controlled with nonsteroidal anti-inflammatory drugs (NSAIDs), although, certainly, there is a place for opioid therapy for severe pain and in cancer-related pain (Gai et al., 2020; Thigpen et al., 2019).

Regarding the latter, illicitly obtained or diverted opioids are highly associated with drug overdose in young people (Nguyen et al., 2020). In addition, leftover, unconsumed opioids that were appropriately prescribed for someone else's pain (e.g., parents) has also led to opioid use in children and adolescents (Yaster et al., 2020). Opioid-misusing youths are at greater risk of driving under the influence, early sexual initiation, and carrying a gun (Bhatia et al., 2020). Although opioid use is decreasing among high school students, in 2016 nearly 4% of the approximately 12 million adolescents aged 12–17 reported misusing opioids over the past year. This usage was even higher, 7%, among older adolescents and young adults aged 18–25. The majority of this misuse was due to prescription drugs, not heroin

In 2017, the FDA issued a warning on codeine and tramadol, stating that codeine should not be used to treat pain or cough, and tramadol should not be used to treat pain in children younger than 12 years or to treat children younger than 18 years for pain after surgery to remove tonsils and adenoids. An additional warning recommended against the use of these two drugs in adolescents between 12 and 18 years who have conditions that may impair breathing, such as obesity, obstructive sleep apnea, or severe lung disease. Breast-feeding parents were also warned not to take codeine or tramadol. Researchers noted a decline, with a 90% reduction in prescriptions for cough and cold medications containing codeine or hydrocodone (Chua and Conti, 2021).

In contrast, the opiate analgesic oxycontin was approved by the FDA in August 2015 for children 11 years or older who are in severe pain and require an opioid for five days or more. In other words, oxycontin was not meant to be administered to children as a first-line option or for a brief, acute pain reaction that might occur, such as the extraction of wisdom teeth. The controversy of how, when, which, and how much opioid should be used in children and adolescents, especially for noncancerous pain, will likely continue. In July 2021, the FDA issued a warning about the inappropriate use of fentanyl patches on children, a possibly fatal event (U.S. Food and Drug Administration, 2021a).

TREATMENT OF ADHD

Attention deficit/hyperactivity disorder (ADHD) is one of the most common neurobehavioral disorders of childhood and can profoundly affect children's academic achievement, well-being, and social interactions (Wolraich et al., 2019). National survey data indicates that about 9% of children 2–17 years of age have had an ADHD diagnosis (Danielson et al., 2018). In that survey, 8.4% of children 2–17 years of age currently had ADHD, representing 5.4 million children, almost two-thirds of whom were taking medication and almost half of whom had received behavioral treatments. Researchers argue that ADHD may be overdiagnosed, especially in children with milder cases (Kazda et al., 2021). Boys are twice as likely as girls to receive a diagnosis of ADHD, possibly because hyperactive behaviors can sometimes be more easily observable and disruptive in boys; these are referred to as externalizing behaviors. Girls are more likely to have internalizing conditions, such as anxiety or depression (Centers for Disease Control and Prevention, 2021b).

ADHD Medications

ADHD is regarded as a chronic illness for which there is effective symptomatic treatment but no cure. Effective medications are available and widely used, along with psychosocial therapies (Posner et al., 2020). In 2011, The American Academy of Pediatrics published a clinical practice guideline for treatment of ADHD. That guideline was revised and updated in 2019 (Wolraich et al., 2019) and recommends that treatment include parent behavioral management training and school supports for 4- to 6-year-olds, parent behavioral management training combined with school supports and medication for 6- to 12-year-olds, and school supports, medications, and transition supports for those over 12 years of age. Teens should be screened for substance abuse. We will discuss specific considerations of certain age groups later in the section.

First we focus on medication. Certainly, medical treatment of ADHD is not new. Amphetamines such as Benzedrine (racemic amphetamine)[1] and dextroamphetamine[2] (Dexedrine) were used to treat ADHD as early as 1937; methylphenidate (Ritalin) was introduced in the United States in 1955 and formally approved by the FDA for use in children in 1961. Since then, multiple formulations of stimulants have been marketed and nonstimulant products have appeared. One example of the latter is viloxazine (Qelbree, discussed later), FDA-approved in 2021.

Stimulant agents are the first-line drug treatments of ADHD. They include the various short- and long-term formulations of **methylphenidate** and amphetamine. Second-tier drugs that have shown benefit are nonstimulants, such as *atomoxetine, guanfacine, and clonidine*. Efforts to compare the stimulant and nonstimulant drugs through meta-analyses are inconsistent, usually concluding that stimulants are more effective than nonstimulants, specifically atomoxetine, guanfacine, and clonidine (Chan et al., 2016; Wolraich et al., 2019).

Methylphenidate

As noted, methylphenidate is likely to be the drug of first choice for the initial treatment of ADHD. Because it is so widely used and because no one dosage regimen is ideal, multiple different dosage forms and methods of delivering methylphenidate to the bloodstream have been devised. Methylphenidate is of rapid onset and short duration and must be administered two or three times daily—but not in the evening—to permit the blood level to drop and allow for normal sleep. The short half-life is a problem in some children who experience an end-of-dose rebound in dysfunctional behavior.

Dependable extended-release preparations have become available. The prototype is Concerta, an osmotic-release preparation that delays absorption and extends duration up to 12 hours. The product is prepared with 22% of the drug in a coating on the outside of the capsule for immediate release of the drug and 78% delivered by an osmotic pump that releases the drug over a 10-hour period in gradually increasing serum concentrations. One daily dose of Concerta yields about the same plasma concentrations as three daily doses of immediate-release methylphenidate and with essentially equal efficacy. Other new formulations of methylphenidate for oral administration are of two types:

1. Single-pulse, sustained-release formulations, such as Ritalin-SR, Metadate ER, and Methylin CD, use a wax matrix to prolong release. Their duration of action is about eight hours, but may be unreliable compared with other preparations.

[1] Near-identical to today's Adderall (mixed amphetamine salts).

[2] The active isomer of racemic amphetamine.

2. Beaded, double-pulse products, such as Ritalin LA, Focalin XR, and Metadate CD, use an extended-release formulation with bimodal release. Ritalin LA and Focalin XR are composed of 50% of an immediate-release formulation and 50% of enteric-coated, delayed-release beads. Metadate CD is composed of 30% immediate release beads and 70% delayed-release beads that are released 4 hours later, eliminating the dose normally taken at midday with lunch.

A transdermal methylphenidate skin patch, sold under the trade name Daytrana, is available. The patch is applied daily, has a clinical onset of effect within 2 hours, and is worn for a maximum of 9 hours. Following removal, the effects of methylphenidate continue for another 3 hours. Patches containing 10, 15, 20, and 30 milligrams are available. If removed before 9 hours, less of the drug is obviously absorbed, and the duration of action is decreased.

A liquid suspension formulation of methylphenidate (Quillivant XR) has also been approved by the FDA for ADHD. In addition, dexmethylphenidate (d-methylphenidate or Focalin), the active D-isomer of methylphenidate, is commercially available. This isomer has twice the potency of methylphenidate, so the dose of dexmethylphenidate is one-half the dose of methylphenidate. Focalin is also available in an extended-release formulation (Focalin XR).

Amphetamines

Amphetamines have been used for the treatment of ADHD since 1937, as previously mentioned. Available amphetamines include dextroamphetamine (Dexedrine), mixed amphetamine salts (Adderall), an extended-release formulation of Adderall (Adderall XR), and lisdexamfetamine (Vyvanse). A transdermal dextroamphetamine preparation was recently FDA-approved and is marketed under the trade name Xelstrym. It is available in four strengths ranging from 4.5 to 18 milligrams. In lisdexamfetamine, a molecule of dextroamphetamine is bonded to L-lysine, a naturally occurring amino acid, resulting in a molecule lacking biological activity, that is, a prodrug. When taken orally, the bond is broken by gastrointestinal enzymes, releasing the amphetamine, which is then absorbed. If crushed and injected, the bond is only slowly broken and, theoretically, diversion to nonmedical use, that is, abuse, may be reduced. Doses of 10, 30, and 70 milligrams of lisdexamfetamine compare to 5–30 milligrams of dextroamphetamine. In 2015, the FDA approved lisdexamfetamine to treat binge-eating disorder, the first drug to be approved for the condition.

New Formulations

Evekeo is a short-term immediate-release amphetamine similar to Adderall, except that it is composed of 50% of the two isomers d- and l-amphetamine, whereas Adderall is 75% d-amphetamine and 25% l-amphetamine. It is approved for the treatment of ADHD in patients 3 years of age and older.

In 2015, two new stimulant formulations were approved for the treatment of ADHD: QuilliChew ER and Dyanavel XR. QuilliChew ER is a long-acting methylphenidate chewable tablet that allows once-daily dosing. It contains approximately 30% immediate-release and 70% extended-release methylphenidate. Methylin CT is also

DR. J'S MUSING 16.1

Why Do Stimulants Calm Hyperactivity in ADHD?

For much of my teaching career, I lectured that using amphetamines to calm children with hyperactivity was a "paradoxical" effect of a drug that usually was associated with psychosis, schizophrenia, and drug abuse. How to explain this paradoxical action? Until recently, it could not be explained, because stimulant drugs given to children with hyperactivity often leads to a decrease in their excessive motor activity (the "paradoxical" effect), with calming of hyperactivity and improved attentional focus. Certainly, dopamine and norepinephrine in the prefrontal cortex are involved, likely maintaining dopamine and norepinephrine in the synaptic cleft (possibly by blocking presynaptic reuptake), thus improving cognition, cognitive processing, and focus.

a methylphenidate formulation available as a chewable tablet. The difference is that Methylin CT is a short-acting formulation, while QuilliChew ER offers the advantage of once-daily dosing.

Dyanavel XR is an extended-release oral suspension, a liquid formulation that contains a 3.2:1 ratio of the D- to L-amphetamine isomer (see Chapter 3), with immediate-release and extended-release components. It is the only extended-release liquid formulation for children 6 years and older.

In 2016, Adzenys, an extended-release amphetamine, was approved by the FDA for patients 6 years and older as the first extended-release drug for ADHD that dissolves in the mouth. That is, the drug is an orally disintegrating tablet, a longer-acting version of amphetamine.

Alternative Medications

About 10–30% of ADHD patients do not respond adequately to stimulants and are considered to be treatment resistant. In addition, some children and their parents may desire that stimulants not be used. Therefore, there is a need for treatment alternatives for patients with ADHD. The three reviewed in this section are now approved for use by the FDA, with a fourth under investigation.

In 2003, the FDA approved **atomoxetine** (Strattera) for the acute treatment of child and adult ADHD. In 2008, the FDA expanded its approval to include indication for the maintenance treatment of ADHD in children and adolescents. That is, the drug has been demonstrated to continue to be effective for long-term treatment, not just for the immediate reduction of symptoms. This is the first selective norepinephrine reuptake inhibitor antidepressant approved for use in treating ADHD in children 6 years of age and older. A British study of 201 children with ADHD reported that atomoxetine was more effective in treatment-naive patients than in patients who had been previously treated with stimulant medication, suggesting that it might be beneficial for patients to try a trial of atomoxetine prior to initiation of stimulants. It may take up to 4 weeks for atomoxetine to be effective and 12 weeks for maximum efficacy (Bushe and Savill, 2014). Atomoxetine has little potential for producing euphoria and has a minimal risk of leading to abuse. Researchers reviewed and confirmed the safety and effectiveness of atomoxetine as monotherapy for pediatric ADHD (Schwartz and Correll, 2014). However, in children and adolescents who had an inadequate response to methylphenidate, atomoxetine was found to be less therapeutically effective than lisdexamfetamine (Nagy et al., 2016).

Two CNS-acting antihypertensive (blood pressure-lowering) alpha-2 agonists in extended release formulation—**clonidine** (Kapvay) and **guanfacine** (Intuniv)—are approved by the FDA for the treatment of ADHD, either as monotherapy or used concomitantly with a stimulant. Researchers compared alpha-2 agonists with stimulants (Harstad et al., 2021). Stimulants were only modestly more effective than alpha-2 agonists (65% vs. 78%). Side effects of alpha-2 agonists were primarily daytime sleepiness (38% vs. 3%), while most common side effects of taking stimulants were moodiness/irritability(50% vs. 29%), appetite suppression (38% vs. 7%), and sleep difficulties (21% vs. 11%).

In 2021, viloxazine-extended release was approved as the first "new" ADHD drug in over a decade (Lamb, 2021). **Viloxazine** (Qelbree) is actually an older drug, first marketed in Europe in 1976 as an antidepressant and then (with arrival of the SSRIs) was withdrawn from sale in 2002. Mechanistically, the drug is an selective norepinephrine reuptake inhibitor with some action at serotonin receptors. As reviewed by researchers "viloxazine modulates serotonergic activity as a selective 5-HT_{2B} receptor antagonist and 5-HT_{2C} receptor agonist and moderately inhibits the norepinephrine transporter, thus blocking the reuptake of norepinephrine" (Edinoff et al., 2021c). Viloxazine closely resembles atomoxetine; however, no comparative studies of atomoxetine and viloxazine have been reported. In at least three Phase 3 manufacturer-sponsored studies, viloxazine-ER reduced ADHD symptoms in children and was well tolerated (Nasser et al., 2020, 2021). Pharmacokinetically, viloxazine's blood concentrations appear to be unaffected by concomitant administration of either lisdexamfetamine (Falson et al., 2021a) or methylphenidate (Falson et al., 2021b). Broader studies should help clarify the role of viloxazine in children with ADHD. Because of the norepinephrine reuptake blockade, the drug might have antidepressant properties. Studies in children with comorbid ADHD and depression might be most welcome.

Centanafadine is an experimental agent under investigation for the treatment of ADHD in adults (Adler et al., 2022; Wigal et al., 2020a) with clinical trials for use in children currently underway. Centanafadine is an inhibitor of norepinephrine, dopamine, and serotonin reuptake. As a triple reuptake blocker, this implies use in the treatment of both ADHD and depression.

ADHD and Specific Age Groups

As mentioned earlier, treatment of ADHD sometimes varies according to age groups. Next, we discuss specific considerations of preschool children, school-age children and adolescents, and even ADHD in adults.

Preschool Children

ADHD appears to occur in about 2.4% of preschool-age children (Harstad et al., 2021). Early recognition can lead to interventions such as parent/teacher-administered behavior therapy, the recommended first-line treatment for preschool patients (Wigal et al., 2020b). Second-line treatments involve use of pharmacological agents. The Preschool ADHD Treatment Study (PATS) has provided the most extensive efficacy and safety data on methylphenidate for treating ADHD in preschoolers, with significant improvement in ADHD symptoms observed with methylphenidate compared with placebo, although adverse event-related discontinuation was higher in PATS compared with studies of methylphenidate for ADHD in school-age children (Greenhill et al., 2006). A 10-year follow-up indicated that stimulant medication was still used by most children, with about 25% off medication and 10% on an antipsychotic medication (Vitelio et al., 2015).

More recently, researchers discuss alpha-2-adrenergic agonists, used in about 25% of preschoolers with ADHD, as perhaps a better first choice over stimulants (Blum et al., 2018; Harstad et al., 2021). While a bit less effective than stimulants, alpha-2 agonists have no known abuse potential. They may be particularly helpful for ADHD with associated aggression and other features of conduct disorder; they may also reduce anxiety and symptoms of posttraumatic stress disorder; and they are somewhat sedating (Mattes, 2016). Use is based on the fact that the two major alpha-2 agonists (guanfacine and clonidine) presumably affect α_{2A} receptors, which are postsynaptic in the frontal cortex. Researchers review the pharmacotherapy of preschool ADHD, noting that not getting treatment early by following a "wait and see" approach "should be avoided, in order to prevent a permanent loss of self-esteem and motivation that may affect some children throughout their lifespan" (Froehlich, 2021; Young et al., 2021).

School-Age Children and Adolescents

According to researchers who reviewed the pharmacological treatment of ADHD in children and adolescents, medications are generally superior to placebo in reducing the severity of inattention, hyperactivity, and impulsivity (Cortese, 2020). As noted, stimulant agents, such as methylphenidate and dextroamphetamine, are the most effective medications for the treatment of core ADHD symptoms and have generally acceptable adverse effect profiles.

There is some evidence that early recognition of ADHD and treatment during childhood will result in a better long-term adult outcome (Fredriksen et al., 2013). Several reviews for the pharmacological treatment of ADHD are available and generally support the use of current medications across the life span (e.g., Caye et al., 2019). Recent reports indicate that medication (especially methylphenidate) helps moderate ADHD behaviors in adolescents with externalizing symptoms (hyperactivity, oppositional defiant, and conduct disorder symptoms), while simultaneously reducing the risk of suicide (Shoval et al., 2021).

Children with ADHD and comorbid aggressive disorders present a special challenge. Researchers performed an eight-week trial in 175 children with ADHD, a disruptive disorder, significant aggressive behaviors, and prior stimulant treatment (Blader et al., 2021). To ongoing stimulant treatment, either risperidone, valproate, or placebo were added along with behavioral therapy. Both antipsychotic medications were effective adjuncts. Risperidone was associated with more unwanted weight gain.

ADHD in Adults

While many children with ADHD outgrow it, about 60% still have the disorder as adults. ADHD in adults is a mental health disorder that includes a combination of persistent problems, such as difficulty paying attention, hyperactivity, and impulsive behavior. Adult ADHD can lead to unstable relationships, poor work or school performance, low self-esteem, and other problems. In some cases, ADHD is not recognized or diagnosed until the person is an adult. Adult ADHD symptoms may not be as clear as ADHD symptoms in children even though symptoms typically start in childhood. In adults, hyperactivity may decrease, but struggles with impulsiveness, restlessness and difficulty paying attention may continue. Adult ADHD seems to affect men and women equally.

Treatment for adult ADHD is similar to treatment for childhood ADHD and includes medications, psychological counseling (psychotherapy), and treatment for any mental health conditions that occur along with ADHD (De Crescenzo et al., 2017). In studies, overall, pharmacological treatments were significantly more efficacious than placebo. The effects of pharmacological treatment for individuals with co-occurring ADHD and substance use disorder are still uncertain. Indeed, over half of young people and adults diagnosed with ADHD also have substance use disorder (Young and Woodhouse, 2021). Viewed slightly differently, one of every four persons with a substance use disorder has ADHD, and this comorbidity is associated with higher severity, more frequent polysubstance dependence, and increased risk of other mental health problems (Vilar-Ribo et al., 2021). As stated by researchers:

> 46% of the chronic drug users studied have symptoms diagnosed as ADHD in adults. Of those who met ADHD criteria in childhood, only 6 did not meet these criteria in adult life, resulting in 89% of ADHD patients maintaining symptoms in adulthood, causing dysfunction in certain life areas. (Rad et al., 2020, 161)

Similarly, others reported:

> Individuals self-reporting a diagnosis of ADD/ADHD were found to have a significantly higher likelihood of engaging in smoking and alcohol binge drinking and were more likely to meet criteria for SUDs than individuals not reporting an ADD/ADHD diagnosis. (Connolly et al., 2019, 1454)

This comorbidity certainly complicates treatment of both disorders, especially since the primary drugs used to treat ADHD are also very significant drugs of compulsive use and abuse.

Adults with ADHD frequently self-medicate with marijuana products. Such use is usually without documentation of efficacy, dosage, or potential side effects. Researchers studied 30 adults with ADHD who were using CBD and reported "nominally statistical improvements" among several domains of ADHD (Cooper et al., 2017). The product studied was Sativex Oromucosal Spray (about 50% THC and 50% CBD). To date, no controlled or comparative trials of CBD for treatment of ADHD in children or adolescents have been published.

Side Effects of ADHD Medications

Common side effects of stimulant medications include sleep disturbances (insomnia), elevations in blood pressure and heart rate, reduction in appetite, abdominal pain, headaches, and possible growth suppression. Rarely, hallucinations and other psychotic symptoms can be seen, and, in general, blood pressure and heart rate are only minimally raised (Wolraich et al., 2019).

There has been concern over stimulant-induced reduction in growth rates and growth velocity, with some conflicting data. One review reported reduced height in adults diagnosed in childhood (Swanson et al., 2017), and other studies found no difference in ultimate height, albeit with a developmental delay in ADHD-treated youth (Harstad et al., 2014). Whether any reductions occur seems to be affected by dose, duration of treatment, and whether the drug is stopped during periods of holiday breaks. Another research group showed that physical maturation was not affected by stimulant medication treatment (Poulton et al., 2016).

An important concern with ADHD medication is whether exposure to stimulants might increase future stimulant abuse. Prescription guidelines for stimulant use advise drug abuse evaluation in ADHD patients of teenage years. As noted earlier, the U.S. Preventive Task Force (2020a) urges screening of persons 18 years of age and older for unhealthy drug use; however, this recommendation makes no mention of screening in persons taking stimulants for ADHD. Drug abuse co-occurring with ADHD is associated with other behavioral problems, such as antisocial behavior, and represents a difficult psychiatric situation (Cunill et al., 2015); interestingly, patients with ADHD who receive consistent stimulant treatment are less likely to start smoking (Schoenfelder et al., 2014). A related concern, which has received extensive attention, is the issue of nonmedical use of diverted stimulants, particularly among college students. Most reviews confirm that such nonmedical use is primarily to improve academic performance rather than recreational.

Although side effects are normally considered to be a negative consequence of drug treatments, there are numerous positive effects of stimulant drugs on the behavior of children and adults that might not be typically appreciated. Lisdexamfetamine has been shown to improve "emotional lability" in children diagnosed with ADHD (Childress et al., 2014). Also, stimulant medications reduce the risk of trauma and injury resulting from vehicular accidents (Chang et al., 2017). In addition, researchers reported that parent-child interactions improved when adults with ADHD were treated with medication. Specifically, parents praised their children more and engaged in less negative talk (Waxmonsky et al., 2014).

CHAPTER REVIEW

1. What are the common addictive substances used by children and adolescents and the long-term effects of substance abuse?
2. Discuss the prevalence of mental health disorders in children and adolescents.
3. Explain the different types of anxiety disorders and methods of treatment for each one.

4. What are the controversies surrounding treatment of depression in children and adolescents? Discuss the preferred methods of treatment today.
5. Explain the use of antipsychotic medication in children and adolescents. What are the overall clinical outcomes of atypical antipsychotics?
6. What medications are most often used to treat bipolar disorder? What are the effects of each one?
7. What types of drugs are used to treat autism spectrum disorders and aggressive behavior in children generally?
8. Describe the use of analgesics in children.
9. Explain the treatment of ADHD in children and adolescents. What medications are most commonly used? Does treatment in children differ from adult treatment?

KEY TERMS

atomoxetine
attention deficit/hyperactivity disorder (ADHD)
autism spectrum disorders (ASDs)
centanafadine
clonidine
guanfacine
methylphenidate
Treatment of Resistant Depression in Adolescents (TORDIA) study
U.S. Preventive Services Task Force (USPSTF)
viloxazine

CHAPTER 17

Geriatric Psychopharmacology

CHAPTER OUTLINE

This chapter reviews how the drugs discussed in earlier chapters are applied in geriatric populations to treat disorders common in older adults, including depression, anxiety disorders, behavioral agitation and aggression, Parkinson's disease, and Alzheimer's disease. First, some general principles concerning the actions and effects of psychoactive drugs administered to older patients:

- Lower doses of medication are often as effective in older adults as higher doses in younger people.
- When initiating drug therapy in older adults, it is wise to "start low and go slow."
- Elimination half-lives are often prolonged in older adults, sometimes to about twice as long as half-lives in younger people, due to pharmacokinetic changes that occur with aging, such as decreased liver enzyme activity. These physiological changes may necessitate adjustment of total daily doses and frequency of dosing of many medications.
- Sedative-hypnotic drugs, especially the long-half-life benzodiazepines and anticholinergics, can cause marked and often prolonged cognitive impairment

presenting as memory deficiencies and possibly even leading to a misdiagnosis of dementia in older adults.

- Sedative-hypnotic drugs can also induce psychomotor incoordination, resulting in an increased incidence of falls, altered driving behaviors, and so on.
- Depression and comorbid anxiety are common in older adults and need to be addressed and treated.
- Psychological therapies can be used effectively to treat anxiety disorders, sleep disorders, and other psychological disorders for which drugs are often prescribed.
- Inappropriate drug use in older adults is a common problem with potentially tragic consequences.
- Substance abuse in older adults often goes undetected and therefore untreated, leading to broader psychological, psychiatric, and physiological morbidities.
- About half of older patients experience chronic or persistent pain and pain is often missed, misdiagnosed, or undertreated (Ali et al., 2018; Schwan et al., 2019).

INAPPROPRIATE DRUG USE IN OLDER ADULTS

Older adults are frequently prescribed medications that they do not need or that cause them significant problems, either because of extensions of expected pharmacological effects or through adverse interactions with other medications (Dahal and Bista, 2022). Inappropriate medication use in older adults is a major functional and safety issue and may cause a substantial proportion of drug-related hospital or care center admissions (Martinot et al., 2018; Motter et al., 2018; Williams et al., 2019). While only 14% of Americans are aged 65 years or older, this group represents the largest per capita consumers of prescription medications. Studies of community-dwelling adults have found that 39% take five or more prescription medications, 38% take at least one or more over-the-counter medications, and 64% take at least one or more dietary supplements (Delara et al., 2022; Qato et al., 2016). To help bring attention to inappropriate drug use in older adults, M. H. Beers in 1997 developed specific criteria for inappropriate use, which included a list of drugs that either were ineffective or posed unnecessarily high risks for people over 65 years of age. This list is updated periodically, and the most recent version (2019) can be found on the American Geriatrics Society Web site.[1] A second tool for identifying inappropriate and potentially harmful medication combinations in older adults is the STOPP/START criteria (Screening Tool of Older Persons' Prescriptions [STOPP] and Screening Tool to Alert to Right Treatment [START]) (O'Mahony, 2020). Other resources have also been developed by specific health care organizations (Baumgartner et al., 2020).

[1]http://www.americangeriatrics.org.

The extent of inappropriate prescription use varies between 14 and 74% (Hukins et al., 2019). Among the psychoactive medicines, benzodiazepines are most commonly inappropriately prescribed, followed by hypnotics, drugs with anticholinergic side effects (such as tricyclic antidepressants), and opioid narcotics. Nonsteroidal anti-inflammatory drugs (NSAIDs) have been implicated as contributing to frailty in older adults (Martinot et al., 2018; Nadiugwu, 2020).

There remains an important question about the risk for dementia from long-term use of benzodiazepines in older adults, as noted in the chapter introduction (Lapeyre-Mestre, 2019). Certainly, benzodiazepines are cognitive inhibitors and are widely and inappropriately used in older adults for treatment of anxiety and insomnia. Many of these same patients eventually develop signs of dementia; however, whether this is related to benzodiazepine use remains elusive (Picton et al., 2018). Today, antipsychotics (such as pimavanserin, soon discussed) are more effective and more widely used (Bessey and Walaszek, 2019; Cummings et al., 2018).

Inappropriate drug use can lead to suboptimal care that is not consistent with evidence-based clinical practice (Maust et al., 2017). All the lists that identify inappropriate drug use in older adults recommend avoiding drugs that produce (1) cognitive inhibition, with drug-induced dementia as the most severe manifestation, (2) unwanted sedation, leading to falls and hip fractures, or (3) bizarre behaviors and/or drug-induced delirium. Tricyclic antidepressants and sedating antihistamines are particular drugs of concern, along with the previously mentioned benzodiazepines and opiates. Drugs with anticholinergic properties are also concerning; in fact, often missed in patient workups are the anticholinergic agents (atropine-like), which are particularly strongly related to cognitive dysfunction. Impairments are demonstrated by declines in memory, psychomotor processing, and reduced cognitive flexibility (Chippa and Roy, 2022). Indeed, discontinuing such medications can often lead to rapid improvements in psychomotor and cognitive functioning, including improved memory and attention.

AGITATION, AGGRESSION, AND PSYCHOSIS IN OLDER ADULTS

Psychosis is common across dementia types (including Parkinsonism and Alzheimer's disease, discussed later), with a prevalence of 20–70% (Ballard et al., 2020; Cummings et al., 2018). Atypical antipsychotic medications (Chapter 11) had become the de facto standard of care for behavioral and psychological symptoms of psychosis in dementia (Bessey and Walaszek, 2019; Gareri et al., 2014) (Table 17.1). These medicines can control agitated and aggressive behaviors in older adults, especially in residents of care centers. However, in 2005, the U.S. Food and Drug Administration (FDA) issued a public health advisory warning of a 1.7-fold risk of all-cause mortality from these medicines compared to placebo. The FDA subsequently issued a black box warning on the use of any antipsychotic for the treatment of agitation and psychosis in patients with dementia. This advisory has been controversial because some studies have failed to verify any increased risk of death (Elie et al., 2009). But other studies confirm some degree of increased risk of mortality in individuals with dementia who are treated

TABLE 17.1 Most Commonly Prescribed Antipsychotic Medications in Nursing Homes

Generic Drug Name	Number of Residents Prescribed Drug	Percent of All Antipsychotic Medication Prescribed
Quetiapine fumarate	1,356,223	31.1
Risperidone	1,061,897	24.4
Olanzapine	570,453	13.1
Haloperidol	402,077	9.2
Aripiprazole	347,900	8.0
Clozapine	232,125	5.3
Ziprasidone	138,881	3.2
Chlorpromazine	65,159	1.5
Fluphenazine	54,867	1.3
All others	109,141	2.9

with antipsychotic medication (Koponen et al., 2017; Norgaard et al., 2022; Zhai et al., 2016). As stated by researchers:

> When dementia is accompanied by psychosis, symptom management is especially challenging. Atypical antipsychotics are used off-label in patients who do not respond to non-pharmacological interventions. However, antipsychotic use is associated with adverse reactions including cognitive impairment, cerebrovascular events, and increased risk of death. (Yunusa et al., 2020)

Indeed, for patients with dementia treated with antipsychotic drugs, the risk for myocardial infarction (MI) was found to be double that for individuals not receiving antipsychotics, and antipsychotics have been shown to increase morbidity risk, including pneumonia (Mehta et al., 2015; Tolppanen et al., 2016). Whether physical fragility or functional impairments affect this data is unclear (Seibert et al., 2021).

As a result of the FDA advisory, the use of atypical antipsychotic medicines seems to be decreasing in older adults with dementia-related psychosis. This is probably good, as these drugs also have the potential to be used indiscriminately and inappropriately to quiet patients who might otherwise not require them. Providers should be educated on behavioral control, with delirium reduced using multicomponent interventions carried out by a multidisciplinary team targeting predisposing and precipitating risk factors for delirium (Bessey and Walaszek, 2019; Morandi and Bellelli, 2020).

Until recently, the two most frequently administered atypical antipsychotics were quetiapine and risperidone (Yunusa and El Helou, 2020), accounting for 55.5% of all antipsychotics prescribed to older adults. Notably, in 2017, the FDA granted Breakthrough Therapy approval to a new atypical antipsychotic, pimavanserin (Nuplazid), for hallucinations and delusions associated with Parkinson's disease psychosis, but it remains an experimental drug in treating dementia-related psychosis (Cummings et al., 2018; Tariot et al., 2021). A second atypical antipsychotic under consideration for use in older adults with dementia-related psychosis that has shown to be effective in treatment of agitation in patients with Alzheimer's disease is brexpiprazole (Rexulti), a drug approved to treat schizophrenia and treatment-resistant depression (Aftab et al., 2021; Grossberg et al., 2020; Marcinkowska et al., 2020). It has been shown to be effective in treatment of agitation in patients with Alzheimer's dementia (Grossberg et al., 2020).

Besides antipsychotics, three other drugs or classes of drugs have shown promise in treating dementia-related delirium: (1) melatonin and the melatonin-receptor agonist ramelteon (Rozerem), (2) the orexin receptor antagonist suvorexant (Belsomra) (Sys et al., 2020), and (3) the antidepressant drug citalopram (Qasim and Simpson, 2022).

Researchers reviewed melatonin-based and ramelteon-based therapies for delirium, most notably in intensive care unit settings (Choy et al., 2018; Lewandowska et al., 2020; Ng et al., 2020). Sleep deprivation has been shown to be a major contributor to delirium (Mo et al., 2016), and melatonin levels are greatly decreased in older adults. Restoring these levels may lead to a decrease in delirium.

A second potential class of agents are the suvorexant-like orexin inhibitor hypnotics (Glass et al., 2020). In a study that included 1298 patients over 65 years of age for a period of 3–12 months, one group of researchers found that suvorexant exerted beneficial effects on multiple sleep patterns (Tampi et al., 2018). Indeed, in patients with mild Alzheimer's and sleep difficulties, suvorexant significantly increased total sleep time and sleep efficiency (Blackman et al., 2021).

Another research team studied 118 intensive care unit patients, 70% of whom were admitted following cardiovascular surgery and who were mechanically ventilated (Masuyama et al., 2018). Suvorexant reduced the incidence of delirium from 59% to 44%. Other researchers reviewed suvorexant as an adjunct for delirium prevention in acutely hospitalized patients (Adams et al., 2020). They noted:

> In acutely hospitalized patients, treatment with suvorexant 15-20 mg alone or in combination with ramelteon resulted in a reduction in development of delirium, time until delirium onset, and length of hospital stay. . . . Adverse effects were no worse than placebo. (1)

Note that most of the reports on both melatonin and suvorexant were based on data from acutely ill, hospitalized patients. We still need studies of these drugs, alone or in combination, in less severely ill patients with dementia-related delirium as well as comparisons with pimavanserin. Whatever medications are used to control dementia-related delirium, the goals are to reduce the following:

- Agitation, such as pacing, wandering, restlessness, or the inability to sit long enough to eat
- Aggression, either verbal or physical, which might be directed at staff or other residents for individuals in care centers

- Physical resistance and noncompliance with care
- Psychosis marked by hallucinations or delusions
- Depressive symptoms, such as apathy or lack of interest
- Inappropriate sexual behaviors that are verbal or physical
- Sleep disturbances, such as day-night reversal

In agitated, aggressive, anxious older adults with dementia, behavioral improvement, if it occurs, may allow the patient to remain in a home environment, delaying admission to a facility with more restrictive care. Thus, the humanitarian benefits of trying antipsychotic medications may outweigh any increase in cardiovascular risk in some patients. These agents should be used with discretion, close monitoring, and only as part of a nonpharmacological, environmental, and behavioral intervention package (Porsteinssona and Antonsdottir, 2017). In addition, when these drugs are used, they should be for the shortest term possible. In some cases, however, drug treatment may need to be continued, as discontinuation may cause an individual to relapse and symptoms such as hallucinations or delusions to re-emerge.

DEPRESSION IN OLDER ADULTS

Untreated depression in older adults can seriously reduce both quality and length of life. Indeed, older individuals with depression "have an elevated risk of persistent depressive symptoms and treatment resistance. They also have higher risk of developing cognitive impairment with progression to dementia and higher rates of medical comorbidity, frailty, and mortality" (Diniz, 2018). However, depression in older adults remains underdiagnosed and often poorly or inadequately treated. The rate of suicide for persons over 65 years of age is more than four times the national average for all persons. White males over the age of 75 years have the highest suicide rate at 48.7 deaths per 100,000 population (Conejero et al., 2018). Other risk factors for suicide in older adults include:

- Prolonged illness
- Ongoing chronic pain
- Untreated depression
- Terminal illness
- Death of a spouse
- Social isolation/loneliness
- Recent change in living situation or work status (retired, move to nursing home, etc.)

No medication alone can solve or even address all these risk factors; psychological interventions are preferred, as is a combination of psychological interventions plus antidepressant medication. One example of the latter is a program called IMPACT (Improving Mood: Promoting Access to Collaborative Treatment), which involves a team composed of a depression case manager, such as a psychologist, social worker, or a nurse; a primary care physician; and a consulting psychiatrist (van Leeuwen et al., 2009). In assessing and endorsing this program, researchers stated (Hunkeler et al., 2006):

> Tailored collaborative care actively engages older adults in treatment for depression and delivers substantial and persistent long-term benefits. Benefits included less depression, better physical functioning, and an enhanced quality of life. The IMPACT model may show the way to less depression and healthier lives for older adults. (259)

Other researchers confirmed that using an evidence-based collaborative treatment model such as IMPACT can produce improved outcomes for older individuals who suffer from late-life depression (Penkunas and Hahn-Smith, 2015).

In further support of this collaborative care model, one group studied patients over the age of 70 who had been diagnosed with major depression (Reynolds et al., 2006). Here, they compared the efficacy of placebo medication, medication alone, psychological therapy alone, and combined medication and psychological therapy. The medication chosen was paroxetine (Paxil); the psychological therapy chosen was weekly interpersonal psychotherapy (IPT). Remarkably, combination therapy improved the percentage of patients achieving remission from 35% with either therapy alone to 58%. Results confirmed that depression in older adults is best treated by a combination of antidepressant medication and psychological interventions (Marvanova and McGrane, 2021).

In terms of specific drugs, for the last 20 years, serotonergic antidepressants have been shown to be effective in treating depression in older adults (Brender et al., 2021; Hsu et al., 2021). Such agents include paroxetine, escitalopram, mirtazapine, and sertraline. Researchers analyzed the results of eight double-blind, randomized controlled trials of antidepressant continuation treatment of depression in older adults using relapse as an outcome indicator (Kok et al., 2011). They found that continuation of antidepressant treatment resulted in fewer relapses when compared to placebo, suggesting that continued treatment with antidepressants is efficacious in maintaining recovery. However, there is still concern about the use of antidepressants in older adults. This primarily involves the low rate of response to antidepressant treatment (treatment-resistant depression, soon discussed) and a slightly increased risk of drug-induced morbidity and mortality, as noted earlier (Gerhard et al., 2020).

The presence of an anxiety disorder comorbid with a depressive disorder correlates with poorer outcome for depression treatment (Saade et al., 2019). Similarly, a high pretreatment level of anxiety increases the risk of nonresponse to antidepressant treatment as well as the risk of recurrence in the first two years of maintenance treatment. Depressed older patients should be screened for anxiety disorders and treated for them, if they are present, as aggressively as for the depressive disorder.

Treatment-resistant depression in older adults presents unique challenges (Knochel et al., 2015), especially as "at least 50 percent of older adults with late-life depression fail to respond to antidepressant pharmacotherapy" (Lenze et al., 2015). In older patients with unipolar depression resistant to selective serotonin reuptake inhibitors (SSRIs), aripiprazole (Abilify) added to an SSRI resulted in a 50% rate of remission in formerly resistant older adults (Lenze et al., 2015). Strategies for patients who are treatment resistant are presumed to be similar to those in younger patients; however, "antidepressant combination or augmentation strategies are less well studied in older people who fail to achieve remission or those with treatment-resistant depression, compared with younger populations" (Marvanova and McGrane, 2021). Brexpiprazole (Rexulti) is a newer atypical antipsychotic that is considered effective in treatment-resistant depression, as noted earlier (Fava et al., 2017). However, as mentioned, like all atypical antipsychotics, its use in older adults is likely associated "with a higher risk of all cause-mortality" and with increased rates of pneumonia. At least in these cases, use likely should be avoided (Chekani et al., 2020). Recently, researchers reported that esketamine failed to demonstrate efficacy in older patients in a Phase 3 trial (Aftab et al., 2021). Two trials have been reported with ketamine, one positive and the other generally negative (reviewed by Gupta et al., 2021). Stimulants have also been tried as augmenting agents for treatment-resistant depression in older adults. Here, methylphenidate appears efficacious, especially when combined with an SSRI such as citalopram and used for short periods of time (Smith et al., 2021). Finally, the comorbidity of depression and chronic pain is strong and needs to be addressed in older adults (Ali et al., 2018; Honda et al., 2022; Schwan et al., 2019).

PARKINSON'S DISEASE

Parkinson's disease is the second most common neurodegenerative disease in older adults after Alzheimer's disease. Parkinson's disease affects one to two per 1000 persons at any time (Tysnes and Storstein, 2017). One million people in the United States and 6 million people worldwide are currently living with Parkinson's disease, and more than 60,000 new cases are diagnosed in the United States each year (Armstrong and Okun, 2020). Although the cause of Parkinson's disease is still being studied, its symptoms are thought to follow from a deficiency in the number and function of dopamine-secreting neurons located primarily in the substantia nigra, a subthalamic area of the brain. Progressive loss of these neurons is a feature of normal aging; however, most people do not lose the huge number of dopamine neurons required to cause Parkinson's disease symptoms.

Parkinson's disease is regarded as a movement disorder with three cardinal signs:

- Bradykinesia (slowness and poverty of movement)
- Muscle rigidity (especially a "cogwheel"-type rigidity)
- Resting tremor, which usually abates during voluntary movement

A revision of the diagnostic criteria excludes postural instability as a previously listed fourth hallmark (Tysnes and Storstein, 2017). The clinical features emerge when about 80% of dopamine neurons are lost.

Current research suggests that Parkinson's disease not only is a motor disorder but also presents with nonmotor symptoms that may actually precede the onset of observable motor deficits by a period of 5–20 years. Some of these nonmotor signs include olfactory loss, bowel and sleep problems, and disorders of mood and cognition (Reich and Savitt, 2019; Sauerbier et al., 2016). Therefore, Parkinson's disease is considered a multisystemic disorder with multiple presentations, each of which may have a unique etiology that includes specific gene variants combined with environmental influences (Delamarre et al., 2017; Ferreira and Massano, 2017).

To that end, progress is being made in the etiology of Parkinson's disease. Mutations in a specific gene that encodes for a specific protein (alpha-synuclein) may be responsible for Parkinsonism with Lewy pathology (Rosborough et al., 2017; Xu et al., 2015). Monoclonal antibodies that bring to this alpha-synuclein protein have been developed and investigated in clinical trial. (To date, these drugs [prasinezumab and cinpanemab] have not led to clinical improvement [Lang et al., 2022; Pagano et al., 2022].)

Recall from Chapter 11 that the first-generation, or traditional, antipsychotic agents, such as haloperidol and chlorpromazine, were used to treat schizophrenia. The most prominent side effects of those drugs are movement disorders that resemble those seen in Parkinson's disease. Mechanistically, these side effects result from drug-induced blockade of dopamine-2 receptors, resulting in a hypo- (or low) dopaminergic state. Parkinson's disease is similarly associated with a hypodopaminergic state but characterized by an irreversible and progressive loss of dopamine neurons, as noted.

Like many neurodegenerative diseases, there are no effective neuroprotective therapies. Currently, patients are treated symptomatically while not addressing the *cause* of loss of dopamine neurons. This involves a combination of dopamine replacement therapies, designed to maintain dopaminergic function and slow the effect of the loss of dopamine neurons, or deep-brain electrical stimulation to combat behavioral symptoms (Hayes, 2019). Replacement of the dopamine or the administration of either dopaminergic agonists or inhibitors of dopamine breakdown can restore function and ameliorate much of the symptomatology. These three approaches—(1) dopamine replacement therapy, (2) administration of a dopaminergic agonist, and (3) administration of dopamine breakdown inhibitors—underlie much of today's treatment of the disease. Increasing dopamine in the brain, however, does bring with it some untoward effects, including impulse control disorders such as pathological gambling, binge eating, reckless driving, and hypersexuality (Armstrong and Okun, 2020), as well as dyskinetic movement disorders.[2]

Without treatment, progression will occur over five to ten years to a state of severe rigidity and loss of movement in which patients cannot care for themselves.[3] However, the availability of effective treatments for Parkinson's disease symptoms has radically altered the prognosis of this disease. In most cases, good functional mobility can be maintained for many years, and the life expectancy of an affected person has been greatly extended.

One medication seems to be offering additional hope. **Nilotinib** (Tasigna) is a drug marketed for the treatment of chronic leukemia. Trials have demonstrated that it is capable of attenuating inflammation in models of Parkinson's disease (Pagan et al., 2021; Simuni et al., 2021). Study results have been controversial, and there is optimism that it might reduce both the motor and the cognitive problems in patients with moderately advanced Parkinson's and mild to severe cognitive impairment. Other researchers, however, reported lack of efficacy of nilotinib and urged that the drug should not be further tested (Simuni et al., 2021).

---

[2]A dyskinesia is an impairment in the ability to control movements, characterized by spasmodic or repetitive motions or lack of coordination.

[3]The 1990 film *Awakenings* depicts this feature of Parkinson's disease.

Levodopa

Levodopa (L-dihydroxyphenylalanine, L-dopa), a precursor drug to dopamine, continues to be the mainstay of therapy for Parkinson's disease, although today it is usually used in combination with other medications (Figure 17.1). Because the loss of dopamine is the primary problem in patients with Parkinson's disease, replacement of the dopamine would be expected to ameliorate the symptoms of the disease. It does, but not by itself, because dopamine poorly crosses the blood-brain barrier from plasma into the central nervous system (CNS). The precursor compound in the biosynthesis of dopamine from the amino acid tyrosine, *dihydroxyphenylalanine* (*dopa*), crosses the blood-brain barrier into the CNS, where it is converted into dopamine, replacing the

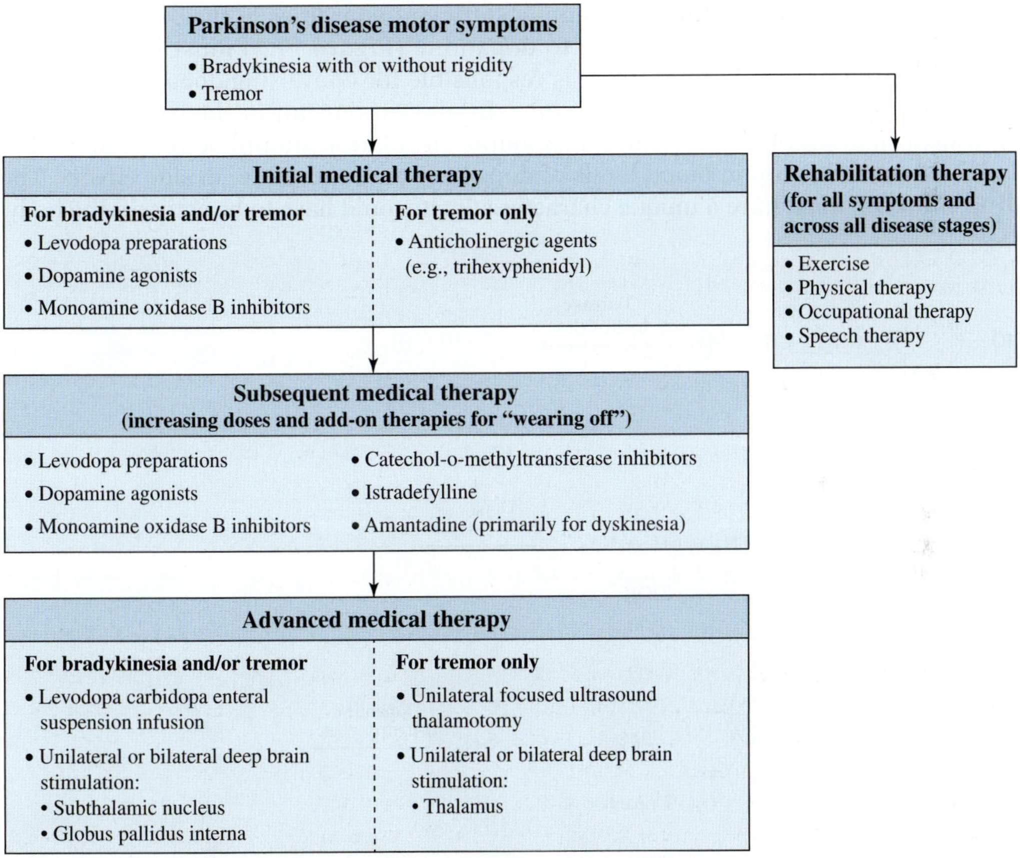

FIGURE 17.1 Parkinson's Disease Therapy. Proposed general approach to treating motor symptoms in Parkinson's disease. Initial treatment can occur with levodopa preparations, dopaminergic agonists, or MAO-B inhibitors, with recent evidence favoring levodopa for many persons. Anticholinergic agents may be used for tremor in young persons who are cognitively intact. Side effects are limiting. Exercise and rehabilitation efforts are needed across all stages. With progression, increasing doses may be necessary and the addition of other therapies with complementary mechanisms of action. [Information from Armstrong and Okun, 2020.]

dopamine that is absent. Therefore, today levodopa—the *levo* isomer being more active than the *dextro* isomer—is the most effective treatment for motor disability.

Mechanism of Action

Administered orally, levodopa is rapidly absorbed into the bloodstream, where most of it (about 95%) is converted to dopamine in the plasma. Although only a small amount (about 1–5%) of levodopa crosses the blood-brain barrier and is converted to dopamine in the brain, it is enough to alleviate the symptoms of Parkinson's disease. In the CNS, levodopa is converted to dopamine, primarily within the presynaptic terminals of dopaminergic neurons in the basal ganglia.

One problem with this therapy is that, when levodopa is administered by itself, it is converted to dopamine in the body, resulting in undesirable side effects such as nausea. One approach to solving the problem is to reduce the high levels of dopamine in the systemic circulation while maintaining sufficient quantities in the brain. To do so, the biosynthetic pathway that leads to dopamine (Figure 17.2) must be examined. Since the enzyme *dopa decarboxylase* is responsible for converting dopa to dopamine, by inhibiting this enzyme in the systemic circulation but not in the brain, systemic biotransformation of any dopa in the systemic circulation should be reduced, with a concomitant reduction in blood levels of dopamine and, therefore, in side effects. The drug, however, must have a unique characteristic: it would have to be active in the body,

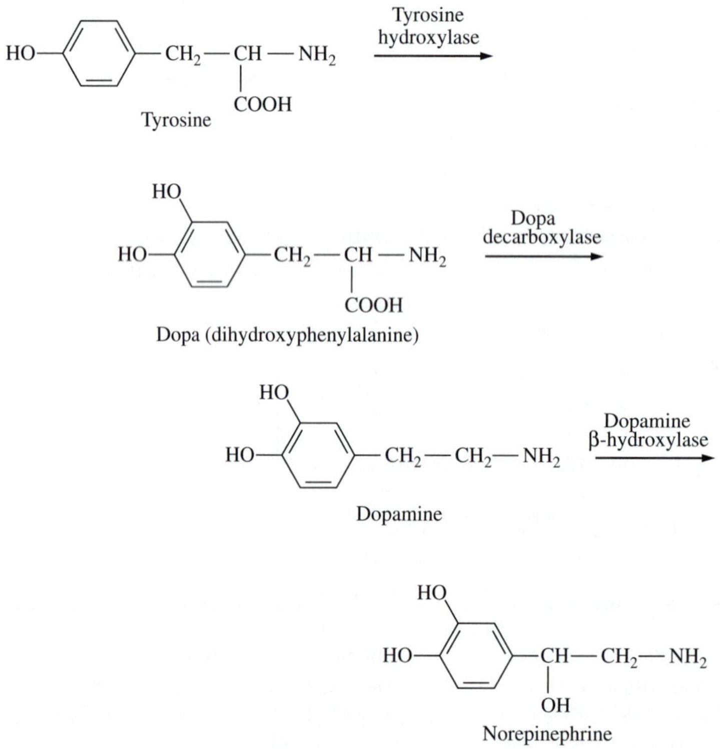

FIGURE 17.2 Synthesis of Dopamine from Tyrosine.

but not cross the blood-brain barrier into the brain. Thus, any dopa that reaches the brain would undergo metabolic conversion in the CNS but not in the periphery.

An example of such a drug is carbidopa in combination with levodopa. The combination is marketed as an immediate-release product (usually generic); a controlled-release version (Sinemet CR); an extended-release version (Rytary); an oral suspension (Duopa); and a carbidopa–levodopa–entacapone combination (Stalevo). The entacapone in Stalevo selectively inhibits the enzyme catechol-o-methyltransferase (COMT) in the periphery, which further protects the levodopa from peripheral degradation and enhances central bioavailability. By combining entacapone and/or carbidopa with levodopa, the dose of levodopa is reduced by 75%, with a concomitant reduction in side effects and no loss of CNS therapeutic effect. (Entacapone and COMT inhibitors will be discussed in more detail in the next section.) The current treatment of Parkinson's disease relies heavily on these products. The combination of levodopa and carbidopa provides near-maximal therapeutic benefit with the fewest side effects (Stocchi et al., 2015).

Side Effects of Levodopa

Unfortunately, as time goes on, each dose of levodopa may become less effective and the patient's symptoms fluctuate dramatically between doses, eventually developing into the "on-off" phenomenon (Figure 17.3). During the "on" phase, symptoms are under good control, but as the medication effect wears off between doses, symptoms become more evident; this is referred to as the "off" phase. Part of the phenomenon is due to the short half-life of levodopa; it can be minimized by increasing the dose and/or by decreasing the interval between doses. This adjustment, however, risks the development of levodopa-induced movement disorders (dyskinesia), which can be as uncomfortable and disabling as the rigidity and akinesia of Parkinsonism. Indeed, within about five years after initiating levodopa treatment, over 50% of patients develop these disabling motor disorders.

The most common side effects of levodopa include hypotension, nausea, dry mouth, dizziness, sedation, and headache early in the course of treatment. Motor symptoms, such as dyskinesias, can develop as the disease progresses. Still later and as the patient ages, confusion, delusions, hallucinations, agitation, and psychosis may be seen. Although psychotic symptoms in other disorders, such as schizophrenia, are treated with antipsychotic medication, using such drugs for patients with Parkinson's disease is problematic, since the drugs block dopamine receptors and would be expected to worsen the core symptoms of the disorder and block the effects of the drugs used to enhance dopamine activity.

Does levodopa therapy adversely accelerate the course of Parkinson's disease? According to most experts, there is no reason to be concerned about advancing the disorder by appropriate use of levodopa, which does not lose its effectiveness over time. But after about five years of treatment, motor complications such as dyskinesias and the "on-off" effect develop as the brain continues to lose dopamine-producing neurons and the remaining neurons make less dopamine. Therefore, it is important to have a comprehensive discussion with patients, spouses, families, and caregivers about the available options and when to start treatment. Although starting treatment early can reduce symptoms, the efficacy may be time limited. Furthermore, waiting too long to start treatment can subject the patient and their loved ones to a significantly reduced quality of life and rising risks of other forms of morbidity, like falling.

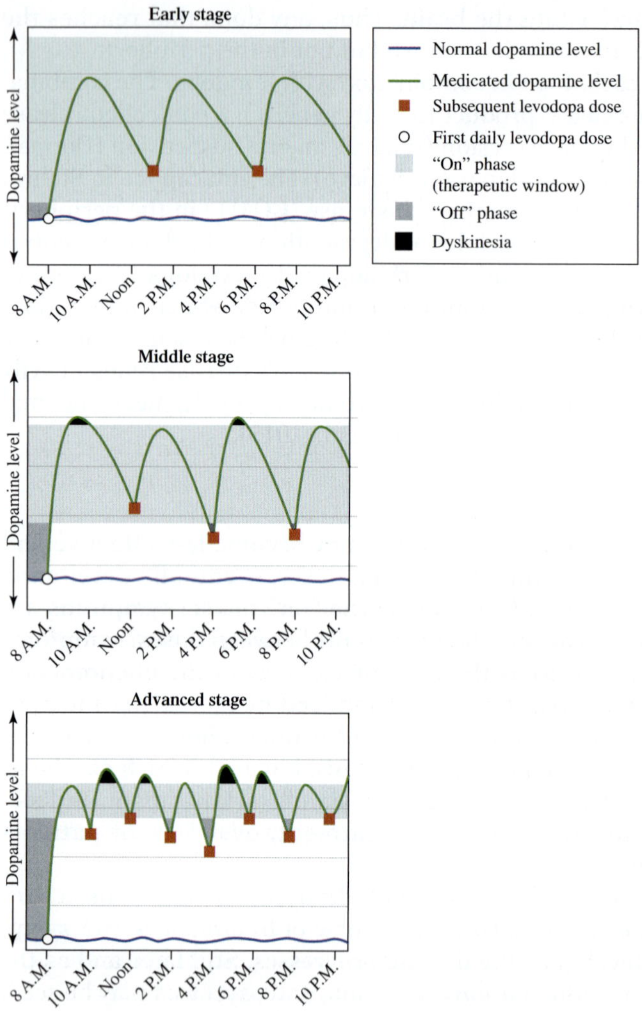

FIGURE 17.3 The "On-Off" Phenomenon with Levodopa. The interaction between medication dosing, the wearing-off phenomenon, and dyskinesias over time. Levodopa is typically dosed three times daily, which provides adequate dopamine concentrations. As the disease progresses, higher and more frequent doses of levodopa are needed. Dyskinesias can also develop. With further progression, the "on" time, when medication helps motor symptoms, narrows. [Information from Armstrong and Okun, 2020.]

Alternatives to Levodopa Therapy

As discussed, levodopa is the most used initial treatment for Parkinson's disease. However, after prolonged or high-dose use, motor complications, such as abnormal involuntary movements and motor fluctuations, can develop. Another drug class can then be added to reduce motor complications and levodopa dose. The most widely used adjuvant drugs are dopamine reuptake inhibitors (DRIs), such as **catechol-o-methyltransferase (COMT) inhibitors** and **monoamine oxidase type B (MAO-B) inhibitors** and dopamine agonists. Researchers addressed the choice of alternative agents and concluded:

> Patient-rated quality of life was inferior when COMT inhibitors were used as adjuvant treatment compared with MAO-B inhibitors or dopamine agonists among people who experienced motor complications that were uncontrolled by levodopa therapy. (Gray et al., 2022, 131)

Here we discuss a variety of alternative agents used to treat Parkinson's disease.

COMT Inhibitors

As noted, one target for the Parkinson's disease therapeutic regimen involves an enzyme called catechol-o-methyltransferase (COMT). Even with the Sinemet combination, much of an oral dose of levodopa is wasted. COMT in the vasculature of the gastrointestinal (GI) tract and liver converts levodopa to an inactive metabolite with no clinical benefit. The half-life and clinical effects of Sinemet can be increased with the addition of a COMT-inhibitory drug. In 1998, the first of these drugs, tolcapone (Tasmar), was introduced; it blocks the COMT enzyme, increasing the half-life of levodopa and prolonging its effect. Unfortunately, tolcapone caused a few cases of serious liver toxicity, so in late 1998 it was withdrawn from the market in Canada and Europe. In the United States, its use is restricted to cases where all other adjunctive therapies have failed, and close monitoring of liver function is required.

A second COMT inhibitor, entacapone (Comtan), became available in 2001 and has not yet been associated with liver toxicity. Like tolcapone, entacapone inhibits peripheral COMT, but does not alter central COMT. Inhibition of peripheral degradation of levodopa increases central levodopa and, therefore, central dopamine concentrations. Coadministration of entacapone with levodopa plus carbidopa potentiates the effects of levodopa in patients with Parkinson's disease and reduces the "off" periods, but use of the COMT inhibitor has also resulted in an increased risk for producing dyskinesias. In 15–20% of patients, the "on-off" phenomenon may be extreme and disabling; doses of levodopa that originally were effective for 8 hours last for only 1 or 2 hours.

In 2004, the FDA approved a fixed combination product, Stalevo, containing levodopa, carbidopa, and entacapone. The combination provides more dopamine to the brain for a longer period of time, providing more "on" time and less "off" time associated with each dose of levodopa. The most common side effects associated with the use of COMT inhibitors like entacapone include dyskinesia, hallucinations, confusion, nausea, diarrhea, orange discoloration of the urine, and low blood pressure after standing up. In fact, in the randomized controlled trial Stalevo Reduction in Dyskinesia Evaluation in Parkinson's Disease (STRIDE-PD), it was found that adding entacapone did indeed reduce the frequency of the "on-off" episodes, but it also increased the frequency of dyskinesias. The results also indicated that there was an increase in the frequency of cardiovascular events such as myocardial infarction and stroke (Stocchi et al., 2015). Thus, there was some concern about the safety of using Stalevo; however, a later analysis of the data from the STRIDE-PD study did not find any increase in myocardial infarctions, stroke, prostate cancer, or death in entacapone-treated patients.

More recently, an alternative COMT inhibitor has become available. As with entacapone, opicapone (Ongentys) decreases L-dopa peripheral metabolism. Taken once daily, it appears to be a safe and effective alternative COMT inhibitor (Rodrigues and Ferreira, 2017; Salamon et al., 2019)

Dopamine Receptor Agonists

Between one and five years after the start of levodopa therapy, most patients gradually become less responsive. One hypothesis for this effect is that the progression of Parkinson's disease may be associated with an increasing inability of dopamine neurons to synthesize and store dopamine. To relieve this problem, attempts have been made to identify drugs that directly stimulate postsynaptic dopamine receptors in the basal ganglia. These drugs do not depend on the ability of existing dopaminergic neurons to synthesize dopamine. As a result, they are increasingly being advocated for use in early stages of Parkinson's disease, especially in patients younger than about 65. These drugs might also be effective in the later stages of Parkinson's disease, when dopamine neurons are largely absent or nonfunctional.

Several dopamine receptor agonists are available in the United States for the treatment of Parkinson's disease: bromocriptine (Parlodel), pramipexole (Mirapex), transdermal rotigotine (Neupro), and ropinirole (Requip). Apomorphine (Apokyn) is an older drug that can be used as an adjunctive treatment for the sudden appearance of the "off" phase. It is injected and its effects are of rapid onset and last about 30 minutes. It is usually used as a "rescue" medication when the levodopa effect wears off between doses. Clinicians must be trained in its administration; it causes significant nausea and is taken with antinausea medication.

Bromocriptine has been available since 1978 and has a structure that closely resembles that of dopamine. Pramipexole and ropinirole were marketed in 1997. They are indicated for use in early-onset Parkinson's disease; their efficacy and safety profiles are much better than that of bromocriptine. Both can increase quality of life in the early stages of the disease by improving motor problems and decreasing fluctuations in response to levodopa. Pramipexole also exerts a beneficial antidepressant effect. Their long half-lives may at least partially explain the reduction in the "on-off" phenomenon of levodopa therapy. Side effects of dopamine agonists include somnolence, dizziness and orthostatic hypotension, nausea and vomiting, hallucinations, confusion, swelling of the legs and feet, insomnia, dyskinesias, and impulse control disorders discussed earlier (Grall-Bronnec et al., 2018; Lizarraga et al., 2020). Pramipexole and probably ropinirole cause what is known as "sleep attacks." These are unpredictable sudden-onset episodes of extreme sedation or drowsiness. Thus, patients must be warned about driving and the increased risk of attack if using other drugs that cause sedation or have other disorders of sleep regulation.

Monoamine Oxidase B Inhibitors

Selegiline (Eldepryl, Zelapar) reduces symptoms of Parkinson's disease through a unique mechanism.[4] The enzyme *monoamine oxidase* (MAO) exists in two isoenzyme

[4]In Chapter 12, selegiline is discussed as the antidepressant transdermal skin patch Emsam.

forms: MAO-A and MAO-B. Although both are present in the brain, MAO-B is the more predominant enzyme, while MAO-A is more predominant in the periphery, especially in the GI tract. MAO-A is more closely involved with tyramine, norepinephrine, serotonin, and, to some extent, dopamine nerve terminals, while MAO-B has preferential affinity for dopamine neurons located in the substantia nigra. Selegiline selectively and irreversibly inhibits MAO-B. As a result, selegiline inhibits the local breakdown of dopamine, thus preserving the small amounts of dopamine that are present. Both actions enhance the therapeutic effect of levodopa. Unlike the older nonselective MAO inhibitors used as clinical antidepressants (Chapter 12), selegiline does not inhibit peripheral metabolism of levodopa; thus, it can safely be taken with levodopa. Selegiline also exhibits fewer drug-food interactions, at least at the lowest dose commercially available of 6 milligrams daily. Unfortunately, in Parkinson's disease, selegiline's usefulness is limited.

Approved by the FDA in 2006, rasagiline (Azilect) is the second selective MAO-B inhibitor FDA-approved for Parkinson's disease. Rasagiline increases "on" times and decreases "off" periods when combined with carbidopa or levodopa. Rasagiline is a centrally acting selective inhibitor of MAO-B that is thought to increase extracellular dopamine in the striatum. Researchers reported a possibly beneficial effect of the early use of rasagiline at a dose of 1 milligram per day but negative findings at a dose of 2 milligrams per day (Olanow et al., 2009). Rasagiline may also possess a potential neuroprotective effect against the progression of Parkinson's disease (Szoko et al., 2018) as well as in Alzheimer's disease (where it increases cerebral blood flow in several brain regions) (Song et al., 2021). Some authors suggest that MAO-B drugs should be used as the initial treatment for Parkinson's disease due to their safety profile (Gray et al., 2022). By using them first, providers can save the use of L-dopa until Parkinsonian symptoms become more severe and disabling. Side effects associated with the selective MAO-B inhibitors include agitation, dizziness, nausea, headache, back pain, and difficulty falling asleep, especially with selegiline. Thus, selegiline should not be given after 1:00 P.M. In older adults with Parkinson disease, selegiline often causes confusion, which may prevent it from being useful in this group. Combining MAO-B inhibitors with drugs that increase dopaminergic activity can sometimes produce dyskinesias, hallucinations, and hypertension.

Recently introduced was a third MAO-B inhibitor, safinamide (Xadago) (Blair and Dhillon, 2017). Safinamide is intended as adjunctive medication to levodopa/carbidopa in patients with mid- to late-stage Parkinson's disease (Bette et al., 2018; Muller, 2018). In addition to improvements in motor activity, safinamide also appears to exert neuroprotective effects that could be beneficial to patients, as it may slow the progression of neuronal loss (Teixeira et al., 2018). Researchers compared selegiline, rasagiline and safinamide, concluding:

> Selegiline and rasagiline are irreversible inhibitors forming a covalent bond with MAO-B. In contrast, safinamide is a reversible inhibitor. . . . Among antiparkinsonian agents, MAO-B inhibitors have the greatest neuroprotective potential because of inhibition of dopamine metabolism, induction of neuroprotective factors, and, with safinamide, inhibition of glutamate release. (Alborghetti and Nicoletti, 2019)

Cholinergic Receptor Antagonists

Although widely used before the introduction of levodopa, anticholinergic agents are now used much less and are considered second-tier agents for the treatment of Parkinsonian symptoms. The use of these drugs was based on an understanding of the control of fine motor movements through the nigrostriatal system. The normal control of movement requires a balance between dopamine and acetylcholine transmission within this system, hence the so-called *dopamine–acetylcholine balance theory* of movement disorders. Any shift in this balance through an increase or decrease in one neurotransmitter relative to the other results in hypo- or hyperkinetic movement disorders. In Parkinson's disease, the dopamine-producing cell bodies in the substantial nigra are being destroyed and dopamine output is decreasing, producing a functional imbalance in the dopamine–acetylcholine transmission in favor of acetylcholine. To restore balance, you can either (1) increase the dopamine transmission by using one of the methods described earlier, such as replacement, postsynaptic stimulation, or inhibition of breakdown, or (2) decrease the effect of acetylcholine by using anticholinergic drugs.

Occasionally, anticholinergic drugs are used as an adjunct to L-dopa in patients with tremors that are difficult to control. Anticholinergic drugs relieve tremor in about 50% of patients, but they do not reduce rigidity or motor slowing. Anticholinergic drugs, however, can produce cognitive dysfunction that limits their use, especially in older adults, who may already have an underlying cognitive disorder (Sheu et al., 2019). Representative agents include trihexyphenidyl (Artane), biperiden (Akineton), and benztropine (Cogentin). Occasionally, the antihistaminic drug diphenhydramine (Benadryl) is also used because diphenhydramine has significant anticholinergic properties. Typical side effects of anticholinergic drugs include dry mouth, blurred vision, constipation, urinary retention, and the already mentioned potential for cognitive impairment.

Amantadine and Memantine

Amantadine (Symmetrel) is an antiviral agent used to treat viral influenza with modest antiparkinsonian actions (to control tremor). Its mechanism of action in Parkinson's disease is unclear; it may alter dopamine release or reuptake, or it may have anticholinergic properties. Its effect is mainly to reduce dyskinesias, but this may only be temporary. Side effects include dry mouth, constipation, urinary retention, swelling of the ankles, confusion, possible visual hallucinations, and a blotchy, purplish skin rash on the extremities. Amantadine and a related drug, **memantine** (Namenda), are active at NMDA-type glutaminergic receptors; this action perhaps offers a degree of "brain protection" that may contribute to its effects. Memantine is used to treat the cognitive and behavioral effects of dementia. Side effects include diarrhea, dizziness, weakness, sleepiness or trouble sleeping, and nausea.

In 2017, an extended-release form of amantadine (Gocovri) was the first drug FDA-approved specifically to treat dyskinesia in Parkinson's disease. This was followed shortly thereafter by a second extended-release form of amantadine (Osmolex-ER). Both are once daily formulations.

THC Analogues

Researchers demonstrated that *nabilone* effectively reduced the nonmotor symptoms in Parkinson's disease (Peball et al., 2020). Nabilone (Chapter 9) is a synthetic analogue of tetrahydrocannabinol (THC) with similar properties to THC, namely, a partial agonist action at both cannabinoid 1 and 2 receptors. Required doses were low. Unexpected side effects included a worsening of motor symptoms.

Researchers also discuss the neuroprotective effects of phytocannabinoids, which may be neuroprotective due to antioxidant and anti-inflammatory effects (Prakash and Carter, 2021). Such agents might be used to ameliorate Parkinson's disease progression and/or provide neuroprotective effects to reduce the risk of development of Parkinsonism. The Parkinson's Foundation has published a consensus statement on the use of medical marijuana for Parkinson's disease (Parkinson's Foundation, 2020). They noted that "The most promising avenue for now seems to be the use of CBD [cannabidiol] for the symptomatic relief of non-motor symptoms associated with Parkinson's disease (anxiety, sleep disturbances, and pain)."

Other Drugs and Formulations

As mentioned earlier, pimavanserin has been approved by the FDA specifically to treat psychosis in Parkinson's disease (Ballard et al., 2020). Pimavanserin is an atypical antipsychotic drug that is an inverse agonist at 5-HT2_A receptors, thus reducing serotonergic activity. It is effective in reducing hallucinations and delusions without causing a worsening of Parkinsonian symptoms (Bozymski et al., 2017; Kianirad and Simuni, 2017).

Other drugs and formulations being used to treat Parkinson's disease include the following:

- New formulations of levodopa. An example is Inbrija, which is an inhaled version of levodopa that is used as a rescue medication for "off" periods.
- New formulations of apomorphine. An example is Apokyn, which is a sublingual formulation also to be used as a rescue medication for "off" periods.
- Adenosine A_{2A} receptor antagonists, which reduce "off" times and suppress dyskinesias. An example is istradefylline (Nourianz), which was FDA-approved in 2019 as an adjunct to levodopa therapy in Parkinson's disease. The adenosine A_{2A} receptor is expressed in the brain and has a role in the regulation of glutamate and dopamine, making it an interesting target for the treatment of Parkinson's disease.
- Droxidopa (Northera) is a prodrug, metabolized to norepinephrine in nerve endings and other tissues. The drug has now been FDA-approved in patients with neurodegenerative diseases such as parkinsonism (Palma and Kaufmann, 2020; Quarracino et al., 2020).

Apathy

Apathy, or lack of motivation, indifference, or general lack of interest, is a significant problem in patients with Parkinson's disease (Pagonabarrage and Kulisevsky, 2017). Not only does it interfere with effectiveness of treatment, but it also poses significant burdens on caregivers, families, and medical costs. Researchers discuss the diagnosis and management of apathy in Parkinson's disease (Mele et al., 2020) and propose that neuronal degeneration in the prefrontal cortex produces symptoms of apathy (van Dyck et al., 2021). They further propose that methylphenidate may ameliorate these symptoms by "boosting norepinephrine and dopamine actions in prefrontal-striatal-thalamocortical circuits."

ALZHEIMER'S DISEASE

Alzheimer's disease is the most common neurodegenerative disease and accounts for 60–80% of all cases of dementia. It is a progressive disease that results in the irreversible loss of cholinergic neurons, particularly in the cerebral cortex and hippocampus, and is characterized by the abnormal accumulation of amyloid-β and tau proteins in the brain (Pirscoveanu et al, 2017; Shepherd et al.,2020). Onset occurs generally after 65 years of age but is being increasingly reported in people between the ages of 34 and 64 years (Hendriks et al., 2021). There are approximately 175,000 persons in the age range of 34–64 years with dementia and more than 6.5 million persons over the age of 65 years with dementia in the United States (Knopman, 2021). The number of people aged 65 and older with Alzheimer's disease is estimated to reach 7.1 million by 2025. By 2050, the number may almost triple to a projected 13.8 million, barring the development of medical breakthroughs to prevent, slow, or stop the disease. Currently, Alzheimer's costs the nation $260 billion. This number is expected to rise to $1.1 trillion by 2050.

Time between symptom onset and death may span four to eight years. Alzheimer's disease is the sixth leading cause of death in the United States. (See the Did You Know? box.) The gradual and continuous decline caused by Alzheimer's disease is characterized by cognitive deterioration, changes in behavior, loss of functional independence, and increasing requirements for care. Hallmarks of prodromal or early onset of Alzheimer's disease include progressive impairment in memory, judgment, decision making, orientation to physical surroundings, and language. **Dementia**, defined as cognitive impairment with the inability to form new memory, is the critical feature of Alzheimer's disease. Diagnosis is based on neurological examination and the exclusion of other causes of dementia. A combined workgroup from the National Institute on Aging and the Alzheimer's Association has established guidelines for an Alzheimer's diagnosis (Jack et al., 2011; McKhann et al., 2011). These diagnostic guidelines expanded upon older guidelines, adding two modifications: (1) the incorporation of biomarker tests[5] and (2) the identification of three stages of the disease. These three stages are (1) a preclinical stage, in which biomarker changes may signal the presence of the disease before any cognitive or behavioral signs or symptoms appear (Jack et al., 2018; Oh and Rabins, 2019); (2) mild cognitive impairment (MCI), which is a stage of the disorder that presents with mild cognitive changes that do not necessarily impair daily functioning or always progress to definitive Alzheimer's disease; and (3) Alzheimer's disease

[5]*Biomarker tests* are clinical tests that can measure some biological change in the body or brain that can be reliably associated with the presence of the disease.

with all of the recognized signs and symptoms (Karlawish et al., 2017). Unfortunately, until recently, a definitive diagnosis could be made only at autopsy, where neuronal loss and accumulation of deposits of protein plaques (amyloid-β) and neurofibrillary tangles, composed of abnormal microtubules (tau), are observed. It is not yet known whether these plaques and tangles might cause Alzheimer's disease or may actually be protective.

Did You Know?

Alzheimer's Disease Age-Adjusted* Death Rates in 2019, by State

In 2019, there were seven states with an age-adjusted death rate from Alzheimer's disease of over 40 per 100,000 population: Mississippi (48.8), Alabama (44.6), Washington (42.2), Georgia (41.9), Louisiana (41.4), Tennessee (41.1), and South Dakota (40.5). At the other end of the scale, six states had an age-adjusted death rate of under 20 per 100,000 population: New York (13.7), Maryland (13.8), Massachusetts (17.7), Connecticut (18.1), Florida (18.3), and Hawaii (19.1). The Centers for Disease Control and Prevention states that the most closely correlated risk factors for Alzheimer's disease are age and genetics. However, a number of modifiable risk factors have been identified that may prevent or delay dementia (Livingston et al., 2020). These include hypertension, untreated hearing impairment, smoking, obesity, depression, diabetes, low social contact, head injury, excessive alcohol consumption, air pollution exposure in later life, and physical activity. Indeed, researchers have noted that regular exercise lowered tau concentrations and slowed the rate of cognitive decline (Desai et al., 2021).

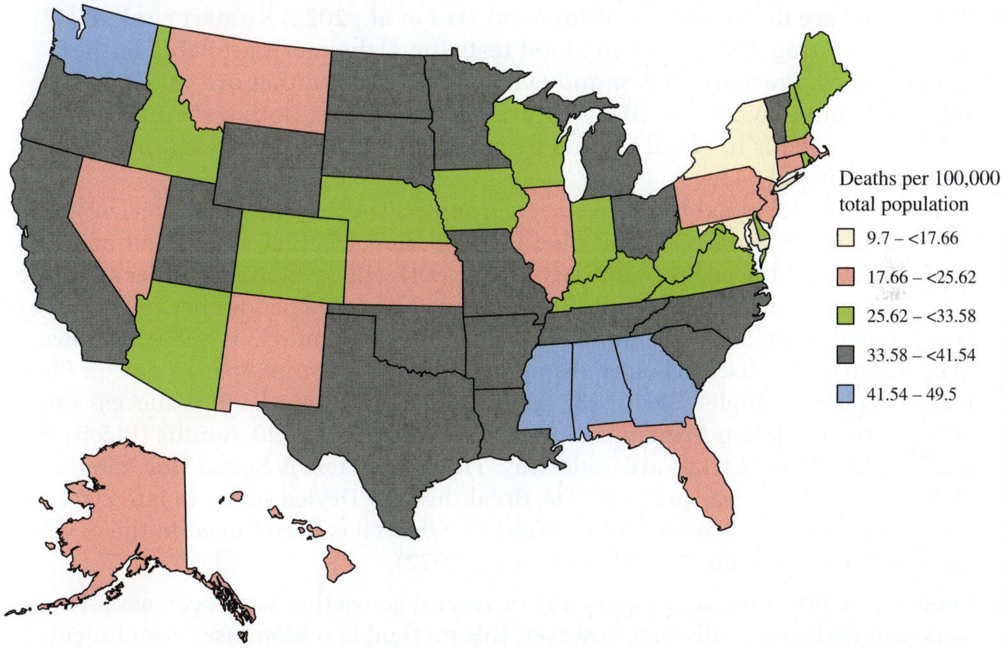

[Data from National Center for Health Statistics, U.S. Centers for Disease Control and Prevention.]

**Age-adjusted* means that the death rates are adjusted for differences in total population and age distribution in the individual states.

Great interest has arisen over early diagnosis of Alzheimer's disease because by the time mental decline is observable, severe brain damage has already occurred. Early diagnosis also can help families plan for the future, take care of financial and legal matters, address safety issues, learn about living options, and develop social networks. To this end, the following biomarkers are being evaluated (Alzheimer's Association, 2022):

1. Structural imaging techniques like magnetic resonance imaging (MRI), computed tomography (CT) scans, functional MRI, and single-photon emission computed tomography (SPECT) can define tissue damage and rule out other illnesses with similar symptoms to Alzheimer's. Researchers studied prognostic markers of early Alzheimer's disease in 1431 persons with varying stages of early cognitive decline and found that tau positron emission tomography (PET) scans were more sensitive for predicting cognitive decline than amyloid scans, and tau PET is "a promising prognostic tool for predicting cognitive decline in preclinical and prodromal stages of Alzheimer's disease" (Ossenkoppele et al., 2021).
2. The study of proteins present in cerebrospinal fluid (CSF), obtained by an invasive procedure called a spinal tap, can link biomarkers, such as total tau, beta-amyloid, and phosphorylated tau, that correlate their presence with early-onset Alzheimer's (Young and Mormino, 2022). This method, the Lumipulse G β-Amyloid Ratio test, has been extensively clinically validated and is now FDA-approved (FDA news release, May 2022; Hansson et al., 2021; Levey, 2021; Rubin, 2022a).
3. Blood tests are under rapid development (Hu et al., 2022; Kumari et al., 2022). As of this writing, there are two blood tests for Alzheimer's available in the United States: *PrecivityAD Test* and *Quest AD-Detect*. Neither are yet FDA-approved, and they are not likely covered by insurance. Both tests measure amyloid-β proteins in blood plasma by measuring the ratio of two amyloid-β proteins, β40 and β42.

   Two additional blood tests have been granted FDA Breakthrough Device status. The first is *AlzoSure Predict*. This blood test predicts whether an asymptomatic patient (having little or no cognitive impairment) will develop Alzheimer's disease in the next six years (Garcia et al., 2021). A protein called p53 is checked along with how it reacts to an antibody and binds to it. High levels of p53 have been shown to be a sign of the disease before the appearance of its symptoms. To date, a Phase 1 trial has been completed with 482 participants and showed a 98% success rate in correctly predicting Alzheimer's disease over a period of 90 months (Piccirella et al., 2022). Phase 2 trials are underway. The second test is *Simoa* (for "single molecule array"). It was granted FDA Breakthrough Device status in late 2021 and it tests for a specific protein called pTau181, which has been linked to the development of Alzheimer's disease (Thomas et al., 2022).
4. Genetic risk profiling can identify any of several genes that have been associated with Alzheimer's disease; however, this method is seldom used for clinical diagnosis.

As testing methods evolve, they will require much public discussion (Musiek and Morris, 2021), as early diagnosis requires serious societal, family, and financial decisions.

Medication Therapy

Most of the drugs currently used for treating patients with Alzheimer's disease only ameliorate symptoms by acting on brain neurotransmitters. These drugs, while clinically useful, do not alter the course or the progression of the disease.

Acetylcholinesterase Inhibitors

The fact that some of the symptoms of Alzheimer's disease are thought to be due to a deficiency of acetylcholine[6] neurotransmission has given rise to a **cholinergic-deficiency theory** of Alzheimer's disease. Indeed, researchers have found that deficits in the functioning of acetylcholine-secreting neurons (cholinergic deficits) are correlated with the cognitive impairments of Alzheimer's disease (Marucci et al., 2021). Consistent with this idea is the observation that patients with severe Alzheimer's disease show acetylcholine and acetylcholinesterase (AChE) levels that are 60–85% lower than normal, which implies very little residual cholinesterase enzyme in the cortex—a condition that is still compatible with life, but no longer optimal for brain function. Therefore, reinforcing cholinergic function by inhibiting the enzyme that breaks down acetylcholine in the synapse (Chapters 2 and 3) is a widespread therapy. In practice, this is accomplished through use of drugs called *acetylcholinesterase inhibitors* (*AChE-I*), which do not alter the course of the dementia but attempt to slow cognitive decline. As Alzheimer's disease progresses and fewer cholinergic neurons remain functional, the effects of these drugs diminish. Currently, there are three FDA-approved AChE inhibitors, each offering modest improvements in cognitive symptoms (Alzheimer's Association, 2022; Blanco-Silvente et al., 2017; Haake et al., 2020).

1. Donepezil (Aricept), approved for all stages of Alzheimer's
2. Rivastigmine (Exelon), approved for mild to moderate Alzheimer's
3. Galantamine (Razadyne), approved for mild to moderate Alzheimer's

Donepezil can provide minimal to moderate stability in cognitive function and behavioral improvement for some patients with Alzheimer's. Maybe about one-third of individuals will derive some benefit and one-fifth will demonstrate much more definitive benefit. A seven-day donepezil patch was shown to be comparable to oral tablets and provides convenience for caregivers (Dinh et al., 2022; Han et al., 2022). The patch (trade name Adlarity) received FDA approval in 2022.

---

[6]It has long been appreciated that acetylcholine is involved in cognitive functioning, memory, learning, attention, and other higher brain functions (Hampel et al., 2018).

Rivastigmine is clinically effective, producing modest improvements in cognitive functioning and activities of daily living. It also causes a very slow reversible inhibition of AChE-I, prolonging its therapeutic action. Also available is a rivastigmine transdermal patch (Exelon Patch). With the patch, 24-hour concentrations remain relatively stable (Khoury et al., 2018). Caregivers may prefer the patch to the oral capsule. Researchers stated:

> Rivastigmine's availability as both a transdermal formulation and oral capsule may improve adherence rates and care giver satisfaction. To date, the data from randomized clinical trials and post marketing observational studies have shown evidence for an impact on cognitive functions in Alzheimer's disease with good safety and tolerability. (Nguyen et al., 2021, 35)

Galantamine appears to have a safety and efficacy profile similar to that of rivastigmine in measures of both cognitive functioning and functional ability. In a study of older patients (average age 84 years) with severe Alzheimer's disease, researchers reported that galantamine moderately improved cognitive functioning, but failed to significantly improve measures of overall activities of daily living (Burns et al., 2009).

In addition, a naturally occurring AChE-I, **huperzine A**, has been studied as a treatment for Alzheimer's disease. This substance, derived from the moss *Huperzia serrata*, has been used for centuries as a Chinese folk medicine. It has modest AChE-I activity, and it may be useful as an alternative medication for treatment of Alzheimer's disease (Damar et al., 2016). Researchers studied huperzine analogues and noted that some had "advantages of easy synthesis, high potency and selectivity, and improved neuroprotection, making it a potential huperzine-type lead compound for Alzheimer's disease drug development" (Miao et al., 2021).

These data imply that AChE inhibitors have modest but positive effects compared with placebo in Alzheimer's disease treatment, affecting cognition, function, and behavioral outcomes, as previously mentioned; however, the effects are not sustained indefinitely, and the disease continues to progress even while patients are receiving treatment. Until new therapies are developed, the AChE inhibitors will remain important Alzheimer's disease treatments.

Memantine

Glutamate is the principal excitatory neurotransmitter in the brain. Glutaminergic overactivity may result in neuronal damage, a phenomenon termed *excitotoxicity*. Excitotoxicity ultimately leads to neuronal calcium overload and has been implicated in neurodegenerative disorders. In addition, glutaminergic NMDA receptor activity appears to be important in memory processes, dementia, and the pathogenesis of Alzheimer's disease. Glutaminergic overstimulation at NMDA receptors is thought to be toxic to neurons, and prevention of this neurotoxicity affords a degree of brain protection to limit further deterioration.

Memantine (discussed earlier in the section on Parkinson's disease) is a noncompetitive NMDA receptor antagonist that has been shown to reduce clinical deterioration in patients with moderate to severe Alzheimer's disease. It seems to promote cellular plasticity, can preserve or enhance memory, and can protect against the excitotoxic destruction of cholinergic neurons. As a "weak" NMDA antagonist, memantine may reduce overactive NMDA receptor activity that would be neurotoxic while sparing the synaptic responsiveness required for normal behavioral functioning, cognition, and memory.

As with the AChE inhibitors, memantine does not attack the root cause of Alzheimer's disease, which is believed to involve brain proteins and peptides rather than neurotransmitters. Thus, these drugs may forestall further functional decline for a limited time, but they have not been shown to slow the disease progression or avoid the ultimate outcome.

Memantine's efficacy is perhaps best when combined with an AChE inhibitor (Kishi et al., 2017). Namzaric is the brand name of a combination product containing memantine and donepezil. Namzaric simplifies administration, although not all studies find that adding a second Alzheimer's drug produces any additional benefit.

Dopaminergic Neurotransmission

In the previous discussions, cholinergic neurotransmission was presented as the major pharmacological target of current treatments (AChE inhibitors); however, as recently discussed by researchers:

> Much evidence has strengthened the idea that impairment of dopaminergic transmission might contribute to cognitive dysfunction in Alzheimer's disease. Dopamine is a key neuromodulator affecting several distinct steps of synaptic transmission, playing an important role in the control of higher cognitive functions, such as memory, learning, and decision making. (Koch et al., 2020)

As a result, researchers have evaluated the efficacy of rotigotine (Neupro), a dopaminergic receptor agonist, to improve cholinergic transmission and cortical plasticity in 94 patients with mild to moderate Alzheimer's disease. A transdermal skin patch administered to patients already on AChE inhibitors, rotigotine failed to improve global cognition but did appear to improve cognitive functions associated with the frontal lobe and in activities of daily living.

Aducanumab, Donanemab, and Related Drugs

In 2021, the FDA gave accelerated approval for **aducanumab** (Aduhelm) for the treatment of mild to moderate cognitive impairment in patients with Alzheimer's disease. Aducanumab does not act on brain neurotransmitters and appears to reduce beta-amyloid plaques in the brain, an action the FDA hopes will "lead to a reduction in the clinical decline of this devastating form of dementia" (Avgerinos et al., 2021; Cavazzoni, 2021; Mukhopadhyay and Banerjee, 2021). According to researchers:

> Aducanumab is the first monoclonal antibody approved for mild Alzheimer's disease. As the definition of Alzheimer's disease has evolved, the amyloid-β (Aβ) pathway has been increasingly implicated in its pathogenesis. The approval of Aducanumab is based on reduction of the Aβ, which forms a surrogate marker for this pathway. (Mukhopadhyay and Banerjee, 2021, 1537)

Aducanumab was the first new Alzheimer's therapy since 2003. Approval was based on two trials sponsored by the manufacturer. One trial was "trending positive while the second showed no benefits" (Alexander et al., 2021; Knopman et al., 2021). Both

DR. J'S MUSINGS 17.1

Was the FDA Objective?

Before a drug is approved for sale, an outside committee of independent, objective scholars reviews the data submitted to the FDA. Almost always, the FDA will follow the expert panel's recommendation. In the case of aducanumab, however, the committee vote was almost unanimously against approval (ten members opposed approval and one member was uncertain) (Manly and Glymour, 2021), yet the drug was still approved. Since that time, at least three committee members have resigned in protest. As a result, the Office of the Inspector General has been asked to investigate whether FDA employees who favored approval may have worked too closely with employees of the drug manufacturer. Several senators and congressional representatives have called for hearings to investigate how the FDA made its decision (Karlawish, 2021). Approval has raised false hopes, despite the enormous cost of the drug. Given the lack of demonstration of efficacy against meaningful improvements in the life of patients with early Alzheimer's, should government insurers be required to pay for the drug, or should it be a self-purchase by the wealthy who might be able to afford the drug, even if it is not effective? To me, the rush to approval by the FDA in the absence of proven efficacy in patients has left too much uncertainty, confusion, and anger to justify current approval.

trials were stopped early, and the manufacturer stated that there was sufficient efficacy signal to justify approval. The FDA apparently concluded that reduction in amyloid load in early Alzheimer's was a valid surrogate end point for potential clinical benefit. The FDA's decision was immediately controversial (see Dr. J's Musings 17.1) and raised multiple questions, including who will pay for this questionably effective drug. Indeed, only after approval did the manufacturer announce the price: aducanumab will come to market at an annual price of $56,000 (Schulman et al., 2021), a value that has now been reduced to $28,200 but which is still overpriced. Researchers estimated that a cost-effective price for the drug ranged from $2,950 to $8,360 per year (Whittington et al., 2022). Because of its expense and as yet unproven efficacy, the Centers for Medicare and Medicaid (CMS) has proposed that they will pay for aducanumab and related drugs only in patients who are enrolled in clinical trials (Centers for Medicare & Medicaid Services, 2022). Even this decision is controversial. Researchers discuss this controversy and state that "definitive results will hopefully be available by the end of 2023" (Shi et al., 2022).

A second, very similar drug, **donanemab**, is under development (Mintun et al., 2021). Donanemab is another monoclonal antibody that uniquely targets amyloid-β (p3-42), a pyroglutamate form of amyloid-β (Aβ) exclusively found in plaques, thereby reducing the excess protein that supposedly causes these abnormal plaques. Researchers reported on a Phase 2 clinical trial of donanemab in patients in the earliest stages of Alzheimer's disease (Mintun et al., 2021). The authors, all affiliated with the manufacturer of the drug, claimed reductions in amyloid plaque levels along with improvements in cognition (compared with non-drug-treated controls) and improvements in activities of daily living at 76 weeks of treatment. In contrast, another researcher criticized the conduct and conclusions of the initial study of donanemab, stating:

> Tau load may be a biomarker of cognition but was not altered by donanemab. As there is no clear evidence that removing cerebral amyloid plaques with Aβ antibodies, such as donanemab, improves cognition and the activities of daily living in Alzheimer's disease, trials with these agents should be abandoned. (Doggrell, 2021, 797)

A Phase 3 clinical trial is underway and is scheduled for completion in November 2025. Donanemab has been reported to be similarly non-cost-effective (Ross et al., 2022). At this time, efficacy in reducing the rate of cognitive impairment and clinical benefit has not been demonstrated (Karlawish, 2021; Rubin, 2021c, 2021b). However, recently other researchers concluded that donanemab cleared abnormal amyloid levels in the brain and such reduction was associated with reductions in tau load and positive effects on disease progression (Shcherbinin et al., 2022).

Under early development is a third monoclonal antibody, **semorinemab**, that targets brain proteins that tend to accumulate in Alzheimer's disease. Specifically, semorinemab targets tau proteins. Early Phase 1 data were encouraging, but in a larger 73-week Phase 2 study in 422 patients with prodromal of early Alzheimer's disease, semorinemab did not slow clinical deterioration or slow tau accumulation (Teng et al., 2022). One researcher reviews the mostly discouraging data on drugs targeting amyloid deposits in the brain, focusing on nonamyloid therapies such as tau neurofibrillary tangles that are a hallmark of Alzheimer's disease (Rubin, 2022a).

Lecanemab is anti-amyloid protofibril antibody that in January 2023 received accelerated FDA approval under the brand name Leqembi for use in early Alzheimer's disease. Administered i.v. every two weeks, the drug significantly reduced brain amyloid levels and exerted positive effects on clinical decline (Swanson et al., 2022). Brain edema is a major side effect occurring in about 12% of patients.

SAGE-718 is a cholesterol derivative that is a positive allosteric modulator of the glutaminergic NMDA receptor and, as such, may improve learning and memory in patients with neurodegenerative diseases such as Alzheimer's (Hill et al., 2022). The drug is currently in Phase 2 clinical testing for treatment of cognitive impairment and executive functioning.

Candesartan

Researchers examined the comparative neurocognitive effects of two mechanistically different antihypertensive medications in older adults (mean age 66 years) with mild cognitive impairment (Hajjar et al., 2020). Compared were an angiotensin receptor blocker, **candesartan** (Atacand), and an angiotensin-converting enzyme inhibitor, lisinopril, in adults with hypertension and cognitive impairment. Of the two, candesartan was associated with improvement in executive cognitive processing as well as in memory processing. Effects appear to be independent of therapeutic effects of the drug on blood pressure.

Omega-3 Fatty Acids

Although they are not traditional medication, early studies on the effects of diets rich in fish oils, such as the omega-3 fatty acids docosahexaenoic acid (DHA) and eicosapentaenoic acid (EPA), reported a 47% reduction in the incidence of Alzheimer's disease in a large population of British older adults (Schaefer et al., 2006). Based on these early findings, it was thought that taking omega-3 fatty acid supplements or eating foods rich in omega-3s might be a good prophylactic intervention. Subsequent studies have not provided a definitive answer to the question of whether omega-3 supplementation may delay or prevent the cognitive decline seen in Alzheimer's disease. Researchers demonstrated that combination treatment of vitamin B together with omega-3 fatty acid was effective in slowing the rate of brain atrophy in older adults with mild cognitive impairment while either treatment alone was ineffective (Jerneren et al., 2015; Oulhaj et al., 2016). While reviewing omega-3 fatty acids for dementia, other researchers stated that omaga-3 fatty acids "might be a promising treatment option for dementia" (Burckhardt et al., 2016). Still others have reiterated conclusions that omega-3 fatty acid treatment "may be beneficial in disease onset, where there is slight impairment of brain function" (Canhada et al., 2018). However, there is no strong evidence that taking EPA and DHA supplements or eating fish and other omega-3-rich foods on a regular basis has any beneficial effect for individuals who currently suffer from dementia. Usefulness would be only in very early, prodromal, and mild states of memory dysfunction (Ajith, 2018; Desale and Chinnathambi, 2020).

In the Pipeline

Researchers discussed the results (and, mostly, lack thereof) of new drugs in the pipeline for use in Alzheimer's disease (Cummings et al., 2022). To date, most trials have been terminated early because of lack of efficacy. As stated, "Effective or disease-modifying drugs for Alzheimer's are still lacking" (Huang et al., 2020). Nevertheless, dozens of drugs are in clinical trials with "agents representing an array of treatment mechanisms and targets" (Cummings et al., 2022).

Sodium benzoate, a D-amino acid oxidase inhibitor, has emerged as a possible treatment for cognitive impairments in Alzheimer's disease. A series of papers document these positive results in later-stage dementia, with results superior in females compared to males (Lane et al., 2021; Lin et al., 2020, 2021).

An older report noted that feeding cinnamon to mice reduced neuronal apoptosis, inhibited glial activation, improved learning and memory, and reduced the amyloid-β burden in the hippocampus (Modi et al., 2015). The authors proposed that cinnamon powder (with its metabolite being sodium benzoate) might be "a promising natural supplement in halting the progression of Alzheimer's disease." Studies from additional investigators seem indicated.

Depression and Apathy

Alzheimer's disease is associated not only with cognitive impairments, but also with a myriad of bothersome mood alterations that pose further challenges to treatment (Cassano et al., 2019; Dyer et al., 2018).

Depression

Depression in older adults was discussed earlier in the chapter, but it's important to mention that depression associated with Alzheimer's disease is common. Some estimates are that between 30 and 50% of patients with Alzheimer's disease are on antidepressants (Lozupone et al., 2020). Certainly, depression in this population should be treated with antidepressant medications that lack anticholinergic side effects because they are better tolerated and produce fewer adverse cognitive effects. In addition, SSRIs can be combined with drugs used to treat Alzheimer's disease with few adverse interactions (Khundakar and Thomas, 2015). Efficacy of antidepressant medication is modest and often debatable (Lozupone et al., 2020).

Apathy

Over the years, psychostimulants have been noted to be effective in reducing apathy in Alzheimer's patients. Recently, reviewers reported that 10 milligrams of methylphenidate administered twice daily reduced apathy (compared to placebo treatment), with the greatest improvement in the first 100 days of the study (Mintzer et al., 2021). It was also proposed that methylphenidate increased "norepinephrine and dopamine actions in prefrontal-striatal-thalamocortical circuits" (van Dyck et al., 2021). Other researchers addressed the treatment of apathy and found that methylphenidate exerted positive effects on apathy scores, with no effect on cognitive functioning. They stated that this suggests that "the effect of the treatment is specific to the treatment of apathy and not a secondary effect of improvements in cognition" (Mintzer et al., 2021).

Alternatives to the use of the psychostimulants for treating apathy include the antidepressant bupropion (which, in one trial, was not superior to placebo treatment; Maier et al., 2020), the dopamine receptor agonist bromocriptine, and memantine (now shown to be noneffective in treating apathy; Rozankovic et al., 2021).

Principles of Care

In 2006, the American Association for Geriatric Psychiatry outlined minimal care standards and principles for patients with Alzheimer's and their caregivers. The association issued a position statement calling on clinicians to treat Alzheimer's disease as part of their typical practice. The statement focuses on the following five important areas of therapy:

- Alzheimer's disease therapies targeting aspects of the current pathophysiological understanding of the disease
- Symptomatic therapies for cognitive symptoms
- Symptomatic therapies for other neuropsychiatric symptoms
- Interventions targeted at and the provision of supportive care for patients
- Interventions targeted at and the provision of supportive care for caregivers

These principles still apply today. Disease therapies include therapies aimed at preventing deposits of amyloid plaques and preventing excitotoxic neuronal damage. As discussed, therapies for cognitive symptoms include the use of AChE-I drugs and memantine and involve methodologies for maintaining adherence to treatments (Campbell et al., 2017). Therapies for other symptoms might include treatments for depression, apathy, agitation, aggression, sleep, and delusions, among other symptoms, and these therapies can be both nonpharmacological and pharmacological.

Supportive care for patients and caregivers should be tailored to the condition, circumstances, and progression of functional and cognitive decline. Caregivers need to be educated about Alzheimer's disease and how their services are essential. They especially need to be given emotional support and respite.

CHAPTER REVIEW

1. Explain the prevalence and dangers of inappropriate drug use in older populations.
2. What are the most common medications used for treatment of psychosis in older adults? Discuss the risks involved with these drugs and possible alternative agents used for treatment.
3. What are some of the risk factors for depression in older adults? Explain the strategies for treatment and some of the specific drugs that are used. Note how treatment-resistant depression is especially challenging.
4. What are some of the symptoms of Parkinson's disease?
5. Discuss the approaches used for treatment of Parkinson's disease, specifically levodopa therapy and other alternatives.
6. Explain the role of biomarkers in evaluating Alzheimer's disease. What tools are currently being developed or used?
7. What are the currently available medications used to treat Alzheimer's disease?
8. Differentiate acetylcholinesterase inhibitors from one another and from memantine.
9. What are some other medical therapies that are being used or are under development for the treatment of Alzheimer's disease?

KEY TERMS

aducanumab
Alzheimer's disease
amantadine
candesartan
catechol-O-methyltransferase (COMT) inhibitors
cholinergic-deficiency theory
dementia
donanemab
donepezil
galantamine
huperzine A
levodopa
memantine
monoamine oxidase type B (MAO-B) inhibitors
nilotinib
rivastigmine
SAGE-718
semorinemab

CHAPTER 18

Challenging Times for Mental Health: The COVID-19 Pandemic and Beyond

CHAPTER OUTLINE

The years 2020–2022 will long be remembered for the unparalleled societal disruption and devastating death toll associated with the COVID-19 pandemic caused by the SARS-CoV-2 coronavirus. In this chapter, we will review some of the factors involved in pandemic-related effects on mental health and consider how and to what extent pharmacological therapies might be used to mitigate these effects, both now and in future pandemics.

LESSONS FROM THE PANDEMIC

At the time of this writing, in the fall of 2022, the number of reported COVID-19 cases in the United States since the start of the pandemic is approaching 100 million, with more than 1 million reported U.S. deaths from the disease (USAFacts, 2022). The COVID-19 pandemic has also resulted in a significant escalation in reported mental health crises, especially in conjunction with the ongoing opioid epidemic (see Chapter 10). To begin, consider the following:

- In the calendar year ending April 2021 (the first full year of the pandemic in the United States), there were over 100,000 drug overdose deaths in the United States, an increase of 28.5% from the 78,056 deaths during the year ending April 2020 (Centers for Disease Control and Prevention, 2021a). Overdose deaths have primarily involved synthetic opioids (e.g., fentanyl and its derivatives) and the psychostimulants cocaine and methamphetamine.

- Early in the COVID-19 pandemic, over 40% of U.S. adults reported at least one adverse mental or behavioral health problem: 31% reported symptoms of anxiety or depression, 26% reported symptoms of trauma- and stress-related disorders, and 3% reported starting or increasing substance abuse as a coping mechanism (Rahman et al., 2020). Pregnant females appear to be particularly vulnerable, especially Black females (Njoroge et al., 2022).
- Adverse mental health effects among older adults during the pandemic may be slightly less prevalent than among younger age groups (Vahla et al., 2020). Nevertheless, older persons are affected (Fischer et al., 2020), with cognitive decline being particularly important (Liu et al., 2022).
- Hispanic people, Black people, essential workers, unpaid caregivers, people living in poverty, and people with preexisting mental health problems experienced high rates of adverse mental health symptoms (Fornaro et al., 2021), and those with preexisting substance abuse disorders were perhaps the worst affected (Barocas, 2021; Friedman et al., 2021).
- COVID-19 has taken an extreme toll on the mental health of children younger than 18 (Centers for Disease Control and Prevention, 2022f; Samji et al., 2022; Solmi et al., 2022). Over 167,000 U.S. youths lost a parent, grandparent, or caregiver during the period April 2020 to December 2021. Other adverse childhood issues and experiences associated with significant mental health problems during the pandemic include depression, posttraumatic stress disorder (PTSD), suicidal ideation and attempts at suicide, increased risk of substance abuse, violence, sexual abuse, and shorter schooling (Ghosh et al., 2020; Slomski, 2021a). About 65% of U.S. children with pandemic-related psychopathology are from minoritized racial and ethnic groups, and children with preexisting mental health disorders may be particularly vulnerable (Jefsen et al., 2021).
- Infection with the COVID-19 virus may involve the central nervous system, with effects that may persist over the long term (Centers for Disease Control and Prevention, 2022e) (see the discussion in the section "Long-Haulers" later in this chapter). (For a discussion of the biological mechanisms—such as neuroinflammation—that may be involved in these effects, see Szczesniak et al., 2020.)

Factors associated with the prevalence of anxiety, depression, and stress during and after a disaster such as the COVID-19 pandemic include the intensity of the disaster, the duration of its impact, the postdisaster level of functioning of the survivors, family disruptions, and the level of social support. Hopefully, educational and social assistance efforts can reduce the mental and emotional impact of a disaster, and pharmaceutical interventions can be limited to the short term.

The use of addictive substances such as alcohol markedly increases during periods of crisis, resulting in increases in the incidence of anxiety, depression, and domestic violence (Evans et al., 2020; Rubin, 2021a; White et al., 2022).). Educational efforts may help to minimize such excessive use, along with any necessary pharmacological interventions. Alcohol use, for example, increased markedly during the pandemic in 2020, especially among women (Pollard et al., 2020), and alcohol-related deaths increased by about 25% during the first year of the pandemic (White et al., 2022). Unfortunately, smoking cessation programs have largely been mired in "lost years" as a result of the pandemic (Bandi et al., 2022; Jaklevic, 2021).

During the COVID-19 pandemic, people with opioid dependence and addiction have had to deal with additional problems created by personal isolation, social distancing, interrupted addiction support, and decreased availability of medication-assisted therapies (e.g., therapies involving administration of methadone or buprenorphine) (Joudrey et al., 2021). The interruptions in support and in the availability of medication-assisted therapies for this population were of course unintended consequences of the well-intended safety measures of personal isolation and social distancing (DiCarlo et al., 2021). Again, among those dealing with problems related to opioid use, Black people, Indigenous peoples, and Hispanic people have been disproportionately affected (Friedman and Hansen, 2022). Innovative programs encompassing telemedicine, online counseling, opioid prescription management programs, take-home naloxone and expanded methadone availability, and even emergency room coordination to deal with suicidality and overdoses have all helped. As noted by one team of researchers:

> Addiction treatment must go beyond "detox" programs to recovery programs based on integrated mental health care, medications for addiction treatment and postdischarge counseling. Critical for the longer term will be decriminalization of the use of illicit opioids and integration of addiction treatment into mainstream health care coverage. (Mason and Heyser, 2021)

Dealing effectively with substance use disorders during a pandemic is a worthy goal but remains problematic. Researchers have proposed five essential steps in using public policy to produce substantial and meaningful gains in public health (Barry and Saloner, 2021); these steps were developed using the opioid crisis as an example but can apply to any complex health care crisis:

- Define the problem
- Publicize the problem to generate interest in solving it
- Weigh policy alternatives
- Implement policies
- Evaluate the effectiveness of policies

Health Care Workers

The factors discussed above that lead to increases in mental health issues in the general population during a pandemic or other societal disaster also affect health care workers. In addition, the increased use of addictive substances such as alcohol in the general population and the consequent increases in the incidence of anxiety, depression, and even domestic violence mean that health care workers are confronted with a situation similar to battlefield conditions, with the associated uncertainty about resources, capacities, and risks, as well as constant exposure to suffering, death, and threats to their own safety. These conditions engender high levels of fear and anxiety in the short term and place health care workers at risk for professional burnout and for developing syndromes caused by persistent exposure to stress (Albott et al., 2020).

A review of research covering 33,000 health care workers found that anxiety and fear occurred in 23.2% of workers, depression in 22.8%, and insomnia in 38.9% (Pappa et al., 2020). In total, 62.5% of health care workers expressed general health concerns, fear, insomnia, psychological distress, burnout, anxiety, depression, symptoms of PTSD, somatization, and stigmatization (de Pablo et al., 2020). Proposed interventions to mitigate the impact of the pandemic on health care workers include mental health crisis lines (Feinstein et al., 2020) and a "battle buddies" model that would include a peer support buddy and a designated health consultant (Albott et al., 2020). A trial in which 300 milligrams of cannabidiol was administered twice daily to treat emotional exhaustion and burnout in 120 participant health care workers over a period of 28 days reported positive results, with few adverse side effects (four participants experienced mild elevations in liver enzymes, and one experienced a severe skin reaction; all recovered after the drug was discontinued) (Crippa et al., 2021).

Children and Adolescents

As noted above, children and adolescents are a particularly vulnerable group and are experiencing a time of difficult transition due to social isolation, lockdowns, disconnection from friends and the consequent loss of peer support, acute and chronic stress, depression, loss of variety in life, and other factors (Centers for Disease Control and Prevention, 2021c, 2022c). As a result of such factors, Internet and social media use has increased, as has persistent worrying about the future, which may later result in significant mental health issues (Guessoum et al., 2020; Loades et al., 2020). A variety of studies have provided examples of such effects:

- A Canadian study reported a high number of new cases of anorexia nervosa during the first wave of the COVID-19 pandemic (Agostino et al., 2021).
- A review of research on the mental health effects of social isolation and loneliness in youth found that these factors increased the risk of depression and possibly anxiety not only at the time of loneliness, but even up to nine years later, and that the duration of loneliness was more strongly correlated with depressive symptoms than was the intensity of loneliness (Loades et al., 2020).
- A study reported a marked increase in child and adolescent anxiety and depression during the pandemic, with about one youth in four or five experiencing symptoms, double the prepandemic prevalence (Racine et al., 2021); another study confirmed that result, finding that childhood and adolescent depression and anxiety doubled during the first year of the pandemic (Slomski, 2021b).

Clearly, the effects of social distancing and economic pressures, along with the identification of risk and resilience factors and even of child maltreatment, need to be studied and addressed. One study discusses telepsychiatry as a possible method for maintaining contact with and professional care for youth (Fegert et al., 2020). Of course, exercise, especially outdoor exercise, is especially valuable.

Adults

The mental health of adults worldwide has been adversely affected by the COVID-19 pandemic, with increases in stress, anxiety, depression, insomnia, denial, anger, and fear (Torales et al., 2020; Vahla et al., 2020). A study of adults in Spain during the pandemic reported that 65% of adults (73% females) had experienced anxiety or symptoms of depression (Fullana et al., 2020). A U.S. study found that the prevalence of depression was more than three times higher during the pandemic than before (see Figure 18.1) and that a higher risk of having symptoms of depression was associated with having lower income, having less than $5,000 in savings, and being exposed to higher levels of stress (e.g., from job loss) (Ettman et al., 2020).

As discussed earlier, social isolation, while beneficial in reducing the spread of the disease, can play a crucial role in increasing people's vulnerability to addiction and in making recovery from addiction more difficult (Volkow, 2020). Although difficult to document, social isolation may also contribute to increases in intimate partner violence, both in men and in women (Evans et al., 2020). A study of older adults (aged 50 or older) found a staggering increase in social isolation, from 14% in 2017 to 61% in 2020 (Escalante et al., 2021).

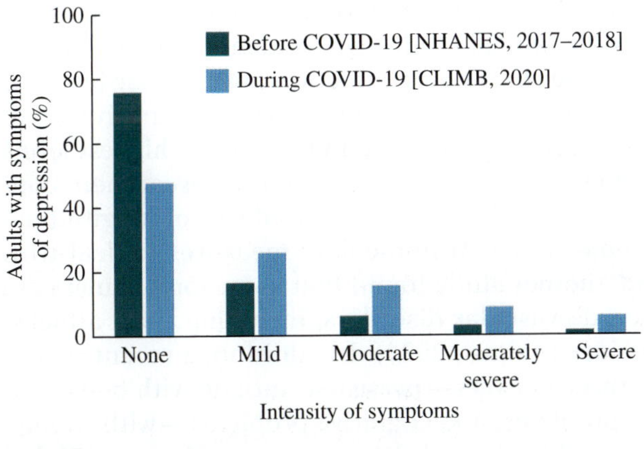

FIGURE 18.1 Prevalence of Depression Symptoms in U.S. Adults, Before (2017–2018) vs. During (2020) the COVID-19 Pandemic. NHANES: National Health and Nutritional Examination Survey (2017–2018). CLIMB: Covid-19 and Life Stressors Impact on Mental Health and Well-Being study (data collected March 31–April 13, 2020). [Comparative data from Ettman et al., 2020.]

On the more hopeful side, another study found that positive family experiences had the beneficial effect of providing resilience buffering (Prime et al., 2020). A program involving layperson-delivered, empathy-oriented telephone calls reported marked reductions in loneliness, depression, and anxiety in a wide population of persons compared with a control group (Kahlon et al., 2021). The average age of persons studied was 65 years, 56% lived alone, 79% were women, 39% were Black, 22% were Hispanic or Latino, and all reported at least one mental health condition. Everyone in the study received telephone calls four times daily at the beginning of the program, which were then reduced in frequency over a four-week period.

Long-Haulers

Addressing the acute consequences of the COVID-19 pandemic is of course an important priority, but so is addressing the long-term mental health issues experienced by many survivors of acute infections (so-called long-haulers). Postinfection syndromes are not new; they have accompanied other pandemics in the past but have been poorly studied and poorly treated. Researchers have called the long-term consequences of COVID-19 infections our "next public health disaster in the making," have advocated for awareness and preparedness and for not dismissing symptoms and complaints (as has occurred after past pandemics), and have noted that "[t]he majority [of long-haulers] will be women; many will have chronic, incapacitating conditions and will bounce around the health care system for years" (Phillips and Williams, 2021). In addition, the personal financial burdens associated with both acute and long-term COVID-19 can be extreme (Graves et al., 2021).

Symptoms experienced by long-haulers include fatigue, cough, chest tightness, breathlessness, palpitations, myalgia (muscle aches and pains), and difficulty in cognitive focusing (brain fog) (Raveendran et al., 2021). Symptoms often resemble those associated with fibromyalgia and chronic fatigue syndrome (Wadehra, 2022). Patients with persistent cognitive impairment after COVID-19 infection have higher levels of inflammatory markers in their cerebrospinal fluid, and those whose cognitive problems developed during acute COVID-19 infection were found to have the highest levels of inflammatory markers (Kousathanas et al., 2022). One team of researchers concluded that "COVID-19 survival was associated with an increased risk of longitudinal cognitive decline, highlighting the importance of immediate measures to deal with this challenge" (Liu et al., 2022), and another study found that some long-haulers are at risk of a broad range of adverse cardiovascular disorders, including heart attacks, ischemic heart disease, and heart failure (Abbasi, 2022). In addition, a recent review grouped long COVID-19 effects into three clusters—persistent fatigue with body pain or mood swings, ongoing respiratory problems, and cognitive problems—with women aged 20 years or older exhibiting the highest rate of these symptom clusters (Global Burden of Disease Long COVID Collaborators, 2022).

A major National Institutes of Health initiative is aimed at identifying the causes, prevention, and treatment of the symptoms experienced by individuals who have been sickened by COVID-19 and do not fully recover over a period of a few weeks (National Institutes of Health, 2021).

DR. J'S MUSINGS 18.1

Long COVID "Brain Cloud"

In the 1990 romantic-comedy film *Joe Versus the Volcano*, Joe Banks (played by Tom Hanks) is diagnosed as having a fatal "brain cloud" and is advised by the doctor, "You have some life left . . . live it well." In the end, however, after jumping into an erupting volcano with his new wife (played by Meg Ryan) and miraculously escaping death, Joe learns that the diagnosis of brain cloud was bogus, and they live happily ever after.

Unfortunately, a real-life diagnosis of brain cloud (or brain fog) is not necessarily bogus. Perhaps 35% of persons infected with the COVID-19 virus report having long-term symptoms (Levine, 2022), in many cases including neuropsychiatric symptoms that can be described as "brain fog": cognitive impairment, sleep difficulties, depression, PTSD, anxiety, fatigue, headache, and substance abuse disorders (Clift et al., 2022; Frontera and Simon, 2022; Hellmuth et al., 2021). Many symptoms of COVID-induced brain impairments may mimic the effects of fibromyalgia, with generalized fatigue and widespread, persistent pain (Ursini et al., 2021). The mechanisms underlying such symptoms remain unclear, but it is known that the COVID-19 virus can reach the brain and cause inflammation, thrombi, and brain damage (Boldrini et al., 2021). The costs associated with these and other symptoms of long COVID are enormous, with one researcher having estimated an eventual total cost of $2.6 trillion (Cutler, 2022). This is not romantic-comedy!

MOVING FORWARD: ADDRESSING INEQUITIES AND PROVIDING MENTAL HEALTH SUPPORT

As discussed above, the increase in the prevalence of mental health disorders in the context of the COVID-19 pandemic has had especially adverse effects among minoritized groups. Inequities in health and health care have led to a situation in which there is an increased need for mental health support not just in society overall but especially among those groups, as well as among those who are more vulnerable because of pre-existing psychiatric disorders. In this section, we will discuss those issues and the uses and limitations of psychopharmacological treatments in managing them.

Inequities in Health and Health Care

With the wide availability of effective vaccines, we seem to be entering a new phase of the COVID-19 pandemic: a time when we must address issues related to inequities in health, frontline health care infrastructure, and community preparedness (Chin, 2021; Galea, 2021; Nuzzo and Gostin, 2022). Low-income communities have been especially hard hit, especially those serving people who are uninsured or are insured mainly by Medicaid (Anderson et al., 2022; Knudsen and Chokshi, 2021; Schwandt et al., 2022). Certainly, compared with white populations, COVID-19 disease severity has been greater in minoritized groups—African Americans, Hispanic people, and Asian Americans—and those groups face a higher risk of testing positive for COVID-19, a higher risk of intensive care unit admission if infected, and a greater likelihood of not having health insurance, of having less access to primary care, and of having more comorbidities (Magesh et al., 2021).

As discussed above, many persons with COVID-19 experience symptoms beyond the acute phase of the disease, primarily fatigue, brain fog, sleep problems, worsening of mental health, and increased risk of psychiatric illness (Abel et al., 2021). These effects suggest that the virus might cause brain damage that might contribute to adverse long-term psychiatric outcomes (Boldrini et al., 2021).

Certainly, the recent pandemic-related influx of large grants to local governments can be used to increase equity while effectively targeting resources to the people in greatest need: the homeless, those with substance use disorders, those with other mental health disorders, the unemployed, those with unsafe living conditions, and so forth (Barry and Saloner, 2021).

Mental Health Support

The COVID-19 pandemic is having an impact on mental health care now and will continue to have an impact for the foreseeable future (Vahratian et al., 2021). Two studies reviewing mental health issues during the current pandemic offer immediate and longer-term strategies to address vital mental health issues, with an emphasis on the urgent need for research on how mental health consequences for vulnerable groups can be mitigated under pandemic conditions (Brown et al., 2020; Holmes et al., 2020). These vulnerable groups include those with past or present mental health issues and those who become unwell in response to anxiety, loneliness, and self-isolation (Smith and Lim, 2020).

Ongoing access to mental health support will continue to be important. Certainly, many patients with preexisting psychiatric disorders have reported a worsening of psychiatric symptoms during the pandemic, both affective symptoms and psychotic or delusional symptoms (Vindegaard and Benros, 2020). Given pandemic-related measures such as isolation and social distancing, this presents special challenges for providers of psychiatric services (Bojdani et al., 2020). One team of researchers noted that "little attention is on mental health" and that "psychological first aid is a crucial early intervention . . . providing psychosocial support during outbreaks like COVID-19" (Shah et al., 2020). These researchers advocate a RAPID model of mental health support with the following five steps:

1. *Rapport and reflective listening*. Using techniques such as paraphrasing with empathy to establish initial contact with the patient and maintain rapport.
2. *Assessment*. Evaluating the patient's psychological and basic physical needs.
3. *Prioritization*. Using triage principles to focus on patients who need emergency care.

4. *Intervention*. Using cognitive and behavioral interventions to reduce the patient's distress and improve the patient's functioning, as well as to meet the patient's basic needs.
5. *Disposition and follow-up*. Regularly monitoring the patient until the patient's situation stabilizes, including the provision of continuing support.

Unfortunately, there is a continuing severe shortage of mental health practitioners: 45% of the U.S. population lives in areas with a shortage of mental health professionals, particularly rural areas; the United States needs about 7500 more mental health professionals to fill those gaps; and there is a particularly acute shortage of mental health professionals to serve children—vast areas of the United States have none (Kuehn, 2022).

Support for the More Vulnerable

There is an association between having a positive COVID-19 test and having a psychiatric comorbidity (Abel et al., 2021). In addition, highly vulnerable persons, such as those with schizophrenia, bipolar disorder, mood disorders, and/or substance abuse disorders, are at increased risk for COVID-19 infection hospitalization and death (Abel et al., 2021; Ceban et al., 2021). The highest risk of adverse effects from COVID-19 infection, including mortality, appears to be in persons with schizophrenia and/or bipolar disorders (Ceban et al., 2021; Fond et al., 2021; Fornaro et al., 2021); caring for people with these and other serious mental health issues during the pandemic is a particular challenge (Druss, 2020; Kahl and Correll, 2020).

In addition, a study of mental health care for immigrants and refugees in the context of the COVID-19 pandemic found that "[s]tigma toward mental disorders and lack of technology literacy were the main challenges in scaling up digital health applications for immigrants and refugees" and that, regardless of these issues, immigrants and refugees receiving telemedicine treatments "reported positive attitudes toward applications of digital health in mental health care, and positive improvement on their anxiety, depression, and PTSD symptoms" (Liem et al., 2021).

Given that the pandemic has had adverse mental health effects in previously healthy people and especially in people with preexisting psychiatric disorders (such effects include exacerbation of symptoms, poorer access to services, alcohol and other drug overuse, and homelessness, all of which exacerbate stress, which in turn exacerbates psychiatric disorders), researchers recommend that these effects should be addressed with good practices that can result in sustained, efficient, and equitable delivery of mental health care (Moreno et al., 2020). The same researchers propose that intermittent monitoring may be of benefit:

> The frequency of face-to-face, video, and telephone contact with different types of mental health providers; rates of prescription and use of psychiatric medication; rates of emergency mental health treatment and the proportion of patients with severe mental disorders should be compared with the corresponding data from before the pandemic. (Moreno et al., 2020, 819)

What is needed? Certainly, needs include more mental health clinics, increased access to mental health medications and nonmedication treatments, training of additional mental health workers, establishment of mental health emergency facilities, more effective provision of services in underserved areas of inner cities, and so forth. (For a discussion of some of the major changes necessary to prepare for the next pandemic, see Emanuel et al., 2022.)

Pharmacological Issues

Pharmacological issues involved in pandemic responses have not been adequately addressed, for reasons that likely range from a shortage of psychiatric prescribers to the limited knowledge of nonprescribers about psychopharmacology. Symptoms that take the form of expressed concerns about stress, anxiety, depression, insomnia, denial, anger, isolation, loneliness, and fear would seem to be amenable, at least partially, to drug therapy, though clinicians must recognize that there is no "magic pill" for treating such maladies. Whatever mental health interventions prove to be therapeutic in the context of the pandemic, clinicians should assure patients that their prepandemic medications will be continued. No patient should be denied ongoing treatments with medications such as antidepressants, mood stabilizers, antipsychotics, or stimulants (e.g., for attention deficit/hyperactivity disorder); acute withdrawal from these prescription psychopharmaceuticals would only add to patents' distress. In line with this principle, a study done during the second year of the pandemic found that the prescription of antianxiety, antidepressant, and hypnotic medications showed modest increases, as did the prescription of benzodiazepines for women (who may experience more social isolation than men do) (Kahlon et al., 2021; Milani et al., 2021).

New stressors such as those associated with the pandemic can bring on or exacerbate affective disorders, with medications plus psychotherapy being the treatment regimen of choice. Antidepressants (see Chapter 12) should be considered for treating extreme sadness, hopelessness, and feelings of isolation (Oskotsky et al., 2021). Bipolar disorder (see Chapter 14) may manifest as irritability, depression, impulsiveness, substance abuse, and aggression, and such symptoms can indicate a need for rapid intervention with patients who might pose a danger to self or others if left untreated. Treatment of anxiety, feelings of isolation, and loneliness is more complicated, and positive outcomes cannot be achieved with medications alone—psychological interventions are also needed. Insomnia is also difficult to treat, and benzodiazepine receptor agonists (such as zolpidem) should generally be avoided in favor of orexin or melatonin receptor antagonists, which may help to normalize sleep-wake cycles. In general, long-term benzodiazepine use should be avoided because of risks of cognitive impairment and dependence. If a benzodiazepine is determined to be necessary, a short-acting agent should be used, in the lowest possible dose and only for a short period of time. (See Chapter 13 for detailed discussion of the treatment of anxiety and insomnia.)

Psychological distress can make it difficult to manage drug treatment of patients with psychotic or delusional disorders. (For reviews of some of the major issues involved in treating people with preexisting psychotic disorders, as well as those who might develop a psychosis as a result of the pandemic, see Brown et al., 2020, and Taquet et al., 2021.)

Limitations of Pharmacological Therapy

Over the past 50 years, psychopharmacology has contributed greatly to improving the mental health of people in our society. The lives of millions with affective or psychotic disorders have improved markedly, and research continues into the development of treatments leading to further improvements (e.g., treatments for slowing the progression of Alzheimer's disease). On the negative side, there are still nearly 60 million U.S. adults with one or more mental illnesses, many psychoactive drugs are prone to compulsive abuse, and nearly 20 million people have a substance use disorder involving licit and/or illicit psychoactive drugs (see Figure 18.2). The ongoing crises resulting from the overuse and illicit use of opioids and benzodiazepines, either individually or in combination, are associated with thousands of unnecessary deaths (Pardo, 2022).

In response, recognition of the limitations of traditional psychopharmacological treatments has reactivated interest and support for nonpharmacological approaches to treating mental illness, particularly psychotherapy but also somatic treatments such as transcranial magnetic stimulation for depression. In addition, the scope of pharmacological research is being extended based on a deeper understanding of basic neurophysiology, such as the circuitry of fear, as opposed to an understanding of specific clinical syndromes, such as anxiety. Finally, there has been a renewal of national investment in research and increased public support for the development of better treatments for mental illness.

While psychoactive medications are not fully the answer to life's problems, they do have utility, and their beneficial effects should not be ignored. Thus, prescribers of medications must learn about psychotherapies, and nonprescribers must learn about psychopharmacology, its uses, and its limitations. What do psychoactive drugs do? They *set the stage* for psychotherapies to be effective. Medications can help reset brain chemistry, and once chemistry gets in line, the patient may be able to stop using medication or reduce the dose while maintaining chemical balance and beginning psychotherapy that might have longer-lasting effects. In the absence of medication, the efficacy of psychotherapy may be much reduced. Highly distressing symptoms such as depression, anxiety, anger, and agitation may need to be addressed with medications

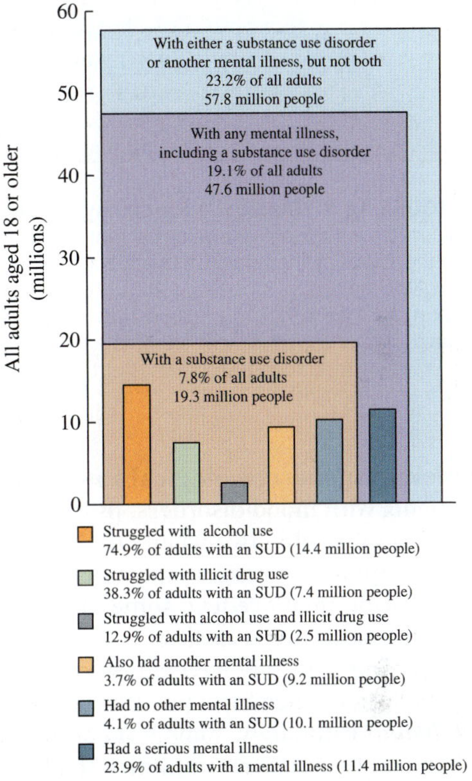

FIGURE 18.2 Mental Illness and Substance Use Disorders in U.S. Adults Aged 18 or Older, 2018. In 2018, 57.8 million U.S. adults had either a substance use disorder or one or more other mental illnesses; 47.6 million had at least one mental illness of any kind, with 11.4 million having at least one serious mental illness; and 19.3 million had a substance use disorder, with 9.2 million also having at least one other mental illness and 10.1 million having no other mental illness (of those 19.3 million, 14.4 million struggled with alcohol use, 7.4 million with illicit drug use, and 2.5 million with both). [Data from Substance Abuse and Mental Health Services Administration, 2019.]

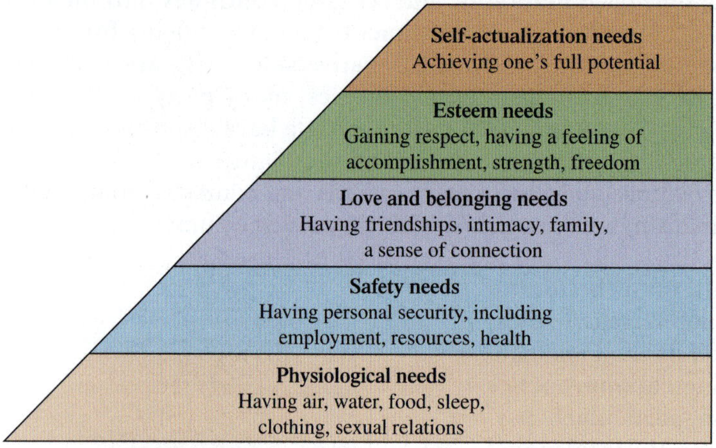

FIGURE 18.3 Maslow's Hierarchy of Needs. The hierarchy illustrates a theory of psychological motivation that was first developed in the 1940s by the American psychologist Abraham Maslow and is still widely cited today. According to this theory, people are motivated to satisfy the needs toward the broad base of the hierarchy before addressing needs higher up (the specific number and descriptions of the needs in the hierarchy vary among researchers, but this basic idea of a motivational hierarchy remains).

before nonpharmacological interventions can be introduced effectively. In some patients with mood disorders, psychotherapy alone may be effective to some degree but may be more effective when combined with pharmacotherapy. For example, a patient with unipolar depression may not have the energy to benefit much from psychotherapy; medication might reduce some of the patient's symptoms to a point where the patient has the energy to go further.

Saying that *only* medication or *only* psychotherapy is enough deprives the patient of the best chance for a positive response to treatment. *The choice is not either/or*, but *both/and*! Ultimately, some level of ongoing drug treatment may be needed to maintain chemical balance and minimize the frequency and severity of relapses. In essence, the combination of medication and psychotherapy may provide the level of lifestyle support needed to help patients find the required energy and motivation to satisfy their human needs, as expressed in Maslow's hierarchy of needs (see Figure 18.3).

CHAPTER REVIEW

1. Discuss the factors involved in the increase in substance abuse during the COVID-19 pandemic. What approaches have been proposed for dealing with this problem now and in future pandemics?
2. Discuss the pandemic-related factors that lead to increases in mental health issues among health care workers. What interventions have been proposed to mitigate the impact of those factors?

3. How has the mental health of children and adolescents been affected by the pandemic?
4. How has the mental health of adults been affected by the pandemic?
5. What is meant by the term "long-haulers"? Describe some of the symptoms experienced by long-haulers.
6. Discuss the factors that have a negative impact on the provision of mental health support services, particularly during the COVID-19 pandemic.
7. Which groups have been especially vulnerable to adverse mental health effects during the pandemic?
8. Discuss the pharmacological issues involved in responses to the pandemic.
9. Explain why treatment of mental health issues should be a combination of pharmacotherapy and psychotherapy.

APPENDIX A

CLINICAL APPLICATIONS OF PSYCHOPHARMACOLOGY AND WHAT THEY TEACH US

The 11 clinical examples discussed in this appendix illustrate the combination of pharmacotherapies and psychological therapies in the treatment of specific, real-life patients' distress. The ultimate choice of treatment strategy is invariably a decision made among the prescriber, the patient, the patient's caregivers, and any relevant nonprescribing therapists—that is, the decision is made by a health care team, keeping in mind that modest alterations in medication choices can make huge differences in a patient's quality of life. Importantly, these clinical examples demonstrate how nonprescribing members of a health care team can contribute to patient care by making suggestions for changes in medications or for incremental adjustments in dosage.

Client A

Client A was a 45-year-old man who had been diagnosed with bipolar II disorder and had been prescribed lithium to treat the condition. He presented with complaints of an 80-pound weight gain and an inability to remember names. Recognizing these problems as side effects of lithium therapy, the therapists advocated for a medication switch from lithium to valproate, having noted a study on the efficacy of valproic acid (a form of valproate) in treating bipolar II. After the switch to valproate, Client A lost about 40 pounds and his memory function improved, allowing him to continue working.

Five years later, however, this same Client A presented with complaints of listlessness, lack of energy, and sexual dysfunction. The health care team learned that the client had been diagnosed with depression and had been prescribed escitalopram, which he was taking in addition to the valproic acid. The team decided to discontinue both of these drugs and to initiate treatment with aripiprazole. Two weeks after the switch to aripiprazole, the client reported that the drug was "intolerable" and complained of aches, myalgias, flulike symptoms, and electric shocks in his head. Fortunately, the team psychologist realized that these symptoms were not side effects of aripiprazole but instead indicated that the client had serotonin discontinuation syndrome due to stopping the escitalopram (a selective serotonin reuptake inhibitor [SSRI] antidepressant). The psychologist counseled the client that he should continue with the aripiprazole and that the distressing symptoms would probably soon disappear. Three weeks later, the symptoms had ceased, the client was more energized, sexual function was improving, and no bipolar symptoms were reported. Continual progress was made over the next few months.

Client B

Client B, a man in his late 20s, was referred by his physician for evaluation of cognitive difficulties. After neuropsychological testing, the client was diagnosed with significant cognitive dysfunction, with the greatest difficulty being word recall. A review of the client's medications revealed that he had recently been prescribed topiramate as treatment for anxiety and posttraumatic stress disorder (PTSD). The team replaced the topiramate with pregabalin, which led to rapid resolution of the cognitive difficulties.

Client C

Client C was a 48-year-old woman who had been diagnosed with depression and anxiety and had been prescribed sertraline. This led to some improvement in her depression and anxiety, but she gradually developed a panic disorder. Further history taking revealed that she had recently undergone surgery for benign breast cysts and that she was a heavy coffee drinker. Sertraline interferes with the metabolism of caffeine, which had resulted in doubling her blood level of caffeine—that is, it had resulted in caffeinism, which is associated with anxiety, panic disorder, and the development of benign breast cysts. She began drinking smaller amounts of caffeinated coffee and eventually drinking decaffeinated coffee only, and the panic disorder resolved.

Client D

Client D was a 28-year-old man, a Gulf War veteran with severe PTSD, with symptoms that included nighttime terrors and acting threateningly toward his wife. Moreover, he was amnestic for these episodes. Medication review revealed that he had been prescribed zolpidem for sleep, and the team thought that the zolpidem might be causing the amnesia and his behaviors during this blackout state. Replacement of zolpidem with gabapentin at bedtime improved his PTSD symptoms and resolved the amnestic episodes.

Client E

Client E was an 88-year-old woman residing in a care center whose family took her to therapy for increasing dementia. Medication review revealed that she had been taking imipramine for depression and diazepam for anxiety and sleep difficulties. Like other tricyclic antidepressants, imipramine has anticholinergic effects and can cause cognitive impairments, and benzodiazepines such as diazepam are widely known to worsen dementia. Replacement of these medications with quetiapine and mirtazapine led to cognitive improvements, reduced anxiety, better sleep patterns, and improvements in appetite.

Client F

Client F was a 5-year-old girl presenting with rages and aggressive behaviors made worse by psychostimulants and antidepressants. She was prescribed valproic acid and showed marked improvement in behavior. She was then referred to a psychologist, and it was decided that the behavioral improvement made it possible to start family therapy to address problems underlying the girl's behaviors. It was thought that effective family therapy might eventually make it possible to stop the valproic acid.

Client G

Client G, a 69-year-old woman, was brought to an emergency room confused and disoriented and suffering from delusions—she did not know where she was and stated that she was a movie star and the hospital was a movie studio. She experienced fluctuating agitation, had not slept in days, and was aggressive and disruptive. She had no history of mental illness, and there was no evidence of illegal drug use or alcohol use. A medical examination revealed a systemic infection; laboratory tests also indicated an elevation in her serum glucose levels. A psychologist thought that the delirium (i.e., the confusion and disorientation) was possibly caused by her systemic infection, so the immediate goal was to treat the source of the infection while stabilizing her behaviorally with an antipsychotic that could be given by intramuscular injection to reduce the agitation quickly and facilitate sleep. Afterward, the drug could be given orally on a regular dosing schedule to maintain stability.

Several antipsychotics have acute intramuscular formulations, including haloperidol, aripiprazole, olanzapine, and risperidone. Haloperidol was excluded because it can have extrapyramidal side effects, which are more likely in the elderly and when the drug is given by intramuscular injection. The hospital formulary did not include aripiprazole. Olanzapine was excluded because its high anticholinergic effect would tend to worsen the delirium; in addition, olanzapine has a risk of producing metabolic side effects that include insulin resistance and can worsen diabetes, and the patient already had increased blood glucose levels. The team's recommendation was to use the second-generation antipsychotic drug risperidone rather than the alternative option of a benzodiazepine; it was felt that risperidone was less risky and would provide more benefit. Risperidone was first given in small doses of 0.5 milligram via intramuscular injection on an as-needed basis and then orally in low doses of 0.5 milligram twice per day. With this regimen, the patient was able to sleep, her delusions subsided, and she became calm and regained her orientation to place. After two days, she was discharged with a referral to an outpatient psychiatrist who could follow her for ongoing treatment as needed.

Client H

Client H was a 55-year-old man who met the criteria for major depressive disorder with some anxiety. He had diabetes, mild hypertension, and painful diabetic neuropathy and had had previous depressive episodes and one suicide attempt. He had been treated with paroxetine, sertraline, and bupropion, and his depression had improved slightly with each of these medications but had never remitted. The team's goal was to reduce the depressive symptoms, the anxiety, and possibly the neuropathic pain. Treatment with one of the tricyclic antidepressants was considered because those drugs can help with neuropathic pain and depression; however, their side effects (including anticholinergic-induced cognitive inhibition) and their lethality in overdose made them not a good choice. The team's recommendation was that the patient be given a serotonin and norepinephrine reuptake inhibitor because he had not achieved remission with the two SSRIs (paroxetine and sertraline). Given his mild hypertension, venlafaxine was rejected in favor of duloxetine, which has an indication for neuropathic pain, depression, and anxiety. This treatment was successful, and the patient was instructed to tell his physician if he took any other medications or supplements because duloxetine is a CYP-2D6 and CYP-1A2 inhibitor and has potential drug-drug interactions.

Client I

Client I was a 33-year-old woman who had been hospitalized with her first episode of mania. She had no previous history of depression, no history of drug or alcohol use, and no medical issues. Because of the manic episode, the team recommended starting her on lithium after first giving her a pregnancy test, discussing her choice of a birth control method, and measuring her baseline serum creatinine and thyroid hormone levels (lithium can produce fetal malformations and can have adverse kidney and thyroid effects). She began lithium with the average starting dose of 300 milligrams twice a day, but after one week, she complained of stomach irritation and some diarrhea. However, these are common side effects of lithium, particularly early in treatment, so she was encouraged to drink adequate fluid while continuing to take the medication. After a short period, the side effects resolved.

Client J

Client J was a 27-year-old man who had been admitted to the hospital after a manic episode. He had been having five to six manic or depressive episodes a year and had struggled on and off with alcohol abuse. Valproic acid treatment was started because the patient was a rapid cycler, with four or more depressive or manic episodes per year, and because of his comorbid alcohol abuse. He began with 250 milligrams twice a day, which was increased to 500 milligrams twice a day. Blood tests then showed a low level of valproic acid and a doubling of his levels of liver enzymes. However, it is not unusual for patients on anticonvulsants to show an increase in liver enzymes, and as long as those levels are not tripled, no change in therapy is indicated. Therefore, the patient continued to take the medication while also continuing to be monitored.

Client K

Client K, a 21-year-old man with symptoms consistent with schizophrenia, was admitted to the hospital because of profound psychotic behavior. He had never been treated, and an antipsychotic was recommended. Blood tests showed that the patient had mildly elevated total cholesterol and low HDL (so-called good cholesterol) for his age. Because of the increased risk of dyslipidemia, olanzapine and quetiapine were ruled out, and risperidone, ziprasidone, and aripiprazole were recommended. But after risperidone was started and then increased to 3 milligrams twice a day, which is a high average dose, the patient complained that he felt "uncomfortable" in his skin, like "I can't sit still." This indicated that he was likely experiencing akathisia, which is not uncommon with risperidone, and because akathisia is associated with an increased risk for suicide, it needs to be addressed; however, current options for dealing with akathisia are often unsatisfactory. The dose of risperidone was reduced, but then the psychosis worsened. The higher dose of risperidone was reinstituted while a low, 15-milligram dose of the 5-HT2 serotoninergic antagonist mirtazapine was added, and the patient's psychotic symptoms improved and the akathisia decreased. The goal was to eventually reduce the risperidone dose and let the adjunct mirtazapine effectively suppress the akathisia.

Going Forward: Patient Compliance, Practitioner Awareness, and the Uses of Telemedicine

The cases described above are in no way unusual: thousands of other cases like them can be found in the literature on treatments with psychotherapeutic medications. Taken together, these cases show how important it is for clinicians to be aware of the following important questions that may affect patients' compliance with specific suggestions for treatment:

- *Can the client afford the prescribed medication?* Patients and physicians alike are susceptible to ads for heavily promoted, expensive, brand-name medications. The medications promoted in such ads are typically new and may have significant advantages over older drugs, but they also have their own constellation of side effects. Fortunately, over time, brand-name psychotherapeutic drugs often become available in less-expensive generic forms.
- *Can the client tolerate weight gain?* Some clients can tolerate a degree of weight gain, while weight gain might lead to noncompliance in others. For example, mirtazapine might be appropriate as an antidepressant for a client who can tolerate weight gain, while duloxetine or bupropion might be appropriate for a client who wants to lose weight. The same considerations apply in recommending medications for the treatment of bipolar disorder and behavioral disorders associated with anger, agitation, and aggression.
- *Can the client tolerate any degree of cognitive dysfunction?* Many psychotherapeutic drugs are associated with drug-induced cognitive dysfunction, including the benzodiazepines, the tricyclic antidepressants, lithium, some anticonvulsant mood stabilizers, and some antipsychotic drugs. Many patients—for example, young people, older adults, and people with traumatic brain injury—might not tolerate agents that have detrimental effects on their cognitive functioning. Other patients, however, might be able to tolerate some degree of cognitive dysfunction if the therapeutic

benefits seem to outweigh that adverse effect. Clinicians prescribing such agents should keep in mind that cognitive dysfunction may interfere not only with the efficacy of cognitive therapies, but also with overall life functioning.

- *Does the client have access to health care?* The COVID-19 pandemic not only severely strained heath care providers and facilities, but also affected access to health care for patients with mental health and substance abuse disorders. Consider, for example, a study that addressed the disparity between federal and state policies for the treatment of opioid use disorder found that, beneficially, 44 states had expanded access to medication for the treatment of opioid use disorder; however, the study also found that no state had implemented all federal policies aimed at comprehensively expanding access to opioid use disorder treatment during the pandemic (Pessar et al., 2021).

Understandably, it is difficult for practitioners to keep up fully with new developments. One major development is that indications for psychoactive drugs have increased to include broader applications, which raises concerns about possibly dangerous drug-drug interactions. Among the factors that may help reduce the often-overwhelming complexity of decision making about drug treatment are the following:

- Internet-based resources—including telemedicine applications—have become more accessible, useful, and comprehensive.
- Communication and collaboration among physicians, counselors, psychologists, and other specialists can be promoted and encouraged—for example, group practices that include experts from several specialties can ensure this collaboration.
- Collaboration can also include greater communication with patients to ensure that they are aware of the issues associated with their medications, especially in regard to polypharmacy.

One positive outcome of the COVID-19 pandemic has been the expansion of telemedicine, allowing conferences among multiple persons with minimal expenditure of time and minimal travel. For example, a three-month study of telemedicine for mental health care in a rural community began by noting that "[f]ifteen million residents living in rural locations in the United States struggle with mental illness, substance dependence, or comorbid conditions, and are not receiving adequate health care" and then noting that "[a]pproximately 55% of the 3,075 rural communities in the United States lack psychiatric providers" (Talarico, 2021); the study reported that the use of telemedicine led to improved medication adherence as well as improved patient satisfaction.

On the negative side, another study noted that, as helpful as telemedicine can be, it has several limitations (Gajarawala and Pelkowski, 2021):

- Telemedicine will not work for every type of visit. Patients still have to go to the doctor's office for imaging tests, blood work, and other procedures, as well as for diagnoses that require a more hands-on approach.
- The security of personal health data transmitted electronically is a concern.

- While insurance companies are increasingly covering the cost of telehealth visits during the COVID-19 pandemic, some services may not be fully covered, leading to out-of-pocket costs.
- Not everyone has easy access to telemedicine conferences via personal computers.
- Prescribing controlled substances may not be possible.

Regardless of such limitations, the use of telemedicine during the COVID-19 pandemic has taught us that telemedicine can significantly help patients access health care. However, telemedicine cannot eliminate face-to-face meetings, especially in the early stages of diagnosis and treatment of serious mental disorders.

APPENDIX B

QUICK REFERENCE TO PSYCHOTHERAPEUTIC DRUGS

The tables in this appendix provide information about the therapeutic doses and the availability of generic formulations of psychotherapeutic drugs encountered in clinical practice, as well as information about some important side effects of those drugs, including sedation, weight gain, and cognitive impairment.[1] The tables cover the following categories of drugs, supplementing the discussions of these drugs in the chapters:

- antidepressant drugs
- drugs used to treat bipolar disorder
- psychostimulant drugs
- drugs used to treat obsessive-compulsive disorder
- antipsychotic drugs
- drugs used to treat insomnia
- antianxiety drugs (anxiolytics)

To the best of my knowledge, the information in these tables is accurate and up to date, but it is important to note that this appendix is only intended as a general reference, not as a guide for prescribing for individual patients. Check the manufacturer's product information sheet or the Physicians' Desk Reference (PDR) for any changes in dosage and for contraindications. Common side effects of psychotherapeutic drugs are shown in the table below, but specific drugs may produce other specific effects.

[1]The tables in this appendix were prepared with information from John Preston, Psy.D. References used as sources for the information in these tables include the *Clinical Handbook of Psychotropic Drugs Online*, 23rd ed. (2019), R. M. Procyshyn et al. (eds.), Hogrefe Publishers, and Epocrates™ (an online application). Brand names in the tables are registered trademarks.

Common Side Effects of Psychotherapeutic Drugs

Anticholinergic Effects (Block Acetylcholine Receptors)
Dry mouth
Constipation
Urinary retention
Blurred vision
Memory impairment
Confusion

Extrapyramidal Effects (Block Dopamine Receptors in Basal Ganglia)
Parkinson-like effects: rigidity, shuffling gait, tremor, flat affect, lethargy
Dystonias: spasms in neck and other muscle groups
Akathisia: intense, uncomfortable sense of inner restlessness
Tardive dyskinesia: often a persistent movement disorder (lip smacking, writhing movements, jerky movements)

Antidepressant Drugs

Names			Side Effects			
Generic	Brand	Therapeutic Dose Range	Sedation	Weight Gain	Cognitive Impairment	Generic Available
Amitriptyline	Elavil	75–300 mg	high	0–low	mid	yes
Amoxapine	Asendin	100–600	mid	0–low	low	yes
Atomoxetine	Strattera	40–100 mg	low	0	0	yes
Brexpiprazole	Rexulti	1–2 mg	low	low	0–low	no
Bupropion-ER	Wellbutrin-ER	150–450 mg	low	0	0	yes
Citalopram	Celexa	10–40 mg	low	low	low	yes
Clomipramine	Anafranil	75–300 mg	high	0–low	mid	yes
Desipramine	Norpramin	75–300 mg	low	0–low	mid	yes
Desvenlafaxine	Pristiq	50 mg	mid	low	0	yes
Dextromethorphan/ bupropion	Auvelity[a]	45 mg / 105 mg	0	0	0	no
Doxepin	Sinequan	75–300 mg	high	0–low	mid	yes
Duloxetine	Cymbalta	60–120 mg	low	low	0	yes
Escitalopram	Lexapro	10–20 mg	low	low	low	yes
Fluoxetine[b]	Prozac	20–80 mg	low	low	low	yes
Fluvoxamine	Luvox	50–300 mg	low	low	low	yes
Imipramine	Tofranil	75–300 mg	mid	mid	mid	yes
Levomilnacipran	Fetzima	40–120 mg	0–low	0–low	0–low	no
Maprotiline	Ludiomil	75–225 mg	high	0–low	low	yes
Mirtazapine	Remeron	15–45 mg	mid	mild	low	yes
Nortriptyline	Aventyl	50–150 mg	mid	0–low	low	yes
Paroxetine	Paxil	20–50 mg	low	low	low	yes

Antidepressant Drugs (continued)

Names			Side Effects			
Generic	Brand	Therapeutic Dose Range	Sedation	Weight Gain	Cognitive Impairment	Generic Available
Protriptyline	Vivactil	5–60 mg	mid	0–low	mid	yes
Sertraline	Zoloft	50–200 mg	low	low	low	yes
Trazodone-XR	Desyrel	50–600 mg	mid	0–low	low–mid	yes
Trimipramine	Surmontil	75–300 mg	high	0–low	mid	yes
Venlafaxine-XR	Effexor-XR	75–225 mg	low	low	0	yes
Vilazodone	Viibryd	20–40 mg	low	low	low	no
Vortioxetine	Trintellix	5–20 mg	low	low	0	no
MAO Inhibitors						
Phenelzine	Nardil	30–90 mg	low	0	0	yes
Rasagiline	Azilect	1–2 mg	low	0	0	yes
Safinamide	Xadago	50–100 mg	0	0	0	no
Selegiline	Emsam	6–12 mg	low	0	0	No
Tranylcypromine	Parnate	20–60 mg	low	0	0	yes

[a]Auvelity is a combination of 45 mg of dextromethorphan and 105 mg of bupropion.
[b]Prozac is available in a 90-mg time-release/weekly formulation.

Drugs Used to Treat Bipolar Disorder

Names			Side Effects		
Generic	Brand	Serum Level	Weight Gain	Cognitive Impairment	Generic Available
Brexpiprazole	Rexulti	—[c]	mid	0–low	no
Carbamazepine	Tegretol	4–10[b]	low	low	yes
Cariprazine	Vraylar	—[c]	low	mid	no
Dexmedetomidine	Precedex	—[c]	high	high	no
Gabapentin	Neurontin	—[c]	low	low	yes
Lamotrigine	Lamictal	—[c]	0	0	yes
Lithium salts	Eskalith	0.8–1.2[a]	high	high	yes
Olanzapine/fluoxetine	Symbyax	—[c]	high	high	yes
Oxcarbazepine	Trileptal	—[c]	low	low	yes
Tiagabine	Gabitril	—[c]	0	0	yes
Topiramate	Topamax	—[c]	0	mid–high	yes
Valproic acid	Depakote	50–100[b]	mid	low	yes

[a]Milliequivalents per liter; blood levels associated with acute treatment.
[b]Micrograms per milliliter.
[c]Serum monitoring not necessary.

Psychostimulant Drugs

Names			
Generic	Brand	Therapeutic Dose Range[a]	Generic Available
Amphetamine	Adzenys XR[b] (ODT[c])	12.5 mg	no
	Dyanavel XR[b] (suspension)	2.5–20 mg	no
	Evekeo	5–40 mg	no
Armodafinil	Nuvigil	150–250 mg	no
D- and L-amphetamine	Adderall	5–40 mg	no
Dexmethylphenidate	Focalin	5–20 mg	yes
Dextroamphetamine	Dexedrine	5–40 mg	yes
	IR	10–30 mg	no
	Mydayis ER[b]	12.5–50 mg	no
	ProCentra (liquid)	5–40 mg	no
Lisdexamfetamine	Vyvanse	30–70 mg	no
Methylphenidate	Aptensio XR[b]	10–60 mg	no
	Concerta[b]	18–72 mg	no
	Daytrana[b] (patch)	10–30 mg	no
	Metadate CD[b]	20–60 mg	no
	Quillivant XR[b]	20–60 mg	no
	Ritalin	10–60 mg	yes
Modafinil	Provigil	100–400 mg	no
Viloxazine	Qelbree	100–200 mg	no

[a]Adult doses.
[b]Sustained release.
[c]ODT = orally disintegrating tablet.

Drugs Used to Treat Obsessive-Compulsive Disorder

Names			
Generic	Brand	Therapeutic Dose Range[a]	Generic Available
Citalopram	Celexa	20–60 mg	yes
Clomipramine	Anafranil	150–250 mg	yes
Duloxetine[b]	Cymbalta	60–120 mg	yes
Escitalopram[b]	Lexapro	10–20 mg	yes
Fluoxetine	Prozac	20–80 mg	yes
Fluvoxamine	Luvox	50–300 mg	yes
Paroxetine	Paxil	20–60 mg	yes
Sertraline	Zoloft	50–200 mg	yes
Venlafaxine[b]	Effexor	75–375 mg	yes

[a]Doses required to control obsessive-compulsive symptoms are often higher than the doses generally used to treat depression.
[b]Off-label.

Antipsychotic Drugs

Names			Side Effects		
Generic	Brand	Therapeutic Dose Range	Weight Gain	Cognitive Impairment	Generic Available
Aripiprazole	Abilify[a]	10–30 mg	low	0	yes
Asenapine	Saphris	5–20 mg	mid	low	no
Brexpiprazole	Rexulti	2–4 mg	low	low	no
Cariprazine	Vraylar	1.5–6 mg	0	low	no
Chlorpromazine	Thorazine	250–1000 mg	high	mid	yes
Clozapine	Clozaril	300–900 mg	high	low	yes
Fluphenazine	Prolixin[a]	2.5–40 mg	high	low	yes
Haloperidol	Haldol[a]	2–20 mg	mid	low	yes
Iloperidone	Fanapt	4–24 mg	mid	low	no
Loxapine	Loxitane	60–250 mg	0	low	yes
Lumateperone	Caplyta	42 mg	0	low	no
Lurasidone	Latuda	40–160 mg	0	low	yes
Molindone	Moban	20–225 mg	low	low	yes
Olanzapine	Zyprexa[a]	5–20 mg	high	low	yes
Paliperidone	Invega[a]	6–12 mg	mid	low	yes
Perphenazine	Trilafon	8–64 mg	mid	low	yes
Pimavanserin	Nuplazid	34 mg	high	high	no
Pimozide	Orap	2–10 mg	low	low	yes
Quetiapine	Seroquel (XR)	400–800 mg	mid	low	yes
Risperidone	Risperdal[a]	2–16 mg	mid	low	yes
Thiothixene	Navane	10–60 mg	mid	low	yes
Thioridazine	Mellaril	150–800 mg	high	mid	yes
Trifluoperazine	Stelazine	4–40 mg	mid	low	yes
Ziprasidone	Geodon	40–160 mg	low	0	yes

[a]Available in a time-release intramuscular formulation.

Drugs Used to Treat Insomnia

Names			
Generic	Brand	Therapeutic Dose Range	Generic Available
Benzodiazepines[a]			
Estazolam	Prosom	1–2 mg	yes
Flurazepam	Dalmane	15–30 mg	yes
Quazepam	Doral	7.5–15 mg	yes
Temazepam	Restoril	7.5–30 mg	yes
Triazolam	Halcion	0.125–0.5 mg	yes
Nonbenzodiazepines			
Chlorohydrate	Noctec	500–1000 mg	yes
Daridorexant	Quviviq	25–50 mg	no
Diphenhydramine	Benadryl	25–50 mg	yes
Doxepin[b]	Silenor	10–50 mg	yes
Eszopiclone	Lunesta	1–3 mg	yes
Hydroxyzine	Vistaril	50–100 mg	yes
Lemborexant	Dayvigo	5–10 mg	no
Ramelteon	Rozerem	8 mg	no
Suvorexant	Belsomra	10–20 mg	no
Tasimelteon	Hetlioz	20 mg	no
Trazodone[b]	Desyrel	25–50 mg	yes
Zaleplon	Sonata	5–10 mg	yes
Zolpidem	Ambien	5–10 mg	yes
	Ambien ER	6.25–12.5 mg	yes

[a]Benzodiazepines used to treat anxiety (see next table) can also be used to treat insomnia.
[b]Also marketed for the treatment of depression.

Antianxiety Drugs (Anxiolytics)

Names			
Generic	Brand	Therapeutic Dose Range	Generic Available
Benzodiazepines[a]			
Alprazolam	Xanax	0.25–4 mg	yes
	Xanax ER	0.5–1 mg	yes
Chlordiazepoxide	Librium	20–100 mg	yes
Clonazepam	Klonopin	0.5–4 mg	yes
Clorazepate	Tranxene	15–60 mg	yes
Diazepam	Valium	8–40 mg	yes
Lorazepam	Ativan	2–10 mg	yes
Oxazepam	Serax	30–120 mg	yes
Nonbenzodiazepines			
Atenolol[b]	Tenormin	25–100 mg	yes
Buspirone	BuSpar	10–60 mg	yes
Clonidine[b]	Catapres	0.1–0.3 mg	yes
Guanfacine[b]	Tenex	0.5–3 mg	yes
Propranolol[b]	Inderal	10–80 mg	yes

[a]Can produce cognitive impairment.
[b]Antihypertensive drug used off-label to treat certain anxiety disorders.

GLOSSARY

Absorption. See **Drug absorption.**

Abstinence syndrome. See **Withdrawal syndrome.**

Acamprosate. The first pharmacological agent specifically designed to maintain abstinence in people with alcoholism after detoxification.

Acetylcholine. A neurotransmitter that activates two types of receptors, muscarinic and nicotinic.

AChE inhibitors. Drugs that block the action of AChE (acetylcholinesterase); used to slow cognitive decline in Alzheimer's disease.

Addiction. An often self-destructive adjustment to one's environment, an adjustment that represents a pattern of coping through habituation; addiction to drugs can be defined as tolerance and dependence plus drug-seeking behaviors that interfere with a normal healthy life.

Adenosine. A neurotransmitter that functions as a neuromodulator that influences the release of several other neurotransmitters in the CNS; adenosine levels usually increase during the day and exert a sleep-inducing effect in the brain.

ADH. See **Alcohol dehydrogenase.**

ADHD. See **Attention deficit/hyperactivity disorder.**

Aducanumab. A monoclonal antibody used for the treatment of mild to moderate cognitive impairment in patients with Alzheimer's disease.

Affinity. The strength with which a drug binds to a receptor.

Agomelatine. A novel antidepressant that acts as a melatonin receptor agonist and has been found to be effective in the treatment of anxiety, including PTSD.

Agonist. A drug that mimics a neurotransmitter by binding to and activating its receptor.

Alcohol. See **Ethyl alcohol.**

Alcohol dehydrogenase (ADH). An enzyme involved in alcohol metabolism; it is a cofactor in the conversion of ethanol to acetaldehyde.

Alcoholism. As viewed by the AMA, a chronic disease with certain well-defined characteristics (which broadly match up with the DSM-5 diagnostic criteria for alcohol use disorder); also, from the perspective of the media and the general public, any regular pattern of excessive drinking.

Alcohol use disorder (AUD). A disorder defined by 11 diagnostic criteria in DSM-5; it can be classified as mild, moderate, or severe depending on how many diagnostic criteria are met in the individual case.

Alzheimer's disease. A progressive neurodegenerative disease that results in the irreversible loss of cholinergic neurons, particularly in the cerebral cortex and hippocampus, and is characterized by the abnormal accumulation of amyloid-beta and tau proteins in the brain.

α-PVP. See **Flakka.**

Amantadine. An antiviral agent used to treat viral influenza and Parkinson's disease (to control tremor).

Amoxapine. An atypical antidepressant that is primarily a norepinephrine reuptake inhibitor but is also a potent blocker of serotonin 5-HT2_A receptors.

Amphetamines. A variety of compounds in the class of phenylethylamines, including amphetamine itself, methamphetamine, and MDMA, among others.

AMT. A serotoninlike psychedelic compound (alpha-methyltryptamine); it is one of the novel psychoactive tryptamines.

Amygdala. An almond-shaped brain structure (part of the limbic system) involved in emotional responses.

Anandamide. The natural neurotransmitter at cannabinoid receptors.

Anesthetics. See **General anesthetics.**

Antagonist. A drug that blocks the action of a neurotransmitter by binding to but not activating its receptor.

Antianxiety drugs. See **Anxiolytic drugs.**

Anticonvulsant drugs. Sedative-hypnotic drugs used to manage epilepsy.

Antidepressant drugs. Drugs used to treat depression.

Antiepileptic drugs. See **Anticonvulsant drugs.**

Antipsychotic drugs. Drugs used to treat a variety of psychiatric disorders, particularly those disorders that present with psychotic, hallucinogenic, or delusional symptoms.

Anxiolytic drugs. Sedative-hypnotic drugs used to alleviate anxiety.

Aripiprazole. An antipsychotic drug that is a partial agonist at D_2 and 5-HT1_A receptors, as well as an antagonist at 5-HT2 receptors.

ASDs. See **Autism spectrum disorders.**

Asenapine. An antipsychotic drug used for the treatment of schizophrenia and manic or mixed episodes of bipolar disorder in adults and adolescents.

Ataxia. A loss of muscle coordination and balance that may affect speech, eye movements, the ability to swallow, walking, picking up objects, and other voluntary movements.

Atomoxetine. A selective norepinephrine reuptake inhibitor antidepressant used for the acute and long-term treatment of child and adult ADHD.

Attention deficit/hyperactivity disorder (ADHD). One of the most common neurobehavioral disorders of childhood, characterized by reduced attention span, impulsivity, and/or hyperactivity; it can profoundly affect children's academic achievement, well-being, and social interactions.

Atypical antidepressants. Drugs that are slight modifications of the basic tricyclic structure of first-generation antidepressants but still exhibit antidepressant efficacy.

Atypical antipsychotics. See **Second-generation antipsychotics.**

AUD. See **Alcohol use disorder.**

Autism spectrum disorders (ASDs). A group of pervasive developmental disorders characterized by severe developmental deficits in social and communication skills and by the presence of repetitive behaviors, highly restricted interests, and/or anomalous sensory behaviors.

Autoreceptors. Receptors located on the presynaptic membrane that bind neurotransmitter molecules released by the presynaptic neuron and serve as a negative feedback mechanism to reduce the synthesis and further release of neurotransmitter molecules.

AXS-05. A noncatecholamine antidepressant that is a combination of bupropion and dextromethorphan; it is also an NMDA receptor antagonist.

Ayahuasca. A hallucinogenic tea brewed from parts of two plants: the vine *Banisteriopsis caapi* and the shrub *Psychotria viridis*, which contain the psychedelic compounds DMT and harmine.

BAC. See **Blood alcohol concentration.**

Baclofen. A drug used in the treatment of neuromuscular spasticity; it was formerly thought to have some efficacy in treating alcoholism.

Barbiturates. A class of chemically related sedative-hypnotic drugs structured around the basic barbiturate nucleus; they can differ significantly from each other in their individual pharmacokinetics, especially in their half-life.

Basal ganglia. A brain structure that includes the caudate nucleus, putamen, and globus pallidus and that is primarily responsible for coordinating and organizing smooth voluntary motor functions.

"Bath salts." See **Synthetic cathinones.**

BDNF. See **Brain-derived neurotrophic factor.**

Benzodiazepines. A class of chemically related sedative-hypnotic drugs structured around the basic benzodiazepine nucleus; first brought to market in 1961, they quickly became the most widely used class of psychotherapeutic drugs.

Binding. See **Drug-receptor binding.**

Binge drinking. Drinking that brings blood alcohol concentration to 0.08% or higher in a span of about 2 hours; for typical adult males, this means consuming five or more drinks in that span, and for typical adult females, it means consuming four or more drinks in that span.

Bioavailability. How much of a drug that is administered actually reaches its target and how long it persists there.

Bipolar CHOICE (Clinical Health Outcomes Initiative in Comparative Effectiveness). A study comparing the effectiveness of lithium and quetiapine in treating bipolar disorder.

Bipolar disorder (manic-depressive disorder). A mental health disorder characterized by extreme shifts in mood, high suicide rate, sleep problems, and dysfunctions of psychological traits like self-esteem.

Bipolar I disorder. A subtype of bipolar disorder characterized by at least one episode of full-blown mania with or without an episode of major depression.

Bipolar II disorder. A subtype of bipolar disorder characterized by less severe manic episodes and more frequent episodes of major depression.

Blackouts. Periods of time during which a person may be awake but of which the person later has little or no memory; most commonly, blackouts result from excessive consumption of alcohol or from large doses of sedative drugs.

Blood alcohol concentration (BAC). The weight of alcohol in a fixed volume of blood, used as a measure of the degree of intoxication; the BAC depends on body weight, the quantity and rate of alcohol ingestion, and the rates of alcohol absorption and metabolism.

Blood-brain barrier. A specialized structural barrier that plays a key role in maintaining a protected environment in the brain.

Brain-derived neurotrophic factor (BDNF). A protein that is one of a group of substances called *neurotrophins*, which are important for the normal development and health of the nervous system.

Brain-disease model of addiction. The theory that addiction is a result of long-term neurophysiological changes in the reward circuit of the brain induced by the continued use of certain drugs.

Brain stem. The part of the brain attached to the top of the spinal cord; it consists of the medulla, the pons, and the midbrain.

Brexanolone. A noncatecholamine antidepressant that is an intravenous formulation of allopregnanolone and a modulator of $GABA_A$ receptors; used for the treatment of postpartum depression.

Brexpiprazole. An atypical antipsychotic drug used for the treatment of schizophrenia, treatment-resistant major depression, and anxiety.

Brivaracetam. An anticonvulsant drug used for the treatment of both partial and major motor seizures; its efficacy does not seem to surpass that of levetiracetam.

Bufotenine. A serotoninlike psychedelic compound (5-hydroxy DMT, or dimethylserotonin).

Buprenorphine. A partial opioid agonist widely used in the treatment of opioid dependence; it has also found use as an analgesic.

Bupropion. An SSRI antidepressant that is a weak reuptake inhibitor of dopamine and norepinephrine.

Butorphanol. A mixed opioid agonist-antagonist analgesic that is available as a nasal spray (the first opioid analgesic so formulated); its use is generally limited to veterinary medicine.

BZP. A catecholaminelike and amphetaminelike psychedelic compound (benzylpiperazine); low doses cause stimulant effects, while hallucinogenic actions predominate at higher doses.

Caffeine. The most widely consumed psychoactive drug in the world; it stimulates the central nervous system, produces diuresis, stimulates the cardiac muscle, and relaxes the bronchi.

Caffeinism. A clinical syndrome resulting from habitual consumption of excessive amounts of caffeine.

cAMP response-element binding protein (CREB). One of the intracellular targets of second-messenger systems; it activates genes that control the production of brain-derived neurotrophic factor.

Candesartan. An antihypertensive medication used to treat mild cognitive impairment in patients with Alzheimer's disease.

Cannabidiol (CBD). A nonpsychedelic agent with various therapeutic application derived from plants of the genus *Cannabis*; it is produced when the cannabinoid cannabidiolic acid undergoes decarboxylation.

Cannabinoid cycling. The process of periodically switching from high-THC, low-CBD strains of medical cannabis to high-CBD, low-THC strains, in order to avoid the development of tolerance to the drug.

Cannabinoid receptors. Receptors in the family of GPCRs that are activated by cannabinoids; there are two types, CB1 and CB2, with CB1 receptors found mainly in the CNS and CB2 receptors found mainly outside the CNS, primarily in tissues of the immune system.

Cannabinoids. Compounds found in plants of the genus *Cannabis*.

Cannabis. A name for the drug marijuana and the genus name of the plant species (principally, *Cannabis sativa* and *Cannabis indica*) from which the drug is derived.

Cannabis use disorder. A disorder defined by seven diagnostic criteria in DSM-5; it can be classified as mild, moderate, or severe depending on how many diagnostic criteria are met in the individual case.

Carbamazepine. An anticonvulsant drug that was introduced in 1963; it perhaps has a less intense sedative effect than do other antiepileptics, but its use risks serious alterations in the cellular composition of blood and increases in the production of drug-metabolizing enzymes in the liver.

Carboxy-THC. An inactive metabolite of THC; urine testing for THC use focuses on identification of carboxy-THC, which is only slowly excreted.

Cariprazine. An antipsychotic drug with a higher affinity for D_3 receptors than for D_2 receptors; it is used for treatment of schizophrenia and for acute treatment of mania in persons with bipolar disorder, bipolar depression, and major depressive disorder.

Carisoprodol. A nonbarbiturate sedative-hypnotic drug that is a precursor compound to meprobamate; after it is absorbed, it is rapidly metabolized to meprobamate, which is the active form of the drug.

Carrier proteins. See **Transporter proteins.**

Catecholamine. A group of neurotransmitters that includes dopamine, norepinephrine, and epinephrine.

Catechol-*O*-methyltransferase (COMT) inhibitors. A class of dopamine reuptake inhibitors used as adjuvant medications with levodopa to reduce motor complications and levodopa dose in patients with Parkinson's disease.

CATIE (Clinical Antipsychotic Trials of Intervention Effectiveness) study. A study of the effectiveness of antipsychotic drugs, conducted in the United States between January 2001 and December 2004.

CBD. See **Cannabidiol.**

Cebranopadol. A mixed NOP and mu opioid receptor agonist with analgesic efficacy similar to that of morphine in treating a variety of pain states, including moderate to severe cancer-related pain.

Ceiling effect. The maximum effect that can be produced by a drug, regardless of dosage.

Cenobamate. An anticonvulsant drug that used for the treatment of partial seizures in adults; it is a sodium channel blocker that is also thought to enhance presynaptic GABA release, thereby increasing GABA's inhibitory effects.

Central nervous system (CNS). Brain and spinal cord.

Cerebellum. A large, bulbous brain structure located behind the brain stem; its function is to coordinate voluntary movements, posture, and balance.

Cerebral cortex. The outer layer of the cerebrum; in each hemisphere, the cerebral cortex is divided into four lobes (occipital, temporal, parietal, and frontal).

Cerebrum. The largest part of the brain, almost completely covering the brain stem and the diencephalon; it is divided into left and right hemispheres, separated by a fissure.

Charlotte's Web. An unusual strain of medical marijuana containing very little THC (i.e., with a very high ratio of CBD to THC); the name comes from its widely reported beneficial use in treating Charlotte Figi, a young child with a refractory form of epilepsy.

Chloral hydrate. A nonbarbiturate sedative-hypnotic drug that was introduced into medicine in the late nineteenth century; the combination of chloral hydrate with alcohol, called a *Mickey Finn*, was an early example of a date rape drug.

Chlorpromazine. A first-generation antipsychotic drug synthesized in 1951; it was first used in anesthesia mixtures and then found to be effective in alleviating the clinical manifestations of psychosis.

Cholinergic-deficiency theory. The theory that symptoms of Alzheimer's disease are due to a deficiency of acetylcholine neurotransmission.

Cingulate cortex. A brain structure (part of the limbic system) involved in integrating sensory, motor, visceral, motivational, and emotional information.

Circadin. A drug for the treatment of insomnia, it is a prolonged-release formulation of melatonin; not available over the counter in the United States, it has been approved for use by prescription in other countries.

Citalopram. An SSRI antidepressant that has been found to be more effective at treating the core emotional symptoms of depression than sleep symptoms or atypical symptoms.

Clinical Antipsychotic Trials of Intervention Effectiveness. See **CATIE study.**

Clobazam. An anticonvulsant drug used for the treatment of seizures associated with Lennox-Gastaut syndrome; it is a benzodiazepine that is also used for the treatment of refractory epilepsy and for the short-term treatment of severe anxiety and agitation seen in psychotic disorders.

Clomipramine. A tricyclic antidepressant that is classified as a mixed serotonin-norepinephrine reuptake inhibitor; it has a greater effect on serotonin reuptake than the classic tricyclic antidepressants, is an effective anxiolytic, and is also used to treat obsessive-compulsive disorder.

Clonidine. An antihypertensive drug used for the treatment of ADHD, either as monotherapy or concomitantly with a stimulant.

Clozapine. The first of the second-generation antipsychotic drugs; it was discovered in 1959 and in 1966 was found to have antipsychotic efficacy without the disabling neurological side effects that were seen with chlorpromazine and other phenothiazine antipsychotics.

Cocaethylene. A pharmacologically active metabolite of cocaine produced in people who use cocaine and ethanol concurrently; it is an ethyl ester of cocaine's main metabolite, benzoylecgonine.

Cocaine. A psychostimulant derived from the leaves of the coca plant; it acts primarily by blocking reuptake of the neurotransmitter dopamine.

Cocaine base. A crystalline compound produced by treating cocaine hydrochloride with an alkaline solution and adding a solvent; it can be heated until the crystals convert to a stable vapor that can be inhaled (smoked).

Cocaine hydrochloride. A compound produced by soaking and mashing coca leaves to form coca paste, which is then treated with hydrochloric acid; it is the powdered form in which cocaine is usually exported.

Codeine. A prodrug that constitutes about 0.5% of the crude exudate from the opium poppy and that is metabolized to morphine by the enzyme CYP-2D6; once widely prescribed as a low-potency opioid, it was usually combined with aspirin or acetaminophen for the relief of mild to moderate pain.

Cognitive-behavioral therapy. A type of psychotherapy in which individuals are taught about their illness, taught how to recognize signs and symptoms, and helped to develop cognitive and behavioral coping strategies.

Combining Medications to Enhance Depression Outcomes (CO-MED) trial. A trial comparing the efficacy of escitalopram monotherapy versus two-antidepressant combinations in the treatment of both acute and long-term major depressive disorder.

Comorbid disorder. A disorder that coexists with another disorder in the same individual (e.g., major depressive disorder and a substance abuse disorder are often comorbid disorders).

Complex sleep-related behaviors. Behaviors such as "sleep driving" and other activities of which the person has no subsequent memory, often due to the use of sedative-hypnotic drugs.

Cost Utility of the Latest Antipsychotic Drugs in Schizophrenia Studies. See **CUtLASS 1.**

Cotinine. The weakly active primary metabolite of nicotine; used as a biomarker for exposure to tobacco smoke.

Cravings. Strong urges to use a drug again, even after long periods of abstinence.

CREB. See **cAMP response-element binding protein.**

Cross-tolerance. Condition in which tolerance of one drug results in a lessened response to another drug.

CUtLASS 1 (Cost Utility of the Latest Antipsychotic Drugs in Schizophrenia Studies). A British study of the effectiveness of antipsychotic drugs, reported in 2006.

Cytochrome P450 enzyme family. A large group of proteins, mostly (but not only) found in the liver, responsible for metabolizing a wide variety of endogenous and exogenous substances.

Dabbing. A method of rapidly inhaling concentrated THC; butane is passed through a tube packed with dried cannabis to produce butane hash oil, with THC concentrations of 80% or more, which is then vaporized and inhaled ("dabbed") through a water pipe.

Dementia. Cognitive impairment with the inability to form new memory; it is the critical feature of Alzheimer's disease.

Depression (major depressive disorder; MDD). A highly prevalent, chronic, recurring, and potentially life-threatening illness characterized by sometimes profound alterations of emotion or mood, decreased interest in pleasurable activities, decreased ability to experience pleasure, sleep difficulties, fatigue or loss of energy, feelings of worthlessness or excessive guilt, and possible thoughts of death or suicide.

Desensitization. See **Downregulation.**

Desomorphine. A designer drug that can be synthesized from codeine with other ingredients; as a homemade mixture it has many contaminants and is very toxic.

Desvenlafaxine. An SNRI antidepressant that is the active metabolite of venlafaxine and thus has the efficacy, safety, and tolerability of venlafaxine.

Dextroamphetamine. A pharmacologically potent isomer of amphetamine.

Dextromethorphan. A common ingredient in over-the-counter cough suppressants; high doses can induce hallucinations, delusions, and paranoia.

Dimethyltryptamine. See **DMT.**

Dissolvable tobacco products. Finely powdered tobacco formed into pellets, strips, or "sticks" that are placed under the tongue, where they dissolve and are swallowed over the course of 15 minutes or so.

Disulfiram. A drug used in the treatment of chronic alcoholism that interferes with the normal metabolic degradation of alcohol in the body, producing an unpleasant reaction when a small quantity of alcohol is consumed.

DMA. Any of a series of six structurally related catecholaminelike and amphetaminelike psychedelic compounds (dimethoxyamphetamine); little is known about the effects, risks, or toxicities associated with their use.

DMAA. A nonamphetamine psychostimulant found in dietary energy products.

DMT. A serotoninlike psychedelic compound (dimethyltryptamine) that produces LSD-like effects and is an agonist at 5-HT2_A receptors; it is the main psychedelic constituent in ayahuasca.

DOM. A catecholaminelike and amphetaminelike psychedelic compound (2,5-dimethoxy-4-methylamphetamine, also known as "STP"); it has effects that are similar to those of mescaline, but it is 100 times more potent than mescaline and is associated with a high incidence of overdose and acute toxic reactions.

Donanemab. A monoclonal antibody used in the treatment of Alzheimer's disease; it targets a form of amyloid-β exclusively found in plaques.

Donepezil. An acetylcholinesterase inhibitor used in the treatment of Alzheimer's disease.

Dopamine. A catecholamine neurotransmitters in the central nervous system, considered to be the primary reward neurotransmitter in the brain and important in mediating voluntary movement (loss of dopamine neurons produces Parkinson's disease).

Dose-response relationship. The relationship between the dose of a drug and the clinical response to the drug at each dose level.

Downregulation. A decrease in the number and sensitivity of postsynaptic receptors and a consequent decrease in the response of the postsynaptic neuron due to the presence in the synaptic cleft of excessive numbers of neurotransmitter molecules and/or an agonist over an extended period of time.

Doxepin. An antihistamine (histamine receptor antagonist) and antidepressant used for the treatment of sleep maintenance insomnia.

Drug. A chemical substance used for its effects on bodily processes.

Drug absorption. Mechanism by which a drug reaches the bloodstream from the skin, lungs, stomach, intestinal tract, or muscle.

Drug administration. Procedures through which a drug enters the body (oral administration of tablets or liquids, inhalation of powders, injection of sterile liquids, and so on).

Drug dependence. State in which the use of a drug is necessary for either physical or psychological well-being.
Drug distribution. Movement of drug between the blood and various tissues of the body.
Drug receptor. See **Receptor.**
Drug-receptor binding. The attachment of a drug to a receptor on the surface of a neuron.
Drug tolerance. Progressively decreasing responsiveness to a drug, meaning that progressively increasing doses of the drug are needed to produce the same effect.
Duloxetine. An SNRI antidepressant that seems to be mildly effective in the treatment of both depression and anxiety.
Dysthymia. See **Persistent depressive disorder.**

Early-onset alcoholism. Alcoholism that develops by age 25 or earlier and is associated with a strong family history of alcoholism and notable antisocial traits.
Ecstasy. See **MDMA.**
Efficacy. The ability of a drug to produce its intended effect.
Electronic cigarettes (e-cigarettes). Cigarette-shaped nicotine-delivery devices; users add a nicotine-containing liquid to the device, which uses battery power to heat the liquid until it emits a nicotine vapor that is inhaled.
Elemicin. A catecholaminelike and amphetaminelike psychedelic compound present in nutmeg and mace.
Endorphins. Opioid peptide neurotransmitters that may be involved in a wide variety of emotional states.
Enkephalins. Opioid peptide neurotransmitters involved in pain perception and in stress responses.
Enzyme induction. Increased production of drug-metabolizing enzymes in the liver, stimulated by certain drugs (inducers).
Ephedrine. A pharmacologically active compound that occurs naturally in the herb *Ephedra sinica*.
Escitalopram. An SSRI antidepressant that is also used for the treatment of generalized anxiety disorder; it is the active isomer of citalopram.
Esketamine. A psychedelic compound that is a glutamate NMDA receptor antagonist; it is the pharmacologically more active isomer of ketamine and is used as an anesthetic and an antidepressant.
Eslicarbazepine. An anticonvulsant drug used as an ancillary medication to treat partial seizures; it is a prodrug to oxcarbazepine, which means it has the same actions as oxcarbazepine.
Eszopiclone. A nonbenzodiazepine agonist at benzodiazepine receptors that is used for the treatment of insomnia.
Ethanol. See **Ethyl alcohol.**
Ethyl alcohol. A sedative-hypnotic intoxicant in various fermented and/or distilled beverages, widely used by humans from at least Neolithic times.
Excessive drinking. As defined by the Centers for Disease Control, "binge drinking, heavy drinking, and any alcohol use by pregnant women or anyone younger than 21."
Exocytosis. The process by which synaptic vesicles fuse with the presynaptic membrane and release neurotransmitter molecules into the synaptic cleft.
Extrapyramidal symptoms . Neurological side effects of antipsychotic drugs similar to symptoms of Parkinson's disease, resulting from the drugs' effects on dopamine neurons in the extrapyramidal motor system.
Ezogabine. An anticonvulsant drug used as an adjunctive treatment for adults with partial-onset seizures.

Family-focused therapy. A type of psychotherapy especially for individuals with bipolar disorder; families are taught about the disorder, how to recognize signs of episodes, how to support the individual's efforts to manage the illness through adherence to the treatment plan, how to avoid negative communication styles that exacerbate or trigger episodes, and other skills.

FAS. See **Fetal alcohol syndrome.**

Fentanyl. A short-acting opioid that is structurally related to meperidine; originally marketed for use after surgery to relieve surgical pain, it is currently widely synthesized in laboratories and contributes significantly to the opioid epidemic.

Fetal alcohol syndrome (FAS). A developmental disorder caused by excessive consumption of alcohol by the mother during pregnancy; it is characterized by deficits in mental development and abnormalities in physical development, particularly of the skull and face of the infant.

First-generation antidepressants. The tricyclic antidepressants and the monoamine oxidase inhibitors, which are effective in the treatment of depression but have adverse side effects.

First-generation antipsychotics. Antipsychotic drugs developed in the 1950s and 1960s; although their antipsychotic actions cannot be separated from their neurological side effects, they continue to be used to treat schizophrenia, as well as bipolar disorder, hyperactivity, agitation, and anxiety.

First-pass metabolism. The breakdown of drugs as they are transported through the gastrointestinal tract or the liver before they reach the rest of the body through the circulatory system.

5-hydroxytryptamine (5-HT). See **Serotonin.**

5-MeO-MiPT. A serotoninlike psychedelic compound (5-methoxy-N-methyl-N-isopropyltryptamine, with the street name "moxy"); it is one of the novel psychoactive tryptamines.

Flakka (α-PVP). A frequently abused synthetic cathinone; it is one of the drugs known as "bath salts."

Flashbacks. Recurring acute effects of LSD and related substances long after the drug has been eliminated from the body; usually short-lasting and nondistressing. See also **Hallucinogen persisting perception disorder.**

Flumazenil. A benzodiazepine that binds to $GABA_A$ benzodiazepine receptors but exhibits no intrinsic pharmacological activity; thus, it competitively blocks the access of pharmacologically active benzodiazepines to the receptors and can be used as an antidote in cases of benzodiazepine overdoses.

Fluoxetine. The first SSRI antidepressant and the first nontricyclic antidepressant that could be considered a first-line treatment; its efficacy is comparable to that of the tricyclics, with few or no anticholinergic or antihistaminic side effects; it is also used in the treatment of persistent depressive disorder, bulimia, alcohol withdrawal, and anxiety disorders.

Fluvoxamine. An SSRI antidepressant that is a structural derivative of fluoxetine; it is comparable in efficacy to imipramine, with fewer serious side effects, and is effective in the treatment of anxiety disorders.

Forebrain. One of the three major divisions of the brain, made up of the telencephalon (which includes the thalamus and hypothalamus) and diencephalon (which includes the cerebrum, the basal ganglia, and the limbic system).

GABA. See **Gamma aminobutyric acid.**

Gabapentin. An anticonvulsant drug that is a structural analogue of GABA; it was synthesized with the aim of developing a specifically GABA-mimetic antiepileptic drug.

Galantamine. An acetylcholinesterase inhibitor used in the treatment of Alzheimer's disease.

Gamma aminobutyric acid (GABA). An inhibitory amino acid neurotransmitter.

Gamma hydroxybutyrate (GHB). A nonbarbiturate sedative-hypnotic drug that is also a natural neurotransmitter; it binds to GHB receptors on both pre- and postsynaptic neurons, with the effect of inhibiting GABA release.

General anesthetics. Drugs that are used to produce amnesia and loss of consciousness during surgery.

Generic name. The name given to a drug by its discoverer or original manufacturer, often an abbreviated form of the structural name; drugs with the same generic name may be marketed under different brand names by different manufacturers.

Glutamate (glutamic acid). An excitatory amino acid neurotransmitter; it is a precursor to GABA, an inhibitory neurotransmitter.

GPCRs (G-protein-coupled receptors). See **Metabotropic receptors.**

G protein. An intraneuronal protein attached to a G-protein-coupled receptor; activation of the receptor leads to release of one component of the G protein, with various effects on the neuron.

G-protein-coupled receptors (GPCRs). See **Metabotropic receptors.**

Guanfacine. An antihypertensive drug used for the treatment of ADHD, either as monotherapy or concomitantly with a stimulant.

Half-life. The time needed for half the amount of drug in the blood to be eliminated.

Hallucinogens. See **Psychedelic drugs.**

Hallucinogen persisting perception disorder (HPPD). A condition characterized by recurring acute effects of LSD and related substances long after the drug has been eliminated from the body; it is usually long-term and distressing. See also **Flashbacks.**

Harmine. A monoamine oxidase inhibitor that seems to potentiate the effects of DMT in ayahuasca.

Heated tobacco products. Devices that are hybrids between tobacco cigarettes and e-cigarettes; they heat tobacco to a high enough temperature to produce a tobacco-flavored vapor without smoke or tar.

Heroin. A semisynthetic opioid produced by a chemical modification of morphine; it is three times more potent than morphine and provides an intense rush when injected intravenously.

Hindbrain. One of the three major divisions of the brain, made up of the myelencephalon (which includes the medulla) and the metencephalon (which includes the cerebellum and the pons).

Hippocampus. A brain structure (part of the limbic system) involved in learning and memory.

Hookahs. Pipes that pass the smoke from burning tobacco through water so the smoke is cooled before inhalation.

Huperzine A. A naturally occurring acetylcholinesterase inhibitor that has been studied as a treatment for Alzheimer's disease; it is derived from the moss *Huperzia serrata*.

Hydrocodone. One of the most commonly prescribed and abused opioid medications; it is a relatively weak analgesic that is converted into the more active compound hydromorphone.

Hydromorphone. An opioid that is structurally related to morphine and is 6–10 times more potent than morphine.

Hypothalamus. A collection of neuronal structures near the junction of the midbrain and the thalamus just above the pituitary gland (whose function it modulates); it regulates body temperature, certain metabolic processes, and other autonomic activities.

Ibogaine. A naturally occurring substance found in the roots of the iboga tree (*Tabernanthe iboga*) in Gabon and Cameroon, where it is used as a psychedelic and for divination; its medical use has been limited because of a poor safety profile, including cardiotoxicity.

Iloperidone. An antipsychotic drug with side effects that include dizziness, dry mouth, fatigue, nasal congestion, somnolence, tachycardia, orthostatic hypotension, some elevation in prolactin, and weight gain.

Imipramine. The prototype tricyclic antidepressant; its antidepressant properties were discovered accidentally in 1950.

Inhalants. Breathable chemical vapors that produce psychoactive effects.

Interpersonal and social rhythm therapy. A type of psychotherapy that stresses the importance of establishing and maintaining a regular life schedule and teaching the individual and their family problem-solving skills that will improve the individual's satisfaction within social situations.

Intramuscular injection. An injection into a muscle.

Intravenous injection. An injection into a vein.

Ionotropic receptors (ion channel receptors). Receptors that form a membrane-spanning ion channel on postsynaptic neurons; when activated by the binding of a neurotransmitter or drug, the ion channel in these fast-acting receptors enlarges to let ions enter the neuron.

Isomers. Two or more molecules with the same molecular formula but different three-dimensional shapes (i.e., different arrangements of their atoms in space).

Ketamine. A psychedelic compound (a racemic mixture, with the street name "Special K") that is a glutamate NMDA receptor antagonist; developed as an anesthetic, it induces a phencyclidinelike anesthetic state in low doses, with similar but less severe psychiatric side effects; its pharmacologically more active isomer is esketamine.

Khat. A flowering shrub (*Catha edulis*) native to East Africa; the leaves and fresh shoots can be chewed or brewed as a tea, with effects similar to, but less powerful than, amphetamine and cocaine.

Kratom. The common name for the plant *Mitragyna speciosa,* the leaves of which contain the alkaloid mitragynine; low doses have a stimulant action, but high doses produce sedation and opioidlike effects.

LAAM. See **Levo-alpha acetylmethadol.**

Lacosamide. An anticonvulsant drug used in the treatment of partial-onset seizures; it modulates sodium channels without affecting fast action potentials.

Lamotrigine. An anticonvulsant drug that acts by inhibiting ion fluxes through sodium channels, stabilizing neuronal membranes, and inhibiting the presynaptic release of neurotransmitters, principally glutamate.

Lemborexant. An orexin receptor antagonist used for the treatment of insomnia.

Levetiracetam. An anticonvulsant drug used for the treatment of partial-onset seizures; its unique mechanism of action makes it suitable for add-on therapy in patients with refractory seizures.

Levo-alpha acetylmethadol (LAAM). An oral opioid analgesic used as a second-line treatment in the management of opioid dependence; it has a slow onset and a longer duration of action than methadone.

Levodopa. A precursor drug to dopamine that is used in the treatment of Parkinson's disease, usually in combination with other medications.

Levomilnacipran. An SNRI antidepressant used for the treatment of major depressive disorder; its typical side effects include sexual dysfunction, tachycardia, palpitations, hypertension, and vomiting.

Limbic system. A group of brain structures involved in memory and emotion.

Lipid solubility. The ability of a chemical compound to dissolve in fats and oils.

Lithium. An alkali metal used as a medication for long-term treatment of bipolar disorder, treatment of acute episodes of bipolar disorder, and augmentation of antidepressant drugs in persons with treatment-resistant depression.

Lithium Treatment Moderate-Dose Use Study (LiTMUS). A study conducted to answer the question of whether combining lithium with other mood stabilizers or second-generation antipsychotics resulted in any greater benefit, relative to the additional side effect risk, than just using the mood stabilizers or antipsychotics alone.

LSD (lysergic acid diethylamide). A synthetic serotoninlike psychedelic compound with intense physiological and psychological effects at very small doses.

Lumateperone. An antipsychotic drug with the prominent side effect of sedation.

Lurasidone. An antipsychotic drug with side effects that include somnolence, nausea, extrapyramidal symptoms, and akathisia.

Lysergic acid amide. A serotoninlike psychedelic compound; it is the psychoactive component in ololiuqui.

Lysergic acid diethylamide. See **LSD.**

Major depressive disorder. See **Depression.**

Manic-depressive disorder. See **Bipolar disorder.**

MAO. See **Monoamine oxidase.**

MAOIs. See **Monoamine oxidase inhibitors.**

Maprotiline. A tricyclic antidepressant that was one of the first clinically available antidepressants with a modification of the basic tricyclic structure; it has a long half-life, blocks norepinephrine reuptake, and is as efficacious as imipramine.

Margin of safety. See **Therapeutic index.**

Marijuana. A drug derived from dried, crushed parts (leaves, flowers, and small branches) of plants of the genus *Cannabis*.

mCPP. A serotoninlike psychedelic compound (meta-chlorophenylpiperazine) that is an agonist at almost all 5-HT receptors; its effects are generally considered to be unpleasant, including depressive symptoms, anxiety, and panic attacks.

MDA. A catecholaminelike and amphetaminelike psychedelic compound (3,4-methylenedioxyamphetamine); it is a metabolite of MDMA and may contribute to MDMA's effects.

MDAI. A catecholaminelike and amphetaminelike psychedelic compound (5,6-methylenedioxy-2-aminoindane); it is a reuptake inhibitor of serotonin, dopamine, and norepinephrine, especially of serotonin, with effects that are reported to include spiritual experiences, euphoria, empathy, and intensified sensory experiences.

MDD (major depressive disorder). See **Depression.**

MDE. A catecholaminelike and amphetaminelike psychedelic compound; its effects in smaller doses resemble those of MDMA and, in larger doses, resemble those of MDA.

MDMA. A catecholaminelike and amphetaminelike psychedelic compound (methylene-dioxymethamphetamine, also known as "ecstasy") initially developed as an appetite suppressant, later used as an aid in psychotherapy, but today frequently abused socially, while also being used for treatment of PTSD.

MDPV. A frequently abused synthetic cathinone; it is one of the drugs known as "bath salts."

Melatonin. A hormone secreted by the pineal gland in a circadian rhythm; it has many functions in the body, including sleep promotion.

Memantine. A medication used to treat the cognitive and behavioral effects of dementia; it is active at NMDA receptors.

Meperidine. A synthetic opioid that is one-tenth as potent as morphine, produces a similar type of euphoria, and is equally likely to cause dependence.

Mephedrone. A frequently abused synthetic cathinone; it is one of the drugs known as "bath salts."

Meprobamate. A nonbarbiturate sedative-hypnotic drug that was marketed in 1955 as an alternative to the barbiturates for daytime sedation and anxiolysis.

Mescaline. A catecholaminelike and amphetaminelike psychedelic; it is a component of the peyote cactus.

Mesolimbic dopamine pathway. The core of the reward circuit in the brain; it begins with a group of dopamine-releasing neurons in the ventral tegmental area that project to brain structures including the nucleus accumbens, amygdala, hippocampus, and prefrontal cortex, where they release dopamine when the ventral tegmental area is activated.

Metabolic syndrome. An array of side effects most often associated with second-generation psychotics, including weight gain, dyslipidemia, and glucose intolerance, which can lead to diabetes.

Metabotropic receptors (G-protein-coupled receptors [GPCRs]). Receptors found in the membrane of both post- and presynaptic neurons; when activated by the binding of a neurotransmitter or drug, these slow-acting receptors have a variety of effects on the neurons, mediated by second messengers.

Methadone. A synthetic opioid very similar to morphine; because it blocks the effects of heroin withdrawal, it is used as an orally administered substitute for heroin in addiction treatment programs.

Methamphetamine. A modified version of dextroamphetamine formed by substituting a methyl group for the hydrogen atom at one end.

Methaqualone. A nonbarbiturate sedative-hypnotic drug that was frequently prescribed in the 1960s and 1970s; during the late 1970s, its popularity as a recreational drug peaked, and its level of abuse rivaled that of marijuana and alcohol.

Methoxetamine. A drug that is structurally and pharmacologically similar to ketamine, with potential for therapeutic use as an antidepressant and an analgesic.

Methylone. A frequently abused synthetic cathinone; it is one of the drugs known as "bath salts."

Methylphenidate. A stimulant medication used for the treatment of ADHD.

Midbrain. One of the three major divisions of the brain, made up of the mesencephalon.

Mirtazapine. A noradrenergic/specific serotonergic antidepressant used for the treatment of major depressive disorder; it increases the presynaptic release of both norepinephrine and serotonin.

Mitragynine. The predominant alkaloid in kratom; it is believed to be a partial agonist at the mu opioid receptor and an antagonist at the delta opioid receptor.

Monoamine oxidase (MAO). An enzyme capable of metabolizing norepinephrine, dopamine, and serotonin to inactive products.

Monoamine oxidase inhibitors (MAOIs). A class of early antidepressant drugs that bind to and block the enzyme monoamine oxidase; along with the tricyclic antidepressants, they constitute the first-generation antidepressants.

Monoamine oxidase type B (MAO-B) inhibitors. A class of dopamine reuptake inhibitors used as adjuvant medications with levodopa to reduce motor complications and levodopa dose in patients with Parkinson's disease.

Morphine. An opioid contained in the resinous exudate from the seed pods of the opium poppy; it is considered the model opioid analgesic against which all others are compared.

Muscarinic receptors. Acetylcholine receptors that are activated by muscarine; they are involved in various complex CNS functions, such as memory, arousal, heart rate, attention, and analgesia.

Myristicin. A catecholaminelike and amphetaminelike psychedelic compound present in nutmeg and mace.

Nalbuphine. An opioid agonist of limited analgesic effectiveness but not likely to produce either respiratory depression or patterns of abuse; it is mainly used as a treatment for morphine-induced pruritus.

Nalmefene. A full opioid antagonist that is a structural derivative of oxymorphone and is used primarily in the treatment of alcoholism but also in the treatment of opioid overdose, addiction, and dependence.

Naloxone. A full opioid antagonist that is a structural derivative of oxymorphone and is used in the treatment of opioid overdose, addiction, and dependence.

Naltrexone. A full opioid antagonist that is a structural derivative of oxymorphone and is used primarily in the treatment of alcoholism but also in the treatment of opioid overdose, addiction, and dependence.

Nefazodone. A serotonin-2 antagonist/reuptake inhibitor antidepressant that is chemically related to trazodone; it is seldom used because of its liver toxicity and the availability of many alternatives.

Negative symptoms (of schizophrenia). Deficits in communication skills, emotion, or affect; social or interpersonal skills; motivation; and psychomotor activity.

Neonatal abstinence syndrome. A condition of newborns characterized by signs and symptoms of drug withdrawal due to drug use by the mother during pregnancy.

Neurogenesis. The birth of new neurons; it is now known that new neurons are produced throughout life in the hippocampus and the frontal cortex.

Neurogenic theory of depression. The theory that depression is a neurodegenerative disorder involving atrophy of neurons in the hippocampus and frontal cortex.

Neuroleptic malignant syndrome (NMS). A potentially lethal side effect of treatment with antipsychotic drugs that increase dopamine transmission; symptoms include fever, severe muscle rigidity of the "lead pipe" type, autonomic changes such as fluctuating blood pressure, and altered consciousness that may progress to stupor or coma.

Neurotransmitter. A chemical that is released by a neuron and that then attaches to receptors on another neuron, altering the activity of that other neuron.

Nicotine. A highly addictive alkaloid that is a behavioral stimulant and the primary psychoactive component in tobacco; it directly stimulates acetylcholine receptors.

Nicotine replacement therapies. Smoking cessation treatments that substitute another source of nicotine for the nicotine inhaled from smoking.

Nicotinic receptors. Acetylcholine receptors that are activated by nicotine; they are divided into two groups, muscle receptors and neuronal receptors.

Nilotinib. A drug marketed for the treatment of chronic leukemia; it has been studied as a treatment for motor and cognitive problems in patients with Parkinson's disease.

Nitrites. A class of inhalants used primarily as sexual enhancers.

Nitrous oxide. An NMDA receptor antagonist that has shown promise as a rapid-acting antidepressant in patients with treatment-resistant depression; it is also used as an anesthetic.

NMDA receptors. A type of glutamate receptors that are blocked by the psychedelic drugs phencyclidine (PCP) and ketamine.

NMS. See **Neuroleptic malignant syndrome.**

Norepinephrine. A catecholamine neurotransmitter involved in alerting, focusing, and orienting responses, in positive feelings of reward, and in analgesia.

Olanzapine. An antipsychotic drug with side effects that can include sedation, weight gain, and the metabolic syndrome, as well as cognitive impairment in at-risk individuals.

Oliceridine. An opioid receptor agonist used intravenously in the treatment of acute pain.

Ololiuqui. A species of morning glory (*Rivea corymbosa*), the seeds of which, when ingested, produce hallucinations and intoxication due to the presence of lysergic acid amide.

Omega-3 polyunsaturated fatty acids. Nutraceuticals used adjunctively for the treatment of psychiatric disorders, including bipolar disorder.

Ondansetron. A drug typically used as an antinausea medication for patients receiving chemotherapy; it has shown some positive results in treating alcohol use disorder, including in reducing alcohol cravings in early-onset alcoholism.

Opioid. Any drug that binds to and acts as an agonist at any of the various types of opioid receptors, producing analgesia and other pharmacological effects.

Opioid peptides. A group of neurotransmitters that includes the endorphins and enkephalins.

Opioid receptors. Receptors that are activated by opioid peptide neurotransmitters and by opioid drugs.

Opium. A drug produced by drying the resinous exudate from the seedpod of the opium poppy; it contains morphine and codeine as active opioids.

Opium poppy (*Papaver somniferum*). The plant that is the source of the natural opioids.

Orexin. A neuropeptide neurotransmitter that has two forms, orexin-A and orexin-B, which bind with two types of orexin receptors; the orexin system has a key role in supporting and maintaining wakefulness as well as effects on appetite.

Oxcarbazepine. An anticonvulsant drug that is a structural derivative of carbamazepine; it is not itself pharmacologically active but is rapidly metabolized to an active molecule and has not been associated with the white blood cell toxicity associated with carbamazepine.

Oxycodone. A semisynthetic opioid similar in action to morphine that was, until recently, widely prescribed for the treatment of acute pain.

Oxymorphone. An opioid that is structurally related to morphine and is six to ten times more potent.

Pain. One of the most common human experiences and one of the most common reasons people seek medical care.

Paliperidone. An antipsychotic drug that is one of the major metabolites of risperidone, with the same side effects as risperidone.

Paraldehyde. A nonbarbiturate sedative-hypnotic drug that was introduced into medicine in the late nineteenth century; it was historically used to treat the severe alcohol withdrawal symptoms known as *delirium tremens*.

Paregoric. A tincture that contains powdered opium; it can be used in treating diarrhea.

Parkinson's disease. A disorder of the motor system characterized by involuntary movements, tremor, and weakness, resulting from the loss of dopamine-producing neurons.

Paroxetine. An SSRI antidepressant used for treating major depression, persistent depressive disorder, various anxiety disorders, and premenstrual dysphoric disorder, as well as for treating generalized anxiety disorder.

Partial nicotine receptor agonist. A drug (most notably, varenicline) that partially stimulates nicotinic receptors while blocking access of nicotine to those receptors.

Pentazocine. A rarely used mixed opioid agonist-antagonist analgesic; when abused by combining it with tripelennamine, it causes serious medical complications.

Peptide neurotransmitters. Neurotransmitters that are peptides (chain-link sequences of amino acids).

Perampanel. An anticonvulsant drug with a wide spectrum of useful anticonvulsant effects; it is a blocker of the AMPA subtype of glutamate receptors.

Peripheral nervous system (PNS). The nerves that originate in the spinal cord and that connect the spinal cord to the rest of the body.

Persistent depressive disorder (dysthymia). A disorder defined as the experiencing of ongoing symptoms of depression of any severity for a period of two years or more.

Peyote. A spineless cactus (*Lophophora williamsii*) that contains mescaline.

Pharmacodynamics. Study of the interactions of a drug and the receptors responsible for the action of the drug in the body.

Pharmacokinetics. Study of the factors that influence the absorption, distribution, metabolism, and excretion of drugs.

Pharmacology. Branch of science that deals with the study of drugs and their actions on living systems.

Phencyclidine. A psychedelic compound (phenylcyclohexyl piperidine, or PCP, with the street name "angel dust") that is a glutamate NMDA receptor antagonist; developed as an anesthetic, it was soon found to have psychedelic effects and to be associated with a high incidence of psychiatric reactions.

Phenobarbital. The first of the barbiturates to be developed, in 1912.

Phenothiazines. A class of compounds that includes the first antipsychotic drugs to be developed, such as chlorpromazine.

Phenytoin. An anticonvulsant drug that was introduced into medicine in 1938; it produces less sedation than the barbiturates but has many other bothersome side effects that limit its use.

Physical dependence. State in which the use of a drug is required for a person's normal physical functioning.

Pimavanserin. An antipsychotic drug used for the treatment of hallucinations and delusions in Parkinson's disease and in dementia-related psychosis.

Placebo effects. Positive clinical outcomes attributable to the psychosocial context and individual treatment expectations rather than to the effects of a medication or an intervention.

Polypharmacy. The practice of combining medications to improve therapeutic outcomes.

Positive symptoms (of schizophrenia). Symptoms including delusions, hallucinations, and thought disorder, the intensity of which are reduced by antipsychotic drugs that block D_2 receptors in the mesolimbic or mesocortical pathways.

Potency. The amount of a drug required to produce a response of a given intensity.

Pramipexole. A norepinephrine and dopamine reuptake inhibitor used to treat symptoms in Parkinsonism and in restless leg syndrome; it also has antidepressant efficacy.

Prazosin. An antagonist at noradrenaline alpha receptors that has shown efficacy in the treatment of PTSD-related symptoms.

Pregabalin. An anticonvulsant drug used for treating adult patients with partial-onset seizures.

Prodrug. A biologically inactive compound that can be metabolized in the body to produce a drug.

Propoxyphene. An analgesic compound that is structurally similar to methadone; less potent than codeine but more potent than aspirin, it has been removed from commercial sale because of concerns about overdoses and heart rhythm abnormalities.

Propranolol. A beta-blocker (an antagonist at noradrenaline beta receptors) that has been effective against a variety of anxiety disorders, particularly phobias.

Psilocin. A serotoninlike psychedelic compound (4-hydroxy-DMT) found in many species of mushrooms of the genera *Psilocybe, Panaeolus, Copelandia,* and *Conocybe.*

Psilocybin. A serotoninlike compound (4-phosphoryl-DMT) found in many species of mushrooms of the genera *Psilocybe, Panaeolus, Copelandia,* and *Conocybe*; after the mushrooms are ingested, psilocybin is enzymatically converted into the psychedelic agent psilocin.

Psychedelic drugs. Drug that act on various neurotransmitter pathways in the brain to produce hallucinatory perceptual experiences, which may be accompanied by marked changes in cognition and mood.

Psychedelic medicine. The use of psychedelic drugs as medicines.

Psychoactive drugs. Chemical substances that alter mood or behavior as a result of alterations in the functioning of the brain.

Psychological dependence. Compulsion to use a drug for its pleasurable effects.

Psychopharmacology. Branch of pharmacology that deals with the effects of drugs on the brain and behavior.

Psychostimulants. Drugs that exert their primary behavioral effects by augmenting the action of the neurotransmitters norepinephrine, epinephrine, and dopamine.

Quetiapine. An antipsychotic drug with side effects that include sedation, postural hypotension, and, rarely, a potentially fatal increase in the QT interval of the electrocardiogram.

Racemic mixture. A mixture of equal quantities of two optical isomers.

Ramelteon. A melatonin receptor agonist used in the treatment of insomnia characterized by difficulty with sleep onset.

Rapid cycler. A person with bipolar disorder who experiences at least four episodes in a 12-month period.

Receptor. A structure in the nervous system where a neurotransmitter or drug binds to exert its characteristic effect; most receptors are members of genetically encoded families of specialized proteins.

Redistribution. The movement of a drug from more perfused organs to less perfused organs.

REL-1017. A noncatecholamine antidepressant that is an NMDA channel blocker that preferentially targets hyperactive channels while maintaining physiological glutaminergic neurotransmission.

Reward circuit. Nerve pathways connecting the brain structures that mediate feelings of pleasure and satisfaction.

Risperidone. An antipsychotic drug that is most likely to produce extrapyramidal symptoms and to be associated with increased prolactin levels; however, it has been effective in treating nonpsychotic disorders such as autism.

Rivastigmine. An acetylcholinesterase inhibitor used in the treatment of Alzheimer's disease.

Rufinamide. An anticonvulsant drug that was FDA approved in 2008 for the treatment of Lennox-Gastaut syndrome in both children and adults.

SAGE-718. A cholesterol derivative that is active at NMDA receptors; it is being studied for possible use in improving learning and memory in patients with neurodegenerative disorders such as Alzheimer's disease.

Salvinorin A. A psychedelic compound found in the leaves of the perennial herb *Salvia divinorum*; it is an opioid kappa receptor agonist.

Schizophrenia. One of the most severe mental diseases, a syndrome characterized by positive symptoms that include hallucinations, delusions, and disorganized speech and behavior, by negative symptoms such as decreased motivation and diminished expressiveness, and by cognitive deficits involving impaired executive functions, memory, and speed of mental processing.

Scopolamine. An anticholinergic drug that is an antagonist at muscarinic receptors; it is one of the two most common naturally occurring muscarinic antagonists, with effects, depending on dosage, that include delirium, drowsiness, euphoria, amnesia, fatigue, dreamless sleep, restlessness, excitement, and hallucinations.

Second-generation antidepressants. Antidepressants that are grouped according to their proposed mechanism of action; they have varying degrees of monoamine uptake blocking properties as well as specific presynaptic receptor blocking properties.

Second-generation antipsychotics. Antipsychotic drugs that have a much lower risk than first-generation antipsychotics of producing neurological and metabolic side effects; like first-generation antipsychotics, block the D_2 receptors, but they also block 5-HT2 receptors.

Second messenger. A molecule produced in G-protein-coupled receptors when the released component of the G protein activates an enzyme in the neuron; second messengers can have a variety of effects within the neuron, including activation of ion channels in ionotropic receptors.

Sedative-hypnotic drugs. A chemically diverse group of substances that act on the central nervous system to depress brain activity, often by increasing the activity of inhibitory neurons.

Selective serotonin reuptake inhibitors (SSRIs). Second-generation antidepressant drugs that block the reuptake of serotonin.

Seltorexant. A dual orexin receptor antagonist that is under investigation for use in the treatment of insomnia and major depression.

Semorinemab. A monoclonal antibody that targets brain proteins that tend to accumulate in Alzheimer's disease.

Sequenced Treatment Alternatives to Relieve Depression (STAR*D) study. A study conducted over a six-year period ending in 2006, with the aim of identifying specific treatment strategies that would improve the long-term outcome of people with depressive disorder.

Serotonin (5-hydroxytryptamine, 5-HT). A neurotransmitter in both the brain and the peripheral nervous system (in the gut) that is involved in depression, appetite, sleep, and sexual responsiveness, among other functions.

Serotonin-norepinephrine reuptake inhibitors (SNRIs). Antidepressants that have efficacy in the treatment of a wide variety of anxiety and depressive disorders, with side effects associated with serotonin overactivity.

Sertraline. The second SSRI antidepressant approved for clinical use in the United States; it is more potent than fluoxetine in blocking serotonin reuptake but also may block the uptake of dopamine.

Side effects. Drug-induced effects that accompany the primary effect for which the drug is administered.

SNRIs. See **Serotonin-norepinephrine reuptake inhibitors.**

Snus. Moist powdered tobacco in small mesh pouches that are held in the mouth under the upper lip for about 30 minutes and then discarded; to get the nicotine, users swallow the by-product rather than spitting it out.

Specificity. A drug's ability to bind to just one type of receptor.

Spice. A street name for synthetic cannabinoids.

Spinal cord. The large group of nerves that run through the center of the spine and carry messages between the brain and the rest of the body.

Standard drink. A portion of any alcoholic beverage containing 0.6 oz of ethyl alcohol.

STAR*D. See **Sequenced Treatment Alternatives to Relieve Depression.**

Steady-state concentration. A plateau in the concentration in blood of a drug administered at regular intervals, reached after a length of time that depends on the drug's half-life.

STEP-BD study (Systematic Treatment Enhancement Program for Bipolar Disorder). A study that compared pharmacological treatments for bipolar disorder in a semicontrolled, real-world environment.

Stiripentol. An anticonvulsant drug used for the treatment of seizures associated with Dravet syndrome in patients 2 years of age and older taking clobazam; it acts by increasing GABA transmission and by limiting GABA synaptic uptake, which prolongs GABA activity.

Striatum. The largest structure of the basal ganglia; it consists of a cluster of neurons critical in the motor and reward systems, as well as in multiple aspects of cognition, decision making, motivation, and reinforcement.

Subcutaneous injection. Injection just under the skin.

Substance P. A peptide neurotransmitter (a gut-brain peptide) that regulates affective behavior, increasing the perception of pain.

Substance use disorder (SUD). As defined in DSM-5, a pattern of problematic symptoms resulting from the regular use of a substance such as a psychoactive drug.

SUD. See **Substance use disorder.**

Suicidality. Suicidal thoughts and behaviors.

Suvorexant. An orexin receptor antagonist used for the treatment of insomnia.

Sympathomimetics. See **Psychostimulants.**

Synapse. A specialized structure at the junction between two neurons, consisting of a presynaptic neuronal membrane, a postsynaptic neuronal membrane, and a minute space between the two (the synaptic cleft).

Synaptic cleft. The gap between the pre- and postsynaptic membranes of a synapse, across which neurotransmitter molecules diffuse.

Synaptic plasticity. Ability of synapses to strengthen or weaken over time, as a result of increases or decreases in their activity.

Synthetic cathinones. Synthesized derivatives of cathinone, in particular the frequently abused derivatives known as "bath salts."

Synthetic nicotine products. Products containing laboratory-produced nicotine; they are available in flavors as disposable vaping products and in pouches advertised as "tobacco-free" that are designed to be held in the mouth like snus.

Tapentadol. A partial opioid agonist with both analgesic and antidepressant effects, similar to tramadol.

Tardive dyskinesia. A movement disorder that appears after months or years of treatment with antipsychotic drugs; symptoms include involuntary hyperkinetic, choreiform movements in single or multiple parts of the body.

Tasimelteon. A melatonin receptor agonist used to treat non-24-hour sleep-wake disorder, a circadian rhythm disorder in which the person's biological clock fails to synchronize to a 24-hour day.

TCAs. See **Tricyclic antidepressants.**

TDM. See **Therapeutic drug monitoring.**

Tetrahydrocannabinol (THC). The major psychoactive agent derived from plants of the genus Cannabis; it is produced when the cannabinoid tetrahydrocannabinolic acid undergoes decarboxylation.

TFMPP. A catecholaminelike and amphetaminelike psychedelic compound (trifluoromethylphenylpiperazine); low doses cause stimulant effects, while hallucinogenic actions predominate at higher doses.

Thalamus. A brain structure that relays information from most sensory systems to the appropriate cortical areas for processing and integration.

THC. See **Tetrahydrocannabinol.**

Therapeutic drug monitoring (TDM). The process of correlating the plasma level of a drug with the therapeutic response.

Therapeutic index. A measure of drug safety: the ratio LD_{50}:ED_{50}.

Therapeutic window. A well-defined range of blood levels associated with an optimal clinical response to a drug.

Tiagabine. An anticonvulsant drug that was introduced in 1998; it prolongs GABA's synaptic action by inhibiting GABA reuptake transporters.

Tianeptine. An atypical antidepressant of the class of tricyclic antidepressants that works by increasing serotonin reuptake in the brain, modulating the system of glutamate NMDA receptors, and functioning as an indirect partial opioid agonist.

TMA. A catecholaminelike and amphetaminelike psychedelic compound (trimethoxyamphetamine); it is reported to elicit a range of emotions, from sadness to empathy and euphoria.

Tolerance. See **Drug tolerance.**

Topiramate. A drug used to prevent relapse in people with alcoholism; it is an effective anticonvulsant and is also a useful adjunct in the treatment of bipolar disorder, especially in cases where bipolar disorder occurs with comorbid substance abuse, binge-eating disorder, or weight gain from other medications.

TORDIA study. See **Treatment of Resistant Depression in Adolescents study.**

Tramadol. A "mixed mechanism" opioid that exerts analgesic effects through inhibition of both ascending and descending pain pathway while also having antidepressant effects.

Tranquilizers. See **Anxiolytic drugs.**

Transdermal patches. Bandagelike therapeutic systems that adhere to the skin and provide continuous, controlled release of a drug from a reservoir through a semipermeable membrane.

Transporter proteins. Structures in the presynaptic membrane that take neurotransmitter molecules back into the presynaptic neuron to be repackaged for later release.

Trazodone. An atypical antidepressant therapeutically as efficacious as the tricyclic antidepressants; its most common side effect is drowsiness, which makes it an attractive sleep aid for depressed patients with comorbid insomnia.

Treatment of Resistant Depression in Adolescents (TORDIA) study. A 2008 study of treatment-resistant depression in adolescents; the study found that combining pharmacological and psychological treatments is more effective than using medication alone.

Treatment-resistant depression. Mild to moderate depression that does not respond to antidepressants that are frequently prescribed despite their poor efficacy and adverse side effects.

Tricyclic antidepressants (TCAs). A class of drugs that all have a characteristic three-ring molecular core; they not only effectively relieve symptoms of depression but also have significant anxiolytic and analgesic actions.

2C-B. A serotoninlike psychedelic compound (4-bromo-2,5-dimethoxyphenethylamine); it is similar to MDMA in its mechanism of action and its effects.

U-47700. A synthetic opioid with 7.5 times greater binding affinity for mu opioid receptors than morphine; its effects are said to be very similar to those of morphine and heroin.

Upregulation. An increase in the number and sensitivity of postsynaptic receptors and a consequent increase in the response of the postsynaptic neuron due to the presence in the synaptic cleft of fewer than normal numbers of neurotransmitter molecules and/or an antagonist over an extended period of time.

U.S. Preventive Services Task Force (USPSTF). An independent agency that reviews medical evidence and makes recommendations about specific preventive care services.

Valproic acid. An anticonvulsant drug that was introduced in 1974; it is effective in treating petit mal seizures but can have serious adverse consequences if used during pregnancy.

Venlafaxine. A mixed serotonin-norepinephrine reuptake inhibitor antidepressant used in the treatment of major depressive disorder; at higher doses, it also inhibits the reuptake of dopamine.

Ventral tegmental area. A brain structure (part of the limbic system) that is a major component of the reward circuit in the brain.

Vigabatrin. An anticonvulsant drug used for treating two forms of severe epilepsy (infantile spasms and refractory partial epilepsy); serious side effects can include loss of peripheral vision and even permanent loss of vision.

Vilazodone. A drug used for the treatment of major depressive disorder; it blocks presynaptic serotonin reuptake, is a weak stimulant at $5\text{-HT}1_A$ receptors and may also have some effect on blocking the presynaptic reuptake of both norepinephrine and dopamine.

Viloxazine. A selective norepinephrine reuptake inhibitor used for the treatment of ADHD; it also has some action at serotonin receptors.

Vortioxetine. An atypical antidepressant used for the treatment of major depressive disorder; it exerts several different actions at various serotonin receptor subtypes.

Withdrawal syndrome. A predictable group of symptoms following the abrupt discontinuation or rapid decrease in dosage of a drug on which the person has become dependent.

Zaleplon. A nonbenzodiazepine agonist at benzodiazepine receptors that is used for the treatment of insomnia.

Ziprasidone. An antipsychotic drug with side effects that can include sedation and a metabolic syndrome, as well as a slight risk for extending the QT interval and for inducing two serious and potentially fatal dermatological reactions.

Zolpidem. A nonbenzodiazepine agonist at benzodiazepine receptors that is used for the treatment of insomnia.

Zuranolone. A noncatecholamine antidepressant used for the treatment of major depressive disorder and postpartum depression.

REFERENCES

Abad, V. C., and Guilleminault, C. (2018). "Insomnia in Elderly Patients: Recommendations for Pharmacological Management." *Drugs & Aging* 35: 791–817.

Abate, G., et al. (2021). "Potential and Limits of Cannabinoids in Alzheimer's Disease Therapy." *Biology (Basel)* 10: 542.

Abbasi, J. (2022). "The Covid Heart—One Year After SARS-CoV-2 Infection. Patients Have an Array of Increased Cardiovascular Risks." *JAMA*, 327: 1113–1114.

Abbott, L. C., and Nigussie, F. (2020). "Adult Neurogenesis in the Mammalian Dentate Gyrus." *Anatomia, Histologia, Embryologia* 19: 3–16.

Abel, K. M., et al. (2021). "Association of SARS-CoV-2 Infection with Psychological Distress, Psychotropic Prescribing, Fatigue, and Sleep Problems Among UK Primary Care Patients." *JAMA Network Open* 4: e2134803.

Abolfazli, R., et al. (2011). "Double-Blind, Randomized, Parallel-Group Clinical Trial of Efficacy of the Combination Fluoxetine Plus Modafinil Versus Fluoxetine Plus Placebo in the Treatment of Major Depression." *Depression and Anxiety* 28: 297–302.

Abou-Khalil, B. W. (2022). "Update on Antiseizure Medications 2022." *Continuum* (Minneapolis, MN) 28: 500–535.

Adam, R., et al. (2020). "Phase II Double-Blind Randomized Controlled Trial of Exogenous Administration of Melatonin in Chronic Pain (DREAM-CP): A Study Protocol." *British Medical Journal Open* 10: e034443.

Adamo, D., et al. (2021). "Vortioxetine as a New Frontier in the Treatment of Chronic Neuropathic Pain: A Review and Update." *Therapeutic Advances in Psychopharmacology* 11: 20451253211034320.

Adams, A. D., et al. (2020). "The Role of Suvorexant in the Prevention of Delirium During Acute Hospitalization: A Systematic Review." *Journal of Critical Care* 59: 1–5.

Adams, A. J., et al. (2017). "'Zombie' Outbreak Caused by the Synthetic Cannabinoid AMB-FUBINACA in New York." *New England Journal of Medicine* 376: 235–242.

Addicott, M. A., et al. (2009). "The Effect of Daily Caffeine Use on Cerebral Blood Flow: How Much Caffeine Can We Tolerate?" *Human Brain Mapping* 3: 3102–3114.

Addy, P. H. (2012). "Acute and Post-Acute Behavioral and Psychological Effects of Salvinorin A in Humans." *Psychopharmacology* 220: 195–204.

Adkins, D. E., et al. (2012). "Genone-Wide Pharmacogenomic Study of Citalopram-Induced Side Effects in STAR*D." *Translational Psychiatry* July 3; 2: e129.

Adler, L. A., et al. (2022). "Efficacy, Safety, and Tolerability of Centanafadine Sustained-Release Tablets in Adults with Attention-Deficit/Hyperactivity Disorder: Results of 2 Phase 3, Randomized, Double-blind, Multicenter, Placebo-Controlled Trials." *Journal of Clinical Psychopharmacology* 10: 1097.

Aftab, A., et al. (2021). "Recent Developments in Geriatric Psychopharmacology." *Expert Review of Clinical Pharmacology* 14: 341–355.

Agarwal, S. D., and Landon, B. E. (2019). "Patterns in Outpatient Benzodiazepine Prescribing in the United States." *JAMA Network Open* 2: e187399.

Agin-Liebes, G. I., et al. (2020). "Long-Term Follow-up of Psilocybin-Assisted Psychotherapy for Psychiatric and Existential Distress in Patients with Life-Threatening Cancer." *Journal of Psychopharmacology* 34: 155–166.

Agostino, H., et al. (2021). "Trends in the Incidence of New-Onset Anorexia Nervosa and Atypical Anorexia Nervosa Among Youth During the COVID-19 Pandemic in Canada." *JAMA Network Open* 4: e2137395.

Ahmadi, J., et al. (2019). "A Randomized Clinical Trial of the Effects of Bupropion and Buprenorphine on the Reduction of Methamphetamine Craving." *Trials* 20: 468.

Aiken, A., et al. (2018). "Age of Alcohol Initiation and Progression to Binge Drinking in Adolescence: A Prospective Cohort Study." *Alcoholism, Clinical and Experimental Research* 42: 100–110.

Aiken, A., et al. (2020). "Parental Supply of Sips and Whole Drinks of Alcohol to Adolescents and Associations with Binge Drinking and Alcohol-Related Harms: A Prospective Cohort Study." *Drug and Alcohol Dependence* 215: 108204.

Ajith, T. A. (2018). "A Recent Update on the Effects of Omega-3 Fatty Acids in Alzheimer's Disease." *Current Clinical Pharmacology* 13: 252–260.

Akbar, M., et al. (2017). "Medications for Alcohol Use Disorders: An Overview." *Pharmacology and Therapeutics* 185: 64–85. https://doi.org/ 10.1016/j.pharmthera.2017.11.007.

Akbar, M., et al. (2018). "Medications for Alcohol Use Disorders: An Overview." *Pharmacology and Therapeutics* 185: 64–85.

Akinsanya, A., et al. (2017). "Prazosin in Children and Adolescents with Posttraumatic Stress Disorder Who Have Nightmares: A Systematic Review." *Journal of Clinical Psychopharmacology* 37: 84–88.

Albertini, E., et al. (2019). "Psychopharmacological Decision Making in Bipolar Disorder During Pregnancy and Lactation: A Case-By-Case Approach to Using Current Evidence." *Focus (American Psychiatric Publications)* 17: 249–258.

American Addiction Centers (2022). "Spiked Substances." Alcohol.org.

Alborghetti, M., and Nicoletti, F. (2019). "Different Generations of Type-B Monoamine Oxidase Inhibitors in Parkinson's Disease: From Bench to Bedside. *Current Neuropharmacology* 17: 861–873.

Albott, C. S., et al. (2020). "Battle Buddies: Rapid Deployment of a Psychological Resilience Intervention for Health Care Workers During the COVID-19 Pandemic." *Anesthesia and Analgesia* 131: 43–54.

Alexander, G. C., et al. (2021). "Evaluation of Aducanumab for Alzheimer's Disease: Scientific Evidence and regulatory Review Involving Efficacy, Safety, and Futility." *JAMA* 325: 1717–1718.

Alexandre, J., et al. (2020). "Synthetic Cannabinoids and Their Impact on Neurodevelopmental Processes." *Addiction Biology* 25: e12824.

Alhowail, A. (2019). "Candidate Mechanisms of Caffeine Improving Memory Dysfunction." *Die Pharmazie* 74: 705–710.

Alhowail, A. (2021). "Molecular Insights into the Benefits of Nicotine on Memory and Cognition (Review)." *Molecular Medicine Reports* 23: 398.

Ali, A., et al. (2018). "Managing Chronic Pain in the Elderly: An Overview of the Recent Therapeutic Advancements." *Cureus* 10: e3293

Ali, Z., et al. (2020). "Evaluating Lurasidone as a Treatment Option for Bipolar Disorder." *Expert Opinion in Pharmacotherapy* 21: 253–260.

Allen, K. B., et al. (2020). "Childhood Anxiety—If We Know So Much, Why Are We Doing So Little?" *JAMA Psychiatry* 77: 887–888.

Allsop, D. J., et al. (2015). "Cannabinoid Replacement Therapy (CRT): Nabiximols (Sativex) as a Novel Treatment for Cannabis Withdrawal." *Clinical Pharmacology and Therapeutics* 97: 571–574.

Almohammed, O. A., et al. (2022). "Antidepressants and Health-Related Quality of Life (HRQoL) for Patients with Depression: Analysis of the Medical Expenditure Panel Survey From the United States." *PLOS ONE* 17: e0265928.

Alsayouf, H. A., et al. (2021). "Risperidone or Aripitprazole Can Resolve Autism Core

Signs and Symptoms in Young Children: Case Study." *Children* (Basel) 8: 318.

Althaus, A. L., et al. (2020). "Preclinical Characterization of Zuranolone (SAGE-217), a Selective Neuroactive Steroid $GABA_A$ Receptor Positive Allosteric Modulator." *Neuropharmacology* 181: 108333.

Alzheimer's Association. (2022). "2022 Alzheimer's Disease Facts and Figures."

Amari, D. T., et al. (2022). "Falls, Healthcare Resources and Costs in Older Adults with Insomnia Treated with Zolpidem, Trazodone, or Benzodiazepines." *BMC Geriatrics* 22: 484.

Amen, D. G., et al. (2017). "Discriminative Properties of Hippocampal Hypoperfusion in Marijuana Users Compared to Healthy Controls: Implications for Marijuana Administration in Alzheimer's Dementia." *Journal of Alzheimer's Disease* 56: 261–273.

American College of Obstetricians and Gynecologists Committee on Obstetric Practice. (2017). "Committee Opinion No. 722: Marijuana Use During Pregnancy and Lactation." *Obstetrics and Gynecology* 130: 205–209.

American Geriatrics Society. (2019). "American Geriatrics 2019 Updated AGS Beers Criteria for Potentially Inappropriate Medication Use in Older Adults." *Journal of the American Geriatrics Society* 67: 674–694.

American Psychiatric Association. (2013). *Diagnostic and Statistical Manual of Mental Disorders,* 5th ed. [DSM-5]. Washington, DC: American Psychiatric Association.

American Psychiatric Association. (2022). *Diagnostic and Statistical Manual of Mental Disorders,* 5th ed., Text Revision [DSM-5-TR]. Arlington, VA: American Psychiatric Association.

Amerio, A., et al. (2018). "Safety and Efficacy of Lithium in Children and Adolescents: A Systematic Review in Bipolar Illness." *European Psychiatry* 54: 85–97.

Ames, F. (1958). "A Clinical and Metabolic Study of Acute Intoxication with *Cannabis sativa* and Its Role in the Model Psychosis." *Journal of Mental Science* 104: 972–999.

Ammerman, S., et al. (2015). "The Impact of Marijuana Policies on Youth: Clinical, Research, and Legal Update." *Pediatrics* 135: e769–e785.

Amram, O., et al. (2021). "Changes in Methadone Take-Home Dosing Before and After COVID-19." *Journal of Substance Abuse Treatment*, in press.

Amram, O., et al. (2022). "Changes in Methadone Take-Home Dosing Before and After COVID-19." *Journal of Substance Abuse Treatment* 133: 108552.

Amsterdam, J. D. (2003). "A Double-Blind, Placebo-Controlled Trial of the Safety and Efficacy of Selegiline Transdermal System without Dietary Restrictions in Patients with Major Depressive Disorder." *Journal of Clinical Psychiatry* 64: 208–214.

Andersen, J. M., et al. (2020). "Prenatal Exposure to Methadone or Buprenorphine and Long-Term Outcomes: A Meta-Analysis." *Early Human Development* 143: 104997.

Andersen, K. A. A., et al. (2021). "Therapeutic Effects of Classic Serotonergic Psychedelics: A Systematic Review of Modern Era Clinical Studies." *Acta Psychiatrica Scandinavica* 143: 101–118.

Anderson, K. N., et al. (2020). "Maternal Use of Specific Antidepressant Medications During Early Pregnancy and the Risk of Selected Birth Defects." *JAMA Psychiatry* 77: 1246–1255.

Anderson, K. N., et al. (2022, March 16). "Changes and Inequities in Adult Mental Health-Related Emergency Department Visits During the COVID-19 Pandemic in the US." *JAMA Psychiatry*, e220164.

Andrade, C. (2012). "Drugs That Escape Hepatic Metabolism." *Journal of Clinical Psychiatry* 73: e889–e890.

Andrade, C. (2015). "Cost of Treatment as a Placebo Effect in Psychopharmacology: Importance in the Context of Generic Drugs." *Journal of Clinical Psychiatry* 67: e534–e536.

Andrade, C. (2016). "A Method for Deciding About the Possible Safety of Modafinil and Armodafinil in Patients with Seizure Disorder." *Journal of Clinical Psychiatry* 77: e25–e28.

Andrade, C. (2017). "Ketamine for Depression, 3: Does Chirality Matter?" *The Journal of Clinical Psychiatry* 78(6): e674–e677.

Andrade, C. (2018a). "Relative Efficacy and Acceptability of Antidepressant Drugs in Adults with Major Depressant Disorder: Commentary on a Network Meta-Analysis." *Journal of Clinical Psychology* 79: 18f12254.

Andrade, C. (2018b). "Valproate in Pregnancy: Recent Research and Regulatory Responses." *Journal of Clinical Psychiatry* 79: 18f12351.

Andrade, C. (2022). "Insights for the Use of Ketamine from Randomized Controlled Trials that Compared Ketamine with Electroconvulsive Therapy in Severe Depression." *Journal of Clinical Psychiatry* 83: 22f14451.

Angerer, V., et al. (2016). "Separation and Structural Characterization of the New Synthetic Cannabinoid JWH-018 Cyclohexyl Methyl Derivative 'NE-CHMIMO' Using Flash Chromatography, GC-MS, IR and NMR Spectroscopy." *Forensic Science International* 266: e93–e98.

Anmella, G., et al. (2019). "Expert Advice on the Management of Valproate in Women with Bipolar Disorder at Childbearing Age." *European Neuropsychopharmacology* 29: 1199–1212.

Anton, R. F. (2008). "Naltrexone for the Management of Alcohol Dependence." *The New England Journal of Medicine* 359: 715–721.

Anton, R. F. (2020). "Efficacy of Gabapentin for the Treatment of Alcohol Use Disorder in Patients with Alcohol Withdrawal Symptoms: A Randomized Clinical Trial." *JAMA Internal Medicine* 180: 728–736.

Anton, R. F., et al. (2020). "Efficacy of Gabapentin for the Treatment of Alcohol Use Disorder in Patients with Alcohol Withdrawal Symptoms: A Randomized Clinical Trial." *JAMA Internal Medicine* 180: 728–736.

Antonoudiou, P., et al. (2022). "Allopregnanolone Mediates Affective Switching, Through Modulation of Oscillatory States in the Basolateral Amygdala." *Biological Psychiatry* 91: 283–293.

Appa, A., et al. (2021). "Drug Overdose Deaths Before and After Shelter-in-Place Orders During the COVID-19 Pandemic in San Francisco." *JAMA Network Open* 4: e2110452.

Apraku, J., and Okoro, C. O. (2019). "Design, Synthesis and Anticonvulsant Evaluation of Fluorinated Benzyl Amino Enaminones." *Biorganic & Medicinal Chemistry* 27: 161–166.

Aran, A., et al. (2019). "Brief Report: Cannabidiol-Rich Cannabis in Children with Autism Spectrum Disorder and Sever Behavioral Problems—A Retrospective Feasibility Study." *Journal of Autism Developmental Disorders* 49: 1284–1288.

Araujo, A. M., et al. (2015). "The Hallucinogenic World of Tryptamines: An Updated Review." *Archives of Toxicology* 89: 1151–1173.

Arfman, I. J., et al. (2020). "Therapeutic Drug Monitoring of Antiepileptic Drugs in Women with Epilepsy Before, During, and After Pregnancy." *Clinical Pharmacokinetics* 59: 427–445.

Arkell, T. R., et al. (2020). "Effect of Cannabidiol and Delta-9-Terrahydrocannabinol on Driving Performance: A Randomized Clinical Trial." *JAMA* 324: 2177–2186.

Armstrong, M. J., and Okun, M. S. (2020). "Diagnosis and Treatment of Parkinson Disease. A Review." *JAMA* 323: 548–560.

Arnaud, A., and Bonthapally, V. (2022). "Zuranoloe Provides a Rapid Response Without Chronic Dosing: Response to Correspondence by ten Doesschate et al." *Journal of Affective Disorders* 301: 445–447.

Arnold, V. K., et al. (2014). "A 9-Week, Randomized, Double-Blind, Placebo-Controlled, Parallel-Group, Dose-Finding Study to Evaluate the Efficacy and Safety of Modafinil as Treatment for Adults with ADHD." *Journal of Attention Disorders* 18: 133–144.

Artukoglu, B. B., et al., (2020). "Pharmacologic Treatment of Tardive Dyskinesia: A Meta-Analysis and Systematic Review." *Journal of Clinical Psychiatry* 81: 19r12798.

Ashok, A. H., et al. (2017). "The Dopamine Hypothesis of Bipolar Affective Disorder: The State of the Art and Implications for Treatment." *Molecular Psychiatry* 22: 666–679.

Ashok, A. H., et al. (2017). "Association of Stimulant Use with Dopaminergic Alterations in Users of Cocaine, Amphetamine, or Methamphetamine: A Systematic Review and Meta-Analysis." *JAMA Psychiatry* 74: 511–519.

Ashton, M. M., et al. (2021). "A Systematic Review of Nutraceuticals for the Treatment of Bipolar Disorder." *Canadian Journal of Psychiatry* 66: 262–273.

Asnis, G. M., et al. (2016). "Pharmacotherapy Treatment Options for Insomnia: A Primer for Clinicians." *International Journal of Molecular Sciences* 17: 50.

Aspvall, K., et al. (2021). "Effect of an Internet-Delivered Stepped-Care Program vs In-Person Cognitive Behavioral Therapy on Obsessive-Compulsive Disorder Symptoms in Children and Adolescents. A Randomized Clinical Trial." *JAMA* 325: 1863–1873.

Asrani, S. K., et al. (2019). "Burden of Liver Diseases in the World." *Journal of Hepatology* 70: 151–171.

Attilia, F., et al. (2018). "Alcohol Withdrawal Syndrome: Diagnostic and Therapeutic Methods." *Rivista di Psychiatria* 53: 118–122.

Avalos, C. B., and Sprecher, S. G. (2021). "Single-Cell Transcriptomic Reveals Dual and Multi-Transmitter Use in Neurons Across Metazoans." *Frontiers in Molecular Neuroscience* 14: 623148.

Avancena, A. L., et al. (2021). "Cost-Effectiveness of Alcohol Use Treatments in Patients with Alcohol-Related Cirrhosis." *Journal of Hepatology* 74: 1286–1294.

Avgerinos, K., et al. (2021). "Effects of Monoclonal Antibodies Against Amyloid-Beta on Clinical and Biomarker Outcomes and Adverse Event Risks: A Systematic Review and Meta-Analysis of Phase III RCTs in Alzheimer's Disease." *Ageing Research Reviews* 68: 10116.

Avila, J. A., et al. (2018). "Chronic Voluntary Oral Methamphetamine Induces Deficits in Spatial learning and Hippocampal Protein Kinase Mzeta with Enhanced Astrogliosis and Cyclooxygenase-2 Levels." *Heliyon* 4: e000509.

Azad, T. D., et al. (2020). "Patterns of Opioid and Benzodiazepine Use in Opioid-Naïve Patients with Newly Diagnosed Low Back and Lower Extremity Pain." *Journal of General Internal Medicine* 35: 291–297.

Azhari, N., et al. (2021). "Ketamine-Facilitated Behavioral Treatment for Cannabis-Use Disorder: A Proof of Concept Study." *American Journal of Drug and Alcohol Abuse* 47: 92–97.

Bachhuber, M. A., et al. (2016). "Increasing Benzodiazepine Prescriptions and Overdose Mortality in the United States, 1996–2013." *American Journal of Public Health* 106: 686–688.

Baehr, C., et al. (2022). "Preclinical Efficacy and Selectivity of Vaccines Targeting Fentanyl, Alfentanil, Sufentanil, and Acetylfentanyl in Rats." *ACS Omega* 7: 16584–16592.

Baggott, M. J., et al. (2019). "Effects of the Psychedelic Amphetamine MDA (3,4-Methylenedioxyamphetamine) in Healthy Volunteers." *Journal of Psychoactive Drugs* 51: 108–117.

Bahji, A., et al. (2020a). "Comparative Efficacy and Tolerability of Pharmacological Treatments for the Treatment of Acute Bipolar Depression: A Systematic Review and Network Meta-Analysis." *Journal of Affective Disorders* 269: 154–184.

Bahji, A., et al. (2020b). "Efficacy of 3,4-methylenedioxymethamphetamine (MDMA)–Assisted Psychotherapy for Posttraumatic Stress Disorder: A Systematic Review and Meta-Analysis." *Progress in Neuropsychopharmacology and Biological Psychiatry* 96: 109735.

Bahji, A., et al. (2020c). "Prevalence of Cannabis Withdrawal Symptoms Among People with Regular or Dependent Use of Cannabinoids." *JAMA Network Open* 3: e202370.

Bailey, T. A., and Panjwani, S. (2018). "Atypical Antipsychotics in Late-Life and Treatment-Resistant Depression." *Consulting Pharmacist* 33: 83–88.

Baillargeon, J., et al. (2019). "Association of Opioid and Benzodiazepine Use with Adverse Respiratory Events in Older Adults with Chronic Obstructive Pulmonary Disease." *Annals of the American Thoracic Society* 16: 1245–1251.

Bais, B., et al. (2020). "Prevalence of Benzodiazepines and Benzodiazepine-Related Drugs Exposure Before, During and After Pregnancy: A Systematic Review and Meta-analysis." *Journal of Affective Disorders* 269: 18–27.

Baisden, K., and Dinatale, M. (2019). "Pregnancy and Lactation Labeling Rule: Four Years In—What's Next?" *Division of Pediatric and Maternal Health. Office of New Drugs, Center for Drug Evaluation and Research, Food and Drug Administration.*

Baker, E., and Stavropoulos, K. K. M. (2020). "The Effects of Oxytocin Administration on Individuals with ASD: Neuroimaging and Behavioural Evidence." *Progress in Molecular Biology and Translational Science* 173: 209–238.

Baker, R. G., et al. (2021). "The Helping to End Addiction Long-term (HEAL) Initiative of the National Institutes of Health." *JAMA Network Open,* in press.

Baker, T. B., et al. (2021). "Effects of Combined Varenicline with Nicotine Patch and of Extended Treatment Duration on Smoking Cessation: A Randomized Clinical Trial." *JAMA* 326: 1485–1493.

Bakhshaie, J., et al. (2016). "Cigarette Smoking and the Onset and Persistence of Panic Attacks During Mid-Adulthood in the United States: 1994–2005." *Journal of Clinical Psychiatry* 77: e21–e24.

Balagura, G., et al. (2020). "Fenfluramine for the Treatment of Dravet Syndrome and Lennox-Gastaut Syndrome." *CNS Drugs* 34: 1001–1007.

Baldessarini, R. J., and Tondo, L. (2000). "Does Lithium Treatment Still Work? Evidence of Stable Responses over Three Decades." *Archives of General Psychiatry* 57: 187–190.

Baldessarini, R. J., et al. (2019). "Pharmacological Treatment of Adult Bipolar Disorder." *Molecular Psychiatry* 24: 198–217.

Baldessarini, R. J., et al. (2020). "Bipolar Depression: A Major Unsolved Challenge." *International Journal of Bipolar Disorders* 8: 1.

Balia, C., et al. (2018). "The Pharmacological Treatment of Aggression in Children and Adolescents with Conduct Disorder. Do Callous–Unemotional Traits Modulate the Efficacy of Medication?" *Neuroscience & Behavioral Reviews* 91: 218–238.

Ball et al. (2022). Xylazine poisoning: a systematic review. *Clinical toxicology (Philadelphia, Pa.)*, *60*(8), 892–901. https://doi.org/10.1080/15563650.2022.2063135

Ballard, C., et al. (2018). "Evaluation of the Safety, Tolerability, and Efficacy of Pimavanserin Versus Placebo in Patients with Alzheimer's Disease Psychosis: A Phase 2, Randomized, Placebo-Controlled, Double-Blind Study." *The Lancet Neurology* 17: 213–222.

Ballard, C., et al. (2020). "Psychosis in Alzheimer's Disease." *Current Neurology and Neuroscience Reports* 20: 57.

Ballard, E., et al. (2020). "Symptom Trajectories in the Months Before and After a Suicide Attempt in Individuals with Bipolar Disorder: A STEP-BD Study." *Bipolar Disorder* 22: 245–254.

Ballester, J., et al. (2017). "Pharmacological Treatments for Methamphetamine Addiction: Current Status and Future Directions." *Expert Reviews in Clinical Pharmacology* 10: 305–314.

Ban, T. A. (2007). "Fifty Years Chlorpromazine: A Historical Perspective." *Neuropsychiatric Disease and Treatment* 3: 495–500.

Bandelow, B. (2017). "Treatment of Anxiety Disorders." *Dialogues in Clinical Neuroscience* 19: 93–107.

Bandi, P., et al. (2022). "Changes in Smoking Cessation-Related Behaviors Among US Adults During the COVID-19 Pandemic." *JAMA Network Open* 5: e2225149.

Barker, S. A. (2018). "N, N-Dimethyltryptamine (DMT), an Endogenous Hallucinogen: Past, Present, and Future Research to Determine Its Role and Function." *Frontiers in Neuroscience* 10: 00536.

Barnett, M. L. (2020). "Opioid Prescribing in the Midst of Crisis—Myths and Realities." *The New England Joirnal of Medicine* 382: 1086–1088.

Barocas, J. A. (2021). "Business Not as Usual—COVID-19 Vaccination in Persons with Substance Use Disorders." *New England Journal of Medicine* 384: e6.

Barreto, G. E., et al. (2015). "Beneficial Effects of Nicotine, Cotinine and Its Metabolites as Potential Agents for Parkinson's Disease." *Frontiers in Aging Neuroscience* 6: Article 340.

Barry, C. L., and Saloner, B. (2021). "Using Policy Tools to Improve Population Health—Combating the U.S. Opioid Crisis." *New England Journal of Medicine* 385: 2113–2116.

Barsky, B. A., et al. (2022). Use of Telemedicine for Buprenorphine Inductions in Patents with Commercial Insurance or Medicare Advantage." *JAMA Network Open.* 5: e2142531.

Barton et al. (2020). Update on weight-gain caused by antipsychotics: a systematic review and meta-analysis, Expert Opinion on Drug Safety, 19:3, 295-314, DOI: HYPERLINK "https://doi.org/10.1080/14740338.2020.1713091"10.1080/14740338.2020.1713091

Bartolucci, G., et al. (1969). "Marijuana Psychosis: A Case Report." *Canadian Psychiatric Association Journal* 14: 77–79.

Baselt, R. (2020). *Disposition of Toxic Drugs and Chemicals in Man*, 12th ed. Seal Beach, CA: Biomedical Publications.

Basu, A., et al. (2018) "Is Tapentadol a Potential Trojan Horse in the Postdextropropoxyphene Era in India?" *Indian Journal of Pharmacology* 50: 44–46.

Battle, C. L., et al. (2014). "Clinical Correlates of Perinatal Bipolar Disorder in an Interdisciplinary Obstetrical Hospital Setting." *Journal of Affective Disorders* 158: 97–100.

Battleday, R. M., and Brem, A.-K. (2015). "Modafinil for Cognitive Neuroenhancement in Healthy Non-Sleep-Deprived Subjects: A Systematic Review." *European Neuropsychopharmacology* 25: 1865–1881.

Bauer, I. (2019). "Travel Medicine, Coca and Cocaine: Demystifying and Rehabilitating *Erythyroxylum*—A Comprehensive Review." *Tropical Diseases, Travel Medicine and Vaccines* 5: 20.

Baumann, M. H., et al. (2014). "Bath Salts, Spice, and Related Designer Drugs: The Science Behind the Headlines." *The Journal of Neuroscience* 34: 15150–15158.

Baumann, M. H., et al. (2020). "U-47700 and Its Analogs: Non-Fentanyl Synthetic Opioids

Impacting the Recreational Drug Market." *Brain Sciences* 10: 895.

Baumeister, A. A., et al. (2003). "The Myth of Reserpine-Induced Depression: Role in the Historical Development of the Monoamine Hypothesis." *Journal of the History of Neuroscience* 12: 207–220.

Baumgartner, A. D., et al. (2020). "Interventions to Deprescribe Potentially Inappropriate Medications in the Elderly: Lost in Translation?" *Journal of Clinical Pharmacology and Therapeutics* 45: 453–461.

Bazzari, A. H., and Parri, H. R. (2019). "Neuromodulators and Long-Term Synaptic Plasticity in Learning and Memory: A Steered-Glutamatergic Perspective." *Brain Sciences.* Published online October 31, 2019.

Bechtold, J., et al. (2016). "Concurrent and Sustained Cumulative Effects of Adolescent Marijuana Use on Subclinical Psychotic Symptoms." *American Journal of Psychiatry* 173: 781–789.

Beck, K., et al. (2020). "Association of Ketamine with Psychiatric Symptoms and Implications for Its Therapeutic Use and for Understanding Schizophrenia: A Systematic Review and Meta-Analysis." *JAMA Network Open* 3: e204693.

Bender, A., et al. (2017). "The Association of Folate and Depression: A Meta-Analysis." *Journal of Psychiatric Research* 95: 9–18.

Benedetti, F., et al. (2016). "Teaching Neurons to Respond to Placebos." *Journal of Physiology* 594: 5647–5660.

Bengalorkar, G. M., et al. (2011). "Fospropofol: Clinical Pharmacology." *Journal of Anaesthesiology and Clinical Pharmacology* 27: 79–83.

Benko, J., and Vrankova, S. (2020). "Natural Psychoplastogens as Antidepressant Agents." *Molecules* 25: 1172.

Ben-Menachem, E., et al. (2016). "Efficacy and Safety of Brivaracetam for Partial-Onset Seizures in 3 Pooled Clinical Studies." *Neurology* 87: 314–323.

Benowitz, N. L., et al. (2009). "Nicotine Chemistry, Metabolism, Kinetics and Biomarkers." *Handbook of Experimental Pharmacology* 192: 29–60.

Bentzley, B. S., et al. (2021). "Comparison of Treatments for Cocaine Use Disorder Among Adults: A Systematic Review and Meta-Analysis." *JAMA Network Open* 4: e218049.

Berard, A., et al. (2017). "Antidepressant Use During Pregnancy and the Risk of Major Congenital Malformations in a Cohort of Depressed Pregnant Women: An Updated Analysis of the Quebec Pregnancy Cohort." *British Medical Journal Open* 7: e013372.

Beresniak, A., et al. (2012). "Relationships Between Black Tea Consumption and Key Health Indicators in the World: An Ecological Study." *BMJ Open* 2: e000648.

Berger, A. A., et al. (2022). "Suvorexant in the Treatment of Difficulty Falling and Staying Asleep (Insomnia). *Psychopharmacology Bulletin* 52: 68–90.

Bergese, S. D., et al. (2019). "ATHENA: A Phase 3, Open-Label Study of the Safety and Effectiveness of Oliceridine (TRV130), A G-Protein Selective Agonist At the mu-Opioid Receptor, in Patients with Moderate to Severe Acute Pain Requiring Parenteral Opioid Therapy." *Journal of Pain Research* 12: 3113–3126.

Berglund, K., et al. (2021). "Bioluminescence–Optogenetics." *Advances in Experimental Medicine and Biology* 1293: 281–293.

Berk, J. (2020, August 20). "A Good Place to Start—Low Threshold Buprenorphine Initiation." *New England Journal of Medicine* 383: 701–703.

Berretta, P., and Vari, M. R. (2020). "The Overwhelming Issue of Drug Facilitated Sexual Assaults (DFSA): The Case of GHB." *Clinical Teratology* 170: e44–e45.

Bessey, L., and Walaszek, A. (2019). "Management of Behavioral and Psychological Symptoms of Dementia." *Current Psychiatry* 21: 66.

Betcher, H., et al. (2019). "Use of Antipsychotic Drugs During Pregnancy." *Current Treatment Options in Psychiatry* 6: 17–31.

Bette, S., et al. (2018). "Safinamide in the Management of Patients with Parkinson's Disease Not Stabilized on Levodopa: A Review of Current Clinical Evidence." *Therapeutics and Clinical Risk Management* 14: 1737–1745.

Bettinger, J. J., and Cleary, J. H. (2020). "The Rise in Tianeptine Abuse: Our next Kratom Problem?" *Practical Pain Management,* March/April: 61–64.

Bettinger, J. J., et al. (2019). "The Potential of the Endocannabinoid System." *Practical Pain Management* 19: 56–62.

Bhatia, D., et al. (2020). "Prescription Opioid Misuse and Risky Adolescent Behavior." *Pediatrics* 145: e2019470.

Bidwell, L. C., et al. (2020). "Association of Naturalistic Administration of Cannabis

Flower and Concentrates with Intoxication and Impairment." *JAMA Psychiatry* 77(8): 787–796.

Bifari et al. (2022). REL-1017 (Esmethadone), A Novel NMDAR Blocker for the Treatment of MDD is Not Neurotoxic in Sprague-Dawley Rats. *Frontiers in pharmacology, 13*, 863959. https://doi.org/10.3389/fphar.2022.863959

Binswanger, I. A., et al. (2020). "The Association Between Opioid Discontinuation and Heroin Use: A Nested Case-Control Study." *Drug & Alcohol Dependence* 217: 108248.

Birnbaum, A. K., et al. (2020). "Antiepileptic Drug Exposure in Infants of Breastfeeding Mothers with Epilepsy." *JAMA Neurology* 77: 441–450.

Biselli, T., et al. (2021). "Optogenetic and Chemogenetic Insights into the Neurocircuitry of Depression-Like Behaviour: A Systematic Review." *European Journal of Neuroscience* 53: 9–38.

Bjork, M.-H., et al. (2022). "Association of Prenatal Exposure to Antiseizure Medication with Risk of Autism and Intellectual Disability." *JAMA Neurology* 79: 672–681.

Bjorkholm, C. and L.M. Monteggia (2018). "BDNF—A Key Transducer of Antidepressant Effects." *Neuropharmacology* 102: 72–79.

Black, N., et al. (2019). "Cannabinoids for the Treatment of Mental Disorders and Symptoms of Mental Disorders: A Systematic Review and Meta-Analysis." *Lancet Psychiatry* 6: 995–1010.

Blackman, J., et al. (2021). "Pharmacological and Non-Pharmacological Interventions to Enhance Sleep in Mild Cognitive Impairment and Mild Alzheimer's Disease: A Systematic Review." *Journal of Sleep Research* 30: e13229.

Blader, J. C., et al. (2021). "Stepped Treatment for Attention-Deficit/Hyperactivity Disorder and Aggressive Behavior: A Randomized, Controlled Trial of Adjunctive Risperidone, Divalproex Sodium, or Placebo After Stimulant Medication Optimization." *Journal of the American Academy of Child & Adolescent Psychiatry* 60: 236–251.

Blair, H. A. (2020). "Lumateperone: First Approval." *Drugs* 80: 417–423.

Blair, H. A., and Dhillon, S. (2017). "Safinamide: A Review in Parkinson's Disease." *CNS Drugs* 31: 169–176.

Blanco-Silvente, L., et al. (2017). "Discontinuation, Efficacy, and Safety of Cholinesterase Inhibitors for Alzheimer's Disease: A Meta-Analysis and Meta-Regression of 43 Randomized Clinical Trials Enrolling 16,106 Patients." *International Journal of Neuropsychopharmacology* 20: 519–528.

Blankers, M., et al. (2021). "Changes in Online Psychoactive Substance Trade via Telegram During the COVID-19 Pandemic." *European Addiction Research* 27: 469–474.

Blanton, H. L., et al. (2021). "Sex Differences and the Endocannabinoid System in Pain." *Pharmacology, Biochemistry, and Behavior* 202: 173107.

Blessing, E. M., et al. (2015). "Cannabidiol as a Potential Treatment for Anxiety Disorders." *Neurotherapeutics* 12: 825–836.

Bloomfield, M. A., et al. (2016). "The Effects of Δ9-Tetrahydrocannabinol on the Dopamine System." *Nature* 539: 369–377.

Bloomfield, M. A. P., et al. (2014). "Dopamine Function in Cigarette Smokers: An [^{18}F]-DOPA PET Study." *Neuropsychopharmacology* 39: 2397–2404.

Bloomfield, M. A. P., et al. (2019). "The Neuropsychopharmacology of Cannabis: A Review of Human Imaging Studies." *Pharmacology and Therapeutics* 195: 132–161.

Blount, B. C., et al. (2020). "Vitamin E Acetate in Bronchoalveolar-Lavage Fluid Associated with EVALI." *New England Journal of Medicine* 382: 697–705.

Blum, N. J., et al. (2018). "Common Use of Stimulants and Alpha-2 Agonists to Treat Preschool Attention-Deficit Hyperactivity Disorder: A DBPNet Study." *Journal of Developmental and Behavioural Pediatrics* 39: 531–537.

Blumberg, M. J., et al. (2020). "Procognitive Effects of Antidepressants and Other Therapeutic Agents in Major Depressive Disorder: A Systematic Review." *Journal of Clinical Psychiatry* 81: 19r13200.

Boas, G. R. V., et al. (2019). "Molecular Aspects of Depression: A Review from Neurobiology to Treatment." *European Journal of Pharmacology* 851: 99–121.

Boehnke, K. F., et al. (2016). "Medical Cannabis Use Is Associated with Decreased Opiate Medication Use in a Retrospective Cross-Sectional Survey of Patients with Chronic Pain." *Journal of Pain* 17, 739–744.

Bogenschutz, M., et al. (2016). "Co-Administration of Disulfiram and Lorazepam in the Treatment of Alcohol Dependence and Co-Occurring Anxiety Disorder." *American Journal of Drug and Alcohol Abuse* 42: 490–499.

Boileau, I., et al. (2016). "Rapid Recovery of Vesicular Dopamine Levels in Methamphetamine Users in Early Abstinence." *Neuropsychopharmacology* 41: 1179–1187.

Bojdani, E., et al. (2020). "COVID-19 Pandemic: Impact on Psychiatric Care in the United States." *Psychiatry Research* 289: 113069.

Boland, E. G., et al. (2020). "Cannabinoids for Adult Cancer-Related Pain: Systematic Review and Meta-Analysis." *British Medical Journal Supportive Palliative Care* 10: 13–24.

Boldrini, M., et al. (2021). "How COVID-19 Affects the Brain." *JAMA Psychiatry* 78: 682–683.

Bonar, E. E., et al. (2014). "Synthetic Cannabinoid Use Among Patients in Residential Substance Use Disorder Treatment: Prevalence, Motives, and Correlates." *Drug and Alcohol Dependence* 143: 268–271.

Bonner, E., et al. (2021). "The Chemistry and Toxicology of Vaping." *Pharmacology and Therapeutics* 225: 107837.

Borgan, F., et al. (2019). "In Vivo Availability of Cannabinoid 1 Receptor Levels in Patients with First-Episode Psychosis." *JAMA Psychiatry* 76: 1074–1084.

Borgan, F., et al. (2019). "The Effects of Cannabinoid 1 Receptor Compounds on Memory: A Meta-Analysis and Systematic Review Across Species." *Psychopharmacology* 236: 3257–3270.

Borras, S., et al. (2021). "Medicinal Plants for Insomnia Related to Anxiety: An Updated Review." *Planta Medica* 87: 738–753.

Botanas, C. J., et al. (2019). "Methoxetamine: A Foe or Friend?" *Neurochemistry International* 122: 1–7.

Botanas, C. J., et al. (2021). "R (-)–Methoxetamine Exerts Rapid and Sustained Antidepressant Effects and Fewer Behavioral Side Effects Relative to S (+)–Methoxetamine." *Neuropharmacology* 193: 108610.

Botsford, S., et al. (2020). "Cannabis and Cannabinoids in Mood and Anxiety Disorders: Impact on Illness Onset and Course, and Assessment of Therapeutic Potential." *American Journal of Addictions* 29: 9–28.

Botteranne, H., et al. (2022, September 28). "Evaluation of Early Ketamine Effects on Belief-Updating Biases in Patients with Treatment Resistant Depression." *JAMA Psychiatry*.

Bourin, M. (2021). "Neurogenesis and Neuroplasticity in Major Depression: Its Therapeutic Implication." *Advances in Experimental Medicine and Biology* 1305: 157–173.

Bousman, C. A., and Hopwood, M. (2016). "Commercial Pharmacogenetic-Based Decision Support Tools in Psychiatry." *Lancet* 3: 585–590.

Bouso, J. C., et al. (2021). "Psychedelic Medicines in Major Depression: Progress and Future Challenges." *Advances in Experimental Medicine and Biology* 1305: 515–533.

Bowden, C. L., et al. (2012). "Aims and Results of the NIMH Systematic Treatment Enhancement Program for Bipolar Disorder (STEP-BD)." *CNS Neuroscience & Therapeutics* 18: 243–249.

Bowen, S. E. (2011). "Two Serious and Challenging Medical Complications Associated with Volatile Substance Misuse: Sudden Sniffing Death and Fetal Solvent Syndrome." *Substance Use and Misuse* 46, Supplement 1: 68–72.

Boychuk, D. G., et al. (2015). "The Effectiveness of Cannabinoids in the Management of Chronic Nonmalignant Neuropathic Pain: A Systematic Review." *Journal of Oral & Facial Pain and Headache* 29: 7–14.

Boyle, J., et al. (2008). "Next-Day Cognition, Psychomotor Function, and Driving-Related Skills Following Nighttime Administration of Eszopiclone." *Human Psychopharmacology* 23: 385–397.

Bozymski, K. M., et al. (2017). "Pimavanserin: A Novel Antipsychotic for Parkinson's Disease Psychosis." *Annals of Pharmacotherapy* 51: 479–487.

Brannan, S.K., et al. (2021). "Muscarinic Cholinergic Receptor Agonist and Peripheral Antagonist for Schizophrenia." *New England Journal of Medicine* 384: 717–726.

Breadon, C., and Kulkarni, J. (2019). "An Update on Medication Management of Women with Schizophrenia in Pregnancy." *Expert Opinions in Pharmacotherapy* 20: 1365–1376.

Brecher, E. M., and the Editors of Consumer Reports Magazine. (1972). *Licit and Illicit Drugs: The Consumers Union Report on Narcotics, Stimulants, Depressants, Inhalants, Hallucinogens, and Marijuana—Including Caffeine, Nicotine, and Alcohol.* New York: Little, Brown.

Breedvelt, J. F., et al. (2021). "Continuation of Antidepressants vs Sequential Psychological Interventions to Prevent Relapse in Depression: An Individual Participant Date Meta-Analysis." *JAMA Psychiatry* 78: 868–875.

Brender, R., et al. (2021). "An Update on Antidepressant Pharmacotherapy in Late-Life Depression." *Expert Opinion on Pharmacotherapeutics* 22: 1909–1917.

Brent, D. A., et al. (2008). "Switching to Another SSRI or to Venlafaxine with or without Cognitive Behavioral Therapy for Adolescents with SSRI-Resistant Depression." *JAMA* 299: 901–913.

Brierley, D. I., and Davisson, C. (2012). "Developments in Harmine Pharmacology—Implications for Ayahuasca Use and Drug-Dependence Treatment." *Progress in Neuropsychopharmacology and Biological Psychiatry* 39: 263272.

Brinkman, H. M. and Fristad, M. A. (2022). "Psychosocial Treatments for Bipolar Disorder in Children and Adolescents." *Annual Reviews of Clinical Psychology* 18: 291–327.

Brodnik, Z. D., et al. (2017). "Reinforcing Doses of Intravenous Cocaine Produce Only Modest Dopamine Reuptake Inhibition." *ACS Chemical Neuroscience* 8: 281–289.

Bromley, R. L., et al. (2019). "Intellectual Functioning in Clinically Confirmed Fetal Valproate Syndrome." *Neurotoxicology and Teratology* 71: 16–21.

Brower, K. J., et al. (2011). "Ramelteon and Improved Insomnia in Alcohol-Dependent Patients: A Case Series." *Journal of Clinical Sleep Medicine* 7: 274–275.

Brown, E., et al. (2020). "The Potential Impact of COVID-19 on Psychosis: A Rapid Review of Contemporary Epidemic and Pandemic Research." *Schizophrenia Research* 222: 79–87.

Brubacher, J. R., et al. (2022). "Cannabis Legalization and Detection of Tetrahydrocannabinol in Injured Drivers." *New England Journal of Medicine* 386: 148–156.

Brunetti, P., et al. (2021). "Designer Benzodiazepines: A Review of Toxicology and Public Health Risks." *Pharmaceuticals (Basel)* 14: 560.

Brunner, E., et al. (2014). "Efficacy and Safety of Olanzapine/Fluoxetine Combination vs Fluoxetine Monotherapy Following Successful Combination Therapy of Treatment-Resistant Major Depressive Disorder." *Neuropsychopharmacology* 39: 2549–2559.

Bschor, T., and Kilarski, L. L. (2018). "Are Antidepressants Effective? A Debate on Their Efficacy for the Treatment of Major Depression in Adults." *Expert Review of Neurotherapeutics* 16: 367–374.

Buck, J. M., and Siegel, J. A. (2015). "The Effects of Adolescent Methamphetamine Exposure." *Frontiers in Neuroscience* 9: 151.

Buoli, M., et al. (2016). "Biological Aspects and Candidate Biomarkers for Psychotic Bipolar Disorder: A Systematic Review." *Psychiatry and Clinical Neurosciences* 70: 227–244.

Burckhardt, M., et al. (2016). "Omega-3 Fatty Acids for the Treatment of Dementia." *Cochrane Database Systems Review* 11: 4.

Burke, T. M., et al. (2015). "Effects of Caffeine on the Human Circadian Clock in Vivo and in Vitro." *Science Translational Medicine* 7: 305ra146.

Burns, A., et al. (2009). "Safety and Efficacy of Galantamine (Reminyl) in Severe Alzheimer's Disease (the SERAD Study): A Randomized, Placebo-Controlled, Double-Blind Trial." *Lancet Neurology* 8: 39–47.

Busardo, F. P., and Jones, A. W. (2015), "GHB Pharmacology and Toxicology: Acute Intoxication, Concentrations in Blood and Urine in Forensic Cases and Treatment of the Withdrawal Syndrome." *Current Neuropharmacology* 13: 47–70.

Bushe, C. J., and Savill, N. C. (2014). "Systematic Review of Atomoxetine Data in Childhood and Adolescent Attention-Deficit Hyperactivity Disorder 2009–2011: Focus on Clinical Efficacy and Safety." *Journal of Psychopharmacology* 28: 204–211.

Buspavanich, P., et al. (2019). "Treatment Response of Lithium Augmentation in Geriatric Compared to Non-Geriatric Patients with Treatment-Resistant Depression." *Journal of Affective Disorders* 251: 136–140.

Butelman, E. R., et al. (2010). "The Discriminative Effects of the Kappa-Opioid Hallucinogen Salvinorin A in Nonhuman Primates: Dissociation from Classic Hallucinogen Effects." *Psychopharmacology* 210: 253–262.

Bymaster, F. P., et al. (2005). "The Dual Transporter Inhibitor Duloxetine: A Review of Its Preclinical Pharmacology, Pharmacokinetic Profile, and Clinical Results in Depression." *Current Pharmaceutical Design* 11: 1475–1493.

Byrne, J. J., et al. (2020). "Evaluation of Drug Labels Following the 2015 Pregnancy and Lactation Labeling Rule." *JAMA Network Open* 3: e2015094.

Cahill, K., et al. (2016). "Nicotine Receptor Partial Agonists for Smoking Cessation."

Cochrane Database of Systematic Reviews 5: CD006103.

Cal Polytechnic State University (2023). "What to do if You have been Sexually Assaulted." Cal Polytechnic State University, San Luis Obispo, California, 93407.

Calabrese, J. R., et al. (2021). "Efficacy and Safety of Lumateperone for Major Depressive Episodes Associated with Bipolar I or Bipolar II Disorder: A Phase 3 Randomized Placebo-Controlled Trial." *American Journal of Psychiatry* 178: 1098–1106.

Calipe-Lopez, C., et al. (2019). "Cannabidiol Treatment Might Promote Resilience to Cocaine and Methamphetamine Use Disorders: A Review of Possible Mechanisms." *Molecules* 24: 2563.

Callaghan, R. C., et al. (2012). "Increased Risk of Parkinson's Disease in Individuals Hospitalized with Conditions Related to the Use of Methamphetamine or Other Amphetamine-Type Drugs." *Drug and Alcohol Dependence* 120: 35–40.

Callisto, S. P., et al. (2020). "Severity of Topiramate-Related Working Memory Impairment Is Modulated by Plasma Concentration and Working Memory Capacity." *Journal of Clinical Pharmacology* 60: 1166–1176.

Calsolaro, V., et al. (2019). "The Use of Antipsychotic Drugs for Treating Behavioral Symptoms in Alzheimer's Disease." *Frontiers in Pharmacology* 10: 1465.

Camden, A., et al. (2022). "Categorization of Opioid Use Among Pregnant People and Association with Overdose Deaths." *JAMA Network Open* 5: e2214688.

Cameron, L., and Olson, D. (2018). "Dark Classics in Chemical Neuroscience: N, N-Dimethyltryptamine (DMT)." *ACS Chemical Neuroscience* 9: 2344–2357.

Cameron, L. P., et al. (2021). "A Non-Hallucinogenic Psychedelic Analog with Therapeutic Potential." *Nature* 589: 474–479.

Campbell, N. L., et al. (2017). "Adherence and Tolerability of Alzheimer's Disease Medications: A Pragmatic Randomized Trial." *Journal of the American Geriatric Society* 65: 1497–1504.

Canhada, S., et al. (2018). "Omega-3 Fatty Acids' Supplementation in Alzheimer's Disease: A Systematic Review." *Nutritional Neuroscience* 21: 529–538.

Cantu, F., et al. (2021). "Augmentation with Atypical Antipsychotics for Treatment-Resistant Depression." *Journal of Affective Disorders* 280: 45–53.

Cantu, P., et al. (2021). "Augmentation with Atypical Antipsychotics for Treatment-Resistant Depression." *Journal of Affective Disorders* 280: 45–53.

Canuso, C. M., et al. (2018). "Efficacy and Safety of Intranasal Eskatamine for the Rapid Reduction of Symptoms of Depression and Suicidality in Patients at Imminent Risk for Suicide: Results of a Double-Blind, Randomized, Placebo-Controlled Study." *American Journal of Psychiatry* 175: 620–630.

Cao, Y., et al. (2015). "Light to Moderate Intake of Alcohol, Drinking Patterns, and Risk of Cancer: Results from Two Prospective US Cohort Studies." *BMJ* 351.

Cappelletti, S., et al. (2015). "Caffeine: Cognitive and Physical Performance Enhancer or Psychoactive Drug?" *Current Neuropharmacology* 13: 77–88.

Carbon, M., et al. (2017). "Tardive Dyskinesia Prevalence in the Period of Second-Generation Antipsychotic Use: A Meta-analysis." *Journal of Clinical Psychiatry* 78: 264–278.

Carey, B. (2012). "Learning from the Spurned and Tipsy Fruit Fly." *New York Times*, March 15. http://www.nytimes.com/2012/03/16/health/male-fruit-flies-spurned-by-females-turn-to-alcohol. html.

Carhart-Harris, R. (2022, April 11). "Psilocybin 'Rewires' the Brain to Alleviate Depression." *Medscape*.

Carhart-Harris, R. L. (2019). "How Do Psychedelics Work?" *Current Opinions in Psychiatry* 32: 161.

Carhart-Harris, R. L., et al. (2016a). "Neural Correlates of the LSD Experience Revealed by Multimodal Neuroimaging." *Proceedings of the National Academy of Sciences* 113: 4853–4858.

Carhart-Harris, R. L., et al. (2016b). "Psilocybin and Psychological Support for Treatment of Resistant Depression: An Open-Label Feasibility Study" *Lancet Psychiatry* 3: 619–627.

Carhart-Harris, R. L., et al. (2021). "Trial of Psilocybin versus Escitalopram for Depression." *New England Journal of Medicine* 384: 1402–1411.

Carlat, D. (2015). *Drug Metabolism in Psychiatry: A Clinical Guide*, 3rd ed. Newburyport, MA: Carlat Publishing, LLC.

Carod-Artal, F. J. (2015). "Hallucinogenic Drugs in Pre-Columbian Mesoamerican Cultures." *Neurologia* 30: 42–49.

Carpenter, J., et al. (2020). "Naloxone Dosing After Opioid Overdose in the Era of Illicitly Manufactured Fentanyl." *Journal of Medical Toxicology* 16: 41–48.

Carradori, S., et al. (2018). "MAO Inhibitors and Their Wider Applications: A Patent Review." *Expert Opinion in Therapeutic Patents* 28: 211–226.

Carvalho, A. F., et al. (2020). "Bipolar Disorder." *The New England Journal of Medicine* 383: 58–66.

Casey, D. E., et al. (2012). "Efficacy of Adjunctive Aripiprazole in Major Depressive Disorder: A Pooled Response Quartile Analysis and the Predictive Value of Week 2 Early Response." *Primary Care Companion CNS Disorders* 14(3).

Cassano, T., et al. (2019). "Pharmacological Treatment of Depression in Alzheimer's Disease: A Challenging Task." *Frontiers in Pharmacology* 10: 1067.

Castellanos, J. P., et al. (2020). "Chronic Pain and Psychedelics: A Review and Proposed Mechanism of Action." *Regional Anesthesia & Pain Medicine* 45: 486–494.

Cavazzoni, P. (2021). "FDA's Decision to Approve New Treatment for Alzheimer's Disease." www.fda.gov/drugs/news-events-human-drugs/fdas-decision-approve-new-treatment-alzheimers-disease.

Caye, A., et al. (2019). "Treatment Strategies for ADHD: An Evidence-Based Guide to Select Optimal Treatment." *Molecular Psychiatry* 24: 390–408.

Cazet, L., et al. (2018). "Interaction Between CYP2D6 Inhibitor Antidepressants and Codeine: Is This Relevant? *Expert Opinion in Drug Metabolism and Toxicology* 14: 879–886.

Ceban, F., et al. (2021). "Association Between Mood Disorders and Risk of COVID-19 Infection, Hospitalization, and Death: A Systematic Review and Meta-Analysis." *JAMA Psychiatry* 78: 1079–1091.

Centers for Disease Control and Prevention (2020a). "Current Cigarette Smoking Among Adults in the United States." National Center for Chronic Disease Prevention and Health Protection, Office of Smoking and Health.

Centers for Disease Control and Prevention. (2020b). "Data and Statistics on Birth Defects." www.CDC.gov/ncbddd/birthdefects/data.html.

Centers for Disease Control and Prevention. (2020c). "Prevalence of Autism Spectrum Disorder Among Children Aged 8 Years—Autism and Developmental Disabilities Monitoring Network, 11 Sites, United States, 2016." *Morbidity and Mortality Weekly Report (MMWR)* 69: 1–12.

Centers for Disease Control and Prevention. (2021a, March 18). "CovEx Results."

Centers for Disease Control and Prevention. (2021b). "Data and Statistics About ADHD." National Center on Birth Defects and Developmental Disabilities.

Centers for Disease Control and Prevention. (2021c, November 17). "Drug Overdose Deaths in the U.S. Top 100,000 Annually." National Center for Disease Control and Prevention.

Centers for Disease Control and Prevention (2022). "Drug Overdose: Prescription Opioid Overdose Death Maps." Centers for Disease Control and Prevention, National Center for Injury Prevention and Control, June 6, 2022.

Centers for Disease Control and Prevention. (2022a). "Adolescent Behaviors and Experiences Survey (ABES)."

Centers for Disease Control and Prevention. (2022b). "Anxiety and Depression in Children." National Center on Birth Defects and Developmental Disabilities/Centers for Disease Control and Prevention.

Centers for Disease Control and Prevention. (2022c). "Fetal Alcohol Spectrum Disorders." National Center on Birth Defects and Developmental Disabilities, Washington, D.C.

Centers for Disease Control and Prevention. (2022d). "Guideline for Prescribing Opioids for Chronic Pain." National Center for Disease Control and Prevention.

Centers for Disease Control and Prevention. (2022e, June 22). "Nearly One in Five American Adults Who Have Had COVID-19 Still Have 'Long COVID'."

Centers for Disease Control and Prevention. (2022f, March 31). "New CDC Dada Illuminate Youth Mental Health Threats During the COVID-19 Pandemic."

Centers for Medicare and Medicaid Services. (2022, April 4). "CMS Finalizes Medicare Coverage Policy for Monoclonal Antibodies Directed Against Amyloid for the Treatment of Alzheimer's Disease."

Cerdá, M., et al. (2016). "Persistent Cannabis Dependence and Alcohol Dependence

Represent Risks for Midlife Economic and Social Problems: A Longitudinal Cohort Study." *Clinical Psychological Science* 4: 1028–1046.

Cerdá, M., et al. (2020). "Association Between Recreational Marijuana Legalization in the United States and Changes in Marijuana Use and Cannabis Use Disorder From 2008 to 2016." *JAMA Psychiatry* 77: 165–171.

Cervesi, C., et al. (2017). "Extent, Time Course, and Moderators of Antipsychotic Treatment in Youth with Mood Disorders: Results of a Meta-Analysis and Meta-Regression Analyses." *Journal of Clinical Psychiatry* 78: 347–357.

Chadi, N., et al. (2019). "Understanding the Implications of the 'Vaping' Epidemic Among Adolescents and Young Adults: A Call for Action." *Substance Abuse* 40: 7–10.

Chakrabarty, T., et al. (2020). "Treatment of Mixed Features in Bipolar Disorder: An Updated View." *Current Psychiatry Reports* 22: 15.

Chaliha, D. et al. (2020). "A Systematic Review of the Valproic-Acid-Induced Rodent Model of Autism." *Developmental Neuroscience* 42: 12–48.

Chaliha, D., et al. (2021). "A Systematic Review of the MDMA Model to Address Social Impairment in Autism." *Current Neuropharmacology* 19: 1101–1154.

Chan, E., et al. (2016). "Treatment of Attention-Deficit/Hyperactivity Disorder in Adolescents: A Systematic Review." *JAMA* 315: 1997–2008.

Chan, J., et al. (2014). "Risks of Untreated Depression in Pregnancy." *Canadian Family Physician* 60: 242–243.

Chan, L. F., et al. (2018). "Is Ketamine the Future Clozapine for Depression? A Case Series and Literature Review on Maintenance Ketamine in Treatment-Resistant Depression with Suicidal Behavior." *Journal of Psychiatric Practice* 24: 279–291.

Chang, A., and Fox, S. H. (2016). "Psychosis in Parkinson's Disease: Epidemiology, Pathophysiology, and Management." *Drugs* 76: 1093–1118.

Chang, W. H., et al. (2020). "Bridging the Associations Between Dopamine, Brain Volumetric Variation and IQ in Drug-Naïve Schizophrenia." *Schizophrenia Research* S: 920–964.

Chang, Z., et al. (2017). "Association Between Medication Use for Attention-Deficit/ Hyperactivity Disorder and Risk of Motor Vehicle Crashes." *JAMA Psychiatry* 74: 597–603.

Chapman, J., et al. (2022, November 30). "Borderline Personality Disorder." *Stat Pearls*.

Charlotte, W., et al. (2019) "Withdrawal Management and Treatment of Crystal Methamphetamine Addiction in Pregnancy: A Review of Clinical Effectiveness and Guidelines [Internet]." *Canadian Agency for Drugs and Technologies in Health*, June 17.

Chaudhary, A. M. D., et al. (2019). "A Review of Samidorphan: A Novel Opioid Antagonist." *Cureus* 11: e5139.

Chekani, F., et al. (2020). "Risk of Mortality Associated with Atypical Antipsychotic Use: A National Cohort Study of Older Adults with Depression and Parkinson's Disease." *American Journal of Geriatric Psychiatry* 28: 1079–1088.

Chekroud, A. M., et al. (2017). "Reevaluating the Efficacy and Predictability of Antidepressant Treatments: A Symptom Clustering Approach." *JAMA Psychiatry* 4: 370–378.

Chen, C. S., et al. (2014). "Clinical Correlates of Zolpidem-Associated Complex Sleep-Related Behaviors: Age Effect." *Journal of Clinical Psychiatry* 75: e1314–e1318.

Chen, M., et al. (2018). "Food–Drug Interactions Precipitated by Fruit Juices Other Than Grapefruit Juice: An Update Review." *Food and Drug Analysis* 26 (2S): S61–S71.

Chen, T., et al. (2020). "Trajectories of Heroin Use Predict Relapse Risk Among Heroin-Dependent Patients: A 5-Year Follow-up." *Journal of Clinical Neurosciences* 76: 134–139.

Cheniaux, E., and Nardi, A. E. (2019). "Evaluating the Efficacy and Safety of Antidepressants I Patients with Bipolar Disorder." *Expert Opinions in Drug Safety* 18: 893–913.

Cherian, S. V., et al. (2021). "Association of Vaping and Respiratory Health Among Youth in the Population Assessment of Tobacco and Health (PATH) Study Wave 3." *International Journal of Environmental Research and Public Health* 18: 8208.

Cheung, A. H., et al. (2018). "Guidelines for Adolescent Depression in Primary Care (GLAD-PC): Part II. Treatment and Ongoing Management." *Pediatrics* 141: e20174082.

Chhabra et al. (2022). *Notes From the Field:* Xylazine-Related Deaths—Cook County, Illinois, 2017–2021. MMWR Morb Mortal Wkly Rep 2022;71:503–504. DOI:

HYPERLINK "http://dx.doi.org/10.15585/mmwr.mm7113a3" http://dx.doi.org/10.15585/mmwr.mm7113a3

Chi, T., and Gold, J. A. (2020). "A Review of Emerging Therapeutic Potential of Psychedelic Drugs in the Treatment of Psychiatric Illnesses." *Journal of Neurological Science* 411: 116715.

Childress, A. C., et al. (2014). "The Effects of Lisdexamfetamine Dimesylate on Emotional Lability in Children 6 to 12 Years of Age with ADHD in a Double-Blind Placebo-Controlled Trial." *Journal of Attention Disorders* 18: 123–132.

Childs, E., and deWit, H. (2012). "Potential Mental Risks." In Yi-Fang Chu, ed., *Coffee: Emerging Health Effects and Disease Prevention*, pp. 293–306. Hoboken, NJ: John Wiley & Sons.

Chin, M. H. (2021). "Uncomfortable Truths—What COVID-19 Has Revealed About Chronic-Disease Care in America." *New England Journal of Medicine* 385: 1633–1636.

Ching, C. R. K., et al. (2022). "What We Learn About Bipolar Disorder from Large-Scale Neuroimaging: Findings and Future Directions from the ENIGMA Bipolar Working Group." *Human Brain Mapping* 43: 56–82.

Chippa, V., and Roy, K. (2022, April 1). "Geriatric Cognitive Decline and Polypharmacy." *StatPearls*.

Choi, Y., et al. (2015). "Coffee Consumption and Coronary Artery Calcium in Young and Middle-Aged Asymptomatic Adults." *Heart* 101: 686–691.

Choy, S. W., et al. (2018). "Melatonin and the Prevention and Management of Delirium: A Scoping Study." *Frontiers in Medicine (Lausanne)* 4: 242.

Christiani, D. C. (2020). "Vaping-Induced Acute Lung Injury." *New England Journal of Medicine* 382: 10.

Christoph, A., et al. (2017). "Cebranopadol, A Novel First-in-Class Analgesic Drug Candidate: First Experience in Patients with Chronic Low Back Pain in a Randomized Clinical Trial." *Pain* 168: 1813–1824.

Chua, K-P., and Conti, R. M. (2021). "Prescriptions for Codeine or Hydrocodone Cough and Cold Medications to US Children and Adolescents Following US Food and Drug Administration Safety Communications." *JAMA Network Open* 4: e2134142.

Chung, Y., et al. (2017). "Ventricular Enlargement and Progressive Reduction of Cortical Gray Matter are Linked in Prodromal Youth Who Develop Psychosis." *Schizophrenia Research* 189: 169–174.

Chye, Y., et al. (2019). "The Endocannabinoid System and Cannabidiol's Promise for the Treatment of Substance Use Disorder." *Frontiers in Psychiatry* 10: 63.

Cicero, T., et al. (2015). "Shifting Patterns of Prescription Opioid and Heroin Abuse in the United States." *New England Journal of Medicine* 373: 1789–1790.

Cichon, L., et al. (2020). "Clinical Picture and Treatment of Bipolar Affective Disorder in Children and Adolescents." *Psychiatria Polska* 54: 35–50.

Cimolai, N. (2017). "Safety with Zopiclone Use: Contemporary Issues." *Current Psychopharmacology* 6: 43–50.

Cipollone, G., et al. (2020). "Exploring the Role of Caffeine Use in Adult-ADHD Symptom Severity of US Army Soldiers." *Journal of Clinical Medicine* 9: 3788.

Cipriani, A., et al. (2016). "Comparative Efficacy and Tolerability of Antidepressants for Major Depressive Disorder in Children and Adolescents: A Network Meta-Analysis." *Lancet* 388: 881–890.

Cipriani, A., et al. (2018). "Comparative Efficacy and Acceptability of 21 Antidepressant Drugs for the Acute Treatment of Adults with Major Depressive Disorder: A Systematic Review and Network Meta-Analysis." *Lancet* 391: 1357–1366.

Citrome, L. (2016). "Vortioxetine for Major Depressive Disorder: An Indirect Comparison with Duloxetine, Escitalopram, Levomilnacipran, Sertraline, Venlafaxine, and Vilazodone, Using Number Needed to Treat, Number Needed to Harm, and Likelihood to be Helped or Harmed." *Journal of Affective Disorders* 196: 225–233.

Citrome, L. L. (2018). "Cariprazine for Acute and Maintenance Treatment of Adults with Schizophrenia: An Evidence-Based Review and Place in Therapy." *Neuro Psychiatric Diseases and Treatment* 14: 2563–2577.

Citrome, L. L. (2020). "Medication Options and Clinical Strategies for Treating Tardive Dyskinesia." *Journal of Clinical Psychiatry* 81: TV18059BR2C.

Citrome, L., et al. (2021). "Cariprazine and Akathisia, Restlessness, and Extrapyramidal

Symptoms in Patients with Bipolar Depression." *Journal of Affective Disorders* 288: 191–198.

Claire, R., et al. (2020). "Pharmacological Interventions for Promoting Smoking Cessation During Pregnancy." *Cochrane Database of Systematic Reviews* 3: CD010078.

Clark, C., et al. (2022). "Lithium Pharmacokinetics in the Perinatal Patient with Bipolar Disorder." *Journal of Clinical Pharmacology* 10: 1002.

Clayton, A. H., et al. (2014). "Antidepressants and Sexual Dysfunction: Mechanisms and Clinical Implications." *Postgraduate Medicine* 126: 91–99.

Clayton, A. H., et al. (2015). "Sexual Dysfunction During Treatment of Major Depressive Disorder with Vilazodone, Citalopram, or Placebo: Results from a Phase IV Clinical Trial." *International Clinical Psychopharmacology* 30: 216–223.

Clayton, H. B., et al. (2017). "Health Risk Behaviors with Synthetic Cannabinoids Versus Marijuana." *Pediatrics* 139: e20162675.

Clift, A. K., et al. (2022). "Neuropsychiatric Ramifications of Severe COVID-19 and Other Severe Acute Respiratory Infections." *JAMA Psychiatry* 79, 690–698.

Clos, S., et al. (2015). "Long-Term Effect of Lithium Maintenance Therapy on Estimated Glomerular Filtration Rate in Patients with Affective Disorders: A Population-Based Cohort Study." *Lancet Psychiatry* 2: 1075–1083.

Coe, M. A., et al. (2019). "Buprenorphine Pharmacology Review: Update on Transmucosal and Long-Acting Formulations." *Journal of Addiction Medicine* 13: 93–103.

Cohen, B. M. (2019) "Evidence-Based Drug Treatment of Acute Depression in Bipolar Disorder." *JAMA Psychiatry* 76: 1314–1315.

Cohen, B. M., and Butler, R. (2011). "BZP-Party Pills: A Review of Research on Benzylpiperazine as a Recreational Drug." *International Journal of Drug Policy* 22: 95–101.

Cohen, B. R., et al. (2020). "FDA Initiative for Drug Facts Label for Over-the-Counter Naloxone." *The New England Journal of Medicine* 382: 2129–2136.

Cohen, J., et al. (2020). "Cannabinoids as an Emerging Therapy for Posttraumatic Stress Disorder and Substance Use Disorders." *Journal of Clinical Neurophysiology* 37: 28–34.

Cohen, L. S., et al. (2016). "Reproductive Safety of Second-Generation Antipsychotics: Current Data from the Massachusetts General Hospital National Pregnancy Registry for Atypical Antipsychotics." *American Journal of Psychiatry* 173: 263–270.

Coleman, J. A., et al. (2016). "X-ray Structures and Mechanism of the Human Serotonin Transporter. *Nature* 532: 334–339.

Colloca, L. (2018). "The Fascinating Mechanisms and Implications of the Placebo Effect." *International Review of Neurobiology* 138: xv–xx.

Colloca, L., and Barsky, A. J. (2020). "Placebo and Nocebo Effects." *The New England Journal of Medicine* 382: 554–561.

Coluzzi, F., et al. (2022). "Current and Future Therapeutic Options in Pain Management: Multi-Mechanistic Opioids Involving Both MOR and NOP Receptor Activation." *CNS Drugs* 10: 1007.

Compton, W. M., and Volkow, N. D. (2021). "Extended-Release Buprenorphine and Its Evaluation with Patient-Reported Outcomes." *JAMA Network Open* 4: e219708.

Compton, W. M., et al. (2016). "Relationship Between Nonmedical Prescription Opioid Use and Heroin Use." *New England Journal of Medicine* 374: 154–163.

Conejero, I., et al. (2018). "Suicide in Older Adults: Current Perspectives." *Clinical Interventions in Aging* 13: 691–699.

Connolly, R. D., et al. (2019). "Probabilities of ADD/ADHD and Related Substance Use Among Canadian Adults." *Journal of Attentional Disorders* 23: 1454–1463.

Conroy, D. A., et al. (2016). "Marijuana Use Patterns and Sleep Among Community-Based Young Adults." *Journal of Addictive Diseases* 35: 135.

Convertino, I., et al. (2016). "Neonatal Adaptation Issues After Maternal Exposure to Prescription Drugs: Withdrawal Syndromes and Residual Pharmacological Effects." *Drug Safety* 39: 903–924.

Cooper, R. E., et al. (2017). "Cannabinoids in Attention-Deficit/Hyperactivity Disorder: A Randomized-Controlled Trial." *European Neuropsychopharmacology* 27: 795–808.

Copeland, W. E., et al. (2015). "Adult Functional Outcomes of Common Childhood Psychiatric Problems: A Prospective

Longitudinal Study." *JAMA Psychiatry* 72: 892–899.

Coplan, P. M., et al. (2016). "The Effect of an Abuse-Deterrent Opioid Formulation (OxyContin) on Opioid Abuse-Related Outcomes in the Postmarketing Setting." *Clinical Pharmacology and Therapeutics* 100: 275–286.

Corkery, J. M. (2018). "Ibogaine as a Treatment for Substance Abuse: Potential Benefits and Practical Dangers." *Progress in Brain Research* 242: 217–257.

Cornelis, M. C., et al. (2006). "Coffee, CYP1A2 Genotype, and Risk of Myocardial Infarction." *JAMA* 295: 1135–1141.

Corponi, F., et al. (2019). "Novel Antipsychotics Specificity Profile: A Clinically Oriented Review of Lurasidone, Brexpiprazole, Cariprazine and Lumateperone." *European Neuropsychopharmacology* 29: 971–985.

Correll, C. U., and Schooler, N. A. (2020). "Negative Symptoms in Schizophrenia: A Review and Clinical Guide for Recognition, Assessment, and Treatment." *Neuropsychiatric Disease and Treatment* 16: 519–534.

Correll, C. U., et al. (2019). "Patient Characteristics, Burden and Pharmacotherapy of Treatment-Resistant Schizophrenia: Results from a Survey of 204 US Psychiatrists." *BMC Psychiatry* 19: 362.

Correll, C. U., et al. (2020). "Efficacy and Safety of Lumateperone for Treatment of Schizophrenia." *JAMA Psychiatry* 77: 349–358.

Correll, C. U., et al. (2021). "Safety and Effectiveness of SEP-363856 in Schizophrenia: Results of a 6-Month, Open-Label Extension Study." *CNS Spectrums* 26: 148–149.

Corriger, A, and Pickering, G. (2019). "Ketamine and Depression: A Narrative Review." *Drug Design and Th*erapy 13: 3051–3067.

Corsi, D. J., et al., (2020). "Association of Material Opioid Use in Pregnancy with Adverse Perinatal Outcomes in Ontario, Canada, from 2012–2018." *JAMA Network Open* 3: e208256.

Cortese, C. (2020). "Pharmacologic Treatment of Attention Deficit-Hyperactivity Disorder." *New England Journal of Medicine* 383: 11.

Cosgrove, L., et al. (2019). "Digital Aripiprazole or Digital Evergreening? A Systematic Review of the Evidence and Its Dissemination in the Scientific Literature and in the Media." *BMJ Evidence Based Medicine* 24: 231–238.

Coskun, M. (2012). "Phenomenology, Psychiatric Comorbidity and Family History in Referred Preschool Children with Obsessive-Compulsive Disorder." *Child and Adolescent Psychiatry and Mental Health* 6: 36.

Costa, G., et al. (2020). "Neuronal and Peripheral Damages Induced by Synthetic Psychoactive Substances: An Update of Recent Findings from Human and Animal Studies." *Neural Regeneration Research* 15: 902–816.

Costa, M. H., et al. (2020). "Clozapine and the Course of Bipolar Disorder in the Systematic Treatment Enhancement Program for Bipolar Disorder (STEP-BD)." *Canadian Journal of Psychiatry* 65: 245–252.

Costandi, M. (2015, May 25). "Uncomfortably Numb: The People Who Feel No Pain." *The Guardian.*

Courtney, R. J., et al, (2021). "Effect of Cytisine vs Vareniciline on Smoking Cessation: A Randomized Clinical Trial." *JAMA* 326: 56–64.

Cranford, J. A., et al. (2017). "Prevalence and Correlates of Sleep-Related Problems in Adults Receiving Medical Cannabis for Chronic Pain." *Drug and Alcohol Dependence* 180: 227–233.

Crippa, J. A. S., et al. (2021). "Efficacy and Safety of Cannabidiol plus Standard Care vs Standard care Alone for the Treatment of Emotional Exhaustion and Burnout Among Frontline Health Care Workers During the COVID-19 Pandemic: A Randomized Clinical Trial." *JAMA Network Open* 4: e2120603.

Cristino, L., et al. (2020). "Cannabinoids and the Expanded Endocannabinoid System in Neurological Disorders." *Nature Reviews Neurology* 16: 9–29.

Crowley, K., et al. (2020). "Valproic Acid for the Management of Agitation and Delirium in the Intensive Care Setting: A Retrospective Analysis." *Clinical Therapeutics* 42: e65–e73.

Cruz, S. L., and Bowen, S. E. (2021). "The Last Two Decades of Preclinical and Clinical Research on Inhalant Effects." *Neurotoxicology & Teratology* 87: 106999.

Cullen, K. A., et al. (2019). "e-Cigarette Use Among Youth in the United States, 2019." *JAMA* 322: 2095–2103.

Cummings, J. L., et al. (2022). "Dementia-Related Psychosis and the Potential Role for Pimavanserin." *CNS Spectrums* 27: 7–15.

Cummings, J., et al. (2018). "Pimavanserin: Potential Treatment for Dementia-Related Psychosis." *The Journal of Prevention of Alzheimer's Disease* 5: 253–258.

Cummings, J., et al. (2022). "Alzheimer's Disease Drug Development Pipeline: 2022." *Alzheimer's & Dementia* 8: e12295.

Cunill, R., et al. (2015). "Pharmacological Treatment of Attention Deficit Hyperactivity Disorder with Co-Morbid Drug Dependence." *Journal of Psychopharmacology* 29: 15–23.

Cunningham, C. W., et al. (2011). "Neuropharmacology of the Naturally Occurring k-Opioid Hallucinogen Salvinorin A." *Pharmacological Reviews* 63: 316–347.

Cuomo, A., et al. (2019). "Clinical Guidance for the Use of Trazodone in Major Depressive Disorder and Concomitant Conditions: Pharmacology and Clinical Practice." *Rivista di Psichiatria* 54: 137–149.

Cuomo, A., et al. (2019). "Drug Safety Evaluation of Aripiprazole in Bipolar Disorder." *Expert Opinion in Drug Safety* 18: 455–463.

Cutler, D. M. (2022). "The Costs of Long COVID." *JAMA Health Forum* 3: e221809.

D'Souza, D. C., et al. (2019). "Efficacy and Safety of a Fatty Acid Amide Hydrolase Inhibitor (PF-04457845).in Treatment of Cannabis Withdrawal and Dependence in Men: A Double-Blind, Placebo-Controlled, Parallel Group, Phase 2a Single-Site Randomized Controlled Trial." *Lancet Psychiatry* 6: 35-45.

D'Souza, I., et al. (2021). "Lumateperone (ITI-007) in the Treatment of Bipolar Depression: Results from a Randomized Clinical Trial." *CNS Spectrums* 26: 10.1017.

D'Souza, M. S. (2016). "Neuroscience of Nicotine for Addition Medicine: Novel Targets for Smoking Cessation Medications." *Progress in Brain Research* 223: 191–214.

Dagani, J., et al. (2016). "Meta-Analysis of the Interval Between the Onset and Management of Bipolar Disorder." *Canadian Journal of Psychiatry* 62: 247–258.

Dahal, R., and Bista, S. (2022). "Strategies to Reduce Polypharmacy in the Elderly. *Stat Pearls.*

Dahan, A., et al. (2020). "Benefit and Risk Evaluation of Biased mu-Receptor Agonist Oliceridine versus Morphine." *Anesthesiology* 133: 559–568.

Dahlgren, M. K., et al. (2021). "Urinary Tetrahydrocannabinol After 4 Weeks of a Full-Spectrum, High Cannabidiol Treatment in an Open-Label Clinical trial." *JAMA Psychiatry* 78: 335–337.

Dai, H. (2020) "Self-Reported Marijuana Use in Electronic Cigarettes Among US Youth, 2017 to 2018." *JAMA* 323: 473–474.

Dai, H., and Richter, K. P. (2019). "A National Survey of Marijuana Use Among US Adults with Medical Conditions, 2016–2017." *JAMA Network Open* 2: e1911936.

Dai, H., and Siahpush, M. (2020). "Use of E-Cigarettes for Nicotine, Marijuana and Just Flavoring Among U.S. Youth." *American Journal of Preventative Medicine* 58: 244–249.

Dakwar, E., et al. (2019). "A Single Ketamine Infusion Combined with Mindfulness-Based Behavioral Modification to Treat Cocaine Dependence: A Randomized Clinical Trial." *American Journal of Psychiatry* 176: published online June 24.

Dakwar, E., et al. (2020). "A Single Ketamine Infusion Combined with Motivational Enhancement Therapy for Alcohol Use Disorder: A Randomized Midazolam-Controlled Pilot Trial." *American Journal of Psychiatry* 177: 125–133.

Daly, E. J., et al. (2019). "Efficacy of Esketamine Nasal Spray Plus Oral Antidepressant Treatment for Relapse Prevention in Patients with Treatment-Resistant Depression: A Randomized Clinical Trial." *JAMA Psychiatry* 76: 893–903.

Damar, U., et al., (2016). "Huperzine A as a Neuroprotective and Antiepileptic Drug: A Review of Preclinical Research." *Expert Review of Neurotherapeutics* 16: 671–680.

Daniel, J., and Haberman, M. (2017). "Clinical Potential of Psilocybin as a Treatment for Mental Health conditions." *The Mental Health Clinician* 7: 24–28.

Danielson, M. L., et al. (2018). "Prevalence of Parent-Reported ADHD Diagnosis and Associated Treatment Among U.S. Children and Adolescents, 2016." *Journal of Clinical Child and Adolescent Psychology* 47: 199–212.

Daniulaityte, R., et al. (2019). "Street Fentanyl Use: Experiences, Preferences, and Concordance Between Self-Reports and Urine Toxicology." *International Journal of Drug Policy* 71: 3–9.

Das, S., et al. (2016). "Lysergic Acid Diethylamide: A Drug of 'Use'?" *Therapeutic Advances in Psychopharmacology* 6: 214–228.

Dashtipour, K., et al. (2021). "Pimavanserin Treatment for Parkinson's Disease Psychosis in Clinical Practice." *Parkinson's Disease* 4: 2603641.

Daugaard, C. A., et al. (2020). "Association of Prenatal Exposure to Valproate and Other Antiepileptic with Intellectual Disability and Delayed Childhood Milestones." *JAMA Network Open* 3: e2025570

Davico, C., et al. (2018). "Anticonvulsants for Psychiatric Disorders in Children and Adolescents: A Systematic Review of Their Efficacy." *Frontiers in Psychiatry* 9: 270.

Davis, A. K., et al. (2021). "Effects of Psilocybin-Assisted Therapy on Major Depressive Disorder: A Randomized Clinical Trial." *JAMA Psychiatry* 78: 481–489.

Davis, M. P., et al. (2018). "Treating Chronic Pain: An Overview of Clinical Studies Centered on the Buprenorphine Option." *Drugs* 78: 1211–1228.

Daws, R. E., et al. (2022). "Increased Global Integration in the Brain After Psilocybin Therapy for Depression." *Nature Medicine* 28: 844–851.

de Bartolomeis, A., et al. (2015). "Update on the Mechanism of Action of Aripiprazole: Translational Insights into Antipsychotic Strategies Beyond Dopamine Receptor Antagonism." *CNS Drugs* 29: 773–799.

De Crescenzo, et. al. (2022). Comparative effects of pharmacological interventions for the acute and long-term management of insomnia disorder in adults: a systematic review and network meta-analysis. *Lancet (London, England)*, *400*(10347), 170–184. https://doi.org/10.1016/S0140-6736(22)00878-9

De Crescenzo, F., et al. (2017). "Pharmacological and Non-Pharmacological Treatment of Adults with ADHD: A Meta-Review." *Evidence Based Mental Health* 20: 4–11.

De Genna, N. M., et al. (2022). "Long-term Effects of Prenatal Cannabis Exposure: Pathways to Adolescent and Adult Outcomes." *Pharmacology, Biochemistry, and Behavior* 214: 173358.

De Gregorio, D., et al. (2021). "Hallucinogens in Mental Health: Preclinical and Clinical Studies on LSD, Psilocybin, MDMA, and Ketamine." *The Journal of Neuroscience* 41: 891–900.

de Martin, S., et al. (2021). "REL-1017 (Esmethadone) Increases Circulating BDNF Levels in Healthy Subjects of a Phase 1 Clinical Study." *Frontiers in Pharmacology* 12: 671859.

de Pablo, G. S., et al. (2020). "Impact of Coronavirus Syndromes on Physical and Mental Health of Health Care Workers: Systematic Review and Meta-Analysis." *Journal of Affective Disorders* 275: 48–57.

De Risio, A., and Lang, A. P. (2014). "History and Therapeutic Rationale of Long Acting Antipsychotics." *Current Clinics in Pharmacology* 9: 39–52.

De Ternay, J., et al. (2019). "Therapeutic Prospects of Cannabidiol for Alcohol Use Disorder and Alcohol-Related Damages on the Liver and the Brain." *Frontiers in Pharmacology* 10: 627–649.

Dea, L., et al. (2016). "Management of Bipolar Disorder." *U.S. Pharmacist* 41: 34–37.

Deacon, G., et al. (2017). "Omega 3 Polyunsaturated Fatty Acids and the Treatment of Depression." *Critical Reviews on Food Science and Nutrition* 57: 212–223.

Deane, K. H. O., et al. (2021). "Omega-3 and Polyunsaturated Fat for Prevention of Depression and Anxiety Symptoms: A Systematic Review and Meta-Analysis of Randomized Trials." *British Journal of Psychiatry* 218: 135–142.

Dedic, N., et al. (2019). "SEP-363856, A Novel Psychotropic Agent with a Unique, Non-D, Receptor Mechanism of Action." *Journal of Pharmacology & Experimental Therapeutics* 371: 1–14.

DeGenna, N. M., et al. (2022). "Long-Term Effects of Prenatal Cannabis Exposure: Pathways to Adolescent and Adult Outcomes." *Pharmacology, Biochemistry and Behavior* 214: 173358.

DeGregorio, D., et al. (2021). "Hallucinogens in Mental Health: Preclinical and Clinical Studies on LSD, Psolocybin, MDMA, and Ketamine." *Journal of Neuroscience* 41: 891–900.

Del Casale, A. D., et al. (2019). "Psychopharmacological Treatment of Obsessive-Compulsive Disorder (OCD)." *Current Neuropharmacology* 17: 710–736.

Del Casale, A., et al. (2021). "Current Clinical Psychopharmacology in Borderline Personality Disorder." *Current Neuropharmacology* 9: 10.2174.

Delamarre, A., and Meissner, W. G. (2017). "Epidemiology, Environmental Risk Factors and Genetics of Parkinson's Disease." *Presse Médicale* 46: 175–181.

Delara, M., et al. (2022). "Prevalence and Factors Associated with Polypharmacy: A Systematic Review and Meta-Analysis." *BMC Geriatrics* 22: 601.

Delgado, A., et al. (2020). "Clozapine in Bipolar Disorder: A Systematic Review and Meta-Analysis." *Journal of Psychiatric Research* 125: 21–27.

Deligiannidis, K. M., et al. (2021). "Effect of Zuranolone vs Placebo in Postpartum Depression: A Randomized Clinical Trial." *JAMA Psychiatry* 78: 951–959.

Deligiannidis, K. M., et al. (2021). "Effect of Zuranolone vs Placebo in Postpartum Depression: A Randomized Clinical Trial." *JAMA Psychiatry* 78: 9590969.

DeLisi, L. E. (2014). "Ethical Issues in the Use of Genetic Testing of Patients with Schizophrenia and Their Families." *Current Opinion in Psychiatry* 27: 191–196.

Delli, P. S., et al. (2016). "GABA Content within the Ventromedial Prefrontal Cortex Is Related to Trait Anxiety." *Social Cognitive & Affective Neuroscience* 11: 758–766.

Demchenko, I., et al. (2022). "Intrinsic Connectivity Networks of Glutamate-Mediated Antidepressant Response: A Neuroimaging Review." *Frontiers in Psychiatry* 13: 864902.

Denny, C. H., et al. (2020). "Trends in Alcohol Use Among Pregnant Women in the U.S., 2011–2018." *American Journal of Preventative Medicine* 59: 768–769.

Desai, P., et al. (2021). "Longitudinal Association of Total Tau Concentrations and Physical Activity with Cognitive Decline in a Population Sample." *JAMA Network Open* 4: E2120398.

Desale, S. E., and Chinnathambi, S. (2020). "Role of Dietary Fatty Acids in Microglial Polarization in Alzheimers's Disease." *Journal of Neuroinflammation* 17: 93.

Devinsky, O., et al. (2018). "Effect of Cannabidiol on Drop Seizures in the Lennox-Gastaut Syndrome." *New England Journal of Medicine* 378: 1888–1897.

Diav-Citrin, O., et al. (2014). "Pregnancy Outcome Following in Utero Exposure to Lithium: A Prospective, Comparative, Observational study." *American Journal of Psychiatry* 171: 785–794.

DiCarlo, F., et al. (2021). "Telepsychiatry and Other Cutting-Edge Technologies in COVID-19 Pandemic: Bridging the Distance in Mental Health Assistance." *International Journal of Clinical Practice* 75: e13716.

Dietz, B. M., et al. (2005). "Valerian Extract and Valerenic Acid Are Partial Agonists of the 5HT-5a Receptor in Vitro." *Brain Research Molecular Brain Research* 18: 191–197.

DiForti, M., et al. (2015). "Proportion of Patients in South London with First-Episode Psychosis Attributable to Use of High Potency Cannabis: A Case-Control Study." *Lancet* 2: 233–238.

Dilley, J. A., et al. (2019). "Prevalence of Cannabis Use in Youths After Legalization in Washington State." *JAMA Pediatrics* 173: 192–193.

Dilley, J. A., et al. (2021). "Trends and Characteristics of Manufactured Cannabis Product and Cannabis Plant Product Exposures Reported to US Poison Control Centers, 2017–2019." *JAMA Network Open* 4: e2110925.

Dingwall, K. M., and Cairney, S. (2011). "Recovery from Central Nervous System Changes Following Volatile Substance Misuse." *Substance Use and Misuse* 46 (Supplement 1): 73–83.

Dinh, L., et al. (2022). "Formulation, Preparation, Characterization, and Evaluation of Dicarboxylic Ionic Liquid Donepezil Transdermal Patches." *Pharmaceutics* 14: 205.

Dinis-Oliveira, R. J., et al. (2019). "Pharmacokinetic and Pharmacodynamic Aspects of Peyote and Mescaline: Clinical and Forensic Repercussions." *Current Molecular Pharmacology* 12: 184–194.

Diniz, B. S. (2018). "The Molecular Intersection Between Senescence and Major Depression in the Elderly." *American Journal of Geriatric Psychiatry* 26: 1097–1105.

Dinoff, A., et al. (2020). "A Meta-Analysis of the Potential Antidepressant Effects of Buprenorphine Versus Placebo as an Adjunctive Pharmacotherapy for Treatment-Resistant Depression." *Journal of Affective Disorders* 271: 91–99.

Dodd, S., et al. (2021). "Trace Amine-Associated Receptor 1 (TAAR1): A New Drug Target for Psychiatry." *Neuroscience and Biobehavioral Review* 120: 537–541.

Doggrell, S. A. (2021). "Still Grasping at Straws: Donanemab in Alzheimer's." *Expert Opinions in Investigative Drugs* 30: 797–801.

Donny, E. C., et al. (2015). "Randomized Trial of Reduced-Nicotine Standards for Cigarettes." *New England Journal of Medicine* 374: 394–397.

Doroudgar, S., et al. (2018). "Effects of Chronic Marijuana Use on Driving Performance." *Traffic Injuries Preview* 19: 680–686.

dos Santos, R. G., and Hallak, J. E. C. (2020). "Therapeutic Use of Serotoninergic Hallucinogens: A Review of the Evidence and of the Biological and Psychological Mechanisms." *Neuroscience and Biobehavioral Reviews* 108: 213–434.

dos Santos, R. G., et al. (2016). "Antidepressive, Anxiolytic and Antiaddictive Effects of Ayahuasca, Psilocybin and Lysergic Acid Diethylamide (LSD): A Systematic Review of Clinical Trials published in the Last 25 Years." *Therapeutic Advances in Psychopharmacology* 6: 193–213.

Doss, M. K., et al. (2020). "The Acute Effects of the Atypical Dissociative Hallucinogen Salvinorin A on Functional Connectivity in the Human Brain." *Nature.com/Scientific Reports* 10: 16392.

Dou, W., et al. (2022). "Family and Psychosocial Functioning in Bipolar Disorder: The Mediating Effects of Social Support, Resilience and Suicidal Ideation." *Frontiers in Psychology* 12: 807546.

Dragioti, E., et al. (2019). "Association of Antidepressant Use with Adverse Health Outcomes—A Systematic Umbrella Review." *JAMA Psychiatry* 76: 1241–1255.

Drug Enforcement Division. (2017). "Schedules of Controlled Substances: Placement of 10 Synthetic Cathinones into Schedule I. Final Rule." *Federal Register* 82: 12171–12177.

Druss, B. G. (2020). "Addressing the COVID-19 Pandemic in Populations with Serious Mental Illness." *JAMA Psychiatry* 77: 891–892.

Duan, J., et al. (2019). "Topiramate Precipitating a Manic Episode in a Bipolar Patient Comorbid with Binge Eating Disorder: A Case Report." *Medicine* 98: e15287.

Dubovicky, M., et al. (2017). "Risks of Using SSRI/SNRI Antidepressants During Pregnancy and Lactation." *Interdisciplinary Toxicology* 10: 30–34.

Duman, R. S., et al. (2021). "Role of BDNF in the Pathophysiology and Treatment of Depression: Activity-Dependent Effects Distinguish Rapid-Acting Antidepressants." *Euro pean Journal of Neuroscience* 53: 126–139.

Dunn, K. E., et al. (2017). "Efficacy of Tramadol Extended-Release for Opioid Withdrawal: A Randomized Cliical Trial." *JAMA Psychiatry* 74: 885–893.

DuPlessis, S. S., et al. (2015). "Marijuana, Phytocannabinoids, the Endocrine System, and Male Fertility." *Journal of Assisted Reproduction and Genetics* 32: 1575–1588.

Durazzo, T. C., et al. (2011). "Cortical Thickness, Surface Area, and Volume of the Brain Reward System in Alcohol Dependence: Relationships to Relapse and Extended Abstinence." *Alcoholism: Clinical and Experimental Research* 35: 1187–1200.

Durgam, S., et al. (2016). "Efficacy and Safety of Adjunctive Cariprazine in Inadequate Responders to Antidepressants: A Randomized, Double-Blind, Placebo-Controlled Study in Adult Patients with Major Depressive Disorder." *Journal of Clinical Psychiatry* 77: 371–378.

Dyer, S. M., et al. (2018). "An Overview of Systematic Reviews of Pharmacological and Non-Pharmacological Interventions for the Treatment of Behavioral and Psychological symptoms of Dementia." *International Psychogeriatrics* 30: 295–230.

Earley, W. R., et al. (2018). "Cariprazine Augmentation to Antidepressant Therapy in Major Depressive Disorder: Results of a Randomized, Double-Blind, Placebo-Controlled Trial." *Psychopharmacology Bulletin* 48: 62–80.

Earley, W., et al. (2019). "Cariprazine Treatment of Bipolar Depression: A Randomized Double-Blind Placebo-Controlled Phase 3 Study." *American Journal of Psychiatry* 176: 439–448.

Eastgate, J. (2021). "Consumers: Beware of Antipsychotics Long-Term Debilitating Effects and More Psychotropic Drugs Used to Treat It." Citizens Commission on Human Rights International, Los Angeles.

Eastlack, S. C., et al. (2020). "Kratom—Pharmacology, Clinical Implication, and Outlook: A Comprehensive Review." *Pain Therapy* 9: 55–69.

Eccles, J. C. (1964). *The Physiology of Synapses.* Academic Press.

Edinoff, A. N., et al. (2021). "Brexpiprazole for the Treatment of Schizophrenia and Major Depressive Disorder: A Comprehensive Review of Pharmacological Considerations in Clinical Practice." *Psychopharmacology Bulletin* 51: 69–95.

Edinoff, A. N., et al. (2021). "Full Opioid Agonists and Tramadol: Pharmacological and Clinical Considerations." *Anesthesiology and Pain Medicine* 11: e119156.

Edinoff, A., et al. (2021a). "Brexanolone, A $GABA_A$ Modulator, in the Treatment of Postpartum Depression in Adults: A Comprehensive Review." *Frontiers in Psychiatry* 12: 699–740.

Edinoff, et al. (2021b). "Full Opioid Agonists and Tramadol: Pharmacological and Clinical Considerations." *Anesthesiology and Pain Medicine* 11: e119156.

Edinoff, A. N., et al. (2021c). "Viloxazine in the Treatment of Attention Deficit Hyperactivity Disorder." *Frontiers in Psychiatry* 12: 789982.

Eerdekens, M-H., et al. (2019). "Cancer-Related Chronic Pain: Investigation of the Novel Analgesic Drug Candidate Cebranopadol in a Randomized, Double-Blind, Noninferiority Trial." *European Journal of Pain* 23: 577–588.

Eggink, E., et al. (2019). "Criminal Offending and Associated Factors in Dual Diagnosis Patients." *Psychiatry Research* 273: 355–362.

Ekstrand, J., et al. (2021). "Racemic Ketamine as an Alternative to Electroconvulsive Therapy for Unipolar Depression: A Randomized, Open-Label, Non-Inferiority Trial (KetECT)." *International Journal of Neuropsychopharmacology* 289: 88–89.

Eldar-Lissai, A., et al. (2020). "Cost-Effectiveness of Brexanolone Versus Selective Serotonin Reuptake Inhibitors for the Treatment of Postpartum Depression in the United States." *Journal of Managed Care & Specialty Pharmacy* 26: 627–638.

Eleftheriou, M. E., and Thomas, E. (2021). "Examining the Potential Synergistic Effects Between Mindfulness Training and Psychedelic-Assisted Therapy." *Frontiers in Psychiatry* 12: 707057.

Elie, M., et al. (2009). "A Retrospective, Exploratory, Secondary Analysis of the Association Between Antipsychotic Use and Mortality in Elderly Patients with Delirium." *International Psychogeriatrics* 21: 588–592.

Elkashef, A., et al. (2008). "Marijuana Neurobiology and Treatment." *Substance Abuse* 29: 17–29.

Ellinger et al. (2010). "Efficacy of Metformin and Topiramate in Prevention and Treatment of Second-Generation Antipyschotic-Induced Weight Gain." *Annals of Pharmacotherapy* vol. 44, 4–8: 1350–1351.

Ellsworth, K. A., et al. (2013). "FKBP5 Genetic Variation: Association with Selective Serotonin Reuptake Inhibitor Treatment Outcomes in Major Depressive Disorder." *Pharmacogenetic Genomics* 23: 156–166.

El-Mallakh, R. S., et al. (2015). "Antidepressants Worsen Rapid-Cycling Course in Bipolar Depression: A STEP-BD Randomized Clinical Trial." *Journal of Affective Disorders* 184: 318–321.

El-Mallakh, R. S., et al. (2020). "Asenapine in the Treatment of Bipolar Depression." *Psychopharmacology Bulletin* 50: 8–18.

el-Seedi, H. R., et al. (2005). "Prehistoric Peyote Use: Alkaloid Analysis and Radiocarbon Dating of Archaeological Specimens of *Lophophora* from Texas." *Journal of Ethnopharmacology* 101: 238–242.

ElSohly, M. A., et al. (2016). "Changes in Cannabis Potency Over the Last 2 Decades (1995–2014): Analysis of Current Data in the United States." *Biological Psychiatry* 79: 613–619.

Emanuel, E. J., et al. (2022). "A National Strategy for the 'New Normal' of Life with COVID." *JAMA* 327: 211–212.

Emanuele, E., et al. (2010). "Elevated Urine Levels of Bufotenine in Patients with Autistic Spectrum Disorders and Schizophrenia." *Neuro Endocrinology Letters* 31: 117–121.

Emslie, G. J., et al. (1997). "A Double-Blind, Randomized, Placebo-Controlled Trial of Fluoxetine in Children and Adolescents with Depression." *Archives of General Psychiatry* 54: 1031–1037.

Englund, A. (2017). "Can We Make Cannabis Safer?" *The Lancet Psychiatry* 4: 543–648.

Englund, A., et al. (2013). "Cannabidiol Inhibits THC-Elicited Paranoid Symptoms and Hippocampal-Dependent Memory Impairment." *Journal of Psychopharmacology* 27: 19–27.

Enteen, L., et al. (2010). "Overdose Prevention and Naloxone Prescription for Opioid Users in San Francisco." *Journal of Urban Health:*

Bulletin of the New York Academy of Medicine 87: 931–941.

Erick, P., and Klosterhalfen, S. (2019). "Placebos and the Placebo Effect in Drug Trials." *Handbook of Experimental Pharmacology* 260: 399–431.

Erick, P., and Zipfel, S. (2019). "Placebo Effects in Psychotherapy: A Framework." *Frontiers in Psychiatry* 10: 456, Published online June 26.

Ersche, K. D., et al. (2011). "Abnormal Structure of Frontostriatal Brain Systems Is Associated with Aspects of Impulsivity and Compulsivity in Cocaine Dependence." *Brain* 134: 2013–2024.

Escalante, E., et al. (2021). "Social Isolation and Loneliness: Imperatives for Health Care in a Post-COVID World." *JAMA* 325: 520–521.

Escalante-Alcalde, D., and Chimal-Monroy, J. (2021). "Insights into the Mechanism of Adult Neurogenesis—An Interview with Arturo Alvarez-Buylla." *International Journal of Developmental Biology* 65: 153–161.

Espay, A. J., et al. (2015). "Placebo Effect of Medication cost in Parkinson Disease: A Randomized Double-Blind Study." *Neurology* 84: 794–802.

Espinoza, R. T., and Kellner, C. H. (2022). "Electroconvulsive Therapy." *The New England Journal of Medicine* 386: 667–672.

Esposito, D. B., et al. (2022). "Characteristics of Prescription Opioid Analgesics in Pregnancy and Risk of Opioid Withdrawal Syndrome in Newborns." *JAMA Network Open* 5: e2228588.

Esser, M. B., et al. (2020). "Deaths and Years of Potential Life Loss from Excessive Alcohol Use—United States, 2011–2015." *Morbidity and Mortality Weekly Report* 69: 781–787.

Esser, M. B., et al. (2021). "Binge Drinking, Other Substance Use, and Concurrent Use in the U.S. 2016–2018." *American Journal of Preventive Medicine.* 60: 169–178.

Ettcheto, M., et al. (2020). "Benzodiazepines and Related Drugs as a Risk Factor in Alzheimer's Disease Dementia." *Frontiers in Aging Neuroscience* 11: 344.

Ettman, C. K., et al. (2020). "Prevalence of Depression Symptoms in US Adults Before and During the COVID-19 Pandemic." *JAMA Network Open* 3(9): e2019686.

Evans, M. L., et al. (2020). "A Pandemic Within a Pandemic—Intimate Partner Violence During COVID-19." *New England Journal of Medicine* 383: 2302–2304.

Faden, J., and Citrome, L. (2019). "Examining the Safety, Efficacy, and Patient Acceptability of Inhaled Loxapine for the Acute Treatment of Agitation Associated with Schizophrenia or Bipolar I Disorder in Adults." *Neuropsychiatric Diseases and Treatment* 15: 2273–2283.

Fairbanks, J., et al. (2020). "Evidence-Based Pharmacotherapies for Alcohol Use Disorder: Clinical Pearls." *Mayo Clinic Proceedings* 95: 1964–1977.

Fairley, M., et al. (2021). "Cost-Effectiveness of Treatments for Opioid Use Disorder." *JAMA Psychiatry* 78(7): 767–777. https://doi.org/10.1001/jamapsychiatry.2021.0247.

Falson, S. L., et al. (2021a). "Pharmacokinetics of Coadministered Viloxazine Extended-Release (SPN-812) and Lisdexamfetamine in Healthy Adults." *Journal of Clinical Psychopharmacology* 41: 155–162.

Falson, S. L., et al. (2021b). "Pharmacokinetics of Coadministered Viloxazine Extended-Release (SPN-812) and Methylphenidate in Healthy Adults." *Clinical Drug Investigations* 41: 149–159.

Farag, H. M., et al. (2022). "Comparison of Amitriptyline and US Food and Drug Administration-Approved Treatments for Fibromyalgia. A Systematic Review and Network Meta-Analysis." *JAMA Network Open* 5: e2212939.

Farah and Madan, (2021). *Open access journals: Peer reviewed journals*. Prime Scholars. Retrieved February 3, 2023, from https://www.primescholars.com/articles/coenzyme-treatment-of-childhood-and-adolescent-depression-a-case-series-104819.html

Fares, J., et al. (2019): "Neurogenesis in the Adult Hippocampus: History, Regulation, and Prospective Roles." *International Journal of Neuroscience* 129: 598–611.

Faria, J., et al. (2018). "Comparative Pharmacology and Toxicology of Tramadol and Tapentadol." *European Journal of Pain* 22: 827–844.

Fava, M., et al. (2017). "Switching from Inadequate Adjunctive or Combination Treatment Options to Brexpiprazole Adjunctive to Antidepressant: An Open-Label Study on the Effects on Depressive Symptoms and Cognitive and Physical Functioning." *International Journal of Neuropsychopharmacology* 20: 22–30.

Fava, M., et al., (2020). "Opioid System Modulation with Buprenorphine/Samidorphan

Combination for Major Depressive Disorder: Two Randomized Controlled Studies." *Molecular Psychiatry* 25: 1580–1591.

Fava, M., et al. (2022). "REL-1017 (esmethadone) as Adjunctive Treatment in Patients with Major Depressive Disorder: A Phase 2a Randomized Double-Blind Trial." *American Journal of Psychiatry* 179: 122–131.

FDA News Release. (2022, May 4). "FDA Permits Marketing for New Test to Improve Diagnosis of Alzheimer's Disease."

Feduccia, A. A., and Mithoefer, M. C. (2018). "MDMA-Assisted Psychotherapy for PTSD: Are Memory Reconsolidation and Fear Extinction Underlying Mechanisms?" *Progress in Neuropharmacology & Biological Psychiatry* 84: 221–228.

Feduccia, A. A., et al. (2019). "Breakthrough for Trauma Treatment: Safety and Efficacy of MDMA-Assisted Psychotherapy Compared to Paroxetine and Sertraline." *Frontiers in Psychiatry* 10: 650.

Fegert, J. M., et al. (2020). "Challenges and Burden of the Coronavirus 2019 (COVID-19) Pandemic for Child and Adolescent Mental Health: A Narrative Review to Highlight Clinical and Research Needs in the Acute Phase and the Long Return to Normalcy." *Child and Adolescent Psychiatry and Mental Health* 14: 20.

Feinstein, R. E., et al. (2020). "A Health Care Workers Mental Health Crisis Line in the Age of COVID-19." *Depression and Anxiety* 37: 1–5.

Feldman. R. S. et al. (1997). *Principles of Neuropsychopharmacology* Sunderland, MA: Sinauer.

Ferguson, J. M., et al. (2012). "High-Dose Desvenlafaxine in Outpatients with Major Depressive Disorder." *CNS Spectrums* 17: 121–130.

Ferland, J., and Hurd, Y. L. (2020). "Deconstructing the Neurobiology of Cannabis Use Disorder." *Nature Neurosciences* 23: 600–610.

Fernandez-Ruiz, J., et al. (2012). "Cannabidiol for Neurodegenerative Disorders: Important New Clinical Applications for This Phytocannabinoid?" *British Journal of Clinical Pharmacology* 75: 323–333.

Ferré, S., et al. (2018). "New Developments on the Adenosine Mechanisms of the Central Effects of Caffeine and Their Implications for Neuropsychiatric Disorders." *Journal of Caffeine and Adenosine Research* 8: 121–128.

Ferreira, M., and Massano, J. (2017). "An Updated Review of Parkinson's Disease Genetics and Clinicopathological Correlations." *Acta Neurological Scandinavica* 135: 273–284.

Ferrer, P., et al. (2014). "Antiepileptic Drugs and Suicide: A Systematic Review of Adverse Effects." *Neuroepidemiology* 42: 107–120.

Fickenscher, A., et al. (2006). "Illicit Peyote Use among American Indian Adolescents in Substance Abuse Treatment: A Preliminary Investigation." *Substance Use and Misuse* 41: 1139–1154.

Figgatt, M. C., et al. (2021). "Take-Home Dosing Experiences Among Persons Receiving Methadone Maintenance Treatment During COVID-19." *Journal of Substance Abuse Treatment* 123: 108276.

Figura, C., and Atkinson, T. J. (2020). "Analgesics of the Future: G-Protein mu-Opioid Receptor Ligands." *Practical Pain Management* 20(5).

Figura, C., et al. (2020). "A Kratom Primer: Miracle Medicine or Herb of Abuse?" *Practical Pain Management* September-October, 20(5).

Filbey, F. M., and DeWitt, S. J. (2012). "Cannabis Cue-Elicited Craving and the Reward Neurocircuitry." *Progress in Neuro-Psychopharmacology & Biological Psychiatry* 38: 30–35.

Finch, A. and P. Pillians (2014). "P-glycoprotein and Its Role in Drug–Drug Interactions." *Australian Prescriber* 37: 137–139.

Findling, R. L., et al. (2015). "Lithium in the Acute Treatment of Bipolar I Disorder: A Double-Blind Placebo-Controlled Study." *Pediatrics* 136: 885–894.

Findling, R. L., et al. (2018). "Progress in Diagnosis and Treatment of Bipolar Disorder Among Children and Adolescents: An International Perspective." *Evidence Based Mental Health* 21: 177–181.

Fine, P. G., and Rosenfeld, M. J. (2013). "The Endocannabinoid System, Cannabinoids, and Pain." *Rambam Maimonides Medical Journal* 4: e0022.

Fink, D. S., et al. (2020). "Medical Marijuana Laws and Driving Under the Influence of Marijuana and Alcohol." *Addiction* 115: 1944–1953.

Finkelstein, M. J., et al. (2019). "Analysis of Acetyl Fentanyl in Postmortem Specimens by Gas Chromatography-Mass Spectrometry (GC-MS): Method Validation and Case Report." *Journal of Analytical Toxicology* 43: 343–348.

Fischer, F., et al. (2020). "COVID-19 and the Elderly: Who Cares?" *Frontiers in Public Health* 8: 151.

Fishbane, S., et al. (2020). "Randomized Controlled Trial of Difelikefalin for Chronic Pruritus in Hemodialysis Patients." *Kidney International Reports* 5: 600–610.

Fitzcharles, M. A., et al. (2019). "Medical Cannabis: Strengthening Evidence in the Face of Hype and Public Pressure." *Canadian Medical Association Journal* 191: e907–908.

Floegel, A., et al. (2012). "Coffee Consumption and Risk of Chronic Disease in the European Prospective Investigation into Cancer and Nutrition (EPIC) Germany Study." *American Journal of Clinical Nutrition* 95: 901–908.

Fluyau, D., and Revadigar, N. (2017). "Biochemical Benefits, Diagnosis and Clinical Risks Evaluation of Kratom." *Frontiers of Psychiatry* 18: 62.

Fond, G., et al. (2021). "Association Between Mental Health Disorders and Mortality Among Patients with COVID-19 in 7 Countries: A Systematic Review and Meta-Analysis." *JAMA Psychiatry* 78: 1208–1217.

Fontanella, C. A., et al. (2021). "Association of Cannabis Use with Self-Harm and Mortality Risk Among Youths with Mood Disorders." *JAMA Pediatrics.*

Fornaro, M., et al. (2019a). "Brexpiprazole for Treatment-Resistant Major Depressive Disorder." *Expert Opinions in Pharmacotherapeutics* 20: 1925–1933.

Fornaro, M., et al. (2019b). "The Emergence of Loss of Efficacy During Antidepressant Drug Treatment for Major Depressive Disorder: An Integrative Review of Evidence, Mechanisms, and Clinical Implications." *Pharmacological Research* 139: 494–502.

Fornaro, M., et al. (2020). "Lithium Exposure During Pregnancy and the Postpartum Period: A Systematic Review and Meta-Analysis of Safety and Efficacy Outcomes." *American Journal of Psychiatry* 177: 76–92.

Fornaro, M., et al. (2021). "Implications of the COVID-19 Pandemic for People with Bipolar Disorders: A Scoping Review." *Journal of Affective Disorders* 295: 740–751.

Fountoulakis, K. N., et al. (2020). "The CINP Guidelines on the Definition and Evidence-Based Interventions for Treatment-Resistant Bipolar Disorder." *International Journal of Neuropsychopharmacology* 23: 230–256.

Fournier, J. C., et al. (2010). "Antidepressant Drug Effects and Depression Severity: A Patient-Level Meta-Analysis." *Journal of the American Medical Association* 303: 47–53.

Frampton, J. E. (2019). "Brexpiprazole: A Review in Schizophrenia." *Drugs* 79: 189–200.

Francescangeli, J., et al. (2019). "The Serotonin Syndrome: From Molecular Mechanisms to Clinical Practice." *International Journal of Molecular Sciences* 20: 2288.

Franchini, L., et al. (2020). "Synaptic GluN2A-Containing NMDA Receptors: From Physiology to Pathological Synaptic Plasticity." *Molecular Sciences.* Published online February 24, 2020.

Franklin, M. E., et al. (2011). "Cognitive Behavior Therapy Augmentation of Pharmacotherapy in Pediatric Obsessive-Compulsive Disorder: The Pediatric OCD Treatment Study II (POTS II) Randomized Controlled Trial." *JAMA* 306: 1224–1232.

Fredriksena, M., et al. (2013). "Long-Term Efficacy and Safety of Treatment with Stimulants and Atomoxetine in Adult ADHD: A Review of Controlled and Naturalistic Studies." *European Neuropsychopharmacology* 23: 508–527.

Freeman, T. P., et al. (2020). "Cannabidiol for the Treatment of Cannabis Use Disorder: A Phase 2a, Double-Blind, Placebo-Controlled, Randomized, Adaptive Bayesian Trial." *Lancet Psychiatry* 7: 865–874.

Freudenmann, R. W., et al. (2006). "The Origin of MDMA (Ecstasy) Revisited: The True Story Reconstructed from the Original Documents." *Addiction* 101: 1241–1245.

Freynhagen, R., et al. (2016). "Pregabalin for the Treatment of Drug and Alcohol Withdrawal Symptoms: A Comprehensive Review." *CNS Drugs* 30: 1191–1200.

Friedman, A. S. (2021). "Association of Vaping-Related Lung Injuries with Rates of e-Cigarette and Cannabis Use Across US States." *Addiction* 116: 651–657.

Friedman, J. H. (2018). "Pimavanserin for Psychotic Symptoms in People with Parkinsonism: A Second Chart Review." *Clinical Neuropharmacology* 41: 156–159.

Friedman, J., and Hansen, H. (2022). "Evaluation of Increases in Drug Overdose

Mortality Rates in the US by Race and Ethnicity Before and During the COVID-19 Pandemic." *JAMA Psychiatry* 79: 379–381.

Friedman, J., et al. (2021). "Racial/Ethnic, Social, and Geographic Trends in Overdose-Associated Cardiac Arrests Observed by US Emergency Medical Services During the COVID-19 Pandemic." *JAMA Psychiatry* 78: 886–895.

Friedman, M. J., and Bernardy, N. C. (2017). "Considering Future Pharmacotherapy for PTSD." *Neuroscience Letters* 649: 181–185.

Friedman, R. A. (2014). "Perspective—Antidepressants' Black-Box Warning—10 Years Later." *New England Journal of Medicine* 371: 1666–1668.

Froehlich, T. E. (2021). "Comparison of Medication Treatments for Preschool Children with ADHD: A First Step Toward Addressing a Critical Gap." *JAMA* 325: 2049–2050.

Frontera, J. A., and Simon, N. M. (2022). "Bridging Knowledge Gaps in the Diagnosis and Management of Neuropsychiatric Sequelae of COVID-19." *JAMA Psychiatry* 79: 811–816.

Fu, D.-J., et al. (2020). "Esketamine Nasal Spray for Rapid Reduction of Major Depressive Disorder Symptoms in Patients Who Have Active Suicidal Ideation with Intent: Double-Blind, Randomized Study (ASPIRE I)." *Journal of Clinical Psychiatry* 81: 19m13191.

Fudin, J. (2020, January–February). "Tapentadol: A Real-World Look at Misuse, Abuse, and Diversion." *Practical Pain Management* 20.

Fudin, J., and Raouf, M. (2016). "A Review of Skeletal Muscle Relaxants for Pain Management: Spasticity and Spasm: 2 Distinct Reactions to Motor Neurons That Require Unique and Sometimes Complementary Therapies." *Practical Pain Management,* June 1.

Fuentes, J. J., et al. (2020). "Therapeutic Use of LSD in Psychiatry: A Systematic Review of Randomized-Controlled Clinical Trials." *Frontiers in Psychiatry* 10: Article 943.

Fugger, G., et al. (2022). "The Socio-demographic and Clinical Profile of Patients with Major Depressive Disorder Receiving SSRIs as First-Line Antidepressant Treatment in European Countries." *European Archives of Psychiatry & Clinical Neuroscience* 114: 110480.

Fullana, M. A., et al. (2020). "Coping Behaviors Associated with Decreased Anxiety and Depressive Symptoms During the COVID-19 Pandemic and Lockdown." *Journal of Affective Disorders* 275: 80–81.

Fusar-Poli, L., et al. (2020). "Cannabinoids for People with ASD: A Systematic Review of Published and Ongoing Studies." *Brain Sciences* 10: e572.

Gaglani, A., and Gross, T. (2018). "Pediatric Pain Management." *Emergency Medical Clinics of North America* 36: 323–334.

Gai, N., et al. (2020). "A Practical Guide to Acute Pain Management in Children." *Journal of Anesthesia* 34: 421–433.

Gajarawala, S. N., and J. N. Pelkowski (2021). "Telehealth Benefits and Barriers." *The Journal for Nurse Practitioners* 17: 218–221.

Galea, S. (2021). "Elevating Dignity as a Goal for Health System Achievement in the COVID-19 Era and in the Future." *JAMA Health Forum* 2: e212803.

Gallo, A. T., and Hulse, G. (2021). "Pharmaceutical Uses of Flumazenil in Benzodiazepine Use Disorders: A Systematic Review of Limited Data." *Journal of Psychopharmacology* 35: 211–220.

Gan, T. J., and Wase, L. (2020). "Oliceridine, a G Protein-Selective Ligand at the mu-Opioid Receptor, for the Management of Moderate to Severe Acute Pain." *Drugs Today* 56: 269–286.

Ganz, M. L., et al. (2021). "Cost-Effectiveness of Valbenazine Compared with Deutrabenazine for the Treatment of Tardive Dyskinesia." *Journal of Medical Economics* 24: 103–113.

Gao, S.-Y., et al. (2018). "Selective Serotonin Reuptake Inhibitor Use During Early Pregnancy and Congenital Malformations: A Systematic Review and Meta-Analysis of Cohort Studies of More Than 9 Million Births." *BMC Medicine* 16: 205.

Garcia, A. M. (2017). "U.S. State Statutes Banning Powdered Alcohol: Exceptions and Penalties." *American Journal of Public Health: Law and Ethics* 107: 880–883.

Garcia, S., et al. (2021). "Unfolded p53 as a Marker of Oxidative Stress in Mild Cognitive Impairment, Alzheimer's and Parkinson's Disease." *Current Alzheimer's Research* 18: 695–700.

Garcia-Romeu, A., et al. (2020). "Kratom (*Mitragyna speciosa*): User Demographics, Use Patterns, and Implications for the Opioid Epidemic." *Drug and Alcohol Dependence* 208: 107849.

Gareri, P., et al. (2014). "Use of Atypical Antipsychotics in the Elderly: A Clinical Review." *Clinical Interventions in Aging* 9: 1363–1373.

Garrison-Desany, H., et al. (2022). "Individual and Combined Association Between Prenatal Polysubstance Exposure and Childhood Risk of Attention-Deficit/Hyperactivity Disorder." *JAMA Network Open* 5: e221957.

Gautam, C. S., et al. (2020). "Repurposing Potential of Ketamine: Opportunities and Challenges." *Indian Journal of Psychological medicine* 42: 22–29.

Gautam, M., et al. (2019). "Levomilnacipram: More of the Same? *The Primary Care Companion for CNS Disorders* 21: 19nr02475.

Geffrey, A. L., et al. (2015). "Drug–Drug Interaction Between Clobazam and Cannabidiol in Children with Refractory Epilepsy." *Epilepsia* 56: 1246–1251.

Gerhard, T., et al. (2020). "Mortality Risk of Antipsychotic Augmentation for Adult Depression." *PLoS One* 15: e0239206.

Gershon, S., et al. (2009). "Lithium Specificity in Bipolar Illness: A Classic Agent for the Classic Disorder." *Bipolar Disorders* 11 (suppl. 2): 34–44.

Gerteis, J., et al. (2011). "Are There Effects of Intrauterine Cocaine Exposure on Delinquency During Early Adolescence? A Preliminary Report." *Journal of Developmental and Behavioral Pediatrics* 32: 393–401.

Geschwind, D. H., and Flint, J. (2015). "Genetics and Genomics of Psychiatric Disease." *Science* 349: 1489–1494.

Ghabrash, M. F., et al. (2020). "Cannabidiol for the Treatment of Psychosis Among Patients with Schizophrenia and Other Primary psychotic Disorders: A Systematic Review with a Risk of Bias Assessment." *Psychiatry Research* 286: 112890.

Ghosh, R., et al. (2020). "Impact of COVID-19 on Children: Special Focus on the Psychosocial Aspect." *Minerva Pediatrica* 72: 226–235.

Giacomo, E. D., et al. (2021). "Cannabis and Pregnancy: A Psychiatric, Medical, or General Population Issue?" *European Addiction Research* 27: 156–160.

Giancola, P. R., et al. (2011). "Alcohol, Violence, and the Alcohol Myopia Model: Preliminary Findings and Implications for Prevention." *Addictive Behaviors* 36: 1019–1022.

Gibbons, R. D., et al. (2012). "Suicidal Thoughts and Behavior with Antidepressant Treatment." *Archives of General Psychiatry* 69: 580–587.

Gibby, B. A., et al. (2017). "Long-Term Outcomes of Youth Treated for an Anxiety Disorder: A Critical Review." *Clinical Child and Family Psychology Review* 20: 201–225.

Gilbert, D. G., et al. (2020). "Nicotine Patch for Cannabis Withdrawal Symptom Relief: A Randomized Controlled Trial." *Psychopharmacology* 237: 1507–1519.

Gillespie, N. A., and Kendler, K. S. (2021). "Use of Genetically Informed Methods to Clarify the Nature of the Association Between Cannabis Use and Risk for Schizophrenia." *JAMA Psychiatry* 78(5): 467–468.

Gimenez, A., et al. ((2019). "Adverse Outcomes During Pregnancy and Major Congenital Malformation in Infants of Patients with Bipolar and Schizoaffective Disorders Treated with Antiepileptic Drugs: A Systematic Review." *Psychiatria Polska* 53: 223–244.

Giroud, C., et al. (2015). "E-Cigarettes: A Review of New Trends in Cannabis Use." *International Journal of Environmental Research and Public Health* 12: 9988–10008.

Gitlin, M. J. (2016). "Lithium Side Effects and Toxicity: Prevalence and Management Strategies." *International Journal of Bipolar Disorders* 4: 27.

Gitlin, M. J. (2018). "Antidepressants in Bipolar Depression: An Enduring Controversy." *International Journal of Bipolar Disorders* 6: 25.

Glasner-Edwards, S., and L. Mooney (2014). "Methamphetamine Psychosis; Epidemiology and Management." *CNS Drugs* 28: 1115–1126.

Glass, O. M., et al. (2020). "Considerations and Current Trends in the Management of the Geriatric Patient on a Consultation-Liaison Service." *Current Psychiatry Reports* 22: 21.

Global Burden of Disease Long COVID Collaborators. (2022, October 10). "Estimated

Global Proportions of Individuals with Persistent Fatigue, Cognitive, and Respiratory Symptom Clusters Following Symptomatic COVID-19 in 2020 and 2021." *JAMA*.

Glogauer, J., and Blay, J. (2022). "Cannabinoids, Their Cellular Receptors, and Effects on the Invasive Phenotype of Carcinoma and Metastasis." *Cancer Reports* 5: e1475.

Gobbi, B., et al. (2019). "Association of Cannabis use in Adolescence and Risk of Depression, Anxiety, and Suicidality in Young Adulthood—A Systematic Review and Meta-Analysis." *JAMA Psychiatry* 76: 426–434.

Goel, R., et al. (2018). "An Update on Pharmacotherapy of Autism Spectrum Disorder in Children and Adolescents." *International Review of Psychiatry* 30: 1080/09540261.

Goff, D. C. (2021). "The Pharmacologic Treatment of Schizophrenia—2021." *JAMA* 325: 175–176.

Goh, K. K., et al. (2019). "Lamotrigine Augmentation in Treatment-Resistant Unipolar Depression: A Comprehensive Meta-Analysis of Efficacy and Safety." *Journal of Psychopharmacology* 33: 700–713.

Gold, M. S. (1997). "Cocaine (and Crack): Clinical Aspects." In J. H. Lowinson, P. Ruiz, R. B. Millman, and J. G. Langrod, eds., *Substance Abuse: A Comprehensive Textbook*, 3rd ed. Williams & Wilkins.

Gold, P. E. (2008). "Protein Synthesis Inhibition and Memory: Formation vs Amnesia." *Neurobiology of Learning and Memory* 89: 201–211.

Goldberg, S. B., et al. (2020). "The Experimental Effects of Psilocybin on Symptoms of Anxiety and Depression: A Meta-Analysis." *Psychiatry Research* 284: 112749.

Gomes, T., et al. (2021). "Measuring the Burden of Opioid-Related Mortality in Ontario Canada During the COVID-19 Pandemic." *JAMA Network Open* 4: e2112865.

Gonçalves, J., et al. (2021). "Psychoactive Substances of Natural Origin: Toxicological Aspects, Therapeutic Properties and Analysis in Biological Samples." *Molecules* 26: 1397.

Gonda, X., et al. (2019). "Vortioxetine: A Novel Antidepressant for the Treatment of Major Depressive Disorder." *Expert Opinions in Drug Discovery* 14: 81–89.

Gonda, X., et al. (2021). "Novel Antidepressant Drugs: Beyond Monoamine Targets." *CNS Spectrums* 30: 1–10.

Good, M. M., et al. (2010). "Methamphetamine Use During Pregnancy." *Obstetrics & Gynecology* 116: 330–334.

Goodman, W. K., et al. (2021). "Harmonizing the Neurobiology and Treatment of Obsessive-Compulsive Disorder." *American Journal of Psychiatry* 178: 17–29.

Gordovez, F. J. A., and McMahon, F. J. (2020). "The Genetics of Bipolar Disorder." *Molecular Psychiatry* 25: 544–559.

Gorelick, D. A., et al. (2013). "Tolerance to Effects of High-Dose Oral Delta-9-Tetrahydrocannabinol and Plasma Cannabinoid Concentrations in Male Daily Cannabis Smokers." *Journal of Analytical Toxicology* 37: 11–16.

Gorman, I., et al. (2020). "Posttraumatic Growth After MDMA-Assisted Psychotherapy for Posttraumatic Stress Disorder." *Journal of Traumatic Stress* 33: 161–170.

Gould, G. S., et al. (2020). "Exposure to Tobacco, Environmental Tobacco Smoke and Nicotine in Pregnancy: A Pragmatic Overview of Reviews of Maternal and Child Outcomes, Effectiveness of Interventions and Barriers and Facilitators to Quitting." *International Journal of Environmental Research in Public Health* 17: 2034.

Grall-Bronnec, M., et al. (2018). "Dopamine Agonists and Impulse Control Disorders: A Complex Association." *Drug Safety* 41: 19–75.

Grande, I., et al. (2016). "Bipolar Disorder." *Lancet* 387: 1561–1572.

Grange, G., et al. (2020). "Smoking and Smoking Cessation in Pregnancy. Synthesis of a Systematic Review." *Journal of Gynecology, Obstetrics and Human Reproduction* June 30: 101847.

Grant, B. F., et al. (2016). "Epidemiology of DSM-5 Drug Use Disorder: Results from the National Epidemiologic Survey on Alcohol and Related Conditions-III." *JAMA Psychiatry* 73: 39–47.

Grant, B., and Salpekar, J.A. (2018). "Using Lithium in Children and Adolescents with Bipolar Disorder: Efficacy, Tolerability, and Practical Considerations." *Paediatric Drugs* 20: 303–314.

Grant, K. S., et al. (2018). "Cannabis Use During Pregnancy: Pharmacokinetics and Effects." *Pharmacology and Therapeutics* 182: 133–151.

Graves, J. A., et al. (2021). "The Financial Effects and Consequences of COVID-19: A Gathering Storm." *JAMA* 326: 1909–1910.

Gray, R., et al. (2022). "Long-Term Effectiveness of Adjuvant Treatment with Catechol-O-Methyltransferase or Monoamine Oxidase B Inhibitors Compared with Dopamine Agonists Among Patients with Parkinson Disease Uncontrolled by Levodopa Therapy: The PD MED Randomized Clinical Trial." *JAMA Neurology* 79: 131–149.

Gray, S. L., et al. (2016). "Benzodiazepine Use and the Risk of Incident Dementia or Cognitive Decline: Prospective Population Based Study." *BMJ* 352: i90.

Green, A., et al. (2015). "Long-Acting Injectable vs Oral Risperidone for Schizophrenia and Co-Occurring Alcohol Use Disorder: A Randomized Trial." *Journal of Clinical Psychiatry* 10: 1359–1365.

Greenhill, L., et al. (2006). "Efficacy and Safety of Immediate-Release Methylphenidate Treatment for Preschoolers with ADHD." *Journal of the American Academy of Child and Adolescent Psychiatry* 45: 1284–1293.

Gress, K., et al. (2020). "A Comprehensive Review of Partial Opioid Agonists for the Treatment of Chronic Pain." *Best Practice and Research. Clinical Anaesthesiology* 34: 449–461.

Groenewald, C. B., et al. (2022). "Prevalence of Pain Management Techniques Among Adults with Chronic Pain in the United States, 2019." *JAMA Network Open* 5: e2146697.

Grof, P., et al. (2009). "A Critical Appraisal of Lithium's Efficacy and Effectiveness: The Last 60 Years." *Bipolar Disorders* 11 (Suppl. 2): 10–19.

Grossberg, G., et al. (2020). "Efficacy and Safety of Brexpiprazole for the Treatment of Agitation in Alzheimer's Dementia: Two 12-Week, Randomized, Double-Blind, Placebo-Controlled Trials." *American Journal of Geriatric Psychiatry* 28: 383–400.

Grosso, G., et al. (2016). "Coffee, Tee, Caffeine and Risk of Depression: A Systematic Review and Dose-Response Meta-Analysis of Observational Studies." *Molecular Nutrition and Food Research* 60: 223–234.

Grosso, G., et al. (2017). "Coffee, Caffeine, and Health Outcomes: An Umbrella Review." *Annual Review of Nutrition* 27: 131–156.

Grunze, H., et al. (2021). "Comorbid Bipolar and Alcohol Use Disorder—A Therapeutic Challenge." *Frontiers in Psychiatry* 12: 660432.

Guarnieri, M. (2021). "Buprenorphine Blood Concentrations: A Biomarker for Analgesia." *Journal of Opioid Management* 17: 15–20.

Gudin, J., et al. (2020). "Long-Term Safety and Tolerability of NKTR-181 in Patients with Moderate to Severe Chronic Low Back Pain or Chronic Noncancer Pain: A Phase 3 Multicenter, Open-Label, 52 Week Study (SUMMIT-08 LTS." *Pain Medicine* 21: 1347–1356.

Guerrieri, E., et al. (2015). "Synthesis and Pharmacological Evaluation of [(3)H]HS665, a Novel, Highly Selective Radioligand for the Kappa Opioid Receptor." *ACS Chemical Neuroscience* 18: 456–463.

Guessoum, S. B., et al. (2020). "Adolescent Psychiatric Disorders During the COVID-19 Pandemic and Lockdown." *Psychiatry Research* 291: 113264.

Guez, P. R., et al. (2020). "A Single Administration of the Atypical Antipsychotic Ibogaine or Its Metabolite Noribogaine Induces an Antidepressant-Like Effect in Rats." *ACS Chemical Neurosciences* 11: 1661–1672.

Guglielmo, R., et al. (2015). "Topiramate in Alcohol Use Disorders: Review and Update." *CNS Drugs* 29: 383–395.

Guimaraes dos Santos, R., et al. (2021). "The Use of Classic Hallucinogens/Psychedelics in a Therapeutic Context: Healthcare Policy Opportunities and Challenges." *Risk Management and Healthcare Policy* 14: 901–910.

Gundez-Bruce, H., et al. (2019). "Trial of SAGE-217 in Patients with Major Depressive Disorder." *New England Journal of Medicine* 381: 903–911.

Gupta, A., et al. (2021). "A Systematic Review of Ketamine for the Treatment of Depression Among Older Adults." *International Psychogeriatrics* 33: 179–191.

Gurnani, T., et al. (2016). "Pharmacotherapy of Aggression in Child and Adolescent Psychiatric Disorders." *Journal of Child and Adolescent Psychopharmacology* 26: 65–73.

Guttmacher Institute. (2022). "Substance Use During Pregnancy." *State Laws and Policies.*

Gutvirtz, G., et al. (2019). "Maternal Smoking During Pregnancy and Long-Term

Neurological Morbidity of the Offspring." *Addictive Behavior* 88: 86–91.

Haake, A., et al. (2020). "An Update on the Utility and Safety of Cholinesterase Inhibitors for the Treatment of Alzheimer's Disease." *Expert Opinions in Drug Safety* 19: 147–157.

Haass-Koffler, C. L., and Bartlett, S. E. (2012). "Stress and Addiction: Contribution of the Corticotropin Releasing Factor (CRF) System in Neuroplasticity." *Frontiers in Molecular Neuroscience* 5: 1–13.

Haddad, P. M., et al. (2015). "Managing Inadequate Antidepressant Response in Depressive Illness." *British Medical Bulletin* 115: 183–201.

Hafeman, D. M., et al. (2020). "Lithium Versus Other Mood-Stabilizing Medications in a Longitudinal Study of Youth Diagnosed with Bipolar Disorder." *Journal of the American Academy of Child & Adolescent Psychiatry* 59: 1146–1155.

Haight, S. C., et al. (2018). "Opioid Use Disorder Documented at Delivery Hospitalization—United States, 1999–2014." *MNWR Morbidity and Mortality Weekly Report* 67: 845–849.

Hajjar, I., et al. (2020). "Effects of Candesartan vs Lisinopril on Neurocognitive Function in Older Adults with Executive Mild Cognitive Impairment." *JAMA Network Open* 3: e2012252.

Hall, K. T., et al. (2012). "Catechol-O-Methyltransferase val158met Polymorphism Predicts Placebo Effect in Irritable Bowel Syndrome." *PLoS One* 7: e48135.

Hall, W., et al., (2015). "The Brain Disease Model of Addiction: Is It Supported by the Evidence and Has It Delivered on Its Promises?" *Lancet Psychiatry* 2: 105–110.

Hall-Flavin, D. K., et al. (2012). "Using a Pharmacogenomic Algorithm to Guide the Treatment of Depression." *Translational Psychiatry* 2: e172.

Halpin, L. E., et al. (2014). "Neurotoxicity of Methamphatamine and 3,4-methylenedi-oxymethamphetamine." *Life Sciences* 97: 37–44.

Hamill, J., et al. (2019). "Ayahuasca: Psychological and Physiologic Effects, Pharmacology and Potential Uses in Addiction and Mental Illness." *Current Neuropharmacology* 17: 108–128.

Hampel, H., et al. (2018). "The Cholinergic System in the Pathophysiology and Treatment of Alzheimer's Disease." *Brain* 141: 1917–1933.

Han, B., et al. (2021a). "Associations of Suicidality Treads with Cannabis Use as a Function of Sex and Depression Status." *JAMA Network Open* 4: e2113025.

Han, B., et al. (2021b). "Methamphetamine Use, Methamphetamine Use Disorder, and Associated Overdose Deaths Among US Adults." *JAMA Psychiatry*, published online September 22, 2010.

Han, B., et al. (2021c). "Trends in and Characteristics of Buprenorphine Misuse Among Adults in the US." *JAMA Network Open* 4: e2129409.

Han, B., et al. (2021d, June 16). "Use of Medications for Alcohol Use Disorder: Results from the 2019 National Survey on Drug Use and Health." *JAMA Psychiatry*.

Han, D. H., et al. (2013). "Adjunctive Aripiprazole Therapy with Escitalopram in Patients with Co-Morbid Major Depressive Disorder and Alcohol Dependence: Clinical and Neuroimaging Evidence." *Journal of Psychopharmacology* 27: 282–291.

Han, H. J., et al. (2022). "A Multinational, Multicenter, Randomized, Double-Blind, Active Comparator, Phase III Clinical Trial to Evaluate the Efficacy and Safety of Donepezil Transdermal Patch in Patients with Alzheimer's Disease." *Journal of Clinical Neurology* 18: 428–436.

Han, Y., et al. (2019). "The Rising Crisis of Illicit Fentanyl Use, Overdose and Potential Therapeutic Strategies. *Translational Psychiatry* 9: 282–291.

Hanes, K. R. (2001). "Antidepressant Effects of the Herb *Salvia divinorum:* A Case Report." *Journal of Clinical Psychopharmacology* 21: 634–635.

Hansson, O., et al. (2021). "The Alzheimer's Association International Guidelines for Handling of Cerebrospinal Fluid for Routine Clinical Measurements of Amyloid B and Tau." *Alzheimer's Dementia* 17: 1575–1582.

Harris, J. C. (2021). "Psychedelic-Assisted Psychotherapy and Carl Jung's Red Book." *JAMA Psychiatry* 78: 815–816.

Harris, K., et al. (2020). "One Single Large Intramuscular Dose of Naloxone Is Effective and Safe in Suspected Heroin Poisoning." *Emergency Medicine Australasia* 32: 88–92.

Harris, M. G., et al. (2020). "Findings from World Mental Health Survey of the Perceived Helpfulness of Treatment for Patients with Major Depressive Disorder." *JAMA Psychiatry* 77: 830–841.

Harrison, P. J., et al. (2018). "The Emerging Neurobiology of Bipolar Disorder." *Trends in Neurosciences* 41: 1.

Harstad, E. B., et al. (2014). "ADHD, Stimulant Treatment, and Growth: A Longitudinal Study." *Pediatrics* 134: e935–e944.

Harstad, E. B., et al. (2021). "Alpha$_2$ Adrenergic Agonists or Stimulants for Preschool-Age Children with Attention-Deficit/Hyperactivity Disorder." *JAMA* 325: 2067–2075.

Hartel-Petri, R., et al. (2017). "Evidence-Based Guidelines for the Pharmacologic Management of Methamphetamine Dependence, Relapse Prevention, Chronic Methamphetamine-Related, and Comorbid Psychiatric Disorders in Post-Acute Settings." *Pharmacopsychiatry* 50: 96–104.

Hartmann-Boyce, J., et al. (2012). "Nicotine Vaccines for Smoking Cessation." *Cochrane Database of Systematic Reviews* 8: CD007072.

Hartnett, K. P., et al. (2020). "Syndromic Surveillance for E-Cigarette, or Vaping, Product Use-Associated Lung Injury." *New England Journal of Medicine* 382: 766–682.

Hasan, A., et al. (2020). "Cannabis Use and Psychosis; A Review of Reviews." *European Archives of Psychiatry and Clinical Neuroscience* 270: 402–412.

Hashimoto, K. (2019). "Rapid-Acting Antidepressant Ketamin, Its Metabolites and Other Candidates: A Historical Overview and Future Perspective." *Psychiatry and Clinical Neurosciences* 73: 613–627.

Hashimoto, K. (2020). "Molecular Mechanisms of the Rapid-Acting and Long-Lasting Antidepressant Actions of (R)-Ketamine. *Biochemical Pharmacology* 177: 13935.

Hashimoto, Y., et al. (2021). "Lamotrigine in the Maintenance Treatment of Bipolar Disorder." *Cochrane Database of Systematic Reviews* 9: CD013575.

Hatta, K., et al. (2014). "Preventive Effects of Ramelteon on Delirium: A Randomized Placebo-Controlled Trial." *JAMA Psychiatry* 71: 397–403.

Haupt, M., et al. (2021). "Lithium Beyond Psychiatric Indications: The Reincarnation of a New Old Drug." *Neural Regenerative Research* 16: 2283–2387.

Hayes, J. F., et al. (2016). "Self-Harm, Unintentional Injury, and Suicide in Bipolar Disorder During Maintenance Mood Stabilizer Treatment: A UK Population-Based Electronic Health Records Study." *JAMA Psychiatry* 73: 630–637.

Hayes, M. T. (2019). Parkinson's Disease and Parkinsonism." *American Journal of Medicine* 132: 802–807.

Healy, J. R., et al. (2013). "Synthesis, Modeling, and Pharmacological Evaluation of UMB 425, a Mixed Mu Agonist/Kappa Antagonist Opioid Analgesic with Reduced Tolerance Liabilities." *ACS Chemical Neuroscience* 4: 1256–1266.

Heberlein, A., et al. (2011). "Serum Levels of BDNF Are Associated with Craving in Opiate-Dependent Patients." *Journal of Psychopharmacology* 25: 1480–1484.

Hecking, J., et al. (2021). "Emerging Therapeutics Based on the Amino Acid Neurotransmitter System: An Update on the Pharmaceutical Pipeline for Mood Disorders." *Chronic Stress* 5: 24705470211020446.

Heifets, B. D, and Malenka, R. C. (2019). "Disruptive Psychopharmacology." *JAMA Psychiatry* 76: 775–776.

Heinz, A., et al. (2009). "Identifying the Neural Circuitry of Alcohol Craving and Relapse Vulnerability." *Addiction Biology* 14: 108–118.

Heinzerling, A., et al. (2020). "Severe Lung Injury Associated with Use of e-Cigarette, or Vaping, Products—California, 2019." *JAMA Internal Medicine* 180(6): 861–869.

Heise, C. W., and Brooks, D. E. (2017). "Ayahuasca Exposure: Descriptive Analysis of Calls to US Poison Control Centers from 2005–2015." *Journal of Medical Toxicology* 13: 245–248.

Helle, A. C., et al. (2019). "Alcohol Use Disorder and Antisocial and Borderline Personality Disorders. *Alcohol Research* 40: arcr.v40.1.05.

Hellerstein, D. J., et al. (2012). "A Randomized Controlled Trial of Duloxetine Versus Placebo in the Treatment of Nonmajor Chronic Depression." *Journal of Clinical Psychology* 73: 984–991.

Hellmuth, J., et al. (2021). "Persistent COVID-19-Associated Neurocognitive Symptoms in

Non-Hospitalized Patients." *Journal of Neurovirology* 27: 191–195.

Hendricks, P. S., et al. (2015). "Classic Psychedelic Use Is Associated with Reduced Psychological Distress and Suicidality in the United States Adult Population." *Journal of Psychopharmacology* 29: 1041–1043.

Hendriks, S., et al. (2021). "Global Prevalence of Young-Onset Dementia—A Systematic Review and Meta-Analysis." *JAMA Neurology* 2161.

Henningfield, H. E., et al. (2020). "Measuring Opioid Withdrawal in a Phase 3 Study of a New Analgesic, NKTR-181 (Oxycodegol), in Patients with Moderate to Severe Chronic Low Back Pain." *Pain Medicine* 21: 1553–1561.

Henssler, J., et al (2022). "Combining Anti-depressants vs Antidepressant Monotherapy for Treatment of Patients with Acute Depression: A Systematic Review and Meta-Analysis." *JAMA Psychiatry* 79: 300–312.

Henter, I. D., et al. (2021). "Novel Glutamatergic Modulators in the Treatment of Mood Disorders: Current Status." *CNS Drugs* 35: 527–543.

Hermans, K., et al. (2021). "Alcohol Consumption, Cigarette Smoking and Cancer of Unknown Primary Risk: Results from the Netherlands Cohort Study." *International Journal of Cancer* 148: 1586–1597.

Hermens, D. F., and J. Lagopoulos (2018). "Binge Drinking and the Young Brain: A Mini Review of the Neurobiological Underpinnings of Alcohol-Induced Blackout." *Frontiers in Psychology* 19: 9–12.

Hernandez-Diaz, S., et al. (2018). "Topiramate Use Early in Pregnancy and the Risk of Oral Clefts—A Pregnancy Cohort Study." *Neurology* 90: e342–e351.

Herring, W. J., et al. (2016). "Suvorexant in Patients with Insomnia: Pooled Analysis of Three-Month Data from Phase-3 Randomized Controlled Clinical Trials." *Journal of Clinical Sleep Medicine* 12: 1215–1225.

Hesdorffer, D. C., et al. (2016). "Occurrence and Recurrence of Attempted Suicide Among People with Epilepsy." *JAMA Psychiatry* 73: 80–86.

Heuschkel, K., and Kuypers, K. P. C. (2020). "Depression, Mindfulness and Psilocybin: Possible Complementary Effects of Mindfulness Meditation and Psilocybin in the Treatment of Depression. A Review." *Frontiers in Psychiatry* 11: 224.

Hibar, D. P., et al. (2018). "Cortical Abnormalities in Bipolar Disorder: An MRI analysis of 6503 Individuals from the ENIGMA Bipolar Disorder Working Group." *Molecular Psychiatry* 23: 932–942.

Higgins, G. A., et al. (2013). "From Obesity to Substance Abuse: Therapeutic Opportunities for 5-HT2C Receptor Agonists." *Trends in Pharmacological Sciences* 34: 560–570.

Hilker, R., et al. (2018). "Heritability of Schizophrenia and Schizophrenia Spectrum Based on the Nationwide Danish Twin Register." *Biological Psychiatry* 83: 492–498.

Hill, M., et al. (2022). "SAGE-718: A First-in-Class N-Methyl-d-Aspartate Receptor Positive Allosteric Modulator for the Potential Treatment of Cognitive Impairment." *Journal of Medicinal Chemistry* 65: 9063–9075.

Hiluy, J. C., et al. (2019). "Effectiveness of Pharmacologic Interventions in the Management of Weight Gain in Patients with Severe Mental Illness: A Systematic Review and Meta-Analysis." *The Primary Care Companion for CNS Disorders.* 21: 19r02483.

Hindley, G., et al. (2020). "Psychiatric Symptoms Caused by Cannabis Constituents: A Systematic Review and Meta-Analysis." *Lancet Psychiatry* 7: 344–353.

Hines, L. A., et al. (2020). "Association of High-Potency Cannabis Use with Mental Health and Substance Use in Adolescence." *JAMA Psychiatry*, 77: 1044–1051.

Hirai, A. H., et al. (2021). "Neonatal Abstinence Syndrome and Maternal Opioid-Related Diagnoses in the US," 2010–2017.

Hirschtritt, M. E., et al. (2021). "Balancing the Risks and Benefits of Benzodiazepines." *JAMA* 325: 347–348.

Hoang, M. T., et al. (2011). "Association Between Low Serum 25-Hydroxyvitamin D and Depression in a Large Sample of Healthy Adults: The Cooper Center Longitudinal Study." *Mayo Clinic Proceedings* 86: 1050–1055.

Hobart, M., et al. (2019). "Adjunctive Brexpiprazole and Functioning in Major Depressive Disorder: A Pooled Analysis of Six Randomized Studies Using the Sheehan Disability Scale." *International Journal of Neuropsychopharmacology* 22: 173–179.

Hofmann, A. (1994). "Notes and Documents Concerning the Discovery of LSD." *Agents and Actions* 43: 79–81.

Hofmann, S. G. (2020). "The Age of Depression and Its Treatments." *JAMA Psychiatry* 77: 667–668.

Højlund, M., et al. (2021). "Association of Low-Dose Quetiapine and Diabetes." *JAMA Network Open* 4: e213209.

Holmes, E. A., et al. (2020). "Multidisciplinary Research Priorities for the COVID-19 Pandemic: A Call for Action for mental Health Science." *Lancet Psychiatry* 7: 547–560.

Holzman, R. S. (1998). "The Legacy of Atropos, the Fate Who Cut the Thread of Life." *Anesthesiology* 89: 241–249.

Honda, H., et al. (2022). "Depression Is Associated with Chronic Pain in Disabled Older Adults." *Experimental Aging Research* 48: 287–294.

Hondebrink, L., et al. (2017). "Neuropharmacological Characterization of The New Psychoactive Substance Methoxetamine." *Neuropharmacology* 123: 1–9.

Horowitz, M. A., and Taylor, D. (2019). "Tapering of SSRI Treatment to Mitigate Withdrawal Symptoms." *Lancet Psychiatry* 6: 538–546.

Horowitz, M. A., et al. (2020). "Tapering Antipsychotic Treatment." *JAMA Psychiatry* 78: 125–126.

Howard, J. T., et al. (2022). "Trends in Binge Drinking and Heavy Alcohol Consumption Among Pregnant Women in the US, 2011–2020." *JAMA Network Open* 5: e2224846.

Howard, M. O., et al. (2011). "Inhalant Use and Inhalant Use Disorders in the United States." *Addiction Science & Clinical Practice* 6: 18–31.

Howes, S., et al. (2020). "Antidepressants for Smoking Cessation." *Cochrane Database of Systematic Reviews* 4: CD00031.

Hsieh, J. H., et al. (2014). "The Neurobiology of Methamphetamine Induced Psychosis." *Frontiers in Human Neuroscience* 8: 537.

Hsu, T-W., et al. (2021). "Efficacy of Serotonergic Antidepressant Treatment for the Neuropsychiatric Symptoms and Agitation in Dementia: A Systematic Review and Meta-Analysis." *Ageing Research Review* 69: 101262.

Hu, Y., et al. (2022). "Assessment of a Plasma Amyloid Probability Score to Estimate Amyloid Positron Emission Tomography Findings Among Adults with Cognitive Impairment." *JAMA Network Open* 5: e228392.

Huang, L-K., et al. (2020). "Clinical Trials of New Drugs for Alzheimer Disease." *Journal of Biomedical Science* 27: 18.

Huang, X., et al. (2017). "Fentanyl-Related Designer Drugs W-18 and W-15 Lack Appreciable Opioid Activity *in vitro* and *in vivo*." *JCI Insight* 2: e97222.

Huang, Y. H., et al. (2015). "An Epidemiologic Review of Marijuana and Cancer: An Update." *Cancer Epidemiology, Biomarkers and Prevention* 24: 15–31.

Huang, Z-D., et al. (2021). "Comparative Efficacy and Acceptability of Pharmaceutical Management for Adults with Post-Traumatic Stress Disorder: A Systematic Review and Meta-Analysis." *Frontiers in Pharmacology* 11: 559.

Huestis, M. A. (2005). "Pharmacokinetics and Metabolism of the Plant Cannabinoids, Delta9-Tetrahydrocannabinol, Cannabidiol, and Cannabinol." *Handbook of Experimental Pharmacology* 168: 657–690.

Huitfeldt, A., et al. (2020). "Associations of Maternal Use of Benzodiazepines or Benzodiazepine-Like Hypnotics During Pregnancy with Immediate Pregnancy Outcomes in Norway." *JAMA Network Open* 3: e205860.

Hukins, D., et al. (2019). "Identifying Potentially Inappropriate Prescribing in Older People with Dementia: A Systematic Review." *European Journal of Clinical Pharmacology* 75: 467–481.

Hunkeler, E. M., et al. (2006). "Long-Term Outcomes from the IMPACT Randomized Trial for Depressed Elderly Patients in Primary Care." *BMJ* 332: 259–263.

Hurd, Y. L. (2020). "Leading the Next D-CBD Wave—Safety and Efficacy." *JAMA Psychiatry* 7(4): 341–342.

Huxley, R., et al. (2009). "Coffee, Decaffeinated Coffee, and Tea Consumption in Relation to Incident Type 2 Diabetes Mellitus: A Systematic Review with Meta-Analysis." *Archives of Internal Medicine* 169: 2053–2063.

Hwang, Y. J., et al. (2021). "Risk of Hospitalization and Death Associated with

Pimavanserin Use in Older Adults with Parkinson Disease." *Neurology* 13: 10.1212.

Ignaszewski, M., and Waslick, B. (2018). "Update on Randomized Placebo-Controlled Trials in the Past Decade for Treatment of Major Depressive Disorder in Child and Adolescent Patients: A Systematic Review." *Journal of Child and Adolescent Psychopharmacology* 28: 668–675.

Imaz, M. L., et al. (2021). "Neonatal Feeding Trajectories in Mothers with Bipolar Disorder Taking Lithium: Pharmacokinetic Data." *Frontiers in Pharmacology* 12: 752022.

Indave, B. I., et al. (2016). "Antipsychotic Medications for Cocaine Dependence." *Cochrane Database of Systematic Reviews* 19: CD006306.

Ingram, R., et al. (2018). "Some Distorted Thoughts About Ketamine as a Psychedelic and a Novel Hypothesis Based on NMDA Receptor-Mediated Synaptic Plasticity." *Neuropharmacology* 142: 30–40.

Inserra, A., et al. (2021). "Psychedelics in Psychiatry: Neuroplastic, Immunomodulatory, and Neurotransmitter Mechanisms." *Pharmacology Reviews* 73: 1–77.

Ishak, W. W., et al. (2012). "Energy Drinks: Psychological Effects and Impact on Well-Being and Quality of Life—A Literature Review." *Innovations in Clinical Neuroscience* 9: 25–34.

Islam, F. A., et al. (2015). "What to Do When Adolescents with ADHD Self-Medicate with Bath Salts." *Current Psychiatry* 14: e3–e4.

Islami, F., et al. (2021). "Cancer Deaths Attributable to Cigarette Smoking in 152 U.S Metropolitan or Micropolitan Statistical Areas, 2013–2017." *Cancer Causes and Control* 32: 311–316.

Izzo, A. A., et al. (2015). "Endocannabinoids and the Digestive Tract and Bladder in Health and Disease." *Handbook of Experimental Pharmacology* 231: 423–447.

Jack, Jr., C. R., et al. (2011). "Introduction to the Recommendations from the National Institute on Aging-Alzheimer's Association Workgroups on Diagnostic Guidelines for Alzheimer's Disease." *Alzheimer's & Dementia* 7: 257–262.

Jack, Jr., C. R., et al. (2018). "NIA-AA Research Framework: Toward a Biological Definition of Alzheimer's Disease." *Alzheimers Dementia* 14: 535–562.

Jackson, J. L. (2021). "The Pursuit and Maintenance of Happiness." *The New England Journal of Medicine* 385: 1327

Jacob, S., et al. (2022). "Efficacy and Safety of Balovaptan for Socialization and Communication Difficulties in Autistic Adults in North America and Europe: A Phase 3, Randomized, Placebo-Controlled Trial." *Lancet Psychiatry* 9: 199–210.

Jacobsen, P., et al. (2019). "Paroxetine, but not Vortioxetine, Impairs Sexual Functioning Compared with Placebo in Healthy Adults: A Randomized, Controlled Trial." *Journal of Sexual Medicine* 16: 1638–1649.

Jaffe, J. H. (1980). Drug addiction and drug abuse. In A. G. Gilman, L. S. Goodman, & A. Gilman (Eds.) *Goodman and Gilman's The Pharmacological Basis of Therapeutics.* New York: Macmillan.

Jain, R., et al. (2013). "A Randomized, Double-Blind, Placebo-Controlled 6-Wk Trial of the Efficacy and Tolerability of 5 mg Vortioxetine in Adults with Major Depressive Disorder." *International Journal of Neuropsychopharmacology* 16: 313–321.

Jaklevic, M. C. (2021). "COVID-19 and the "Lost Year" for Smokers Trying to Quit." *JAMA* 325: 1929–1930.

James, B. J., et al. (2019). "Bumetanide (Bumex) for Autism Spectrum Disorder in Children: A Review of Randomized Controlled Trials." *Annals of Psychotherapy* 53: 537–544.

Jann, M. W. (2014). "Diagnosis and Treatment of Bipolar Disorders in Adults: A Review of the Evidence on Pharmacologic Treatments." *American Health and Drug Benefits* 7: 489–499.

Jarienski, M. P., et al. (2020). "Polysubstance Use Among Pregnant Women with Opioid Use Disorder in the United States, 2007–2016." *Obstetrics and Gynecology* 136: 556–564.

Jaso, B. A., et al. (2017). "Therapeutic Modulation of Glutamate Receptors in Major Depressive Disorder." *Current Neuropharmacology* 15: 57–70.

Jeffers, A. M., et al. (2021). "Sociodemographic Characteristics Associated with and Prevalence and Frequency of Cannabis Use Among Adults in the US." *JAMA Network Open* 4: e2136571.

Jefsen, O. H., et al. (2021). "Editorial Perspective: COVID-19 Pandemic-Related Psychopathology in Children and Adolescents with Mental Illness." *Journal of Child Psychology and Psychiatry and Allied Disciplines* 62: 798–800.

Jensen, B., et al. (2015). "Medical Marijuana and Chronic Pain: A Review of Basic Science and Clinical Evidence." *Current Pain and Headache Reports* 19: 50.

Jerneren, F., et al. (2015). "Brain Atrophy in Cognitively Impaired Elderly: The Importance of Long-Chain w-3 Fatty Acids and B Vitamin Status in a Randomized Controlled Trial." *American Journal of Clinical Nutrition* 102: 215–221.

Jerome, L., et al. (2020). "Long-Term Follow-up Outcomes of MDMA-Assisted Psychotherapy for Treatment of PTSD: A Longitudinal Pooled Analysis of Six Phase 2 Trials." *Psychopharmacology* 237: 2485–2497.

Jha, M. K. (2022). "Selective Orexin Receptor Antagonists as Novel Augmentation Treatments for Major Depressive Disorder: Evidence for Safety and Efficacy from a Phase 2B Study of Seltorexant." *International Journal of Neuropsychopharmacology* 25: 85–88.

Jiang, Q., et al. (2020). "Effect of Nalbuphine on Patient Controlled Intravenous Analgesia After Radical Resection of Colon Cancer." *Oncology Letters* 19: 2533–2538.

Jing, E., et al. (2016). "Sexual Dysfunction in Selective Serotonin Reuptake Inhibitors (SSRIs) and Potential Solutions: A Narrative Literature Review. *The Mental Health Clinician* 6: 191–196.

Jochim, J., et al. (2019). "Valproate for Acute Mania." *Cochrane Database Systematic Reviews* 10: CD004052.

Johal, H., et al. (2020). "Cannabinoids in Chronic Non-Cancer Pain: A Systematic Review and Meta-Analysis." *Clinical Medicine Insights: Arthritis and Musculoskeletal Disorders* 13.

Johannessen, L. C., et al. (2016). "The Impact of Pharmacokinetic Interactions with Eslicarbazepine Acetate versus Oxcarbazepine and Carbamazepine in Clinical Practice." *Therapeutic Drug Monitoring* 38: 499–505.

John, M. E., et al. (2017). "Bath Salts Abuse leading to New-Onset Psychosis and Potential for Violence." *Clinical Schizophrenia and Related Psychoses* 11: 120–124.

Johnson, B. A., et al. (2000). "Ondansetron for Reduction of Drinking Among Biologically Predisposed Alcoholic Patients: A Randomized Controlled Trial." *JAMA* 284: 963–971.

Johnson, B. A., et al. (2003). "Ondansetron Reduces Mood Disturbance Among Biologically Predisposed, Alcohol-Dependent Individuals." *Alcoholism: Clinical and Experimental Research* 27: 1773–1779.

Johnson, M. W., and Griffiths, R. R. (2017). "Potential Therapeutic Effects of Psilocybin." *The American Society for Experimental NeuroTherapeutics* 14: 734–740.

Johnson, M. W., et al. (2008). "Human Hallucinogen Research: Guidelines for Safety." *Journal of Psychopharmacology* 22: 603–620.

Johnson, M. W., et al. (2011). "Human Psychopharmacology and Dose-Effects of Salvinorin A, a Kappa Opioid Agonist Hallucinogen Present in the Plant *Salvia Divinorum*." *Drug and Alcohol Dependence* 115: 150–155.

Johnson, M. W., et al. (2018). "The Abuse Potential of Medical Psilocybin According to the 8 Factors of the Controlled Substances Act." *Neuropharmacology* 142: 143–166.

Johnson, W. M., et al. (2020). "Bipolar Disorder: Managing the Peaks and Valleys." *International Journal of Psychiatry in Medicine* 55: 349–356.

Johnston, L. D., et al. (2018). "Monitoring the Future National Survey Results on Drug Use 1975–2017: Overview and Key Findings on Adolescent Drug Use." Ann Arbor: Institute for Social Research, The University of Michigan.

Jonas, D. E., et al. (2014). "Pharmacotherapy for Adults with Alcohol Use Disorders in Outpatient Settings: A Systematic Review and Meta-Analysis." *JAMA* 311: 1889–1900. https://doi.org/10.1001/jama.2014.3628.

Jonas, K., et al. (2022): "The Course of General Cognitive Ability in Individuals with Psychotic Disorders." *JAMA Psychiatry* 79: 659–666.

Jones, A. W. (2019). "Forensic Drug Profile: Cocaethylene." *Journal of Analytical Toxicology* 43: 155–160.

Jones, A. W., and L. Andersson (2003). "Comparison of Ethanol Concentrations in Venous Blood and Expired Breath during a Controlled Drinking Study." *Forensic Sciences International* 132: 1825.

Jones, E. J. and Kraft, W. K. (2019). "Analgesia, Opioids, and Other Drug Use

During Pregnancy and Neonatal Abstinence Syndrome." *Clinical Perinatology* 46: 349–366.

Jones, P. B., et al. (2006). "Randomized Controlled Trial of the Effect on Quality of Life of Second- vs First-Generation Antipsychotic Drugs in Schizophrenia: Cost Utility of the Latest Antipsychotic Drugs in Schizophrenia Study (CUtLASS 1)." *Archives of General Psychiatry* 63: 1079–1087.

Jorenby, D. E., et al. (2006). "Efficacy of Varenicline, an $\alpha_4\beta_2$ Nicotinic Acetylcholine Receptor Partial Agonist, vs Placebo or Sustained-Release Bupropion for Smoking Cessation: A Randomized Controlled Trial." *JAMA* 296: 56–63.

Jorgenrud, B., et al. (2021). "The Association Between the Alcohol Biomarker Phosphatidylethanol (Peth) and Self-Reported Alcohol Consumption Among Russian and Norwegian Medical Patients." *Alcohol and Alcoholism.* In press.

Joseph, H., et al. (2000). "Methadone Maintenance Treatment (MMT): A Review of Historical and Clinical Issues." *Mount Sinai Journal of Medicine* 67: 347–364.

Joshi, A., et al. (2019). "Pharmacological Therapies in Bipolar Disorder: A Review of Current Treatment Options." *Psychiatria Danubina* 31: 595–603.

Joshi, P. S., et al., (2019). "Nonclinical Safety Assessment of PF614: A Novel TAAP Prodrug of Oxycodone for Chronic Pain Indication." *Regulatory Toxicology and Pharmacology* 108: 104433.

Joudrey, P. J., et al. (2020). "Methadone for Opioid Use Disorder—Decades of Effectiveness but Still Miles Away in the U.S." *JAMA Psychiatry* 77(11): 1105–1106.

Joudrey, P. J., et al. (2021): "Methadone Access for Opioid Use Disorder During the COVID-19 Pandemic Within the United States and Canada." *JAMA Network Open* 4: e2118223.

Journey, J. D., et al. (2020). "Dextromethorphan Toxicity." *StatPearls Publishing*, Treasure Island (FL).

Juteau, L-C., et al. (2018). "Examining the Association Between Psychiatric Disorders and Cocaine Binges: Results from the COSMO Study." *Journal of Addiction Medicine* 12: 136–142.

Jyri, J., et al. (2010). "Midlife Alcohol Consumption and Later Risk of Cognitive Impairment: A Twin Follow-up Study." *Journal of Alzheimer's Disease* 22: 939–948.

Kaelen, M., et al. (2016). "P.3.039 Effects of LSD and Music on Brain Activity." *European Neuropsychopharmacology* 26: Supplement 1: S80–S81.

Kahl, K. G., and Correll, C. U. (2020). "Management of Patients with Severe Mental Illness During the Coronavirus Disease 2019 Pandemic." *JAMA Psychiatry* 77: 977–978.

Kahlon, M. K., et al. (2021). "Effect of Lay-Person-Delivered, Empathy-Focused Program of Telephone Calls on Loneliness, Depression, and Anxiety Among Adults During the COVID-19 Pandemic: A Randomized Clinical Trial." *JAMA Psychiatry* 78: 616–622.

Kalivas, P. W. (2009). "The Glutamate Homeostasis Hypothesis of Addiction." *Nature Reviews Neuroscience* 10: 561–572.

Kalivas, P. W., et al. (2006). "Animal Models and Brain Circuits in Drug Addiction." *Molecular Interventions* 6: 339–344.

Kalk, N. J., and A. R. Lingford-Hughes (2014). "The Clinical Pharmacology of Acamprosate." *British Journal of Clinical Pharmacology* 77: 315–323.

Kalmoe, M. C., et al. (2020). "Ketamine and Nitrous Oxide: The Evolution of NMDA Receptor Antagonists as Antidepressant Agents." *Journal of the Neurological Sciences* 412: 116778.

Kampman, K. M. (2019). "The Treatment of Cocaine Use Disorder." *Science Advances* 5: eaax1532.

Kane, J. M., and Correll, C. U. (2010). "Past and Present Progress in the Pharmacologic Treatment of Schizophrenia." *Journal of Clinical Psychiatry* 71: 1115–1124.

Kane, J. M., et al. (2020). "185 The Safety and Tolerability of Lumateperone 42 Mg for the Treatment of Schizophrenia: A Polled Analysis of 3 Randomized Placebo-Controlled Trials." *CNS Spectrums* 25: 316–317.

Kanner, A. M., and Bicchi, M. M. (2022). "Antiseizure Medications for Adults with Epilepsy: A Review." *JAMA* 327: 1269–1281.

Kaplan, Y. C. and Demir, O. (2021). "Use of Phenytoin, Phenobarbital, Carbamazepine, Levetiracetam, Lamotrigine and Valproate in Pregnancy and Breastfeeding: Risk of Major Malformations, Dose-Dependency,

Monotherapy vs. Polytherapy, Pharmacokinetics and Clinical Implications." *Current Neuropharmacology* 19: 1805–1824.

Kaptchuk, T. J., and Miller, F. G. (2015). "Placebo Effects in Medicine." *New England Journal of Medicine* 373: 8–9.

Kar, N., et al. (2016). "Clozapine Monitoring in Clinical Practice: Beyond the Mandatory Requirement." *Clinical Psychopharmacology and Neuroscience* 14: 323–329.

Karey, E. (2021). "Ongoing Difficulty of Characterizing Nicotine Product Risks." *JAMA Network Open* 4: e2119888.

Karila, L., et al. (2015). "Synthetic Cathinones: A New Public Health Problem." *Current Neuropharmacology* 13: 12–20.

Karlawish, J. (2021). "Aducanumab and the Business of Alzheimer Disease—Some Choice." *JAMA Neurology* 78: 1103–1104.

Karlawish, J., et al. (2017). "Alzheimer's Disease: The Next Frontier—Special Report 2017." *Alzheimer's & Dementia* 13: 374–380.

Kato, T. (2019). "Current Understanding of Bipolar Disorder: Toward Integration of Biological Basis and Treatment Strategies." *Psychiatry Clinics of Neuroscience* 73: 526–540.

Katz, E. G., et al. (2022). "U.S. Food and Drug Administration's Patient-Focused Drug Development Initiative: Experience with Integration of Patient-Experience Data in a New Drug Application for Esketamine Nasal Spray Plus and Newly Initiated Oral Antidepressant for Treatment-Resistant Depression." *Therapeutic Innovation & Regulatory Science* 56: 38–46.

Katz, I. R., et al. (2022). "Lithium Treatment in the Prevention of Repeat Suicide-Related Outcomes in Veterans with Major Depression or Bipolar Disorder: A Randomized Clinical Trial." *JAMA Psychiatry* 79: 24–32.

Kazda, L., et al. (2021). "Overdiagnosis of Attention-Deficit/Hyperactivity Disorder in Children and Adults." *JAMA Network Open* 4: e215335.

Keefe, J. R., et al. (2021). "Treatment Selection in Borderline Personality Disorder Between Dialectical Behavior Therapy and Psychodynamic Psychiatric Management." *Psychological Medicine* 51: 1829–1837.

Keks, N., et al. (2020). "Comparative Tolerability of Dopamine D 2/3 Receptor Partial Agonists for Schizophrenia." *CNS Drugs* 34: 473–507.

Kelly, B. F., and Nappe, T. M. (2021, January). "Cannabinoid Toxicity." *StatPearls*.

Kendler, K. S. (2020). "The Origin of Our Modern Concept of Depression—The History of Melancholia from 1780–1880: A Review." *JAMA Psychiatry* 77: 863–868.

Kennard, B. D., et al. (2014). "Sequential Treatment with Fluoxetine and Relapse-Prevention CBT to Improve Outcomes in Pediatric Depression." *American Journal of Psychiatry* 171: 1083–1090.

Kessler, D. S., et al. (2018). "Mirtazapine Added to SSRIs or SNRIs for Treatment Resistant Depression in Primary Care: Phase III Randomized Placebo Controlled Trial (MIR)." *British Medical Journal* 363: k4218.

Kessler, R. C., et al. (2022). "Estimated Prevalence of and Factors Associated with Clinically Significant Anxiety and Depression Among US Adults During the First Year of the COVID-19 Pandemic." *JAMA Network Open* 5: e2217223.

Khoraminya, N., et al. (2013). "Therapeutic Effects of Vitamin D as Adjunctive Therapy to Fluoxetine in Patients with Major Depressive Disorder." *Australian & New Zealand Journal of Psychiatry* 47: 271–275.

Khoramizadeh, M., et al. (2019). "Treatment of Amphetamine Abuse/Use Disorder: A Systematic Review of Recent Health Concern." *DARU Journal of Pharmaceutical Sciences* 27: 743–753.

Khosravi, M., et al. (2020). "The Relationship Between Dietary Patterns and Depression Mediated by Serum Levels of Folate and Vitamin B12." *BMC Psychiatry* 20: 63.

Khoury, R. (2022). "Deuterated Dextromethorphan/Qunidine for Agitation in Alzheimer"s Disease." *Neural Regeneration Research* 17: 1013–1014.

Khoury, R., et al. (2018). "An Update on the Safety of Current Therapies for Alzheimer's Disease: Focus on Rivastigmine." *Therapeutic Advances in Drug Safety* 9: 171–178.

Khundakar, A. A., and Thomas, A. J. (2015). "Neuropathology of Depression in Alzheimer's Disease: Current Knowledge and the Potential for New Treatments." *Journal of Alzheimer's Disease* 44: 27–41.

Kianirad, Y., and Simuni, T. (2017). "Pimavanserin, A Novel Antipsychotic for Management of Parkinson's Disease Psychosis."

Expert Review of Clinical Pharmacology 10: 1161–1168.

Kiguchi, N., and Ko, M-C. (2019). "Effects of NOP-Related Ligands in Nonhuman Primates." *Handbook of Experimental Pharmacology* 254: 323–343.

Kiguchi, N., et al. (2022). "Therapeutic Potentials of NOP and MOP Receptor Coactivation for the Treatment of Pain and Opioid Abuse." *Journal of Neuroscience Research* 100: 191–202.

Kilmer, B. (2019). "How Will Cannabis Legalization Affect Health, Safety and Social Equity Outcomes? It Largely Depends on the 14 Ps." *The American Journal of Drug and Alcohol Abuse* 45: 664–672.

Kim, J., et al. (2019). "Esketamine for Treatment-Resistant Depression—First FDA-Approved Antidepressant in the New Class." *The New England Journal of Medicine* 381: 1–4.

Kim, J., et al. (2020). "Insight and Medication Adherence in Schizophrenia: An Analysis of the CATIE Trial.' *Neuropharmacology* 168: 107634.

Kim, K., et al. (2020). "Structure of a Hallucinogen-Activated Gq-Coupled 5-HT_{2A} Serotonin Receptor." *Cell* 182: 1574–1588.

Kim, S., et al. (2016). "Association Between Alcohol Drinking Behaviour and Cognitive Function: Results from a Nationwide Longitudinal Study of South Korea." *BMJ Open* 6: e010494.

Kim, S., et al. (2021). "A Systematic Review of Therapeutic Ketamine Use in Children and Adolescents with Treatment-Resistant Mood Disorders." *European Child & Adolescent Psychiatry* 30: 1485–1501.

Kind, S., and Otis, J. D. (2019). "The Interaction Between Chronic Pain and PTSD." *Current Pain and Headache Reports* 23: 91.

Kinrys, G., et al. (2019). "Tachyphylaxis in Major Depressive Disorder: A Review of the Current State of Research." *Journal of Affective Disorders* 245: 488–497.

Kirby, L. G., et al. (2011). "Contributions of Serotonin in Addiction Vulnerability." *Neuropharmacology* 61: 421–432.

Kishi, T., et al. (2017). "Memantine for Alzheimer's Disease: An Updated Systematic Review and Meta-Analysis." *Journal of Alzheimer's Disorders* 60: 401–425.

Kishi, T., et al. (2020a). "Aripiprazole vs. Brexpiprazole for Acute Schizophrenia: A Systematic Review and Network Meta-Analysis." *Psychopharmacology* 237: 1459–1470.

Kishi, T., et al. (2020b). "Lemborexant vs Suvorexant for Insomnia: A Systematic Review and Network Meta-Analysis." *Journal of Psychiatric Research* 128: 68–74.

Kishi, T., et al. (2021). "Evidence-Based Insomnia Treatment Strategy Using Orexin Antagonists: A Review." *Neuropsychopharmacology Reports* 41: 450–458.

Kishi, T., et al. (2022). "Pharmacological Treatment for Bipolar Mania: A Systematic Review and Network Meta-Analysis of Double-Blind Randomized Controlled Trials. *Molecular Psychiatry* 27: 1136–1144.

Kivimaki, M., et al. (2020). "Association of Alcohol-Induced Loss of Consciousness and Overall Alcohol Consumption with Risks for Dementia." *JAMA Network Open* 3: e2016084.

Klebanoff, M. A., et al. (2021). "Marijuana Use During Pregnancy and Preterm Birth: A Prospective Cohort Study." *American Journal of Perinatology* 38(S01): e146–e154.

Klein, P. K., et al. (2021). "Suicidality Risk of Newer Antiseizure Medications: A Meta-Analysis." *JAMA Neurology* 78: 1118–1127.

Kleinman, R. A. (2020). "Comparison of Driving Times to Opioid Treatment Programs and Pharmacies in the U.S." *JAMA Psychiatry* 77: 1163–1171.

Knable, M. B. (2020). "Promising New Medications for Schizophrenia." *Treatment-Advocacy-Center,* May 12.

Knight, R., et al. (2021). "Neurodevelopmental Outcomes in Children Exposed to Newer Antiseizure Medications: A Systematic Review." *Epilepsia* 62: 1765–1779.

Knochel, C., et al. (2015). "Treatment-Resistant Late-Life Depression: Challenges and Perspectives." *Current Neuropsychopharmacology* 13: 577–591.

Knopman, D. S., et al. (2021). "Failure to Demonstrate Efficacy of Aducanumab: An Analysis of the EMERGE and ENGAGE Trials as Reported by Biogen, December 2019." *Alzheimer's Dementia* 17: 696–701.

Knudsen, J., and Chokshi, D. A. (2021). "Covid 19 and the Safety Net—Moving from Straining to Sustaining." *New England Journal of Medicine* 385: 2209–2211.

Ko, J. Y., et al. (2020). "Characteristics of Marijuana Use During Pregnancy—Eight States, Pregnancy Risk Assessment Monitoring System, 2017." *Morbidity and Mortality Weekly Report*, Centers for Disease Control and Prevention 69: 1058–1063.

Koblan, K. S., et al. (2020a). "A Non-D2-Receptor-Binding Drug for the Treatment of Schizophrenia." *The New England Journal of Medicine* 382: 1497–1505.

Koblan, K. S., et al. (2020b). "138 Efficacy and Safety of SEP-363856: A Novel Psychotropic Agent with a Non-D2 Mechanism of Action, in the Treatment of Schizophrenia." *CNS Spectrums* 25: 287–288.

Koch, G., et al. (2020). "Effect of Rotigotine vs Placebo on Cognitive Functions Among Patients with Mild to Moderate Alzheimer Disease. A Randomized Clinical Trial." *JAMA Network Open* 3: e2010372.

Kohler-Forsberg, O., et al. (2021). "Adjunctive Antidepressant Treatment Among 763 Outpatients with Bipolar Disorder: Findings from the Bipolar CHOICE and LITMUS Trials." *Depression & Anxiety* 38: 114–123.

Kohler-Forsberg, O., et al. (2022). "Association of Lithium Treatment with the Risk of Osteoporosis in Patients with Bipolar Disorder." *JAMA Psychiatry* 79: 454–463.

Kok, R. M., et al. (2011). "Continuing Treatment of Depression in the Elderly: A Systematic Review and Meta-Analysis of Double-Blinded Randomized Controlled Trials with Antidepressants." *American Journal of Geriatric Psychiatry* 19: 249–255.

Kolaczynska, K., et al. (2019). "Receptor Interaction Profiles of 4-Alkozy-Substituted 2,5-Dimethoxyphenethylamines and Related Amphetamines." *Frontiers in Pharmacology* 10: 1423.

Kolahdouzan, M., and M. J. Hamadeh. (2017). "The Neuroprotective Effects of Caffeine in Neurodegenerative Diseases." *CNS Neuroscience & Therapeutics* 23: 272–290.

Kolanos, R., et al. (2013). "'Deconstruction' of the Abused Synthetic Cathinone Methylene-dioxypyrovalerone (MDPV) and an Examination of Effects at the Human Dopamine Transporter." *ACS Chemical Neuroscience* 4: 1524–1529.

Kolikonda, M. K., et al. (2016). "Medical Marijuana for Epilepsy?" *Innovations in Clinical Neuroscience* 13: 23–26.

Kong, L., et al. (2018). "The Risks Associated with the Use of Lamotrigine During Pregnancy." *International Journal of Psychiatry in Clinical Practice* 22: 2–5.

Konstantakopoulos, G., et al. (2020, June 22). "The Preclinical Discovery and Development of Agomelanine for the Treatment of Depression." *Expert Opinion on Drug Discovery* 1–12.

Koob, G. F. (2015). "The Dark Side of Emotion: The Addiction Perspective." *European Journal of Pharmacology* 753: 73–87.

Koob, G. F., and Mason, B. J. (2016). "Existing and Future Drugs for the Treatment of the Dark Side of Addiction." *Annual Review of Pharmacology and Toxicology* 56: 299–322.

Koponen, M., et al. (2017). "Risk of Mortality Associated with Antipsychotic Monotherapy and Polypharmacy Among Community-Dwelling Persons with Alzheimer's Disease." *Journal of Alzheimer's Disease* 56: 107–118.

Koren. G. (2018). Special Aspects of Perinatal & Pediatric Pharmacology, Chapter 59 in B. G. Katzung, *Basic and Clinical Pharmacology*, 14 ed. (New York: McGraw-Hill Education).

Kotzalidis, G. D., et al. (2021). "Vortioxetine vs. Other Antidepressants in Patients with Major Depressive Episode with or Without Substance Abuse Disorder." *Current Neuropharmacology* 19: 2296–2307.

Kourouni, I., et al. (2020). "Critical Illness Secondary to Synthetic Cannabinoid Ingestion." *JAMA Network Open* 3: e208516.

Kousathanas, A., et al. (2022). "Whole-Genome Sequencing Reveals Host Factors Underlying Critical COVID-19." *Nature* 607: 97–103.

Kozela, E., et al. (2020). "Cannabidiol Improves Cognitive Impairment and Reverses Cortical Transcriptional Changes Induced by Ketamine, in Schizophrenia-Like Model in Rats." *Molecular Neurobiology* 57: 1733–1747.

Kozor, R., et al. (2014). "Regular Cocaine Use Is Associated with Increased Blood Pressure, Aortic Stiffness, and Ventricular Mass in Young Otherwise Healthy Individuals." *PLos One* 9: e89710.

Kranzler, H. R., and Soyka, M. (2018). "Diagnosis and Pharmacotherapy of Alcohol Use Disorder: A Review." *JAMA* 320: 815–824.

Krauss, G. L., et al. (2020). "Safety and Efficacy of Adjunctive Cenobamate (YKP3089) in Patients with Uncontrolled Focal Seizures: A Multicentre, Double-Blind, Randomized, Placebo-Controlled, Dose-Response Trial." *The Lancet Neurology* 19: 38–48.

Krebs, E. E., et al. (2018). "Effect of Opioid vs Nonopioid Medications on Pain-Related Function in Patients with Chronic Back Pain or Hip or Knee Osteoarthritis Pain." *JAMA* 319: 872–882.

Krediet, E., et al. (2020). "Reviewing the Potential of Psychedelics for the Treatment of PTSD." *International Journal of Neuropsychopharmacology* 23: 385–400.

Kreutzwiser, D., and Tawfic, Q. A. (2019). "Expanding Role of NMDA Receptor Antagonists in the Management of Pain." *CNS Drugs* 33: 347–374.

Kronstrand, R., et al. (2011). "Unintentional Fatal Intoxications with Mitragynine and O-desmethyltramadol from the Herbal Blend Krypton." *Journal of Analytical Toxicology* 35: 242–247.

Kruegel, A. C., and Grundmann, O. (2018) "The Medicinal Chemistry and Neuropharmacology of Kratom: A Preliminary Discussion of the Promising Medicinal Plant and Analysis of Its Potential for Abuse." *Neuropharmacology* 134: 108–120.

Kryst, J., et al. (2020). "Efficacy and Safety of Intranasal Esketamine for the Treatment of Major Depressive Disorder." *Expert Opinions in Pharmacotherapeutics* 21: 9–20.

Kuehn, B. M. (2022). "Clinician Shortage Exacerbates Pandemic-Fueled 'Mental Health Crisis'." *JAMA* 327: 2179–2181.

Kuehn, B. M. (2022). "Gabapentin Increasingly Implicated in Overdose Deaths." *JAMA* 327: 2387.

Kumar, A., et al. (2016). "Emerging Role of Orexin Antagonists in Insomnia Therapeutics: An Update on SORAs and DORAs." *Pharmacology Reports* 68: 231–242.

Kumar, B., et al. (2018). "Lumateperone: A New Treatment Approach for Neuropsychiatric Disorders." *Drugs Today* 54: 713–719.

Kumari, S., et al. (2022). "Circulatory GSK-3beta: Blood-Based Biomarker and Therapeutic Target for Alzheimer's Disease." *Journal of Alzheimer's Disease* 85: 249–260.

Kuo, S. S., et al. (2022). "Developmental Variability in Autism Across 17,000 Autistic Individuals and 4,000 Siblings Without an Autism Diagnosis." *JAMA Pediatrics* 10.1001.

Kuriyama, A., et al. (2014). "Ramelteon for the Treatment of Insomnia in Adults: A Systematic Review and Meta-Analysis." *Sleep Medicine* 15: 385–392.

Kushner, M. G., et al. (2011). "Vulnerability to the Rapid ("Telescoped") Development of Alcohol Dependence in Individuals with Anxiety Disorder." *Journal of Studies on Alcohol and Drugs* 72: 1019–1027.

Kushner, M. G., et al. (2012). "Alcohol Dependence Is Related to Overall Internalizing Psychopathology Load Rather than to Particular Internalizing Disorders: Evidence from a National Sample." *Alcoholism: Clinical and Experimental Research* 36: 325–331.

Kuypers, K., et al. (2020). "Intoxicated Aggression: Do Alcohol and Stimulants Cause Dose-Related Aggression?: A Review." *European Neuropsychopharmacology* 30: 114–147.

Lahteenvuo, M., and Tiihonen, J. (2021). "Antipsychotic Polypharmacy for the Management of Schizophrenia: Evidence and Recommendations." *Drugs* 81: 1273–1284.

Lake, E. P., et al. (2019). "Buprenorphine for the Treatment of Posttraumatic Stress Disorder." *American Journal of Addiction* 28: 86–91.

Lake, S., et al. (2019). "Frequency of Cannabis and Illicit Opioid Use Among People Who Use Drugs and Report Chronic Pain: A Longitudinal Analysis." *PLoS Medicine* 16: e1002967.

Lake, S., et al. (2020). "Evidence Shows That Cannabis Has Fewer Relative Harms Than Opioids." *Canadian Medical Association Journal* 192: e166–e167.

Lamb, V., et al. (2021). "Viloxazine: Pediatric First Approval." *Paediatric Drugs*. 23: 403-409.

Lancaster, C. L., et al. (2016). "Posttraumatic Stress Disorder: Overview of Evidence-Based Assessment and Treatment." *Journal of Clinical Medicine* 5: 105.

Lancman, M. E., et al. (2016). "The Effects of Lacosamide on Cognition, Quality-of-Life Measures, and Quality of Life in Patients with Refractory Partial Epilepsy." *Epilepsy & Behavior* 61: 27–33.

Landmark, C. J., et al. (2020). "Therapeutic Drug Monitoring of Antiepileptic Drugs: Current Status and Future Prospects." *Expert Opinion on Drug Metabolism and Toxicology* 16: 227–238.

Landry, I., et al. (2020). "Pharmacokinetics, Pharmacodynamics, and Safety of the Dual Orexin Receptor Antagonist Lemborexant: Findings from Single-Dose and Multiple Ascending-Dose Phase 1 Studies in Healthy Adults." *Clinical Pharmacology and Drug Development* 10: 153–165.

Lane, H-Y, et al. (2021). "Brain Activity of Benzoate, a D-Amino Acid Oxidase Inhibitor, in Patients with Mild Cognitive Impairment in a Randomized, Double-Blind, Placebo-Controlled Clinical Trial." *International Journal of Neuropsychopharmacology* 24: 392–399.

Lang, A., et al. (2022). "Trial of Cinpanemab in Early Parkinson's Disease." *The New England Journal of Medicine* 387: 408–420.

Lang, E., et al. (2022). "Recommendation on Instrument-Based Screening for Depression During Pregnancy and the Postpartum Period." *Canadian Medical Association Journal* 194: 981–989.

Lanham, H. J., et al. (2022). "Survey of Barriers and Facilitators to Prescribing Buprenorphine and Clinician Perceptions on the Drug Addiction Treatment Act of 2000 Waiver." *JAMA Network Open* 5: e2212419.

Lanza, H. I., et al. (2020). "Trajectories of Nicotine and Cannabis Vaping and Polyuse from Adolescence to Young Adulthood." *JAMA Network Open* 3: e2019181.

Lapeyre-Mestre, M. (2019). "Benzodiazepines, Cognitive Decline and Dementia: A Review of Causality Criteria from Published Observational Studies." *Therapie* 74: 407–419.

Larsen, C., and Shahinas, J. (2020). "Dosage, Efficacy and Safety of Cannabidiol Administration in Adults: A Systematic Review of Human Trials." *Journal of Clinical Medical Research* 12: 129–141.

Latalova, K., et al. (2014). "Suicide in Bipolar Disorder: A Review." *Psychiatria Danubina* 26: 108–114.

Latimer, D. R., et al. (2021). "Cenobamate, a Sodium Channel Inhibitor and Positive Allosteric Modulator of $GABA_A$ Ion Channels, for Partial Onset Seizures in Adults: A Comprehensive Review and Clinical Implications." *Neurology International* 13: 252–265.

Lattanzi, S., et al. (2018). "Efficacy and Safety of Cannabidiol in Epilepsy: A Systematic Review and Meta-Analysis." *Drugs* 78: 1791–1804.

Laurent, C., et al. (2014). "Beneficial Effects of Caffeine in a Transgenic Model of Alzheimer's Disease-like Tau Pathology." *Neurobiology of Aging* 35: 2079–2090.

Lavretsky, H., et al. (2015). "Citalopram, Methylphenidate, or Their Combination in Geriatric Depression: A Randomized, Double-Blind, Placebo-Controlled Trial." *American Journal of Psychiatry* 172: 561–569.

Lawn, W., et al. (2017). "Well-Being, Problematic Alcohol Consumption and Acute Subjective Drug Effects in Past Year Ayahuasca Users: A Large, International, Self-Selecting Online Survey." *Scientific Reports* 7: 15201.

Le Berre et al. (2017). "Executive Functions, Memory, and Social Cognitive Deficits and Recovery in Chronic Alcoholism: A Critical Review to Inform Future Research." *Alcoholism, Clinical & Experimental Research* 41: 1432–1443.

Le Foll, B., et al. (2014). "Elevation of Dopamine Induced by Cigarette Smoking: Novel Insights from a [^{11}C]-(+)-PHNO PET Study in Humans." *Neuropsychopharmacology* 39: 415–424.

Le Noury, J., et al. (2015). "Restoring Study 329: Efficacy and Harms of Paroxetine and Imipramine in Treatment of Major Depression in Adolescence." *BMJ* 351: h4320.

Leader, L. D., et al. (2019). "Brexanolone for Postpartum Depression: Clinical Evidence and Practical Considerations." *Pharmacotherapy* 39: 1105–1112.

Leas, E. C., et al. (2020). "Self-Reported Cannabidiol (CBD) Use for Conditions with Proven Therapies." *JAMA Network Open* 3: e2020977.

Lebrun-Harris, L. A., et al. (2022). "Five-Year Trends in US Children's Health and Well-being, 2016–2020." *JAMA Pediatrics* 10.1001.

Lee, H., et al. (2009). "Alcohol-Induced Blackout." *International Journal of Environmental Research and Public Health* 6: 2783–2792.

Leen, J. L. S., and Juurlink, D. N. (2019). "Carfentanil: A Narrative Review of Its Pharmacology and Public Health Concerns." *Canadian Journal of Anaesthesia* 66: 414–412.

Lees, B., et al. (2020). "Association of Prenatal Alcohol Exposure with Psychological,

Behavioral, and Neurodevelopmental Outcomes in Children from the Adolescent Brain Cognitive Development Study." *American Journal of Psychiatry* 177: 1060–1072.

Lees, R., et al. (2021). "Psychosocial and Pharmacological Treatments for Cannabis Use Disorder and Mental Health Comorbidities: A Narrative Review." *Psychological Medicine* Feb. 4: 1–12.

Leiman, D., et al. (2021). "Pharmacokinetics and Safety of INL-001 (Bupivacaine HCL) Implants Compared with Bupivacaine HCL Infiltration After Open Unilateral Inguinal Hernioplasty." *Advances in Therapy* 38: 691–706.

Lemelin, M., et al. (2021). "Maternal ADHD Medication Use During Pregnancy and the Risk of ADHD in Children: Importance of Genetic Predispositions and Impact of Using a Sibling Analysis." *European Neuropsychopharmacology* 44: 66–78.

Lenze, E. J., et al. (2015). "Efficacy, Safety, and Tolerability of Augmentation Pharmacotherapy with Aripiprazole for Treatment-Resistant, Depression in Late Life: A Randomised, Double-Blind, Placebo-Controlled Trial." *Lancet* 386: 2404–2412.

Lerman, C., et al. (2015). "Use of the Nicotine Metabolite Ratio as a Genetically Informed Biomarker of Response to Nicotine Patch or Varenicline for Smoking Cessation: A Randomized, Double-Blind Placebo-Controlled Trial." *Lancet Respiratory Medicine* 3: 131–138. https://doi.org/10.1016/S2213-2600(14)70294-2.

Leucht, S., et al. (2020). "Dose-Response Meta-Analysis of Antipsychotic Drugs for Acute Schizophrenia." *American Journal of Psychiatry* 177: 342–353.

Levey, A. (2021). "Progress with Treatments for Alzheimer's Disease." *New England Journal of Medicine* 384: 1762–1763.

Levine, J., et al. (1978). "The Mechanism of Placebo Analgesia." *Lancet* 2: 654–657.

Levine, R. L. (2022). "Addressing the Long-Term Effects of COVID-19." *JAMA* 328: 823–824.

Levinthal, C. F. (2013). *Drugs, Behavior and Modern Society,* 8th ed. New York: Allyn & Bacon.

Levy, S. J. L., et al. (2016). "Substance Use Screening, Brief Intervention, and Referral to Treatment." *Pediatrics* 138: e20161211.

Lewandowska, K., et al. (2020). "The Role of Melatonin and Melatonin Receptor Agonist in the Prevention of Sleep Disturbances and Delirium in Intensive Care Unit—A Clinical Review." *Sleep Medicine* 69: 127–134.

Leweke, F. M., et al. (2012). "Cannabidiol Enhances Anandamide Signaling and Alleviates Psychotic Symptoms of Schizophrenia." *Translational Psychiatry* 2: e94.

Lewis, G., et al. (2021). "Maintenance or Discontinuation of Antidepressants in Primary Care." *The New England Journal of Medicine* 385: 1257–1267.

Li, J., et al. (2022). "Trends in Use of Melatonin Supplements Among US Adults, 1999–2018." *JAMA* 327: 483–485.

Li, L., et al. (2020). "Analysis of US Teen Driving After Using Marijuana, 2017." *JAMA Network Open* 3: e2030473

Li, L., et al. (2022). "Selective Activation of Cannabinoid Receptor-2 Reduces White Matter Injury via PERK Signaling in a Rat Model of Traumatic Brain Injury." *Experimental Neurology* 347: 113899.

Lieberman, J., A., et al. (2005). "Effectiveness of Antipsychotic Drugs in Patients with Chronic Schizophrenia." *New England Journal of Medicine* 353: 1209–1223.

Liem, A., et al. (2021). "Digital Health Applications in Mental Health Care for Immigrants and Refugees: A Rapid Review." *Telemedicine and e-Health* 27: 3–16.

Likhitsathian, S., et al. (2012). "Cognitive Changes in Topiramate-Treated Patients with Alcoholism: A 12-Week Prospective Study in Patients Recently Detoxified." *Psychiatry and Clinical Neurosciences* 66: 235–241.

Lin, C-H., et al. (2020). "Precision Medicine of Sodium Benzoate for the Treatment of Behavioral and Psychological Symptoms of Dementia (BPSD)." *Neuropsychiatric Disease & Treatment* 16: 509–518.

Lin, C-H., et al. (2021). "Effect of Sodium Benzoate on Cognitive Function Among Patients with Behavioral and Psychological Symptoms of Dementia: Secondary Analysis of a Randomized Clinical Trial." *JAMA Network Open* 4: e216156.

Lin, F.-Y., et al. (2014). "Retrospective Population Cohort Study on Hip Fracture Risk Associated with Zolpidem Medication." *Sleep* 37: 673–679.

Lin, J. C., et al. (2011). "Subjective Effects in Humans Following Administration of Party

Pill Drugs BZP and TFMPP Alone and in Combination." *Drug Testing and Analysis* 3: 582–585.

Lin, Y. L., et al. (2019). "Teratogenicity of Valproic Acid and Its Constitutional Isomer, Amide Derivative Valnoctamide in Mice." *Birth Defect Research* 111: 1013–1023.

Ling, S., et al. (2022). "Molecular Mechanisms of Psilocybin and Implications for the Treatment of Depression." *CNS Drugs* 36: 17–30.

Ling, W., et al. (2020). "Effects of Monthly Buprenorphine Extended-Release Injections on Patient-Centered Outcomes: A Long-Term Study." *Journal of Substance Abuse Treatment* 110: 1–8.

Lintzeris, N., et al. (2021). "Patient-Reported Outcomes of Treatment of Opioid Dependence with Weekly and Monthly Subcutaneous Depot vs Daily Sublingual Buprenorphine: A Randomized Clinical Trial." *JAMA Network Open* 4: e219041.

Liossi, C., and Howard, R. F. (2016). "A Biopsychosocial Framework for Assessing and Managing Chronic Pain in Children." *Pediatrics* 138: 1–11.

Lira, M. C., et al. (2020). "Alcohol Policies and Motor Vehicle Crash Deaths Involving Blood Alcohol Concentrations Below 0.08." *American Journal of Preventive Medicine* 58: 622–629.

Lisdahl, K. M., et al. (2018). "Adolescent Brain Cognitive Development (ABCD) Study: Overview of Substance Use Assessment Methods." *Developmental Cognitive Neuroscience* 32: 80–96.

Liu, B., et al. (2020). "Maternal Cigarette Smoking Before and During Pregnancy and the Risk of Preterm Birth: A Dose-Response Analysis of 25 Million Mother–Infant Pairs." *PLoS Medicine* 17: e1003158.

Liu, J., and Wang, L. N. (2012). "Ramelteon in the Treatment of Chronic Insomnia: Systematic Review and Meta-Analysis." *International Journal of Clinical Practice* 66: 867–873

Liu, J., et al. (2016). "MT1 and MT2 Melatonin Receptors: A Therapeutic Perspective." *Annual Reviews of Pharmacology and Toxicology* 56: 361–383.

Liu, J., et al. (2019). "The Role of NMDA Receptors in Alzheimer's Disease." *Frontiers in Neuroscience*. Published online February 8, 2019.

Liu, K., et al. (2011). "Tea Consumption Maybe an Effective Active Treatment for Adult Attention Deficit Hyperactivity Disorder (ADHD)." *Medical Hypotheses* 4: 461–463.

Liu, S., et al. (2021). "Trends in Nonfatal and Fatal Overdoses Involving Benzodiazepines—38 States and the District of Columbia, 2019–2020." *Center for Disease Control and Prevention, Weekly* 70: 1136–1141.

Liu, Y.-H., et al. (2022). "One-Year Trajectory of Cognitive Changes in Older Survivors of COVID-19 in Wuhan, China: A Longitudinal Cohort Study." *JAMA Neurology* 79: 509–517.

Liu, Z.-P., et al. (2017). "Delta Subunit-Containing Gamma-Aminobutyric Acid Receptor Disinhibits Lateral Amygdala and Facilitates Fear Expression in Mice." *Biological Psychiatry* 81: 990–1002.

Livingston, G., et al. (2020). "Dementia Prevention, Intervention, and Care: 2020 Report of the Lancet Commission." *Lancet* 396: 413–446.

Lizarraga, K. J., et al. (2020). "Hallucinations, Delusions and Impulse Control Disorders in Parkinson Disease." *Clinics in Geriatric Medicine* 36: 105–118.

Loades, M. E., et al. (2020, June 3). "Rapid Systematic Review: The Impact of Social Isolation and Loneliness on the Mental Health of Children and Adolescents in the Context of COVID-19." *Journal of the American Academy of Child and Adolescent Psychiatry* 59: 1218–1239.

LoConte, N. K., et al. (2018). "Alcohol and Cancer: A Statement of the American Society of Clinical Oncology." *Journal of Clinical Oncology* 36: 83–93.

Lodge, D., et al. (2019). "The 1980s: D-AP5 and a Decade of NMDA Receptor Discoveries." *Neurochemical Research* 44: 516–530.

Loften, A., et al. (2021). "An Acetylcholine-Dopamine Interaction in the Nucleus Accumbens and its Involvement in Ethanol's Dopamine-Releasing Effect." *Addiction Biology* 26: e12959.

Logrip, M. L., et al. (2015). "Corticostriatal BDNF and Alcohol Addiction." *Brain Research* 1628: 60–67.

Loland, C. J., et al. (2012). "R-Modafinil (Armodafinil): A Unique Dopamine Uptake Inhibitor and Potential Medication for Psychostimulant Abuse." *Biological Psychiatry* 72: 405–413.

Londhe, S., et al. (2020). "Efficacy and Safety of Buprenorphine Transdermal Patch for Immediate Postoperative Analgesia After Tot Knee Arthroplasty Surgery." *Journal of Arthroplasty* 35: S178–S181.

Long, A. S., et al. (2021). "Evaluation of Trials Comparing Single Enantiomer Drugs to Their Racemic Precursors: A Systematic Review." *JAMA Network Open* 4: e215731.

Lopez-Munoz, F., et al. (2018). "A History of the Pharmacological Treatment of Bipolar Disorder." *International Journal of Molecular Science* 19: 2143.

Lopez-Pelayo, H., et al. (2020). "Safety of Nalmefene for the Treatment of Alcohol Use Disorder: An Update." *Expert Opinion on Drug Safety* 19: 9–17.

Lord, C., et al. (2020). "Autism Spectrum Disorder." *Nature Reviews Disease Primers* 6: 5.

Lorenz, T., et al. (2016). "Antidepressant-Induced Female Sexual Dysfunction." *Mayo Clinic Proceedings* 91: 1280–1286.

Loscher, W. and P. Klein (2021). "The Pharmacology and Clinical Efficacy of Antiseizure Medications: From Bromide Salts to Cenobamate and Beyond." *CNS Drugs* 35: 935–963.

Losifescu, D. V., et al. (2022). "Efficacy and Safety of AXS-05 (Dextromethorphan-Bupropion) in Patients with Major Depressive Disorder: A Phase 3 Randomized Clinical Trial (GEMINI)." *Journal of Clinical Psychiatry* 83: 21m14345.

Lowe, H., et al. (2022). "Psychedelics: Alternative and Potential Therapeutic Options for Treating Mood and Anxiety Disorders." *Molecules* 27: 2520.

Lozupone, M., et al. (2020). "The Challenge of Antidepressant Therapeutics in Alzheimer's Disease." *Advances in Experimental Medicine and Biology* 1260: 267–281.

Lu, C., et al. (2014). "Changes in Antidepressant Use by Young People and Suicidal Behavior After FDA Warnings and Media Coverage: Quasi-Experimental Study." *BMJ* 348: g3596.

Lu, W., et al. (2021). "Trends and Disparities in Treatment for Co-Occurring Major Depression and Substance Use Disorders Among US Adolescents from 2011 to 2019." *JAMA Network Open* 4: e2130280.

Lucchetta, R. C., et al. (2018). "Association Between Development of Dementia and Use of Benzodiazepines: A Systematic Review and Meta-Analysis." *Pharmacotherapy* 38: 1010–1020.

Luft, M. J., et al. (2021). "Pharmacologic Interventions for Antidepressant-Induced Sexual Dysfunction: A Systematic Review and Network Meta-Analysis of Trials Using the Arizona Sexual Experience Scale." *CNS Spectrums* 12: 1–10.

Luscher, B., and Mohler, H. (2019). "Brexanolone, A Neurosteroid Antidepressant, Vindicates the GABAergic Deficit Hypothesis of Depression and May Foster Resilience." *F1000 Research* 8: 751.

Lyman, G. H., and Moses, H. L. (2016). "Biomarker Tests for Molecularly Targeted Therapies—The Key to Unlocking Precision Medicine." *New England Journal of Medicine* 375: 4–6.

Lytle, S., et al. (2017). "Long-Acting Injectable Antipsychotics in Children and Adolescents." *Journal of Child and Adolescent Psychopharmacology* 27: 2–9.

MacDonald, K., and Pappas, K. (2016). "Why Not Pot? A Review of the Brain-Based Risks of Cannabis." *Innovations in Clinical Neuroscience* 13: 13–22.

Madison, C. A., and Eitan, S. (2020). "Buprenorphine: Prospective Novel Therapy for Depression and PTSD." *Psychological Medicine* 50: 881–893.

Madsen, H. B., et al. (2012). "Neuroplasticity in Addiction: Cellular and Transcriptional Perspectives." *Frontiers in Molecular Neuroscience* 5: 1–16.

Magesh, S., et al. (2021). "Disparities in COVID-19 Outcomes by Race, Ethnicity, and Socioeconomic Status: A Systematic Review and Meta Analysis." *JAMA Network Open* 4: e2134147.

Maier, F., et al. (2020). "Bupropion for the Treatment of Apathy in Alzheimer's Disease: A Randomized Clinical Trial." *JAMA Network Open* 3: e206027.

Maj, M. (2020). "Helpful Treatment of Depression—Delivering the Right Messages." *JAMA Psychiatry* 77: 784–786.

Majeed, A., et al. (2021). "Efficacy of Dextromethorphan for the Treatment of Depression: A Systematic Review of

Preclinical and Clinical Trials." *Expert Opinion on Emerging Drugs* 26: 63–74.

Malberg, J. E., et al. (2021). "Adult Neurogenesis and Antidepressant Treatment: The Surprise Finding by Ron Duman and the Fiels 20 Years Later." *Biological Psychiatry* 90: 96–101.

Malcolm, R., et al. (2000). "Recurrent Detoxification May Elevate Alcohol Craving as Measures by Obsessive Compulsive Drinking Scale." *Alcohol* 20: 181–185.

Maldonado, J. R. (2017). "Novel Algorithms for the Prophylaxis and Management of Alcohol Withdrawal Syndromes—Beyond Benzodiazepines." *Critical Care Clinics* 33: 559–599.

Malek, A. (2012). "Effects of Prenatal Cocaine Exposure on Human Pregnancy and Postpartum." *Pharmaceutica Analytica Acta* 3: 1–8.

Malhi, G. S., et al. (2020). "The 2020 Royal Australian and New Zealand College of Psychiatrists Clinical Practice Guidelines for Mood Disorders: Bipolar Disorder Summary." *Bipolar Disorder* 22: 805–821.

Mallete, J. R., et al. (2016). "Geographically Sourcing Cocaine's Origin—Delineation of the Nineteen Major Coca Growing Regions in South America." *Scientific Reports* 6: 23520.

Manhapra, A., et al. (2019). "Topiramate Pharmacotherapy for Alcohol Use Disorder and Other Addictions: A Narrative Review." *Journal of Addiction Medicine* 13: 7–22.

Manly, J. J., and Glymour, M. M. (2021). "What the Aducanumab Approval Reveals About Alzheimer Disease Research." *JAMA Neurology* 78: 1305–1306.

Marazziti, D., et el. (2019). "Asenapine for the Treatment of Bipolar Disorder." *Expert Opinions in Pharmacotherapy* 20: 1321–1330.

Marchand, G., et al. (2022). "Birth Outcomes of Neonates Exposed to Marijuana in Utero: A Systematic Review and Meta-Analysis." *JAMA Network Open* 5: e2145653.

Marcinkiewcz, C. A., et al. (2016). "Serotonin's Complex Role in Alcoholism: Implications for Treatment and Future Research." *Alcoholism: Clinical and Experimental Research* 40: 1192–1201.

Marcinkowska, M., et al. (2020). "Management of Dementia-Related Psychosis, Agitation and Aggression: A Review of the Pharmacology and Clinical Effects of Potential Drug Candidates." *CNS Drugs* 34: 243–268.

Marcotte, T. D., et al. (2022). "Driving Performance and Cannabis Users' Perception of Safety: A Randomized Clinical Trial." *JAMA Psychiatry* 79(3): 201–209.

Marder, A. R., and Cannon, T. D. (2019). "Schizophrenia." *New England Journal of Medicine* 18: 1753–1761.

Mariani, J. J., et al. (2012). "Extended Release Mixed Amphetamine Salts and Topiramate for Cocaine Dependence: A Randomized Controlled Trial." *Biological Psychiatry* 72: 950–956.

Mariani, J. J., et al. (2021). "An Open-Label Pilot Study of Pregabalin Pharmacotherapy for Alcohol Use Disorder." *American Journal of Drug and Alcohol Abuse* 47: 467–475.

Mariottini, C., et al. (2021). "Concomitant Drugs with Buprenorphine User Deaths." *Drug & Alcohol Dependence* 218: 108345.

Markham, A. (2020). "Oliceridine: First Approval." *Drugs* 80: 1739–1744.

Marta, L. O. (2019). "Metabolism of Lysergic Acid Diethylamide (LSD): An Update. *Drug Metabolism Reviews* 51: 378–387.

Marti, M., et al. (2021). "New Insights into Methoxetamine Mechanisms of Action: Focus on Serotonergic 5-HT_2 Receptors in Pharmacological and Behavioral Effects in the Rat." *Experimental Neurology* 345: 113836.

Martinak, B., et al. (2017). "Dextromethorphan in Cough Syrup: The Poor Man's Psychosis." *Psychopharmacology Bulletin* 47: 59–63.

Martinez, C., et al. (2010). "Use of Venlafaxine Compared with Other Antidepressants and the Risk of Sudden Cardiac Death or Near Death: A Nested Case-Control Study." *BMJ* 340: c249.

Martinot, P., et al. (2018). "Association Between Potentially Inappropriate Medications and Frailty in the Early Old Age: A Longitudinal Study in the GAZEL Cohort." *Journal of the American Medical Directors Association* 19: 967–973.

Martinotti, G., et al. (2018). "Hallucinogen Persisting Perception Disorder: Etiology, Clinical Features, and Therapeutic Perspectives." *Brain Sciences* 8: 47.

Martins, C. P., et al. (2022). "Pramipexole, a Dopamine D3/D2 Receptor-Preferring Agonist,

Attenuates Reserpine-Induced Fibromyalgia-Like Model in Mice." *Neural Regeneration Research* 17: 450–458.

Martucci, H. F. H., et al. (2018). "Distribution of Furanyl Fentanyl and 4-ANPP in an Accidental Acute Death: A Case Report." *Forensic Science International* 283: e13–e17.

Marucci, G., et al. (2021). "Efficacy of Acetylcholinesterase Inhibitors in Alzheimer's Disease." *Neuropharmacology* 190: 108352.

Marusich, J. A., et al. (2016). "Pharmacological Effects of Methamphetamine and Alpha-PP Vapor and Injection." *Neurotoxicology* 55: 83–91.

Marvanova, M., and McGrane, I. R. (2021). "Treatment Approach and Modalities for Management of Depression in Older People." *Senior Care Pharmacist* 336: 11–21.

Marzani, G. M., and Neff, A. P. (2021). "Bipolar Disorders: Evaluation and Treatment." *American Family Physician* 103: 227–239.

Masi, G., et al. (2010). "Aripiprazole Augmentation in 39 Adolescents with Medication-Resistant Obsessive-Compulsive Disorder." *Journal of Clinical Psychopharmacology* 30, 688–693.

Maslej, M. M., et al. (2020). "Individual Differences in Response to Antidepressants: A Meta-Analysis of Placebo-Controlled Randomized Clinical Trials." *JAMA Psychiatry* 77: 1–12.

Mason, B. J., and Heyser, C. (2021). "Alcohol Use Disorder: The Role of Medication in Recovery." *Alcohol Research* 41(1): 1–17.

Mason, K., et al. (2021). "Effectiveness of a 2-Year Treatment with Aripiprazole Long-Acting Injectable and Comparison with Paliperidone Palmitate." *Therapeutic Advances in Psychopharmacology* 11: 20451253211029490.

Masuda, T., et al. (2019). "Association with Hospitalization and All-Cause Discontinuation among Patients with Schizophrenia on Clozapine vs Other Oral Second-Generation Antipsychotics. A Systematic Review and Meta-Analysis of Cohort Studies." *JAMA Psychiatry* 76: 1052–1062.

Masuyama, T., et al. (2018). "Suvorexant Is Associated with a Low Incidence of Delirium in Critically Ill Patients: A Retrospective Cohort Study." *Psychogeriatrics* 18: 209–215.

Mathai, D. S., et al. (2022). "Toward Synergies of Ketamine and Psychotherapy." *Frontiers in Psychology* 13: 868103.

Matson, T. E., et al. (2021). "Prevalence of Medical Cannabis Use and Associated Health Conditions Documented in Electronic Health Records Among Primary Care Patients in Washington State." *JAMA Network Open* 4: e219375.

Mattes, J. A. (2016). "Treating ADHD in Prison: Focus on Alpha-2 Agonists (Clonidine and Guanfacine)." *The Journal of the American Academy of Psychiatry and the Law* 44: 151–157.

Mattick, R. P., et al. (2018). "Association of Parental Supply of Alcohol with Adolescent Drinking, Alcohol-Related Harms, and Alcohol Use Disorder Symptoms: A Prospective Cohort Study." *The Lancet, Public Health* 3: e64–e71.

Mauro, P. M., et al. (2022). "Use of Medication for Opioid Use Disorder Among US Adolescents and Adults with Need for Opioid Treatment, 2019." *JAMA Network Open* 5: e223821.

Maust, D. T., et al. (2017). "Trends in Central Nervous System-Active Polypharmacy Among Older Adults Seen in Outpatient Care in the United States." *JAMA: Internal Medicine* 177: 583–585.

McAllister, S. D., et al. (2015). "The Antitumor Activity of Plant-Derived Non-Psychoactive Cannabinoids." *Journal of Neuroimmune Pharmacology* 10: 255–267.

McCarthy, M. J., et al. (2021). "A Prospective Study to Determine the Clinical Utility of Pharmacogenetic Testing of Veterans with Treatment-Resistant Depression." *Journal of Psychopharmacology* 35: 992–1002.

McCloud, T., et al. (2015). "Ketamine and Other Glutamate Receptor Modulators for Depression in Bipolar Disorder in Adults." *Cochrane Database of Systematic Reviews* 29: CD011611.

McCutcheon, R. A., et al. (2020a). "Dopamine and Glutamate in Schizophrenia: Biology, Symptoms and Treatment." *World Psychiatry* 19: 15–33.

McCutcheon, R. A., et al. (2020b). "Schizophrenia—An Overview." *JAMA Psychiatry* 77: 201–210.

McGinnis, E., and Kessler, S. K. (2016). "Lacosamide Use in Children with Epilepsy:

Retention Rate and Effect of Concomitant Sodium Channel Blockers in a Large Cohort." *Epilepsia* 57: 1416–1425.

McGinty, E. E., and Barry, C. L. (2020). "Stigma Reduction to Combat the Addiction Crisis—Developing an Evidence Base." *The New England Journal of Medicine* 382: 1291–1292.

McGowan, K. E., et al. (2021). "The Hunger for Mirtazapine: A Discontinuation Syndrome." *Journal of Pain & Palliative Care Pharmacotherapy* 35: 113–116.

McIntyre, R. S., et al. (2017). "The Efficacy of Psychostimulants in Major Depressive Episodes: A Systematic Review and Meta-Analysis." *Journal of Clinical Psychopharmacology* 37: 412–418.

McIntyre, R. S., et al. (2020). "Bipolar Disorders." *Lancet* 396: 1841–1856.

McKetin, R., et al. (2013). "Dose-Related Psychotic Symptoms in Chronic Methamphetamine Users: Evidence from a Prospective Longitudinal Study." *JAMA Psychiatry* 70: 319–324.

McKhann, G. M., et al. (2011). "The Diagnosis of Dementia Due to Alzheimer's Disease: Recommendations from the National Institute on Aging-Alzheimer's Association Workgroups on Diagnostic Guidelines for Alzheimer's Disease." *Alzheimer's & Dementia* 7: 263–269.

McMurray, R., and Striano, P. (2016). "Treatment of Adults with Lennox–Gastaut Syndrome: Further Analysis of Efficacy and Safety/Tolerability of Rufinamide." *Neurology and Therapeutics* 5: 35–43.

Meador, K. J. (2013). "Fetal Antiepileptic Drug Exposure and Cognitive Outcomes at Age 6 Years (NEAD Study): A Prospective Observational Study." *Lancet Neurology* 12: 244–252.

Meador, K. J., et al. (2020). "Fetal Loss and Malformations in the MONEAD Study of Pregnant Women with Epilepsy." *Neurology* 94: e1502–e1511.

Meariman, J. K., et al. (2022). "Nalfurafine, A G-Protein-Based KOR (Kappa Opioid Receptor) Agonist, Enhances the Diuretic Response and Limits Electrolyte Losses to Standard-of-Care Diuretics. *Hypertension* 79: 379–390.

Mechoulam, R. (2010, May 7). Qtd. in "Dr. Raphael Mechoulam." *Medical Marijuana 411.*

Mehta, S., et al. (2015). "Comparative Safety of Atypical Antipsychotics and the Risk of Pneumonia in the Elderly." *Pharmacoepidemiology and Drug Safety* 24: 1271–1280.

Meinhofer, A., et al. (2022). "Association of Comorbid Behavioral and Medical Conditions with Cannabis Use Disorder in Pregnancy." *JAMA Psychiatry* 79: 50–58.

Melas, P. A., et al. (2021). "Cannabidiol as a Potential Treatment for Anxiety and Mood Disorders: Molecular Targets and Epigenetic Insights from Preclinical Research." *International Journal of Molecular Science* 22: 1863.

Melbourne, J. K., et al. (2021). "Primed for Addiction: A Critical Review of the Role of Microglia in the Neurodevelopmental Consequences of Adolescent Alcohol Drinking." *Alcoholism, Clinical and Experimental Resources* 45: 1908–1926.

Mele, B., et al. (2020). "Diagnosis, Treatment and Management of Apathy in Parkinson's Disease: A Scoping Review." *BMJ Open* 10: e037632.

Melton, S. (2017, June 8). "Stirring the Pot: Potential Drug Interactions with Marijuana." *Medscape.*

Meltzer, H. Y. (2012). "Clozapine: Balancing Safety with Superior Antipsychotic Efficacy." *Clinical Schizophrenia & Related Psychoses* 6: 134–144.

Mendez-Millar, M., et al. (2022). "Borderline Personality Disorder." *American Family Physician* 105: 156–161.

Meng, H., et al. (2020). "Cannabis and Cannabinoids in Cancer Pain Management." *Current Opinion in Supportive and Palliative Care* 14: 87–93.

Meredith, S. E., et al. (2013). "Caffeine Use Disorder: A Comprehensive Review and Research Agenda." *Journal of Caffeine Research* 3: 114–130.

Mertens, L. J., and Preller, K. H. (2021). "Classical Psychedelics as Therapeutics in Psychiatry—Current Clinical Evidence and Potential Therapeutic Mechanisms in Substance Use and Mood Disorders." *Pharmacopsychiatry* 54: 176–190.

Mertens, L. J., et al. (2020). "Therapeutic Mechanisms of Psilocybin: Changes in Amygdala and Prefrontal Functional Connectivity During Emotional Processing

After Psilocybin for Treatment-Resistant Depression" *Journal of Psychopharmacology* 34: 167–180.

Metz, T. D., and Borgelt, L. M. (2018). "Marijuana Use in Pregnancy and While Breastfeeding." *Obstetric Gynecology* 132: 1198–1210.

Metz, T. D., and Stickrath, E. H. (2015). "Marijuana Use in Pregnancy and Lactation: A Review of the Evidence." *American Journal of Obstetrics and Gynecology* 213: 761–778.

Mi, W-F., et al. (2020). "Effects of Agomelanine and Mirtazapine on Sleep Disturbances in Major Depressive Disorder: Evidence from Polysomnographic and Resting-State Functional Connectivity Analyses." *Sleep* 43: zsaa092.

Miao, S-X., et al. (2021). "Pd-Catalyzed Direct Diversification of Natural Anti-Alzheimer's Disease Drug: Synthesis and Biological Evaluation of *N*-Aryl Huperzine A Analogues." *Journal of Natural Products* 84: 2374–2379.

Micallef, J., et al. (2018). "Cannabis Smoking Impairs Driving Performance on the Simulator and Real Driving: A Randomized, Double-Blind, Placebo-Controlled, Crossover Trial." *Fundamental & Clinical Pharmacology* 32: 558–570.

Mignogna, K. M., and Goes, F. S. (2022). "Characterizing the Longitudinal Course of Symptoms and Functioning in Bipolar Disorder." *Psychological Medicine* 14: 1–11.

Mignot, E., et al. (2022). "Safety and Efficacy of Daridorexant in Patients with Insomnia Disorder: Results from Two Multicentre, Randomized, Double-Blind, Placebo-Controlled, Phase 3 Trials." *Lancet Neurology* 21: 125–139.

Mihaljevic, S., et al. (2020). "Therapeutic Mechanisms of Ketamine." *Psychiatria Danubina* 32: 325–333.

Milani, S. A., et al. (2021). "Trends in the Use of Benzodiazepines, Z-Hypnotics, and Serotonergic Drugs Among US Women and Men Before and During the COVID-19 Pandemic." *JAMA Network Open* 4: e2131012.

Miliano, C., et al. (2016). "Neuropharmacology of New Psychoactive Substances (NPS): Focus on the Rewarding and Reinforcing Properties of Cannabimimetics and Amphetamine-Like Stimulants." *Frontiers in Neuroscience* 10: 153.

Miller, A. H., and Raison, C. L. (2016). "The Role of Inflammation in Depression: From Evolutionary Imperative to Modern Treatment Target." *Nature Reviews: Immunology* 16: 22–34.

Miller, J. N. and Black, D. W. (2020). "Bipolar Disorder and Suicide: A Review." *Current Psychiatry Reports* 22: 6.

Miller, L., and Campo, J. V. (2021). "Depression in Adolescents." *The New England Journal of Medicine* 385: 445–449.

Milosavljevic, F., et al. (2021). "Association of CYP2C19 and CYP2D6 Poor and Intermediate Metabolizer Status with Antidepressant and Antipsychotic Exposure: A Systematic Review and Meta-Analysis." *JAMA Psychiatry* 78: 270–280.

Minjello, A., et al. (2015). "Identification and Management of Alcohol Withdrawal Syndrome." *Drugs* 75: 353–365.

Minozzi, S., et al. (2015a). "Anticonvulsants for Cocaine Dependence." *Cochrane Database of Systematic Reviews*. 4: CD0006754.

Minozzi, S., et al. (2015b). "Dopamine Agonists for the Treatment of Cocaine Dependence." *Cochrane Database of Systematic Reviews* 5: CD0033524.

Minozzi, S., et al. (2018). "Baclofen for Alcohol Use Disorder." *Cochrane Database of Systematic Reviews* 11(11): CD012557.

Mintun, M. A., et al. (2021). "Donanemab in Early Alzheimer's Disease." *New England Journal of Medicine* 384: 1691–1704.

Mintzer, J., et al. (2021). "Effect of Methylphenidate on Apathy in Patients with Alzheimer Disease. The ADMET 2 Randomized Clinical Trial." *JAMA Neurology* 78: 1324–1332.

Mion, G. (2017). "History of Anaesthesia: The Ketamine Story—Past, Present and Future." *European Journal of Anaesthesiology* 34: 571–575.

Mitchell, J. M., et al. (2012). "Alcohol Consumption Induces Endogenous Opioid Release in the Human Orbitofrontal Cortex and Nucleus Accumbens." *Science Translational Medicine* 11, January 4: 116ra6.

Mitchell, J. M., et al. (2021). "MDMA-Assisted Therapy for Severe PTSD: A Randomized, Double-Blind, Placebo-Controlled Phase 3 Study." *Nature Medicine* 27: 1025–1033.

Mizoguchi, H., and Yamada, K. (2019). "Methamphetamine Use Causes Cognitive Impairment and Altered Decision-Making." *Neurochemistry International* 124: 106–113.

Mizrak, A., et al. (2010). "Pretreatment with Desmedetomidine or Thiopental Decreases Myoclonus After Etomidate: A Randomized, Double-Blind Controlled Trial." *Journal of Surgical Research* 159: e11–e16.

Mizushima, J., et al. (2017). "Early Improvement in Specific Symptoms Predicts Subsequent Recovery in Bipolar Depression: Reanalysis of the Systematic Treatment Enhancement Program for Bipolar Disorder (STEP-BD) Data." *Journal of Clinical Psychiatry* 78: e146–e151.

Mo, Y., et al. (2016). "Emerging Role of Melatonin and Melatonin Receptor Agonists in Sleep and Delirium in Intensive Care Unit Patients." *Journal of Intensive Care Medicine* 31: 451–455.

Moavero, R., et al. (2017). "Cognitive and Behavioral Effects of New Antiepileptic Drugs in Pediatric Epilepsy." *Brain Development* 39: 464–469.

Modi, K. K., et al. (2015). "Cinnamon and Its Metabolite Sodium Benzoate Attenuate the Activation of p21rac and Protect Memory and Learning in an Animal Model of Alzheimer's Disease." *PLoS One* 10: e0130398.

Mojtabai, R., et al. (2016). "National Trends in the Prevalence and Treatment of Depression in Adolescents and Young Adults." *Pediatrics* 138(6).

Mojtabai, R., and Olfson, M. (2020). "National Trends in Mental Health Care for US Adolescents." *JAMA Psychiatry* 77: 703–714.

Molero, P., et al. (2018). "Antidepressant Efficacy and Tolerability of Ketamine and Esketamine: A Critical Review." *CNS Drugs* 32: 411–420.

Mollajani, R., et al. (2019). "Bumetanide Therapeutic Effect in Children and Adolescents with Autism Spectrum Disorder." *Basic and Clinical Neuroscience* 10: 433–441.

Molloy, J. W., et al. (2012). "Association of Coffee and Caffeine Consumption with Fatty Liver Disease, Nonalcoholic Steatohepatitis, and Degree of Hepatic Fibrosis." *Hepatology* 55: 429–436.

Moncrieff, J. et al. (2022). "The Serotonin Theory of Depression: A Systematic Umbrella Review of the Evidence." *Molecular Psychiatry*, In Press.

Montero-Oleas, N., et al. (2020). "Therapeutic Use of Cannabis and Cannabinoids; An Evidence Mapping and Appraisal of Systematic Reviews." *BMC Complementary Medicine and Therapies* 20: 12.

Moody, M. T., et al. (2018). "Analysis of Fentanyl Analogs and Novel Synthetic Opioids in Blood, Serum/Plasma, and Urine in Forensic Casework." *Drug Test Analysis* 10: 1658–1367.

Morandi, A., and Bellelli, G. (2020). "Delirium Superimposed on Dementia." *European Geriatric Medicine* 11: 53–62.

Moreno, C., et al. (2020). "How Mental Health Care Should Change as a Consequence of the COVID-19 Pandemic." *Lancet Psychiatry* 7: 813–824.

Mores, K. L., et al. (2019). "A Review of the Therapeutic Potential of Recently Developed G Protein-Biased Kappa Agonists." *Frontiers in Pharmacology* 10: 407.

Morgan, C. J. A., and Curran, H. V. (2011). "Ketamine Use: A Review." *Addiction* 107: 27–38.

Morley, K.C., et al. (2017). "Pharmaco-therapeutic Agents in the Treatment of Methamphetamine Dependence." *Expert Opinions on Investigative Drugs* 26: 563–578.

Morris, N. P. (2022, January). "Opioid Use Disorder Treatment in the Age of Fentanyl." *JAMA Internal Medicine* 182(4).

Moseley, B. D., et al. (2016). "Efficacy, Safety, and Tolerability of Adjunctive Brivaracetam for Secondarily Generalized Tonic-Clonic Seizures: Pooled Results from Three Phase III Studies." *Epilepsy Research* 127: 179–185.

Motov, S., et al. (2016). "Is There a Role for Intravenous Subdissociative-Dose Ketamine Administered as an Adjunct or as a Single Agent for Acute Pain Management in the Emergency Department? *Journal of Emergency Medicine* 51: 752–757.

Motter, F. R., et al. (2018). "Potentially Inappropriate Medication in the Elderly: A Systematic Review of Validated Explicit Criteria." *European Journal of Clinical Pharmacology* 74: 679–700.

Moussa, M. N., et al. (2015). "Long-Term Moderate Alcohol Consumption Does Not

Exacerbate Age-Related Cognitive Decline in Healthy, Community-Dwelling Older Adults." *Frontiers in Aging Neuroscience* 6: 341.

Moustafa, R. E., et al. (2021). "Designer Benzodiazepines versus Prescription Benzodiazepines: Can Structural Relation Predict the Next Step?" *Critical Reviews in Toxicology* 51: 249–263.

Moykkynen, T., and Korpi, E. R. (2012). "Acute Effects of Ethanol on Glutamate Receptors." *Basic Clinical Pharmacology and Toxicology* 111: 4–13.

Muehlan, C., et al. (2020). "Clinical Pharmacology, Efficacy, and Safety of Orexin Receptor Antagonists for the Treatment of Insomnia Disorders." *Expert Opinion on Drug Metabolism and Toxicology* 16: 1063–1078.

Muir, J., et al. (2019). "Wiring the Depressed Brain: Optogenetic and Chemogenetic Circuit Interrogation in Animal Models of Depression." *Neuropsychopharmacology* 44: 1013–1026.

Mukhopadhyay, S., and Banerjee, D. (2021). "A Primer on the Evolution of Aducanumab: The First Antibody Approved for Treatment of Alzheimer's Disease." *Journal of Alzheimer's Disease* 83: 1537–1552.

Mula, M., and Sander, J. W. (2015). "Suicide and Epilepsy: Do Antiepileptic Drugs Increase the Risk?" *Expert Opinions on Drug Safety* 14: 553–558.

Mularski, R. A., et al. (2006). "Measuring Pain as the 5th Vital Sign Does Not Improve Quality of Pain Management." *Journal of General Medicine* 21: 607–612.

Mullen, J. M., et al. (2021). "Amphetamine Related Psychiatric Disorders." *StatPearls*, July 19, 2021.

Muller, T. (2018). "Safinamide: An Add-On Treatment for Managing Parkinson's Disease." *Clinical Pharmacology* 10: 31–41.

Müller, U., et al. (2013). "Effects of Modafinil on Non-Verbal Cognition, Task Enjoyment and Creative Thinking in Healthy Volunteers." *Neuropharmacology* 64: 490–495.

Muneer, A. (2016). "Pharmacotherapy of Acute Bipolar Depression in Adults: An Evidence Based Approach." *Korean Journal of Family Medicine* 37: 137–148.

Munk-Olsen, T., et al. (2018). "Maternal and Infant Outcomes Associated with Lithium Use in Pregnancy: An International Collaborative Meta-analysis of Six Cohort Studies." *Lancet Psychiatry* 5: 644–652.

Munoz-Negro, J. E., et al. (2021). "A Retrospective Naturalistic Study on the Psychopharmacological Treatment of Schizoaffective Disorder." *International Clinics in Psychopharmacology* 36: 257–263.

Murnane, K. S. (2019). "Serotonin 2A Receptors Are a Stress Response System: Implications for Post-Traumatic Stress Disorder." *Behavioral Pharmacology* 30 (2 and 3 Special Issue): 151–162.

Murphy, P., et al. (2020). "Safety of Lemborexant versus Placebo and Zolpidem: Effects on Auditory Awakening Threshold, Postural Stability, and Cognitive Performance in Healthy Older Participants in the Middle of the Night and Upon Morning Awakening." *Journal of Clinical Sleep Medicine* 16: 765–773.

Murrough, J. W., et al. (2013). "Rapid and Longer-Term Antidepressant Effects of Repeated Ketamine Infusions in Treatment-Resistant Major Depression." *Biological Psychiatry* 74: 250–256.

Murru, A., et al. (2015). "Management of Adverse Effects of Mood Stabilizers." *Current Psychiatry Reports* 17(8): 1–10.

Murthy, P., et al. (2019). "Treatment of Substance Use Disorders with Co-Occurring Severe Mental Health Disorders." *Current Opinions in Psychiatry* 32: 293–299.

Musiek, E. S., and Morris, J. C. (2021). "Possible Consequences of the Approval of a Disease-Modifying Therapy for Alzheimer's Disease." *JAMA Neurology* 78: 141–142.

Musil, R., et al. (2015). "Weight Gain and Antipsychotics: A Drug Safety Review." *Expert Opinion on Drug Safety* 14: 73–96.

Mustafa, A. A., et al. (2018). "A Review of the Opioid Analgesic Benzhydrocodone-Acetaminophen." *Cureus* 10: e2844.

Muthumalage, T., et al. (2020). "Chemical Constituents Involved in E-Cigarette, or Vaping Product Use-Associated Lung Injury (EVALI)." *Toxics* 8: e25.

Muttoni, S., et al. (2019). "Classical Psychedelics for the Treatment of Depression and Anxiety: A Systematic Review" *Journal of Affective Disorders* 258: 11–24.

Nadiugwu, M. C. (2020, June). "Frailty and the Risk of Polypharmacy in the Older Person:

Enabling and Preventative Approaches." *Journal of Aging Research* 6759521.

Nagele, P., et al. (2018). "Exploring Nitrous Oxide as Treatment for Mood Disorders: Basic Concepts." *Journal of Clinical Psychopharmacology* 38: 144–148.

Naglich, A., et al. (2017). "Pharmacological Treatment of Bipolar Disorder with Comorbid Alcohol Use Disorder." *CNS Drugs* 31: 665–674.

Naglich, A. C., et al. (2019). "Systematic Review of Preclinical, Clinical, and Post-Clinical Evidence of Bupropion Misuse Potential." *American Journal of Drug and Alcohol Abuse* 45: 341–354.

Naguy, A., and Al-Enezi, N. (2019). "Lamotrigine Uses in Psychiatric Practice." *American Journal of Therapeutics* 26: e96–e102.

Nagy, P., et al. (2016). "Functional Outcomes from a Head-to-Head, Randomized, Double-Blind Trial of Lisdexamfetamine Dimesylate and Atomoxetine in Children and Adolescents with Attention-Deficit/Hyperactivity Disorder and an Inadequate Response to Methylphenidate." *European Child & Adolescent Psychiatry* 25: 141–149.

Najam, B., et al. (2022). "COVID-19 and Anxiety in Perinatal Women." *Journal of Caring Science* 11: 40–45.

Nakawaki, B., and Crano, W. (2015). "Patterns of Substance Use, Delinquency, and Risk Factors Among Adolescent Inhalant Users." *Substance Use & Misuse* 50: 114–122.

Nasir, M., and Bloch, M. H. (2019). "Trim the Fat: The Role of Omega-3 Fatty Acids in Psychopharmacology." *Therapeutic Advances in Psychopharmacology* 9: 2045125319869791.

Nasser, A., et al. (2020). "A Phase III, Randomized-Controlled Trial to Assess the Efficacy and Safety of Once-Daily SPN-812 (Viloxazine Extended-Release) in the Treatment of Attention-Deficit/Hyperactivity Disorder in School-Age Children." *Clinical Therapeutics* 42: 1452–1466.

Nasser, A., et al. (2021). "The Effect of Viloxazine Extended-Release Capsules on Functional Impairments Associated with Attention-Deficit/Hyperactivity Disorder (ADHD) in Children and Adolescents in Four Phase 3 Placebo-Controlled Trials." *Neuropsychiatric Diseases and Treatment* 17: 1751–1762.

National Center for Health Statistics. (2021, December). *Data Brief No. 428*.

National Institute on Drug Abuse. (2010). *Research Reports: Cocaine Abuse and Addiction.* NIH Publication Number 10–4166. September.

National Institute on Drug Abuse. (2011). "Preventing Drug Use Among Children and Adolescents (In Brief)." *National Institute on Drug Abuse* June 2011.

National Institute on Drug Abuse. (2019). "Marijuana as Medicine." *National Institutes of Health.* Published online.

National Institute on Drug Abuse. (2020a). "Common Comorbidities with Substance Abuse Disorders Research, Part 1. The Connection between Substance Use Disorders and Mental Illness." Available at: https://www.drugabuse.gov/publications/research-reports/common-comorbidities-substance-abuse.

National Institute on Drug Abuse. (2020b). "Is Marijuana Addictive?" *National Institutes of Health.* Published online.

National Institute on Drug Abuse. (2020c). "Monitoring the Future: Trends & Statistics." Available at: https://www.drugabuse.gov/drug-topics/trends-statistics/monitoring-future.

National Institute on Drug Abuse. (2022a, April 21). "Benzodiazepines and Opioids."

National Institute on Drug Abuse. (2022b, January 20). "Overdose Death Rates." Published online.

National Institutes of Health. (2021, February 23). "NIH Launches New Initiative Study (Long COVID)."

Navarrete, F., et al. (2021). "Role of Cannabidiol in the Therapeutic Intervention for Substance Use Disorders." *Frontiers in Pharmacology* 12: 626010.

Nazeer, A., et al. (2014). "ADHD and Adolescent Athletes." *Frontiers in Public Health* 2: 1–7.

Nenn, K. (2022). "Meet the 5 Most Commonly Abused Stimulants." *Substance Abuse and Mental Health Services Administration* March 23, 2022.

Nestler, E. (2005). "Is There a Common Molecular Pathway for Addiction?" *Nature Neuroscience* 8: 1445–1449.

Nestsiarovich, A., et al. (2021). "Preventing New Episodes of Bipolar Disorder in Adults: Systematic Review and Meta-Analysis of Randomized Controlled Trials." *European Neuropsychopharmacology* 3: S0924–977X.

Newton-Howes, G., and Foulds, J. (2018a). "Personality Disorder and Treatment Outcome in Alcohol Use Disorder." *Current Opinions in Psychiatry* 31: 50–56.

Newton-Howes, G., and Foulds, J. (2018b). "Personality Disorder and Alcohol Use Disorder: An Overview." *Psychopathology* 51: 130–136.

Ng, K. T., et al. (2020). "The Effect of Melatonin on Delirium in Hospitalized Patients: A Systematic Review and Meta-Analyses with Trial Sequential Analysis." *Journal of Clinical Anesthesia* 59: 74–81.

Ng, Q. X., et al. (2017). "Clinical Use of Hypericum Perforatum (St. John's Wort) in Depression: A Meta-Analysis." *Journal of Affective Disorders* 210: 211–221.

Ng, Q. X., et al. (2021). "A Systematic Review of the Clinical Use of Gabapentin and Pregabalin in Bipolar Disorder." *Pharmaceuticals* 14: 834.

Nguyen, A. P., et al. (2020). "Association of Opioids Prescribed to Family Members with Opioid Overdose Among Adolescents and Young Adults." *JAMA Network Open* 3: e201018.

Nguyen, K., et al. (2021). "Evaluation of Rivastigmine in Alzheimer's Disease." *Neurodegenerative Disease Management* 11: 35–48.

Nguyen, T., et al. (2022). "Racial and Ethnic Disparities in Buprenorphine and Extended-Release Naltrexone Filled Prescriptions During the COVID-19 Pandemic." *JAMA Network Open* 5(6): e2214765.

Nguyen, V. H., and Harley, K. G. (2022). "Prenatal Cannabis Use and Infant Birth Outcomes in the Pregnancy Risk Assessment Monitoring System." *Journal of Pediatrics* 240: 87–93.

Nguyen, V., and Harley, K. (2022). "Prenatal Cannabis Use and Infant Birth Outcomes in the Pregnancy Risk Assessment Monitoring System." *Journal of Pediatrics* 240: 87–93.

NICE Guideline Updates Team (UK). (2019). "Psychological Interventions for the Treatment of Depression: Depression in Children and Young People, 2019 Evidence Review." National Institute for Health and Care Excellence (UK).

Nicholson, P. J., et al. (2015). "Correspondence Arising: Modafinil for Cognitive Neuroenhancement in Healthy Non-Sleep-Deprived-Subjects." *European Neuropsychopharmacology* 26: 390.

Nielsen, S., et al. (2019). "Pharmacotherapies for Cannabis Dependence." *Cochrane Database System Reviews* 1: CD008940.

Nierenberg, A. A., et al. (2016). "Bipolar CHOICE (Clinical Health Outcomes Initiative in Comparative Effectiveness): A Pragmatic 6-Month Trial of Lithium Versus Quetiapine for Bipolar Disorder." *Journal of Clinical Psychiatry* 77: 90–99.

Nikayin, S., et al. (2022, May 11). "Evaluation of the Trajectory of Depression Severity with Ketamine and Esketamine Treatment in a Clinical Setting." *JAMA Psychiatry.*

Ninnemann, A. L., et al. (2017). "Longitudinal Predictors of Synthetic Cannabinoid Use in Adolescents." *Pediatrics* 138: 1–7.

Nishimon, S., et al. (2021), "Advances in the Pharmacological Management of Non-24-h Sleep-Wake Disorder." *Expert Opinion on Pharmacotherapy* 22: 1039–1049.

Njoroge, W. F. M., et al. (2022). "Association of COVID-19 and Endemic Systemic Racism with Postpartum Anxiety and Depression Among Black Birthing Individuals." *JAMA Psychiatry* 79: 600–609.

Nordh, M., et al. (2021). "Therapist-Guided Internet-Delivered Cognitive Behavioral Therapy vs Internet-Delivered Supportive Therapy for Children and Adolescents with Social Anxiety Disorder. A Randomized Clinical Trial." *JAMA Psychiatry* 10: 1001.

Norgaard, A., et al. (2022). "Effect of Antipsychotics on Mortality Risk in Patients with Dementia with and without Comorbidities." *Journal of American Geriatrics Society* 70: 1169–1179.

Norman, J. L., and Anderson, S. L. (2016). "Novel Class of Medications, Orexin Receptor Antagonists, in the Treatment of Insomnia—Critical Appraisal of Suvorexant." *Nature and Science of Sleep* 14: 239–247.

Norman, T. R., and Olver, J. S. (2019). "Agomelatine for Depression: Expanding the Horizons?" *Expert Opinions in Pharmacotherapy* 20: 647–656.

Nunez, N. A., et al. (2022). "Augmentation Strategies for Treatment-Resistant Major Depression: A Systematic Review and Network Meta-Analysis." *Journal of Affective Disorders* 302: 385–400.

Nutt, D. (2019). "Psychedelic Drugs—A New Era in Psychiatry?" *Dialogues in Clinical Neuroscience* 21: 139–147.

Nutt, D. J., and Rehm, J. (2014). "Doing It by Numbers: A Simple Approach to

Reducing the Harms of Alcohol." *Journal of Psychopharmacology* 28: 3–7.

Nutt, D. J., et al. (2015). "The Dopamine Theory of Addiction: 40 Years of Highs and Lows." *Nature Reviews Neuroscience* 16: 305–312.

Nutt, D., and Carhart-Harris, R. (2020). "The Current Status of Psychedelics in Psychiatry." *JAMA Psychiatry,* June 29, Published online.

Nuzzo, J. B., and Gostin, L. O. (2022). "The First 2 Years of COVID-19: Lessons to Improve Preparedness for the Next Pandemic." *JAMA* 327: 217–218.

O'Donnell, J., et al. (2021, December 17). "Trends in and Characteristics of Drug Overdose Deaths Involving Illicitly Manufactured Fentanyls—United States, 2019–2020." *Morbidity and Mortality Weekly Report* 70: 1740–1746.

O'Keefe, J., et al. (2018). "Coffee for Cardioprotection and Longevity." *Progress in Cardiovascular Disease* 61: 38–42.

O'Mahony, D. O. (2020). "STOPP/START Criteria for Potentially Inappropriate Medications/Potential Prescribing Omissions in Older People: Origin and Progress." *Expert Reviews in Clinical Pharmacology* 13: 15–22.

Ochs-Ross, R., et al. (2021). "Comparison of Long-Term Efficacy and Safety of Esketamine Nasal Spray Plus Oral Antidepressant in Younger Versus Older Patients with Treatment-Resistant Depression: Post-Hoc Analysis of SUSTAIN-2, a Long-Term Open-Label Phase 3 Safety and Efficacy Study." *American Journal of Geriatric Psychiatry* 30: 541–556.

Odendaal, H., et al. (2021). "Association of Prenatal Exposure to Maternal Drinking and Smoking with the Risk of Stillbirth." *JAMA Network Open* 4: e2121726.

Oei, J. L. (2020). "Alcohol Use in Pregnancy and Its Impact on the Mother and Child." *Addiction* 115: 2148–2163.

Ogilvie, B. W., et al. (2015). "Clinical Assessment of Drug-Drug Interactions of Tasimeltion, a Novel Melatonin Receptor Agonist." *Journal of Clinical Pharmacology* 55: 1004–1011.

Oh, E. S., and Rabins, P. V. (2019). "Dementia." *Annals of Medicine* 171: ITC48.

Okereke, O., et al. (2021). "Effect of Long-Term Supplementation with Marine Omega-3 Fatty Acids vs Placebo on Risk of Depression or Clinically Relevant Depressive Symptoms and on Changes in Mood Scores: A Randomized Clinical Trial." *JAMA* 326: 2385–2394.

Olanow, C. W., et al. (2009). "A Double-Blind, Delayed-Start Trial of Rasagiline in Parkinson's Disease." *New England Journal of Medicine* 361: 1268–1278.

Olds, J., and Milner, P. (1954). "Positive Reinforcement Produced by Electrical Stimulation of Septal Area and Other Regions of Rat Brain." *Journal of Comparative and Physiological Psychology* 47: 419–427.

Olfson, M., et al. (2015). "Treatment of Young People with Antipsychotic Medications in the United States." *JAMA Psychiatry* 72: 867–874.

Olsen, V., et al. (2021). "Overcoming Barriers to Treatment of Opioid-Use Disorder." *JAMA* 325(12): 1149–1150.

Olson, S. (2015). "New Designer Drug Flakka Works Like Bath Salts, Causes 'Excited Delirium.'" *Medical Daily*. April 6. http://www.medicaldaily.com/new-designer-drug-flakka-works-bath-salts-causes-excited-delirium-328224.

Ooms, M., et al. (2020). "Effects of Multiple Detoxifications on Withdrawal Symptoms, Psychiatric Distress and Alcohol-Craving in Patients with an Alcohol Use Disorder." *Behavioral Medicine* 12: 15.

Orhurhu, V., et al. (2019). "Ketamine Infusions for Chronic Pain: A Systematic Review and Meta-Analysis of Randomized Controlled Trials." *Anesthesia & Analgesia*: 129: 241–254.

Ornoy, A. (2018). "Pharmacological Treatment of Attention Deficit Hyperactivity Disorder During Pregnancy and Lactation." *Pharmaceutical Research* 35: 46.

Ornoy, A., and Koren, G. (2021) "The Effects of Drugs Used for the Treatment of Attention Deficit Hyperactivity Disorder (ADHD) on Pregnancy Outcome and Breast-feeding: A Critical Review." *Current Neuropharmacology* 19: 1794–1804.

Ornoy, A., et al. (2017). "Antidepressants, Antipsychotics, and Mood Stabilizers in Pregnancy: What Do We Know and How Should We Treat Pregnant Women with Depression." *Birth Defects Research* 109: 933–956.

Orsolini, L., et al. (2019). "Use of Medicinal Cannabis and Synthetic Cannabinoids, Post-Traumatic Stress disorder (PTSD): A Systematic Review." *Medicina* 55: 525.

Orsolini, L., et al. (2020a). "How Does Ayahuasca Work from a Psychiatric Perspective? Pros and Cons of the Entheogenic Therapy." *Human Psychopharmacology,* e2728.

Orsolini, L., et al. (2020b). "New/Designer Benzodiazepines: An Analysis of the Literature and Psychonauts Trip Reports." *Current Neuropharmacology* 18: 809–837.

Oskotsky, T., et al. (2021). "Mortality Risk Among Patients with COVID-19 Prescribed Selective Serotonin Reuptake Inhibitor Antidepressants." *JAMA Network Open* 4: e2133090.

Oslin, D. W. et al. (2022). Effect of Pharmacogenomic Testing for Drug-Gene Interactions on Medication Selection and Remission of Symptoms in Major Depressive Disorder: The PRIME Care Randomized Clinical Trial. *JAMA*, 328(2), 151–161. https://doi.org/10.1001/jama.2022.9805

Ossenkoppele, R., et al. (2021). "Accuracy of Tau Positron Emission Tomography as a Prognostic Marker in Preclinical and Prodromal Alzheimer Disease: A Head-to-Head Comparison Against Amyloid Positron Emission Tomography and Magnetic Resonance Imaging." *JAMA Neurology* 78: 961–971.

Oulhaj, A., et al. (2016). "Omega-3 Fatty Acid Status Enhances the Prevention of Cognitive Decline by B Vitamins in Mild Cognitive Impairment." *Journal of Alzheimers Disease* 50: 547–557.

Owen, M. J., et al. (2016). "Schizophrenia." *Lancet* 388: 86–97.

Owji, S., and Shoja, M. M. (2020). "The History of Discovery of Adult Neurogenesis." *Clinical Anatomy* 33: 41–55.

Ozdemir, Z., et al. (2021). "Monoamine Oxidase-B (MAO-B) Inhibitors in the Treatment of Alzheimer's and Parkinson's Disease." *Current Medicinal Chemistry* 28: 6045–6065.

Özerdem, A., et al. (2016). "Neurobiology of Risk for Bipolar Disorder." *Current Treatment Options in Psychiatry* 3: 315–329.

Pacchiarotti, I., et al. (2016). "Mood Stabilizers and Antipsychotics During Breastfeeding: Focus on Bipolar Disorder." *European Neuropsychopharmacology* 76: 1562–1578.

Pacchiarotti, I., et al. (2019). "Long-Acting Injectable Antipsychotics (LAIs) for Maintenance Treatment of Bipolar and Schizoaffective Disorders: A Systematic Review." *European Neuropsychopharmacology* 20: 457–470.

Pacheco, D., et al. (2019). "Ketamine Induces Central Antinociception Mediated by Endogenous Cannabinoids and Activation of CB-1 Receptors." *Neuroscience Letters* 699: 140–144.

Pacher, P., et al. (2020). "Beyond THC and Endocannabinoids." *Annual Review of Pharmacology and Toxicology* 60: 637–659.

Pacifico, S., et al. (2021). "Novel Mixed NOP/Opioid Receptor Peptide Agonists." *Journal of Medicinal Chemistry* 64: 6656–6669.

Pagan, F. L., et al. (2021). "Long-Term Safety and Clinical Effects of Nilotinib in Parkinson's Disease." *Movement Disorders* 36: 740–749.

Pagano, G., et al. (2022). "Trial of Prasinezumab in Early-Stage Parkinson's Disease." *The New England Journal of Medicine* 387: 421–432.

Pagonabarrage, J., and Kulisevsky, J., (2017). "Apathy in Parkinson's Disease." *International Review of Neurobiology* 133: 657–678.

Pahwa, M., et al. (2021). "New Antipsychotic Medications in the Last Decade." *Current Psychiatry Reports* 23: 87.

Paige, K. J., and Colder, C. R. (2020). "Long-Term Effects of Early Adolescent Marijuana Use on Attentional and Inhibitory Control." *Journal on Studies of Alcohol and Drugs* 81: 64–172.

Paille, F., and Martini, H. (2014). "Nalmefene: A New Approach to the Treatment of Alcohol Dependence." *Substance Abuse and Rehabilitation* 5: 87–94.

Palenicek, T., et al. (2016). "Emerging Toxicity of 5,6-Methylenedioxy-2-Animoindane (MDAI): Pharmacokinetics, Behaviour, Thermoregulation and LD50 in Rats." *Progress in Neuropsychopharmacology& Biological Psychiatry* 69: 49–59.

Palma, J-A., and Kaufmann, H. (2020). "Orthostatic Hypotension in Parkinson Disease." *Clinical Geriatric Medicine* 36: 53–67.

Palpacuer, C., et al. (2018). "Pharmacologically Controlled Drinking in the Treatment of Alcohol Dependence: A Systematic Review with Direct Network Meta-Analysis on Nalmefene, Naltrexone, Acamprosate, Baclofen and Topiramate." *Addiction* 113: 220–237.

Panenka, W. J., et al. (2013). "Methamphetamine Use: A Comprehensive Review of Molecular, Preclinical and Clinical Findings." *Drug and Alcohol Dependence* 129: 167–179.

Pani, P. P., et al. (2011). "Antidepressants for Cocaine Dependence and Problematic Cocaine Use." *Cochrane Database of Systematic Reviews* CD0002950.

Papanti, D., et al. (2013). "'Spiceophrenia': A Systematic Overview of 'Spice'-Related

Psychopathological Issues and a Case Report." *Human Psychopharmacology* 28: 379–389.

Papaseit, E., et al. (2018a). "Acute Pharmacological Effects of 2C-B in Humans: An Observational Study." *Frontiers in Pharmacology* 9: 206.

Papaseit, E., et al. (2018b). "Key Interindividual Determinants in MDMA Pharmacodynamics." *Expert Opinion in Drug Metabolism and Toxicology* 14: 183–195.

Papoutsis, I., et al. (2016). "Benzodiazepines and Driving: Pharmacological and Legal Aspects." *European Journal of Forensic Sciences* 3: 26–34.

Pappa, S., et al. (2020). "Prevalence of Depression, Anxiety, and Insomnia Among Healthcare Workers During the COVID-19 Pandemic: A Systematic Review and Meta-Analysis." *Brain, Behavior and Immunity* 88: 901–907.

Pappagallo, M., et al. (2022). "Comment on Novel Glutamatergic Modulators for the Treatment of Mood Disorders: Current Status." *CNS Drugs* 36: 203–204.

Pardo, B. (2022). "Insights into Mixing Fentanyl and Benzodiazepines from Canadian Drug Seizures." *JAMA Psychiatry* 79: 81–83.

Parikh, S. V., et al. (2015). "Combined Treatment: Impact of Optimal Psychotherapy and Medication in Bipolar Disorder." *Bipolar Disorders* 17: 86–96.

Park, K., et al. (2016). "Effects of Coffee Consumption on Serum Uric Acid." *Seminars in Arthritis and Rheumatism* 45: 580–586.

Park, S-C. (2019). "Neurogenesis and Antidepressant Action." *Cell and Tissue Research.* 377: 95–106.

Park, T. W., et al. (2015). "Benzodiazepine Prescribing Patterns and Deaths from Drug Overdose Among US Veterans Receiving Opioid Analgesics: Case-Cohort Study." *BMJ* 350: h2698.

Parker, G. (2018). "Risks Associated with Lamotrigine Prescription: A Review and Personal Observations" *Australasian Psychiatry* 26: 640–642.

Parker, G., et al. (2021). "A Single-Blind Randomized Comparison of Lithium and Lamotrigine as Maintenance Treatments for Managing Bipolar II Disorder." *Journal of Clinical Psychopharmacology* 41: 381–388.

Parkinson's Foundation. (2020, May). "Parkinson's Foundation Consensus Statement on the Use of Medical Cannabis for Parkinson's Disease."

Passie, T., and Benzenhofer, U. (2018). "MDA, MDMA, and Other 'Mescaline-like' Substances in the US Military's Search for a Truth Drug (1940s to 1960s)." *Drug Testing and Analysis* 10: 72–80.

Patel, A. K., and Balasanova, A. A. (2021). "Treatment of Alcohol Use Disorder." *JAMA* 325: 596.

Patel, K., et al. (2016). "Bupropion: A Systematic Review and Meta-Analysis of Effectiveness as an Antidepressant." *Therapeutic Advances in Psychopharmacology* 6: 99–144.

Patel, M., et al. (2021). "Efficacy of Cariprazine in Bipolar I Depression Across Patient Characteristics: A Post Hoc Analysis of Pooled Randomized, Placebo-Controlled Studies." *International Clinics of Psychopharmacology* 36: 76–83.

Patel, R., et al. (2015). "Do Antidepressants Increase the Risk of Mania and Bipolar Disorder in People with Depression? A Retrospective Electronic Case Register Cohort Study." *British Medical Journal* 5: e008341.

Paterniti, S., et al. (2002). "Long-Term Benzodiazepine Use and Cognitive Decline in the Elderly: The Epidemiology of Vascular Aging Study." *Journal of Clinical Psychopharmacology* 22: 285–293.

Pathan, H., and Williams, J. (2012). "Basic Opioid Pharmacology: An Update." *British Journal of Pain* 6: 11–16.

Patnode, C. D., et al. (2015). "Behavioral Counseling and Pharmacotherapy Interventions for Tobacco Cessation in Adults, Including Pregnant Women: A Review of Reviews for the U.S. Preventive Services Task Force (Internet)." *Annals of Internal Medicine* 163: 608–621.

Patocka, J., et al. (2020). "Flakka: New Dangerous Synthetic Cathinone on the Drug Scene." *International Journal of Molecular Sciences* 21: 8185.

Patsalos, P. N., et al. (2018). "Therapeutic Drug Monitoring of Antiepileptic Drugs in Epilepsy: A 2018 Update." *Therapeutic Drug Monitoring* 40: 526–548.

Patti, F., et al. (2016). "Efficacy and Safety of Cannabinoid Oromucosal Spray for Multiple Sclerosis Spasticity." *Journal of Neurology, Neurosurgery & Psychiatry* 87: 944–951.

Paul, S. E., et al. (2021). "Associations Between Prenatal Cannabis Exposure and Childhood Outcomes: Results from the ABCD Study." *JAMA Psychiatry* 78: 64–76.

Paulus, M. P., and Stewart, J. L. (2020). "Neurobiology, Clinical Presentation, and Treatment of Methamphetamine Use Disorder: A Review." *JAMA Psychiatry.* Published online April 8.

Pava, M. J., and Woodward, J. J. (2012). "A Review of the Interactions Between Alcohol and the Endocannabinoid System: Implications for Alcohol Dependence and Future Directions for Research." *Alcohol* 46: 185–204.

Pavkovic, B., et al. (2018). "Double Screening for Dual Disorder, Alcoholism and Depression." *Psychiatry Research* 270: 483-489.

Pawlik, M. J., et al. (2021). "Selected Molecular Targets for Antiepileptogenesis." *International Journal of Molecular Science* 22: 9737.

Payer, D. E., et al. (2014). "Heightened D3 Dopamine Receptor Levels in Cocaine Dependence and Contributions to the Addiction Behavioral Phenotype: A Positron Emission Tomography Study with [11C]-(+)-PHNO." *Neuropsychopharmacology* 39: 321–328.

Payne, J. L. (2021). "Evaluating Brexanolone for the Treatment of Postpartum Depression." *Expert Opinion on Pharmacotherapy* 22: 959–964.

Peacock, A., et al. (2020). "Opioid Use and Harms Associated with a Sustained-Release Tapentadol Formulation: A Post-Marketing Surveillance Study." *Drug and Alcohol Dependence* 206: 107697.

Pearce, M., et al. (2022). "Association Between Physical Activity and Risk of Depression: A Systematic Review and Meta-Analysis." *JAMA Psychiatry* 79: 550–559.

Peball, M., et al. (2020). "Non-Motor Symptoms in Parkinson's Disease Are Reduced by Nabilone." *Annals of Neurology* 88: 712–722.

Peng, L., et al. (2022). "Complex Persistent Benzodiazepine Dependence—When Benzodiazepine Deprescribing Goes Awry." *JAMA Psychiatry* 79: 639–640.

Penkunas, M. J., and Hahn-Smith, S. (2015). "An Evaluation of IMPACT for the Treatment of Late-Life Depression in a Public Mental Health System." *Journal of Behavioral Health Services & Research* 42: 334–345.

Pereira, V. S., and Hiroaki-Sato, V.A. (2018). "A Brief History of Antidepressant Drug Development: From Tricyclics to Beyond Ketamine. *Acta Neuropsychiatrica* 30: 307–322.

Peritogiannis, V., et al. (2009). "Duloxetine-Induced Hypomania: Case Report and Brief Review of the Literature on SNRIs-Induced Mood Switching." *Journal of Psychopharmacology* 23: 592–596.

Perlis, R. H., and Fava, M. (2022). "Is It Time to Try Sequenced Treatment Alternatives to Relive Depression (STAR*D) Again?" *JAMA Psychiatry* 79: 281–282.

Perlis, R. H., et al. (2006). "Predictors of Recurrence in Bipolar Disorder: Primary Outcomes from the Systematic Treatment Enhancement Program for Bipolar Disorder (STEP-BD)." *American Journal of Psychiatry* 163: 217–224.

Pernia, S., and DeMaafd, G. (2016). "The New Pregnancy and Lactation Labeling Rule." *P & T.* 41: 713–715.

Perry, P. J., et al. (2006). "The Association of Alcohol-Induced Blackouts and Grayouts to Blood Alcohol Concentrations." *Journal of Forensic Science* 51: 896–899.

Pertwee, R. G. (2006). "Cannabinoid Pharmacology: The First 66 Years." *British Journal of Pharmacology* 147: S163–S171.

Pertwee, R. G. (2015). "Endocannabinoids and Their Pharmacological Actions." *Handbook of Experimental Pharmacology* 231: 1–37.

Pessar, S. C., et al. (2021). "Assessment of State and Federal Health Policies for Opioid Use Disorder Treatment During the COVID-19 Pandemic and Beyond." *JAMA Health Forum* 2: e213833.

Peters, A. T., et al. (2011). "Stepping Back to Step Forward: Lessons from the Systematic Treatment Enhancement Program for Bipolar Disorder (STEP-BD)." *Journal of Clinical Psychiatry* 72: 1429–1431.

Peters, E. M., et al. (2021). "Melancholic Features in Bipolar Depression and Response to Lamotrigine: A Pooled Analysis of Five Randomized Placebo-Controlled Trials." *Journal of Clinical Psychopharmacology* 41: 315–319.

Petersen, I., et al. (2016). "Risks Associated with Antipsychotic Treatment in Pregnancy: Comparative Cohort Studies Based on Electronic Health Records." *Schizophrenia Research* 176: 349–356.

Pettinati, H. M., et al. (2010). "A Double-Blind, Placebo-Controlled Trial that Combines Sertraline and Naltrexone for Treating Co-Occurring Depression and Alcohol Dependence." *American Journal of Psychiatry* 167: 668–675.

Phelps, J., et al. (2022). "The Rapid Rise in Investment in Psychedelics: Cart Before the Horse." *JAMA Psychiatry,* Published online January 19.

Philbin, M. M., et al. (2019) "Associations Between State-Level Policy Liberalism, Cannabis, Use, and Cannabis Use Disorder from 2004 to 2012: Looking Beyond Medical Cannabis Law Status." *International Journal of Drug Policy* 65: 97–103.

Phillips, S., and Williams, M. A. (2021). "Confounding Our Next National Health Disaster—Long-Haul Covid." *New England Journal of Medicine* 385: 577–579.

Pianca, T. G., et al. (2016). "Crack Cocaine Use in Adolescents: Clinical Characteristics and Predictors of Early Initiation." *Journal of Clinical Psychiatry* 77: e1205–e1210.

Piccirella, S., et al. (2022). "A Conformational Variant of p53 (U-p53AZ) as Blood-Based Biomarker for the Prediction of the Onset of Symptomatic Alzheimer's Disease." *The Journal of Prevention of Alzheimer's Disease* 9: 469–479.

Picton, J. D., et al. (2018). "Benzodiazepine Use and Cognitive Decline in the Elderly." *America Journal of Health System Pharmacy* 75: e6–e12.

Pierce, J. P., et al. (2021). "Influence of Cigarette Smoking Relapse Among Individuals Who Switched to e-Cigarettes or Other Tobacco Products." *JAMA Network Open* 4: e2128810.

Pigott, E. H. (2015). "The STAR*D Trial: Is it Time to Reexamine the Clinical Beliefs that Guide the Treatment of Major Depression?" *The Canadian Journal of Psychiatry* 60: 9–13.

Pillay, J., et al. (2017). "First- and Second-Generation Antipsychotics in Children and Young Adults: Systematic Review Update." *Comparative Effectiveness Review* 184: 1–567.

Pinto, J. V., et al. (2020). "Cariprazine in the Treatment of Bipolar Disorder: A Systematic Review and Meta-Analysis." *Bipolar Disorder* 22: 360–371.

Piper, B. J., et al. (2017). "Substitution of Medical Cannabis for Pharmaceutical Agents for Pain, Anxiety, and Sleep." *Journal of Psychopharmacology* 31: 569–575.

Pirscoveanu, D., et al. (2017). "Tau Protein in Neurodegenerative Diseases—A Review." *Romanian Journal of Morphology and Embryology* 58: 1141–1150.

Pisano, S., et al. (2019). "Putative Mechanisms of Action and Clinical Use of Lithium in Children and Adolescents: A Critical Review." *Current Neuropharmacology* 17: 318–341.

Pitsillou, E., et al. (2020). "The Cellular and Molecular Basis of Major Depressive Disorder; Towards a Unified Model for Understanding Clinical Depression." *Molecular Biology Reports* 47: 753–770.

Planchez, B., et al. (2020). "Adult Hippocampal Neurogenesis and Antidepressant Effects." *Currect Opinions in Pharmacology* 50: 88–95.

Podgorny, O., and Gulyaeva, N.V. (2021). "Glucocorticoid-Mediated Mechanisms of Hippocampal Damage: Contribution of Subgranular Neurogenesis." *Journal of Neurochemistry* 157: 370–392.

Poleg, S., et al. (2019) "Cannabidiol as a Suggested Candidate for Treatment of Autism Spectrum Disorder." *Progress in Neuropsychopharmacology, Biology and Psychiatry* 89: 90–96.

Pollan, M. (2021). "This Is Your Mind on Plants." Penguin Group (USA).

Pollard, M. S., et al. (2020). "Changes in Adult Alcohol Use and Consequences During the COVID-19 Pandemic in the US." *JAMA Network Open* 3: e2022942.

Popova, S., et al. (2017). "Prevalence of Alcohol Consumption During Pregnancy and Fetal Alcohol Spectrum Disorders Among the General and Aboriginal Populations in Canada and the United States." *European Journal of Medical Genetics* 60: 32–48.

Porsteinssona, A. P., and Antonsdottir, I. M. (2017). "An Update on the Advancements in the Treatment of Agitation in Alzheimer's Disease." *Expert Opinion on Pharmacotherapy* 18: 611–620.

Posner, J., et al. (2020). "Attention-Deficit Hyperactivity Disorder." *Lancet* 395: 450–462.

Post, R. M., et al. (2019). "Beyond Evidence-Based Treatment of Bipolar Disorder: Rational Pragmatic Approaches to Management." *Bipolar Disorder* 21: 650–659.

Potts, A. J., et al. (2020). "Synthetic Cannabinoid Receptor Agonists: Classification and Nomenclature." *Clinical Toxicology* 58: 82–98.

Poulton, A. S., et al. (2016). "Stimulant Medication Effects on Growth and Bone Age in Children with Attention-Deficit/Hyperactivity

Disorder: A Prospective Cohort Study." *International Clinical Psychopharmacology* 31: 93–99.

Pourmand, A., et al. (2017). "Low Dose Ketamine Use in the Emergency Department, a New Direction in Pain Management." *American Journal of Emergency Medicine* 35: 918–921.

Pow, J. L., et al. (2015). "Deinstitutionalization of American Public Hospitals for the Mentally Ill Before and After the Introduction of Antipsychotic Medications." *Harvard Review of Psychiatry* 23: 176–187.

Powell, J. G., et al. (2020). "Brexanolone (Zulresso): Finally, An FDA-Approved Treatment for Postpartum Depression." *Annals of Pharmacotherapy* 54: 157–163.

Prakash, S., and Carter, W. G. (2021). "The Neuroprotective Effects of Cannabis-Derived Phytocannabinoids and Resveratrol in Parkinson's Disease: A Systematic Literature Review of Pre-Clinical Studies." *Brain Science* 11: 1573.

Preskorn, S. H., et al. (2022). "Effect of Sublingual Dexmedetomidine vs. Placebo on Acute Agitation Associated with Bipolar Disorder: A Randomized Clinical Trial." *JAMA* 327: 727–736.

Pressman, M. R. (2011). "Sleep Driving: Sleepwalking Variant or Misuse of Z-Drugs? *Sleep Medicine Reviews* 15: 285–292.

Preuss, U. W., et al. (2020). "A Prospective Comparison of Bipolar I and II Subjects With and Without Comorbid Alcohol Dependence from the COGA Dataset." *Frontiers in Psychiatry* 11: 522228.

Prime, H., et al. (2020). "Risk and Resilience in Family Well-Being During the COVID-19 Pandemic." *American Psychologist* 75: 631–643.

Prince, V., and Bowling, K. C. (2018). "Topiramate in the Treatment of Cocaine Use Disorder." *American Journal of Health-System Pharmacy* 75: e13–e22.

Pulgar, V. M. (2019). "Transcytosis to Cross the Blood Brain Barrier, New Advances and Challenges." *Frontiers in Neuroscience* 12, Article 1019.

Purcell, C., et al. (2019). "Reduction of Benzodiazepine Use in Patients Prescribed Medical Cannabis." *Cannabis and Cannabinoid Research* 4: 214–218.

Qasim, H.S., and Simpson, M.D. (2022). "A Narrative Review of Studies Comparing Efficacy and Safety of Citalopram with Atypical Antipsychotics for Agitation in Behavioral and Psychological Symptoms of Dementia (BPSD)" *Pharmacy (Basel, Switzerland).* 10: 61.

Qato, D. M., et al. (2016). "Changes in Prescription and Over-the-Counter Medication and Dietary Supplement Use Among Older Adults in the United States, 2005 vs 2011." *JAMA: Internal Medicine* 176: 473–482.

Quagliato, L. A., et al. (2018). "Risks and Benefits of Medications for Panic Disorder: A Comparison of SSRIs and Benzodiazepines." *Expert Opinion on Drug Safety* 17: 315–324.

Quan, L., et al. (2021). "Dose-Dependent Efficacy of Aripiprazole in Treating Patients with Schizophrenia or Schizoaffective Disorder: A Systematic Review and Meta-Analysis of Randomized Controlled Trials." *Frontiers in Psychiatry* 12: 717715.

Quarracino, C., et al. (2020). "State-of-the-Art Pharmacotherapy for Autonomic Dysfunction in Parkinson's Disease." *Expert Opinion in Pharmacotherapy* 21: 445–457.

Quera-Salva, M-A., and Claustrat, B. (2018). "Melatonin: Physiological and Pharmacological Aspects Related to Sleep. The Interest of a Prolonged-Release Formulation (Circadin) in Insomnia." *Encephale* 44: 548–557.

Quinn, N. J., et al. (2021). "Prescribing Practices of Valproic Acid for Agitation and Delirium in the Intensive Care Unit." *Annuals of Pharmacotherapy* 55: 311–317.

Racine, N., et al. (2021). "Global Prevalence of Depressive and Anxiety Symptoms in Children and Adolescents During COVID-19: A Meta-Analysis. *JAMA Pediatrics* 175: 1142–1150.

Rad, F., et al. (2020). "Adult ADHD Symptoms in a Group of Patients with Substance Abuse." *Rivista di Psichiatria* 55: 161–167.

Radcliff, J. A., et al. (2018). "A Retrospective Chart Review of Outcomes Resulting from a Three-Day Tramadol Taper for Acute Opioid Withdrawal." *Journal of Addictive Diseases* 37: 252–258.

Ragguett, R-M., and McInTyre, R. S. (2019). "Cariprazine for the Treatment of Bipolar Depression." *Expert Review of Neurotherapeutics* 19: 317–323.

Ragguett, R-M., et al. (2018). "Pharmacodynamic and Pharmacokinetic Evaluation of buprenorphine + Samidorphan for the Treatment of Major Depressive Disorder." *Expert Opinion on Drug Metabolism and Toxicology* 14: 475–482.

Ragguett, R-M., et al. (2019). "Keeping Up with the Clinical Advances: Depression." *CNS Spectrums* 24(S1): 25–37.

Rahman, J., et al. (2020). "Neurological and Psychological Effects of Coronavirus (COVID-19): An Overview of the Current Era Pandemic." *Cureus* 12: e8460.

Raivenius, W. T., et al. (2016). "The Clobazam Metabolite N-desmethyl Clobazam Is an Alpha2 Preferring Benzodiazepine with an Improved Therapeutic Window for Antihyperalgesia." *Neuropharmacology* 109: 366–375.

Raja, S. N., et al. (2020). "The Revised International Association for the Study of Pain Definition of Pain: Concepts, Challenges, and Compromises." *Pain* 16: 1976–1982.

Ramachandraiah, C. T., et al. (2009). "The Story of Antipsychotics: Past and Present." *Indian Journal of Psychiatry* 51: 324–326.

Ramaswamy, S., et al. (2017). "A Double-Blind, Placebo-Controlled Trial of Vilazodone in the Treatment of Posttraumatic Stress Disorder and Comorbid Depression." *Primary Care Companion for CNS Disorders* 19: 17m02138.

Ramos, K. M., et al. (2019). "The NIH BRAIN Initiative: Integrating Neuroethics and Neuroscience." *Neuron* 101: 394–398.

Rando, K., et al. (2013). "Prenatal Cocaine Exposure and Gray Matter Volume in Adolescent Boys and Girls." *Biological Psychiatry* 74: 482–489.

Rang, H. P., and Dale, M. M. (1991). *Pharmacology,* 2nd ed. Edinburgh: Churchill Livingstone.

Ranganathan, S., and Gupta, V. (2020). "Postcoital Contraception." *Stat Pearls* June 5.

Rantala, M. J., et al. (2021). "Bipolar Disorder: An Evolutionary Psychoneuroimmunological Approach." *Neuroscience and Biobehavioral Reviews* 122: 28–37.

Rapino, C., et al. (2018). "Neuroprotection by (endo)Cannabinoids in Glaucoma and Retinal Neurodegenerative Diseases." *Current Neuropharmacology* 16: 959–970.

Rapoport, S. I., et al. (2009). "Bipolar Disorder and Mechanisms of Action of Mood Stabilizers." *Brain Research Reviews* 61: 185–209.

Rasmussen, I. N. (2008). "America's First Amphetamine Epidemic 1929–1971." *American Journal of Public Health* 98: 974–985.

Rausgaard, N. L. K., et al. (2020). "Management and Monitoring of Opioid Use in Pregnancy." *Acta Obstetrica et Gynecologica Scandinavica* 99: 7–15.

Raveendran, A. V., et al. (2021, May–June). "Long COVID: An Overview." *Diabetes & Metabolic Syndrome: Clinical Research & Reviews* 15(3(: 869–875.

Ray, L. A., et al. (2020). "Combined Pharmacotherapy and Cognitive Behavioral Therapy for Adults with Alcohol or Substance Use Disorders: A Systematic Review and Meta-analysis." *JAMA Network Open* 3(6): e208279.

Rehm, J. (2015). "Light or Moderate Drinking Is Linked to Alcohol-Related Cancers, Including Breast Cancer." *BMJ* 351: h4400.

Reich, S. G., and Savitt, J. M. (2019). "Parkinson's Disease." *Medical Clinics of North America* 103: 337–350.

Reiff, C. M., et al. (2020). "Psychedelics and Psychedelic-Assisted Psychotherapy." *American Journal of Psychiatry* 177: 391–410.

Reissig, C. J., et al. (2012). "High Doses of Dextromethorphan, an NMDA Antagonist, Produce Effects Similar to Classic Hallucinogens." *Psychopharmacology* 223: 1–15.

Renelli, M., et al. (2020). "An Exploratory Study of Experiences with Conventional Eating Disorder Treatment and Ceremonial Ayahuasca for the Healing of Eating Disorders." *Eating and Weight Disorders* 25: 437–444.

Renfro, M. L., et al. (2020). "Lofexidine for Acute Opioid Withdrawal: A Clinical Case Series." *The Mental Health Clinician* 10: 259–263.

Rengarajan, A., and Mullins, M. (2013). "How Often Do False-Positive Phencyclidine Urine Screens Occur with Use of Common Medications?" *Clinical Toxicology* 51: 493–396.

Renner, U., et al. (2005). "Pharmacokinetics and Pharmacodynamics in Clinical Use of Scopolamine." *Therapeutic Drug Monitoring* 27: 655–665.

Reyad, A. A., et al. (2020). "Efficacy and Safety of Brexpiprazole in Acute Management of Psychiatric Disorders: A Meta-Analysis of Randomized Controlled Trials." *International Clinical Psychopharmacology* 35: 119–128.

Reynolds, C. F., et al. (2006). "Maintenance Treatment of Major Depression in Old Age." *New England Journal of Medicine* 354: 1130–1138.

Rhee, T. G., and Rosenheck, R. A. (2019). "Does Improvement in Symptoms and Quality of Life in Chronic Schizophrenia Reduce Family Caregiver Burden?" *Psychiatry Research* 271: 402–404.

Rhee, T. G., et al. (2020). "20-Year Trends in the Pharmacologic Treatment of Bipolar Disorder by Psychiatrists in Outpatient Care Settings." *American Journal of Psychiatry* 177: 706–715.

Ricaurte, G. A., et al. (2005). "Amphetamine Treatment Similar to That Used in the Treatment of Attention-Deficit/Hyperactivity Disorder Damages Dopaminergic Nerve Endings in the Striatum of Adult Nonhuman Primates." *Journal of Pharmacology & Experimental Therapeutics* 315: 91–98.

Richardson, J. D., et al. (2011). "Aripiprazole Augmentation in the Treatment of Military-Related PTSD with Major Depression: A Retrospective Chart Review." *BMC Psychiatry* 11: 86.

Richter, L. H., et al. (2019). "Cytotoxicity of New Psychoactive Substances and Other Drugs of Abuse Studied in Human HepG2 Cells Using an Adopted High Content Screening Assay." *Toxicology Letters* 301: 79–89.

Rickels, K., et al. (2012). "Adjunctive Therapy with Pregabalin in Generalized Anxiety Disorder Patients with Partial Response to SSRI or SNRI Treatment." *International Clinical Psychopharmacology* 27: 142–150.

Rickli, A., et al. (2016). "Receptor Interaction Profiles of Novel Psychoactive Tryptamines Compared with Classic Hallucinogens." *European Neuropsychopharmacology* 26: 1327–1337.

Robb, A. S., et al. (2010). "Sertraline Treatment of Children and Adolescents with Posttraumatic Stress Disorder: A Double-Blind, Placebo-Controlled Trial." *Journal of Child and Adolescent Psychopharmacology* 20: 463–471.

Roberson, S. W., et al. (2019). "Antiepileptic Drugs and Suicidality in Veterans with Seizures." *Neurology* 11: In press.

Roberti, R., et al. (2021). "Pharmacology of Cenobamate: Mechanism of Action, Pharmacokinetics, Drug-Drug Interactions and Tolerability." *CNS Drugs* 35: 609–618.

Roberts, C. A., et al. (2016). "Meta-analysis of Executive Functioning in Ecstasy/Polydrug Users." *Psychological Medicine* 46: 1581–1596.

Robillard, R., et al. (2015). "Sleep Is More Sensitive to High Doses of Caffeine in the Middle Years of Life." *Journal of Psychopharmacology* 29: 688–697.

Robinson, J. D., et al. (2020). "Very Low Nicotine Content Cigarettes Disrupt the Feedback Loop of Affective States and Smoking Behavior." *Nicotine and Tobacco Research* 22: 1294–1300.

Rodrigues, F. B., and Ferreira, J. J. (2017). "Opicapone for the Treatment of Parkinson's Disease." *Expert Opinion on Pharmacotherapy* 18: 445–453.

Roemer, A., and Stockwell, T. (2017). "Alcohol Mixed with Energy Drinks and Risk of Injury: A Systematic Review." *Journal of Studies on Alcohol and Drugs* 78: 175–183.

Rohrig, T. P., et al. (2021). "Driving Impairment Cases Involving Etizolam and Flubromazolam." *Journal of Analytical Toxicology* 45: 93–98.

Romano, B., et al. (2014). "Inhibition of Colon Carcinogenesis by a Standardized Cannabis Sativa Extract with a High Content of Cannabidiol." *Phytomedicine* 21: 631–639.

Rommel, A.-S., et al. (2020). "Long-Term Effects of Intrauterine Exposure to Antidepressants on Physical, Neurodevelopmental, and Psychiatric Outcomes: A Systematic Review." *Journal of Clinical Psychiatry* 81: 19r12965.

Romoli, M., et al. (2019). "Valproic Acid and Epilepsy: From Molecular Mechanisms to Clinical Evidences." *Current Neuropharmacology* 17: 926–946.

Romolo, F. S., et al. (2017). "Volatile Lipophilic Substances Management in Case of Fatal Sniffing." *Journal of Forensic and Legal Medicine* 52: 35–39.

Romualdi, P., et al. (2019). "Pharmacological Rationale for Tapentadol Therapy: A Review of New Evidence." *Journal of Pain Research* 12: 1513–1520.

Roncero, C., et al. (2020). "Cannabis Use During Pregnancy and Its Relationship with Fetal Developmental Outcomes and Psychiatric Disorders. A Systematic Review." *Reproductive Health* 17: 25–34.

Rong, C., et al. (2018). "Predictors of Response to Ketamine in Treatment Resistant Major Depressive Disorder and Bipolar Disorder." *International Journal of Environmental Research and Public Health* 15: 771.

Rosborough, K., et al. (2017). "α-Synuclein and Parkinsonism: Updates and Future Perspectives" *Current Neurology and Neuroscience Reports* 17: 31.

Rosenbaum, C. D., et al. (2012). "Here Today, Gone Tomorrow . . . and Back Again? A Review of Herbal Marijuana Alternatives (K2, Spice), Synthetic Cathinones (Bath Salts), Kratom, Salvia Divinorum, Methoxetamine, and Piperazines." *Journal of Medical Toxicology* 8: 15–32.

Rosenberg, R., et al. (2019). "Comparison of Lemborexant with Placebo and Zolpidem Tartrate Extended Release for the Treatment of Older Adults with Insomnia Disorder: A Phase 3 Randomized Clinical Trial." *JAMA Network Open* 2: e1918254.

Ross, E. A., et al. (2011). "Bath Salts Intoxication." *The New England Journal of Medicine* 365: 967–968.

Ross, E. L., et al. (2022, March 28). "Cost-Effectiveness of Aducanumab and Donanemab for Early Alzheimer's Disease in the US." *JAMA Neurology* e220315.

Roth, B. L., et al. (2002). "Salvinorin A: A Potent Naturally Occurring Nonnitrogenous Opioid Selective Agonist." *Proceedings of the National Academy of Sciences* 99: 11934–11939.

Rothschild, A. J., et al. (2012). "Vortioxetine (Lu AA21004) 5 mg in Generalized Anxiety Disorder: Results of an 8-Week Randomized, Double-Blind, Placebo-Controlled Clinical Trial in the United States." *European Neuropsychopharmacology* 22: 858–866.

Rozankovic, P. B., et al. (2021). "Impact of Donepezil and Memantine on Behavioral and Psychological Symptoms of Alzheimer's Disease: Six-Month Open-Label Study." *Cognitive and Behavioral Neurology* 34: 288–294.

Ruberto, V. L., et al. (2020), "Pharmacological Treatments for Patients with Treatment-Resistant Depression." *Pharmaceuticals* 13: E116.

Rubi, L., et al. (2017). "Anti-Addiction Drug Ibogaine Prolongs the Action Potential in Human Induced Pluripotent Stem Cell-Derived Cardiomyocytes." *Cardiovascular Toxicology* 17: 215–218.

Rubin, R. (2021a). "Alcohol-Related Disease Increased as Some People Drank More During the COVID-19 Pandemic." *JAMA* 326: 209–211.

Rubin, R. (2021b). "CMS Considers Controversial Alzheimer Drug Coverage." *JAMA* 326: 690.

Rubin, R. (2021c). "Recently Approved Alzheimer Drug Raises Questions That Might Never Be Answered." *JAMA* 326: 469–472.

Rubin, R. (2022a). "Much Anticipated Alzheimer Disease Prevention Trial Finds No Clinical Benefit from Drug Targeting Amyloid; Highlights Need to Consider Other Approaches." *JAMA* 328: 416–419.

Rubin, R. (2022b, June 21). "New Test to Help Diagnose Alzheimer Disease." *JAMA*.

Rubino, A., et al. (2020). "Association of the US Food and Drug Administration Antipsychotic Drug Boxed Warning with Medication Use and Health Outcomes in Elderly Patients with Dementia." *JAMA Network Open* 3: e203630.

Rucker, J., et al. (2018). "Psychiatry and the Psychedelic Drugs: Past, Present and Future." *Neuropharmacology* 142: 200–218.

Ruder, K. (2022). "Vaping's Cardiopulmonary Associations in Adolescents Examined." *JAMA* July 27.

Rush, A. J., et al. (2011). "Combining Medications to Enhance Depression Outcomes (CO-MED): Acute and Long-Term Outcomes of a Single-Blind Randomized Study." *American Journal of Psychiatry* 168: 689–701.

Rush, A. J., et al. (2020). "What to Expect when Switching to a Second Antidepressant Medication Following an Ineffective Initial SSRI: A Report from the Randomized Clinical STAR*D Study." *Journal of Clinical Psychiatry* 81: 19m12949.

Ruthirakuhan, M., et al. (2019). "Natural and Synthetic Cannabinoids for Agitation and

Aggression in Alzheimer's Disease: A Meta-Analysis." *Journal of Clinical Psychiatry* 80: 18r12617.

Rybakowski, J. K. (2014). "Response to Lithium in Bipolar Disorder: Clinical and Genetic Findings." *ACS Chemical Neuroscience* 5: 413–421.

Rybakowski, J. K. (2018). "Clinical Perspectives of Lithium's Neuroprotective Effect." *Pharmacopsychiatry* 5: 194–199.

Saade, Y. M., et al. (2019). "Comorbid Anxiety in Late-Life Depression: Relationship with Remission and Suicidal Ideation on Venlafaxine Treatment." *Depression and Anxiety* 36: 1125–1134.

Sachs, G. S., et al. (2003). "Rationale, Design, and Methods of the Systematic Treatment Enhancement Program for Bipolar Disorder (STEP-BD)." *Journal of Clinical Psychiatry* 53: 1028–1042.

Sadeghniiat-Haghighi, K., et al. (2016). "Melatonin Therapy in Shift Workers with Difficulty Falling Asleep: A Randomized, Double-Blind, Placebo-Controlled Crossover Field Study." *Work* 55: 225–230.

Sague-Vilavella, M., et al. (2022). "Obstetric Outcomes Regarding the Use of Lithium in Pregnant Women with Bipolar Disorders: A Prospective Cohort Study." *Archives of Women's Mental Health* 25: 729–737.

Salamon, A., et al. (2019). "Opicapone for the Treatment of Parkinson's Disease: An Update." *Expert Opinion in Pharmacotherapy* 20: 2201–2207.

Salas-Wright, C. P., et al. (2015). "Substance Use and Teen Pregnancy in the United States: Evidence from the NSDUH 2002–2012." *Addictive Behaviors* 45: 218–225.

Samji, H., et al. (2022). "Review: Mental Health Impacts of the COVID-19 Pandemic on Children and Youth—A Systematic Review." *Child and Adolescent Mental Health* 27: 173–189.

Sanacora, G. (2020). "Is This Where We Stand After Decades of Research to Develop More Personalized Treatments for Depression?" *JAMA Psychiatry* 77: 560–562.

Sandstrom, A., et al. (2019). "Offspring of Parents with Schizophrenia, Bipolar Disorder, and Depression: A Review of Familial High-Risk and Molecular Genetics Studies." *Psychiatrics & Genetics* 29: 160–169.

Sankaran, D., et al. (2022). "Methamphetamine: Burden, Mechanism and Impact on Pregnancy, the Fetus, and Newborn." *Journal of Perinatology* 42: 293–299.

Sansone, R. A., and Sansone, L. A. (2014). "Marijuana and Body Weight." *Innovations in Clinical Neuroscience* 11: 50–54.

Saraf, G., et al. (2019). "Efficacy and Safety of Cariprazine in the Treatment of Bipolar Disorder." *Expert Opinions in Pharmacotherapies* 20: 2063–2072.

Saraf, G., et al. (2021). "Early Intervention for People at High Risk of Developing Bipolar Disorder: A Systematic Review of Clinical Trials." *Lancet Psychiatry* 8: 64–75

Sari, Y., et al. (2011). "Role of the Serotonergic System in Alcohol Dependence: From Animal Models to Clinics." *Progress in Molecular Biology and Translational Sciences* 98: 401–443.

Sarris, J., et al. (2013). "Plant-Based Medicines for Anxiety Disorders, Part 2: A Review of Clinical Studies with Supporting Preclinical Evidence." *CNS Drugs* 27: 301–319.

Sarris, J., et al. (2020). "Medicinal Cannabis for Psychiatric Disorders: A Clinically-Focused Systematic Review." *BMC Psychiatry* 20: 24.

Sarris, J., et al. (2020). "S-Adenosylmethionine (SAMe) Monotherapy for Depression: An 8-Week Double-Blind, Randomized, Controlled Trial." *Psychopharmacology* 237: 209–218.

Sartim, A. G., et al. (2021). "Co-administration of Cannabidiol and Ketamine Induces Antidepressant-Like Effects Devoid of Hyperlocomotor Side-Effects." *Neuropharmacology* 195: 108679.

Sauerbier, A., et al. (2016). "New Concepts in the Pathogenesis and Presentation of Parkinson's Disease." *Clinical Medicine* 16: 365–370.

Savitz, A., et al. (2021). "Efficacy and Safety of Seltorexant as Adjunctive Therapy in Major Depressive Disorder: A Phase 2B, Randomized, Placebo-Controlled, Adaptive Dose-Finding Study." *International Journal of Neuropsychopharmacology* 24: 965–976.

Sayson, L. V., et al. (2019). "The Novel Methoxetamine Analogs N-Ethylnorketamine Hydrochloride (NENK), 2-MeO-N-Ehthylkeatmine Hydrochloride (2-MeO-NEK), and 4-MeO-N-Ethylketamin Hydrochloride (4-MeO-NEK) Elicit Rapid Antidepressant Effects via Activation of AMPA and 5-HT_2

Receptors." *Psychopharmacology* 236: 2201–2210.

Scammell, T. E., and Winrow, C. (2011). "Orexin Receptors: Pharmacology and Therapeutic Opportunities." *Annual Review of Pharmacology and Toxicology* 51: 243–266. https://doi.org/10.1146/annurev-pharmtox-010510-100528

Schacht, J. P., et al. (2012). "Associations Between Cannabinoid Receptor-1 (CNR1) Variation and Hippocampus and Amygdala Volumes in Heavy Cannabis Users." *Neuropsychopharmacology* 37: 2368–2376.

Schaefer, E. J., et al. (2006). "Plasma Phosphatidyine Docosahexaenoic Acid Content and Risk of Dementia and Alzheimer's Disease." *Archives of Neurology* 63: 1545–1550.

Schedlowski, M., et al. (2015). "Neuro-Bio-Behavioral Mechanisms of Placebo and Nocebo Responses: Implications for Clinical Trials and Clinical Practice." *Pharmacological Review* 67: 697–730.

Scherrer, J. F., et al. (2020). "Comparison of Opioids Prescribed for Patients at Risk for Opioid Misuse Before and After Publication of the Centers for Disease Control and Prevention's Opioid Prescribing Guidelines." *JAMA Network Open* 3: e2027481.

Schifano, F., et al. (2021). "Focus on Over-the-Counter Drugs' Misuse: A Systematic Review on Antihistamines, Cough Medicines, and Decongestants." *Frontiers in Psychiatry* 12: 657397.

Schleider, L. B-L., et al. (2019). "Real Life Experience of Medical Cannabis Treatment in Autism: Analysis of Safety and Efficacy." *Scientific Reports* 9: 200.

Schmid, E., et al. (2016). "Overnight Switching from Oxcarbazepine to Eslicarbazepine Acetate: An Observational Study." *Acta Neurologica Scandinavica* 135: 449–453.

Schneider, J. (2019). "What's in a Name? In This Case, that which We Call Addiction Is Not Dependence." *Practical Pain Management* 18(5): 6–7.

Schnider, P., et al. (2020). "Discovery of Balovaptan, a Vasopressin 1a Receptor Antagonist for the Treatment of Autism Spectrum Disorder." *Journal of Medicinal Chemistry* 63: 1511–1525.

Schoenfelder, E. N., et al. (2014). "Stimulant Treatment of ADHD and Cigarette Smoking: A Meta-Analysis." *Pediatrics* 133: 1070–1080.

Schoevers, J., et al. (2020). "Cannabidiol as a Treatment Option for Schizophrenia: Recent Evidence and Current Studies." *Current Opinions in Psychiatry* 33: 185–191.

Schou, M. (1997). "Forty Years of Lithium Treatment." *Archives of General Psychiatry* 54: 9–23.

Schulman, K.K. et al. (2021). "Will CMS Find Aducanumab Reasonable and Necessary for Alzheimer Disease After FDA Approval?" *JAMA* 326: 383–384.

Schulz, M., et al. (2012). "Therapeutic and Toxic Blood Concentrations of Nearly 1,000 Drugs and Other Xenobiotics." *Critical Care* 16R136.

Schwan, J., et al. (2019). "Chronic Pain Management in the Elderly." *Anesthesiology Clinics* 37: 547–560.

Schwandt, H., et al. (2022). "Changes in the Relationship Between Income and Life Expectancy Before and During the COVID-19 Pandemic, California, 2015–2021." *JAMA* 328: 360–366.

Schwartz, S., and Correll, C. U. (2014). "Efficacy and Safety of Atomoxetine in Children and Adolescents with Attention-Deficit/Hyperactivity Disorder: Results from a Comprehensive Meta-Analysis and Metaregression." *Journal of the American Academy of Child and Adolescent Psychiatry* 53: 174–187.

Schwarzkopf, N., et al. (2018). "Caffeine as an Adulterant of Coca Paste Seized Samples: Preclinical Study on the Rat Sleep–Wake Cycle." *Behavioral Pharmacology* 29: 519–529.

Schweitzer, A. (2014). "A Treasury of Albert Schweitzer." *Open Road Media*, p. 66.

Schwenk, E. S., et al., (2018). "Consensus Guidelines on the Use of Intravenous Ketamine Infusions for Acute Pain Management from the American Society of Regional Anesthesia and Pain Medicine, the American Academy of Pain Medicine and the American Society of Anesthesiologists." *Regional Anesthesia and Acute Pain* 43: 456–466.

Schwitzer, T., et al. (2016). "The Endocannabinoid System in the Retina: From Physiology to Practical and Therapeutic Applications." *Neural Plasticity* 16: 2916732.

Scott, E. C., et al. (2018). "Association of Cannabis with Cognitive Functioning in

Adolescents and Young Adults: A Systematic Review and Meta-Analysis." *JAMA Psychiatry* 75: 585–595.

Scott, J. R., et al. (2018). "Moderate Alcohol Consumption Is Associated with Reduced Pain and Fibromyalgia Symptoms in Chronic Pain Patients." *Pain Medicine* 19: 2525–2527.

Scott, L. J. (2020). "Lemborexant: First Approval." *Drugs* 80: 425–432.

Sealock, T., and Sharma, S. (2020). "Smoking Cessation." *Stat Pearls* January 30.

Seely, K. A., et al. (2011). "Marijuana-Based Drugs: Innovative Therapeutics Designer Drugs of Abuse?" *Molecular Interventions* 11: 36–50.

Segraves, R. T., and Balon, R. (2014). "Antidepressant-Induced Sexual Dysfunction in Men." *Pharmacology, Biochemistry, and Behavior* 121: 132–137.

Seibert, M., et al. (2021). "Efficacy and Safety of Pharmacotherapy for Alzheimer's Disease and for Behavioural and Psychological Symptoms of Dementia in Older Patients with Moderate and Severe Functional Impairments: A Systematic Review of Controlled Trials." *Alzheimers Research & Therapy* 13: 131.

Sekar, A., et al. (2016). "Schizophrenia Risk from Complex Variation of Complement Component 4." *Nature* 530: 177–183.

Selby, P., and Zawertailo, L. (2022). "Tobacco Addiction." *The New England Journal of Medicine* 387: 345–354.

Selph, S. S., and McDonagh, M. S. (2019). "Depression in Children and Adolescents: Evaluation and Treatment." *American Family Physician* 100: 609–617.

Sengpiel, V., et al. (2013). "Maternal Caffeine Intake During Pregnancy Is Associated with Birth Weight but Not with Gestational Length: Results from a Large Perspective Observational Study." *BMC Medicine* 11: 42.

Serna, M., et al. (2015). "Benzodiazepines and Drugs with Anticholinergic Activity Increase Mortality in Patients with Delirium." Annual Meeting of the American Psychiatric Association. Abstract P2–85.

Serowik, K. L., et al. (2021). "Substance Use Disorder Detection Rates Among Providers of General Medical Inpatients." *Journal of General Internal Medicine* 36: 668–675.

Seshachala, B. B., et al. (2021). "Valproate Usage in Pregnancy: An Audit from the Kerala Registry of Epilepsy and Pregnancy." *Epilepsia* 62: 1141–1147.

Sessa, B., et al. (2019). "A Review of 3,4-Methylenediosymethamphetamine (MDMA)-Assisted Psychotherapy." *Frontiers in Psychiatry* 10: 138.

Setien-Suero, E., et al. (2019). "Stopping Cannabis Use Benefits Outcome in Psychosis: Findings from 10-Year Follow-Up Study in the PAFIP-Cohort." *Acta Psychiatrica Scandinavica* 140: 349–359.

Shabir, A., et al. (2018). "The Influence of Caffeine on Sport, Exercise, and Cognitive Performance." *Nutrients* 10: 1528.

Shaerzadeh, F., et al. (2018). "Methamphetamine Neurotoxicity, Microglia, and Neuroinflammation." *Journal of Neuroinflammation* 15: 341.

Shah, K., et al. (2020). "Focus on Mental Health During the Coronavirus (COVID-19) Pandemic: Applying Learnings from the Past Outbreaks. *Cureus* 12: e7405.

Shah, N., et al. (2017). "Clinical Practice Guidelines for Management of Bipolar Disorder." *Indian Journal of Psychiatry* 59: 51–66.

Shah, T., et al. (2021). "Pretreatment Screening and Counseling on Prolonged Erections for Patients Prescribed Trazodone." *Investigative and Clinical Urology* 62: 85–89.

Shalit, N., et al. (2016). "Characteristics of Synthetic Cannabinoid and Cannabis Users Admitted to a Psychiatric Hospital: A Comparative Study." *Journal of Clinical Psychiatry* 77: e989–e995.

Shannon, S., et al. (2019). "Cannabidiol in Anxiety and Sleep: A Large Case Series." *The Permanente Journal* 23: 18–41.

Sharma, R., et al. (2022). "N-Acetyl Cysteine in the Treatment of Cannabis Use Disorder: A Systematic Review of Clinical Trials." *Addictive Behaviors* 129: 107283.

Sharma, T., et al. (2016). "Suicidality and Aggression During Antidepressant Treatment: Systematic Review and Meta-Analyses Based on Clinical Study Reports." *British Medical Journal* 352: i65.

Sharma, V. (2019). "Understanding Antidepressant Tachyphylaxis." *Pharmacological Research* 141: 619.

Shcherbinin, S., et al. (2022). "Association of Amyloid Reduction After Donanemab Treatment with Tau Pathology and Clinical Outcomes: The TRAILBLAZER-ALZ Randomized Clinical Trial." *JAMA Neurology* 2022.2793, In Press.

Shelton, R. C. (2019). "Serotonin and Norepinephrine Reuptake Inhibitors." *Handbook of Experimental Pharmacology* 250: 145–180.

Shen, W. W. (2018). "Anticraving Therapy for Alcohol Use Disorder: A Clinical Review." *Neuropsychopharmacology Reports* 38: 105–116.

Shepherd, C., et al. (2020). "Alzheimer's Amyloid-β and Tau Protein Accumulation Is Associated with Decreased Expression of the LDL Receptor-Associated Protein in Human Brain Tissue." *Brain and Behavior* 10: e01672.

Sherman, B. J., and McRae-Clark, A. L. (2016). "Treatment of Cannabis Use Disorder: Current Science and Future Outlook." *Pharmacotherapy* 36: 511–535.

Sherwood, A. M., et al. (2020). "An Improved, Practical, and Scalable Five-Step Synthesis of Psilocybin." *Synthesis* 52: 688–694.

Sheu, J-J., et al. (2019). "Association Between Anticholinergic Medication Use and Risk of Dementia Among Patients with Parkinson's Disease." *Pharmacotherapy* 39: 798–808.

Shi, M., et al. (2022). "Impact of Anti-amyloid-B Monoclonal Antibodies on the Pathology and Clinical Profile of Alzheimer's Disease: A Focus on Aducanumab and Lecanemab." *Frontiers in Aging Neuroscience* 14: 870517.

Shiffman, S., et al. (2019). "Very-Low-Nicotine-Content Cigarettes and Dependence Among Non-Daily Smokers." *Drug and Alcohol Dependence* 197: 1–7.

Shine, B., et al. (2015). "Long-Term Effects of Lithium on Renal, Thyroid, and Parathyroid Function: A Retrospective Analysis of Laboratory Data." *Lancet* 386: 461–468.

Shoaib, M., and Buhidma, Y. (2018). "Why Are Antidepressant Drugs Effective Smoking Cessation Aids?" *Current Neuropharmacology* 16: 426–437.

Shouan, A., and Grover, S. (2018). "Adjunctive Intranasal Esketamine in Treatment-Resistant Depression." *JAMA Psychiatry* 75: 654.

Shoval, G., et al. (2021). "Evaluation of Attention-Deficit/Hyperactivity Disorder Medications, Externalizing Symptoms, and Suicidality in Children." *JAMA Network Open* 4: e2111342.

Shover, C. L., et al. (2020). "Association of State Policies Allowing Medical Cannabis for Opioid Use Disorder with Dispensary Marketing for This Indication." *JAMA Network Open* 3: e2010001.

Shukla, L., et al. (2017). "Value of Ethyl Glucuronide and Ethyl Sulfate in Serum as Biomarkers of Alcohol Consumption." *Indian Journal of Psychological Medicine* 39: 481–487.

Shyken, J. M., et al. (2019). "Benzodiazepines in Pregnancy." *Clinical Obstetrics and Gynecology* 62: 156–167.

Siegel, A. N., et al. (2021). "Registered Clinical Studies Investigating Psychedelic Drugs for Psychiatric Disorders." *Journal of Psychiatry Research* 139: 71–81.

Sikich, L., et al. (2021). "Intranasal Oxytocin in Children and Adolescents with Autism Spectrum Disorder." *The New England Journal of Medicine* 10: 1056.

Silins, E., et al. (2014). "Young Adult Sequelae of Adolescent Cannabis Use: An Integrative Analysis." *Lancet Psychiatry* 1: 286–293.

Sills, G. J., and Rogawski, M. A. (2020). "Mechanisms of Action of Currently Used Antiseizure Drugs." *Neuropharmacology* 168: 107966.

Silva de Miranda, A., et al. (2019). "Lamotrigine as a Mood Stabilizer: Insights from the Pre-Clinical Evidence." *Expert Opinions in Drug Discovery* 14: 179–190.

Simons, P. (2019). "'Flimsy Evidence' for Esketamine as Depression Treatment." *British Medical Journal* 176, published online October 15.

Simuni, T., et al. (2021). "Efficacy of Nilotinib in Patients with Moderately Advanced Parkinson Disease: A Randomized Clinical Trial." *JAMA Neurology* 78: 312–320.

Singa, R. M. (2016). "Genetic Testing: Adjunct in the Medical Management of Chronic Pain." *Practical Pain Management* 16: 28–31.

Singal, A. K. and Mathurin, P. (2021). "Diagnosis and Treatment of Alcohol-Associated Liver Disease: A Review." *JAMA* 326: 165–176.

Singer, J. A., et al. (2019). "Today's Nonmedical Opioid Users Are Not Yesterday's Patients: Implications of Data Indicating

Stable Rates of Nonmedical Use and Pain Reliever Use Disorder." *Journal of Pain Research* 12: 617–620.

Siemens, W., and Becker, G. (2016). "Methylnaltrexone for Opioid-Induced Constipation: Review and Meta-Analysis for Objective plus Subjective Efficacy and Safety Outcomes." *Therapeutic and Clinical Risk Management* 12: 401–412.

Sindrup, S. H., et al. (2005). "Antidepressants in the Treatment of Neuropathic Pain." *Basic and Clinical Pharmacology and Toxicology* 96: 399–409.

Singh, B., et al. (2016). "Efficacy of Prazosin in Posttraumatic Stress Disorder: A Systematic Review and Meta-Analysis." *Primary Care Companion CNS Disorders* 18.

Sinha, S., et al. (2021). "A Phase III Prospective Active and Placebo-Controlled Randomized Trial of Vilazodone in the Treatment of Major Depressive Disorder." *Cureus* 13: e16689.

Sivilotti, M. L. A. (2016). "Flumazenil, Naloxone, and the 'Coma Coctail'" *British Journal of Clinical Pharmacology* 81: 428–436.

Skinner, M. D., et al. (2014). "Disulfiram Efficacy in the Treatment of Alcohol Dependence: A Meta-Analysis." *PLOS One* 9: e87366.

Skolnick, P. (2021). "Treatment of Overdose in the Synthetic Opioid Era." *Pharmacology & Therapeutics* 9: 108019.

Slade, T., et al. (2016). "Birth Cohort Trends in the Global Epidemiology of Alcohol Use and Alcohol-Related Harms in Men and Women: Systematic Review and Metaregression." *BMJ Open* 6: e011827. http://bmjopen.bmj.com/content/6/10/e011827.full.

Slater, M. E., and Alpert, H. R. (2021), "Surveillance Report #117. Apparent Per Capita Alcohol Consumption: National, State, and Regional Trends, 1977–2019." U.S. Department of Health and Human Services, Public Health Service, National Institutes of Health.

Slomski, A. (2021a). "Thousands of US Youths Cope with the Trauma of Losing Parents to COVID-19." *JAMA* 326: 2117–2119.

Slomski, A. (2021b). "Pediatric Depression and Anxiety Doubled During the Pandemic." *JAMA* 326: 1246.

Smid, M. C., et al. (2019). "Stimulant Use in Pregnancy—An Under-Recognized Epidemic Among Pregnant Women." *Clinical Obstetrics and Gynecology* 62: 168–184.

Smigielski, L., et al. (2019). Psilocybin-Assisted Mindfulness Training Modulates Self-Consciousness and brain Default Mode Network Connectivity with Lasting Effects." *Neuroimage* 196: 207–215.

Smith, B. J., and Lim, M. H. (2020). "How the COVID-19 Pandemic Is Focusing Attention on Loneliness and Social Isolation." *Public Health Research and Practice* 30: 3022008.

Smith, K. R., et al. (2021). "Methylphenidate Use in Geriatric Depression: A Systematic Review." *International Journal of Geriatric Psychiatry* 36: 1304–1312.

Smith, M. J., et al. (2015). "Cannabis-Related Episodic Memory Deficits and Hippocampal Morphological Differences in Healthy Individuals and Schizophrenic Subjects." *Hippocampus* 25: 1042–1051.

Smith, P. (2015). "Can the Bacteria in Your Gut Explain Your Mood?" *New York Times*, September 23, 2015.

Smith, T. T., et al. (2019). "The Impact of Gradual and Immediate Nicotine Reduction on Subjective Cigarette Ratings." *Nicotine and Tobacco Research* 21 (Supplement 1): S73–S80.

Smith, W. R., and Appelbaum, P. S. (2021). "Two Models of Legalization of Psychedelic Substances: Reason for Concern." *JAMA*. Published online August 20.

Smolyakova, A., et al. (2020). "The Endo-cannabinoid System and Synthetic Cannabinoids in Preclinical Models of Seizure and Epilepsy." *Journal of Clinical Neurophysiology* 37: 15–27.

Soares, V. P., and Campos, A. C. (2017). "Evidence for the Anti-Panic Actions of Cannabidiol." *Current Neuropharmacology* 15: 291–299.

Soderstrom, K., et al. (2017). "Cannabinoids Modulate Neuronal Activity and Cancer by CB1 and CB2 Receptor-Independent Mechanisms." *Frontiers in Pharmacology* 8: 720.

Soeter, M., and Kindt, M. (2015). "An Abrupt Transformation of Phobic Behavior After a Post-Retrieval Amnesic Agent." *Biological Psychiatry* 78: 880–886.

Solmi, M., et al. (2020). "Safety of 80 Antidepressants, Antipsychotics, Anti-Attention-Deficit/Hyperactivity Medications and Mood Stabilizers in Children and Adolescents with Psychiatric Disorders: A Large Scale Systematic Meta-Review of 78 Adverse Effects." *World Psychiatry* 19: 214–232.

Solmi, M., et al. (2022). "Physical and Mental Health Impact of COVID-19 on Children, Adolescents, and Their Families: The Collaborative Outcomes Study on Health and Functioning during Infection Times—Children and Adolescents (COH-FIT-C&A)." *Journal of Affective Disorders* 299: 367–376.

Song, I-U., et al. (2021). "Possible Neuroprotective Effects of Rasagiline in Alzheimer's Disease: A SPECT Study." *Acta Radiologica* 62: 784–790.

Song, J., et al. (2017). "Suicidal Behavior During Lithium and Valproate Treatment: A Within-Individual 8-Year Prospective Study of 50,000 Patients with Bipolar Disorder." *American Journal of Psychiatry* 174: 795–802.

Song, X. et. al. (2019). A meta-analysis of naldemedine for the treatment of opioid-induced constipation. *Expert review of clinical pharmacology*, *12*(2), 121–128. https://doi.org/10.1080/17512433.2019.1570845

Sowell, E. R., et al. (2010). "Differentiating Prenatal Exposure to Methamphetamine and Alcohol Versus Alcohol and Not Methamphetamine Using Tensor-Based Brain Morphometry and Discriminant Analysis." *Journal of Neuroscience* 30: 3876–3885.

Soyka, M. (2017). "Treatment of Benzodiazepine Dependence." *New England Journal of Medicine* 376: 1147–1157.

Sparacino, G., et al. (2022). "Existing and Emerging Pharmacological Approaches to the Treatment of Mania: A Critical Overview." *Translational Psychiatry* 12: 169.

Specchio, N., et al. (2021). "Is Cenobamate the Breakthrough We Have Been Wishing For?" *International Journal of Molecular Science* 22: 9339.

Spijker, J., et al. (2020). "Advice for Clinicians on How to Treat Comorbid Anxiety and Depression." *JAMA Psychiatry* 77: 645–646.

Sprenger, J. J., et al. (2020). "Bumetanide for Core Symptoms of Autism Spectrum Disorder (BAMBI): A Single Center, Double-Blinded, Participant-Randomized, Placebo-Controlled, Phase Two, Superiority Trial." *Journal of American Academy of Child and Adolescent Psychiatry* 60: 937–938.

Squeglia, L. M., et al. (2015). "Brain Development in Heavy-Drinking Adolescents." *American Journal of Psychiatry* 172: 531–542.

Srivastava, A. B., et al. (2020). "New Directions in the Treatment of Opioid Withdrawal." *Lancet* 395: 1938–1948.

Stahl, S. M., et al. (2017). "Guidelines for the Recognition and Management of Mixed Depression." *CNS Spectrum* 22: 203–219.

Stahl, S. M., et al. (2020). "Cariprazine as a Treatment Across the Bipolar 1 Spectrum from Depression to Mania: Mechanism of Action and Review of Clinical Data." *Therapeutic Advances in Psychopharmacology* 10: 1–11.

Stanciu, C. N., et al. (2021). "Evidence for Use of Cannabinoids in Mood Disorders, Anxiety Disorders, and PTSD: A Systematic Review." *Psychiatric Services* 72: 429–436.

Steenen, S. A., et al. (2016). "Propranolol for the Treatment of Anxiety Disorders: Systematic Review and Meta-Analysis." *Journal of Psychopharmacology* 30: 128–139.

Stein, D. J., et al. (2014). "Agomelatine in Generalized Anxiety Disorder: An Active Comparator and Placebo-Controlled Study." *Journal of Clinical Psychiatry* 75: 362–368.

Stein, D. J., et al. (2021). "Efficacy of Agomelanine 25-50 mg for the Treatment of Anxious Symptoms and Functional Impairment in General Anxiety Disorder: A Meta-Analysis of Three Placebo-Controlled Studies." *Advances in Therapeutics* 38: 1567–1583.

Steinhoff, B. J. (2021). "Cenobamate Tablets as a Treatment for Focal-Onset Seizures in Adults: *Expert Reviews in Clinical Pharmacology* 14: 161–172.

Stephenson, J. (2022). "Commission Outlines New Strategies to Combat Opioid Crisis." *JAMA Health Forum* 3: e220382.

Stocchi, F., et al. (2015, February 25). "How to Optimize the Treatment of Early Stage Parkinson's Disease." *Translational Neurodegeneration* 4: 4.

Strand, M. C., et al. (2019). "A Clinical Trial on the Acute Effects of Methadone and Buprenorphine on Actual Driving and Cognitive Function of Healthy Volunteers." *British Journal of Clinical Pharmacology* 85: 442–453.

Strang, J., et al. (2019). "Take-Home Naloxone for the Emergency Interim Management of Opioid Overdose: The Public Health Application of an Emergency Medicine." *Drugs* 79: 1395–1418.

Straub, L., et al. (2022). "Association of Antipsychotic Drug Exposure in Pregnancy with Risk of Neurodevelopmental Disorders: A National Birth Cohort Study." *JAMA Internal Medicine* 182: 522–533.

Strawn, J. R., et al. (2010). "Psychopharmacological Treatment of Posttraumatic Stress Disorder in Children and Adolescents: A Review." *Journal of Clinical Psychiatry* 71: 932–941.

Strong, D. R., et al. (2021). "Effect of Graphic Warning Labels on Cigarette Packs on US Smokers' Cognitions and Smoking Behavior After 3 Months: A Randomized Clinical Trial." *JAMA Network Open* 4: e2121387, August 4.

Stuyt, E. (2018). "The Problem with the Current High Potency THC Marijuana from the Perspective of an Addiction Psychiatrist." *Missouri Medicine* 115: 482–486.

Subodh, R. N., et al. (2017). "Prevalence of Dual Diagnosis among Clinic Attending Patients in an Addiction Centre of a Tertiary Care Hospital." *Asian Journal of Psychiatry* Feb. 25: 169–174.

Substance Abuse and Mental Health Services Administration [SAMHSA]. (2014, August 7). Emergency Department Visits Attributed to Overmedication That Involved the Insomnia Medication Zolpidem." *Dawn Report*.

Substance Abuse and Mental Health Services Administration [SAMHSA. (2019). "Key Substance Use and Mental Health Indicators in the United States: Results from the 2018 National Survey on Drug Use and Health." Rockville, MD. Center For Behavioral Health Statistics and Quality, Substance Abuse and Mental Health Services Administration. Health & Human Services Publication No. PEP-19-5068.

Substance Abuse and Mental Health Services Administration [SAMHSA]. (2020). "Key Substance Use and Mental Health Indicators in the United States: Results from the 2019 National Survey on Drug Use and Health. *Center for Behavioral Health Statistics and Quality, Substance Abuse and Mental Health Services Administration.*

Substance Abuse and Mental Health Services Administration [SAMHSA]. (2021a). "Prescription Stimulant Misuse and Prevention Among Youth and Young Adults." Publication No. PEP21-06-01-003.

Substance Abuse and Mental Health Services Administration [SAMHSA]. (2021b). "Tip 63: Medications for Opioid Use Disorder." SAMHSA Publications and Digital Products, PEP21-02-01-002.

Substance Abuse and Mental Health Services Administration [SAMHSA. (2022). "Prevention of Substance Use and Mental Disorders."

Sun, A. Y., et al. (2019). "Safety Considerations in the Psychopharmacology of Pediatric Bipolar Disorder." *Expert Opinions in Drug Safety* 18: 777–794.

Sun, J. W., et al. (2022). "Comparison Rate of Type-2 Diabetes in Adults and Children Treated with Anticonvulsant Mood Stabilizers." *JAMA Network Open* 5: e226484.

Sun, R., et al. (2021). "Trends in Nicotine Product Use Among US Adolescents, 1999–2020." *JAMA Network Open* 4: e2118788.

Sun, Y., et al. (2019). "Trend of Antidepressants Before, During, and After Pregnancy Across Two Decades—A Population-Based Study." *Brain and Behavior* 9: e01441.

Suthoff, E., et al. (2022). "Patient-Reported Health-Related Quality of Life from a Randomized, Placebo-Controlled Phase 2 Trial of Zuranolone in Adults with Major Depressive Disorder." *Journal of Affective Disorders* 308: 19–26.

Svatikova, A., et al. (2015). "A Randomized Trial of Cardiovascular Responses to Energy Drink Consumption in Healthy Adults." *JAMA* 314: 2079–2082.

Swanson, C. J., et al. (2022). "Correction to: A Randomized, Double-Blind, Phase 2b Proof-of-Concept Trial in Early Alzheimer's Disease with Lecanemab, an Anti-AB Protofibril Antibody." *Alzheimer's Research & Therapy* 14: 70.

Swanson, J. M., and MTA Cooperative Group. (2017). "Young Adult Outcomes in the Follow-Up of the Multimodal Treatment Study of Attention-Deficit/Hyperactivity Disorder: Symptom Persistence, Source Discrepancy, and Height Suppression." *Journal of Child Psychology and Psychiatry and Allied Disciplines* 58: 663–678.

Syed, A. B., and Brasic, J. R. (2021). "The Role of Lumateperone in the Treatment of Schizophrenia." *Therapeutic Advances in Psychopharmacology* 11: 20451253211034019.

Sys, J., et al. (2020). "Efficacy and Safety of Non-Benzodiazepine and Non-Z-Drug Hypnotic Medication for Insomnia in Older People: A Systematic Literature Review." *European Journal of Clinical Pharmacology* 76: 363–381.

Szczesniak, D., et al. (2020). "The SARS-CoV-2 and Mental Health: From Biological Mechanisms to Social Consequences."

Progress in Neuropsychopharmacology and Biological Psychiatry 104: 110046.

Szoko, E., et al. (2018). "Pharmacological Aspects of the Neuroprotective Effects of Irreversible MAO-B Inhibitors, Selegiline and Rasagiline, in Parkinson's Disease." *Journal of Neural Transmission* 125: 1735–1749.

Tabi, T., et al. (2020). "Selegiline: A Molecule with Innovative Potential." *Journal of Neural Transmission* 127: 831–842.

Tabuteau, H., et al. (2022). "Effect of AXS-05 (Dextromethorphan-Bupropion) in Major Depressive Disorder: A Randomized Double-Blind Controlled Trial." *American Journal of Psychiatry* 179: 490–499.

Tai, S. J., et al. (2021). "Development and Evaluation of a Therapist Training Program for Psilocybin Therapy for Treatment-Resistant Depression in Clinical Research." *Frontiers in Psychiatry* 12: 586682.

Taipale, H., et al. (2018). Antipsychotics and Mortality in a Nationwide Cohort of 29,823 Patients with Schizophrenia, *Schizophrenia Research* 197: 274-280.

Taipale, H., et al., (2020). "20-Year Follow-Up Study of Physical Morbidity and Mortality in Relationship to Antipsychotic Treatment in a Nationwide Cohort of 62,250 Patients with Schizophrenia (FIN20)." *World Psychiatry* 19: 61–68.

Talal, A. H., et al. (2020). "Toward Precision Prescribing for Methadone: Determinants of Methadone Deposition." *PLos One* 15: e0231467.

Talarico, G., et al. (2019). "Modulation of the Cannabinoid System: A New Perspective for the Treatment of the Alzheimer's Disease." *Current Neuropharmacology* 17: 176–183.

Talarico, I. (2021). "The Use of Telehealth to Increase Mental Health Services Access and Promote Medication Adherence in Rural Locations." *Journal of the American Association of Nurse Practitioners* 33: 1074–1079.

Talati, A., et al. (2016). "Changing Relationships Between Smoking and Psychiatric Disorders Across Twentieth Century Birth Cohorts: Clinical and Research Implications." *Molecular Psychiatry* 21: 464–471.

Tamminga, C. A., et al. (2012). "Glutamate Dysfunction in Hippocampus: Relevance of Dentate Gyrus and CA3 Signaling." *Schizophrenia Bulletin* 38: 927–935.

Tampi, R. R., et al. (2018). "Suvorexant for Insomnia in Older Adults: A Perspective Review." *Drugs in Context* 7: 212517.

Tampi, R. R., et al. (2019). "Evidence for Using Pimavanserin for the Treatment of Parkinson's Disease Psychosis." *World Journal of Psychiatry* 9: 47–54.

Tan, C. H., et al. (2015). "Alcohol Use and Binge Drinking Among Women of Childbearing Age—United States, 2011–2013." *Morbidity and Mortality Weekly Report* (MMWR) 64: 1042–1046.

Tan, S. N., and Tan, C. (2021). "Vortioxetine Improves Cognition in Mild Cognitive Impairment." *International Clinical Psychopharmacology* 36: 279–287.

Taquet, M., et al. (2020). "Mood Homeostasis, Low Mood, and History of Depression in 2 Large Population Samples." *JAMA Psychiatry* 77: 944–951.

Taquet, M., et al. (2021). "6-Month Neurological and Psychiatric Outcomes in 236,379 Survivors of COVID-19: A Retrospective Cohort Study Using Electronic Health Records." *Lancet Psychiatry* 8: 416–427.

Targum, S. D. (2014). "Identification and Treatment of Antidepressant Tachyphylaxis." *Innovations in Clinical Neuroscience* 11: 24–28.

Tariot, P. N., et al. (2021). "Trial of Pimavanserin in Dementia-Related Psychosis." *New England Journal of Medicine* 385: 309–319.

Tau, G. Z., et al. (2014). "Neural Correlates of Reward-Based Spatial Learning in Persons with Cocaine Dependence." *Neuropsychopharmacology* 39: 545–555.

Taylor, L., et al. (2020). "Abrupt Withdrawal of Cannabidiol (CBD): A Randomized Trial." *Journal of Epilepsy and Behavior* 104: 106938.

Taylor, M. J., et al. (2020). "Etiology of Autism Spectrum Disorders and Autistic Traits Over Time." *JAMA Psychiatry,* 77: 936–943.

Teixeira, F. G., et al. (2018). "Safinamide: A New Hope for Parkinson's Disease?" *Drug Discoveries Today* 23: 736–744.

Teixeira-Gomez, A., et al. (2015). "The Neurotoxicity of Amphetamines During the Adolescent Period." *International Journal of Developmental Neurosciences* 41: 44–62.

Teng, E., et al. (2022). "Safety and Efficacy of Semorinemab in Individuals with Prodromal to Mild Alzheimer Disease: A Randomized Clinical Trial." *JAMA Neurology.* 79: 758–767.

Tennant, F. (2016). "Genetic Testing in High-Dose Opioid Patients." *Practical Pain Management* 16: 10–18.

Tenore, G. C., et al. (2015). "Coffee and Depression: A Short Review of Literature." *Current Pharmaceutical Design* 21: 5034–5040.

Thakrar, A. P. (2022). "Short-Acting Opioids for Hospitalized Patients with Opioid Use Disorder." *JAMA Internal Medicine* 182(3): 247–248.

Thase, M. E., et al. (2019). "Results from a Long-Term Open-Label Extension Study of Adjunctive Buprenorphine/Samidorphan Combination in Patients with Major Depressive Disorder." *Neuropsychopharmacology* 44: 2268–2276.

Thase, M. E., et al. (2020). "Improving Cost-Effectiveness and Access to Cognitive Behavior Therapy for Depression: Providing Remote-Ready Computer-Assisted Psychotherapy in Times of Crisis and Beyond." *Psychotherapeutics and Psychosomatics* 89: 307–313.

Thesing, C. S., et al. (2020). "Fatty Acids and Recurrence of Major Depressive Disorder: Combined Analysis of Two Dutch Clinical Cohorts." *Acta Psychiatrica Scandinavica* 141: 362–373.

Thien, C. (2021). "Forgotten Analgesics: The Drugs Pain Practitioners Need to Reconsider." *Practical Pain Management* 21: VH0024790.

Thigpen, J. C., et al. (2019). "Opioids: A Review of Pharmacokinetics and Pharmacodynamics in Neonates, Infants and Children." *European Journal of Drug Metabolism and Pharmacokinetics* 44: 591–609.

Thomas, A. J., et al. (2022). "A Longitudinal Study of Plasma pTau181 in Mild Cognitive Impairment with Lewy Bodies and Alzheimer's Disease." *Movement Disorders: Official Journal of the Movement Disorder Society* 37: 1495–1504.

Thomas, J. M., et al. (2018). "The 5-HT2C Receptor Agonist Meta-chlorophenylpiperazine (mCPP) Reduces Palatable Food Consumption and BOLD fMRI Responses to Food Images in Healthy Female Volunteers." *Psychopharmacology* 235: 257–267.

Thompson, P. M., et al. (2004). "Structural Abnormalities in the Brains of Human Subjects Who Use Methamphetamine." *Journal of Neuroscience* 24: 6028–6036.

Thompson, R. H. (2000). *The Brain: A Neuroscience Primer,* 3rd ed. New York: Worth.

Thong, B. Y-U. (2020). "Drug Hypersensitivity Reactions in Asia: Regional Issues and Challenges." *Asia Pacific Allergy* 10: e8.

Tiihonen, J., et al. (2019). "Association of Antipsychotic Polypharmacy vs Monotherapy with Psychiatric Rehospitalization among Adults with Schizophrenia." *JAMA Psychiatry* 76: 499–507.

Tiihonen, J., et al. (2022). "Long-Term Treatment with Clozapine and Other Antipsychotic Drugs and the Risk of Haematological Malignancies in People with Schizophrenia: A Nationwide Case-Control and Cohort Study in Finland." *Lancet Psychiatry* 9: 353–362.

Tirado-Munoz, J., et al. (2018). "Dual Diagnosis in Depression: Treatment Recommendations." *Adicciones* 30: 66–76.

Toffol, E., et al. (2015). "Lithium Is Associated with Decrease in All-Cause and Suicide Mortality in High-Risk Bipolar Patients: A Nationwide Registry-Based Prospective Cohort Study." *Journal of Affective Disorders* 183: 159–165.

Tohen, M. (2021). "Cariprazine as a Treatment Option for Depressive Episodes Associated with Bipolar I Disorder in Adults: An Evidence-Based Review of Recent Data." *Drug Design, Development and Therapy* 15: 2005–2012.

Tolppanen, A-M., et al. (2016). "Antipsychotic Use and Risk of Hospitalization or Death Due to Pneumonia in Persons with and Those Without Alzheimer Disease." *Chest* 150: 1233–1241.

Tomson, T., and Battino, D. (2009). "Teratogenic Effects of Antiepileptic Medications." *Neurology Clinics* 27: 993–1002.

Tomson, T., et al. (2019). "Teratogenicity of Antiepileptic Drugs." *Current Opinions in Neurology* 32: 246–252.

Tondo, L., et al. (2019). "Clinical Use of Lithium Salts: Guide for Users and Prescribers." *International Journal of Bipolar Disorders* 7: 16.

Tonstad, S., et al. (2011). "Dianicline, a Novel $\alpha_4\beta_2$ Nicotinic Acetylcholine Receptor Partial Agonist, for Smoking Cessation: A Randomized Placebo-Controlled Clinical Trial." *Nicotine and Tobacco Research* 13: 1–6.

Torales, J., et al. (2020). "The Outbreak of COVID-19 Coronavirus and Its Impact on Global Mental Health." *International Journal of Social Psychiatry* 66: 317–320.

Tormoehlen, L. M., et al. (2014). "Hydrocarbon Toxicity: A Review." *Clinical Toxicology* 52: 479–489.

Torpy, J. M., and Livingston, P. H. (2013). "Energy Drinks." *JAMA* 309: 297.

Torrance, N., et al. (2020). "Trends in Gabapentinoid Prescribing, Co-Prescribing of Opioids and Benzodiazepines, and Associated Deaths in Scotland." *British Journal of Aneasthesiology* 125: 159–167.

Torres, C. A., et al. (2020). "Totality of the Evidence Suggests Prenatal Cannabis Exposure Does Not Lead to Cognitive Impairments: A Systematic and Critical Review." *Frontiers in Psychology* 11: 816.

Torres, C., et al. (2021). "Response: Commentary: Totality of the Evidence Suggests Prenatal Cannabis Exposure Does Not Lead to Cognitive Impairments: A Systematic and Critical Review." *Frontiers in Psychology* 12: 651064.

Tran, K., and Ford, C. (2020). "Lurasidone Hydrochloride for Bipolar Disorder; A Review of Clinical Effectiveness, Cost-Effectiveness, and Guidelines [Internet]." *Canadian Agency for Drugs and Technologies in Health, Feb. 20, CADTH Rapid Response Reports.*

Trauer, J. M., et al. (2015). "Cognitive-Behavioral Therapy for Chronic Insomnia: A Systematic Review and Meta-Analysis." *Annals of Internal Medicine* 163: 191–204.

Treatment for Adolescents with Depression Study (TADS) Team. (2004). "Fluoxetine, Cognitive-Behavioral Therapy, and Their Combination for Adolescents with Depression: Treatment for Adolescents with Depression Study (TADS) Randomized Controlled Trial." *JAMA* 292: 807–820.

Trecki, J., et al. (2015). "Synthetic Cannabinoid—Related Illnesses and Deaths." *New England Journal of Medicine* 373: 103–107.

Tsai, D. H., et al. (2021). "Comparison of Water Pipes vs Other Modes of Cannabis Consumption and Subsequent Illicit Drug Use in a Longitudinal Cohort of Young Swiss Men." *JAMA Network Open* 4: e213220.

Tsai, H.-H., et al. (2012). "Evaluation of Documented Drug Interactions and Contraindications Associated with Herbs and Dietary Supplements." *International Journal of Clinical Practice* 66: 1056–1078.

Tundo, A., et al. (2022a). "Efficacy and Safety of 24-Week Pramipexole Augmentation in Patients with Treatment Resistant Depression: A Retrospective Cohort Study." *Progress in Neuropsychopharmacology & Biological Psychiatry* 112: 110425.

Tundo, A., et al. (2022b). "Serotonin Reuptake Inhibitor–Cognitive Behavioural Therapy–Second Generation Antipsychotic Combination for Severe Treatment-Resistant Obsessive-Compulsive Disorder: A Prospective Observational Study." *International Journal of Psychiatry in Clinical Practice* 24: 1–6.

Tupper, K. W., et al. (2015). "Psychedelic Medicine: A Re-emerging Therapeutic Paradigm." *Canadian Medical Association Journal* 187: 1054–1059.

Turcotte, C., et al. (2016). "Impact of Cannabis, Cannabinoids, and Endocannabinoids in the Lungs." *Frontiers in Pharmacology* 7: 317.

Turna, J., et al. (2019). "Cannabidiol as a Novel Candidate Alcohol Use Disorder Pharmacotherapy: A Systematic Review." *Alcoholism: Clinical and Experimental Research* 43: 550–563.

Turnbull, D., et al. (2017). "Caffeine and Cardiovascular Health." *Regulatory Toxicology and Pharmacology* 89: 165–185.

Turner, R., and Agrawal, S. (2020, April 27). "Marijuana." *StatPearls*.

Tysnes, O-B., and Storstein, A. (2017). "Epidemiology of Parkinson's Disease." *Journal of Neural Transmission* 124: 901–905.

U.S. Department of Health and Human Services. (1964). "Smoking and Health: A Report of the Advisory Committee to the Surgeon General of the Public Health Service." Centers for Disease Control and Prevention, Office of Smoking and Health. U.S. Government Printing Office.

U.S. Department of Health and Human Services. (1988). "The Health Consequences of Smoking—Nicotine Addiction: A Report of the Surgeon General." Centers for Disease Control and Prevention, Office of Smoking and Health. U.S. Government Printing Office.

U.S. Department of Health and Human Services. (2001). "Women and Smoking: A Report of the Surgeon General." Centers for Disease Control and Prevention, Office of Smoking and Health. U.S. Government Printing Office.

U.S. Department of Health and Human Services. (2004). "The Health Consequences of Smoking: A Report of the Surgeon General." Centers for Disease Control and Prevention, Office of Smoking and Health. U.S. Government Printing Office.

U.S. Department of Health and Human Services. (2006). "The Health Consequences of Involuntary Exposure to Tobacco Smoke: A Report of the Surgeon General." Centers for Disease Control and Prevention, Office of Smoking and Health. U.S. Government Printing Office.

U.S. Department of Health and Human Services. (2012). "Preventing Tobacco Use Among Youth and Young Adults: A Report of the Surgeon General." Centers for Disease Control and Prevention, Office of Smoking and Health. U.S. Government Printing Office.

U.S. Department of Health and Human Services. (2016a). *"E-Cigarette Use Among Youth and Young Adults*, Chapter 1. Introduction, Conclusions, and Historical Background Relative to E-Cigarettes." Centers for Disease Control and Prevention, Office of Smoking and Health.

U.S. Department of Health and Human Services. (2016b). *Facing Addiction in America: The Surgeon General's Report on Alcohol, Drugs, and Health.*

U.S. Department of Health and Human Services. (2020). "Smoking Cessation: A Report of the Surgeon General." Centers for Disease Control and Prevention, Office of Smoking and Health. U.S. Government Printing Office.

U.S. Department of Health and Human Services. (2021). "Medication Treatment for Autism." National Institutes of Health.

U.S. Food and Drug Administration. (2017). "Want to Quit Smoking? FDA-Approved Products Can Help." *FDA Drug Safety Communication*. http://www.fda.gov/consumers/consumer-updates/want-quit-smoking-fda-approved-products-can-help

U.S. Food and Drug Administration. (2018). "FDA Revises Description of Mental Health Side Effect s of the Stop-Smoking Medicines Chantix (varenicline) and Zyban (bupropion) to Reflect Clinical Trial Findings." *FDA News Release,* April 30.

U.S. Food and Drug Administration. (2019a). "FDA Permits Sale of IQOS Tobacco Heating System Through Premarket Tobacco Product Application Pathway." *FDA Drug Safety Communication*, 2018.

U.S. Food and Drug Administration. (2019b). "FDA Permits Sale of Two New Reduced Nicotine Cigarettes Through Premarket Tobacco Product Application Pathway." *FDA News Release*, December 17.

U.S. Food and Drug Administration. (2019c). "FDA Grants First-Ever Modified Risk Orders to Eight Smokeless Tobacco Products." *FDA News Release,* October 22.

U.S. Food and Drug Administration. (2021a). "Accidental Exposure to Fentanyl Patches Continue to Be Deadly to Children." www.fda.gov/cmsumers/consumer-updates/accidental-exposures-fentanyl-patches-continue-be-deadly-children

U.S. Food and Drug Administration. (2021b, December 2). "FDA Is Temporarily Exercising Enforcement Discretion with Respect to Certain Clozapine REMS Program Requirements to Ensure Continuity of Care for Patients Taking Clozapine."

U.S. Food and Drug Administration. (2022). "Youth and Tobacco." June 29.

U.S. Preventive Services Task Force. (2020a). "Screening for Unhealthy Drug Use: US Preventive Services Task Force Recommendation Statement." *JAMA* 323: 2301–2309.

U.S. Preventive Services Task Force. (2020b). "Primary Care Based Interventions to Prevent Illicit Drug Use in Children, Adolescents, and Young Adults: US Preventive Services Task Force Recommendation Statement." *JAMA* 323: 2060–2066.

U.S. Preventive Services Task Force. (2020c). "Primary Care Interventions for Prevention and Cessation of Tobacco Use in Children and Adolescents: US Preventive Services Task Force Recommendation Statement." *JAMA* 323: 1590–1598.

U.S. Preventive Services Task Force. (2022a). "Screening for Anxiety in Children and Adolescents: US Preventive Services Task Force Recommendation Statement." *JAMA* 328: 1438–1444.

U.S. Preventive Services Task Force. (2022b). "Screening for Depression and Suicide Risk in Children and Adolescents: US Preventive Services Task Force Recommendation Statement." *JAMA* 328: 1534–1542.

Uguz, F., and Sharma, V. (2016). "Mood Stabilizers During Breast-Feeding: A

Systematic Review of the Recent Literature." *Bipolar Disorder* 18: 325–333.

Ursini, F., et al. (2021). "Fibromyalgia: A New Facet of the Post-COVID-19 Syndrome Spectrum? Results from a Web-Based Survey." *Rheumatic & Musculoskeletal Diseases Open* 7: e001735.

USAFACTS. (2022). "US COVID-19 Cases and Deaths by State." USAfacts.org/visualizations/coronavirus-covid-19-spread-map/.

Uspal, N., et al. (2019). "Pediatric Pain Management in the Emergency Department." *Pediatric Emergency Medicine Practice* 16: 1–24.

Vahla, I. V., et al. (2020). "Older Adults and the Mental Health Effects of COVID-19." *JAMA* 324: 2253–2254.

Vahratian, A., et al. (2021). "Symptoms of Anxiety or Depressive Disorder and Use of Mental Health Care Among Adults During the COVID-19 Pandemic—United States, August 2020–February 2021." Centers for Disease Control and Prevention, *Morbidity and Mortality Weekly Report* 70: 490–494.

Vaillant, G. E. (1996). "A Long-Term Follow-Up of Male Alcohol Abuse." *Archives of General Psychiatry* 53: 243–249.

Vajda, F. J., et al. (2017). "Antiepileptic Drugs, Foetal Malformations and Spontaneous Abortions." *Acta Neurologic Scandinavica* 135(3): 360–365.

van Dam, R. M., et al. (2020). "Coffee, Caffeine, and Health." *NEJM* 383: 369–378.

Van den Elsen, G., et al. (2015). "Tetrahydrocannabinol for Neuropsychiatric Symptoms in Dementia: A Randomized Controlled Trial." *Neurology* 84: 2338–2346.

van Dyck, C. H., et al. (2021). "Neurobiologic Rationale for Treatment of Apathy in Alzheimer's Disease with Methylphenidate." *American Journal of Geriatric Psychiatry* 29: 51–62.

van Leeuwen, W. E., et al. (2009). "Collaborative Depression Care for the Old-Old: Findings from the IMPACT Trial." *American Journal of Geriatric Psychiatry* 17: 1040–1049.

Van Schalkwyk, G. I., et al. (2017). "Efficacy of Antipsychotics for Irritability and Aggression in Children: A Meta-Analysis." *Expert Reviews in Neurotherapeutics* 17: 1045–1053.

Váradi, A., et al. (2016). "Mitragynine/Corynantheidine Pseudoindoxyls as Opioid Analgesics with Mu Agonism and Delta Antagonism, Which Do Not Recruit β-Arrestin-2." *Journal of Medical Chemistry* 59(18): 8381–8397.

Vargas, A. S., et al. (2020). "Psilocybin as a New Approach to Treat Depression and Anxiety in the Context of Life-Threatening Diseases—A Systematic Review and Meta-Analysis of Clinical Trials." *Biomedicines* 8: 331.

Varker, T., et al. (2021). "Efficacy of Psychoactive Drugs for the Treatment of Posttraumatic Stress Disorder: A Systematic Review of MDMA, Ketamine, LSD and Psilocybin." *Journal of Psychoactive Drugs* 53: 85–95.

Vassallo, N., et al. (2014). "Good Things in Life: Can Coffee Consumption Reduce the Risk of Developing Alzheimer's Disease?" Institute for Scientific Information on Coffee, from 24th Annual Alzheimer Europe Conference, October 23, 2014.

Vega, M. L., et al. (2020). "Implementation of Advanced Methods for Reproductive Pharmacovigilance in Autism: A Meta-Analysis of the Effects of Prenatal Antidepressant Exposure." *American Journal of Psychiatry* 177: 506–517.

Velayudhan, L., et al. (2021). "Evaluation of THC-Related Neuropsychiatric Symptoms Among Adults Aged 50 Years and Older. A Systematic Review and Metaregression Analysis." *JAMA Network Open* 4: e2035913.

Velosa, J., et al. (2020). "Risk of Dementia in Bipolar Disorder and the Interplay of Lithium: A Systematic Review and Meta-Analyses." *Acta Psychitrica Scandinavica* 141: 510–521.

Verdolini, N., et al. (2021). "Long-Term Treatment of Bipolar Disorder Type I: A Systematic and Critical Review of Clinical Guidelines with Derived Practice Algorithms." *Bipolar Disorder*. 23: 324–340.

Veroniki, A. A., et al. (2017). "Comparative Safety of Anti-Epileptic Drugs During Pregnancy: A Systematic Review and Network Meta-Analysis of Congenital Malformations and Prenatal Outcomes." *BMC Medicine* 15: 95.

Vetreno, R. P., and Crews, F. T. (2015). "Binge Ethanol Exposure During Adolescence Leads to a Persistent Loss of Neurogenesis in the Dorsal and Ventral Hippocampus That Is Associated with Impaired Adult Cognitive Functioning." *Frontiers in Neuroscience* 9: 35.

Vieta, E., and Montes, J. M. (2018). "A Review of Asenapine in the Treatment of Bipolar Disorder." *Clinical Drug Investigations* 38: 87–99.

Vieta, E., et al. (2021). "Two Randomized, Double-Blind, Placebo Controlled Trials and One Open-Label, Long-Term Trial of Brexpiprazole for the Acute Treatment of Bipolar Mania." *Journal of Psychopharmacology* 35: 971–982.

Vilar-Ribo, L., et al. (2021). "Genetic Overlap and Causality Between Substance Use Disorder and Attention-Deficit and Hyperactivity Disorder." *American Journal of Medical Genetics, Part B Neuropsychiatric Genetics* 186: 140–150.

Vindegaard, N., and Benros, M. E. (2020). "COVID-19 Pandemic and Mental Health Consequences: Systematic Review of the Current Evidence." *Brain, Behavior and Immunity* 89: 531–542.

Viswanathan, M., et al. (2020). "Treatment of Depression in Children and Adolescents: A Systematic Review [Internet]." *AHRQ Comparative Effectiveness Reviews* Report No. 20-EHC005-EF.

Voineskos, D., et al. (2020). "Management of Treatment-Resistant Depression: Challenges and Strategies." *Neuropsychiatric Disease and Treatment* 16: 221–234.

Volkmann, C., et al. (2020). "Lithium Treatment Over the Lifespan in Bipolar Disorders." *Frontiers in Psychiatry* 11: 377.

Volkow, N. (2021). "The Federal Responses to the Drug Overdose Epidemic." Testimony presented to the Senate Caucus on International Narcotics Control. *National Institute on Drug Abuse*, July 20.

Volkow, N. D. (2020). "Stigma and the Toll of Addiction." *The New England Journal of Addiction* 382: 1289–1290.

Volkow, N. D., and Blanco, C. (2021). "The Changing Opioid Crisis: Development, Challenges and Opportunities. *Molecular Psychiatry* 26: 218–233.

Volkow, N. D., and McLellan, A. T. (2016). "Opioid Abuse in Chronic Pain: Misconceptions and Mitigation Strategies." *New England Journal of Medicine* 374: 1253–1263.

Volkow, N. D., and Morales, M. (2015). "The Brain on Drugs: From Reward to Addiction." *Cell* 162: 712–725.

Volkow, N. D., et al. (1997). "Relationship Between Subjective Effects of Cocaine and Dopamine Transporter Occupancy." *Nature* 386: 827–830.

Volkow, N. D., et al. (2004). "The Addicted Human Brain Viewed in the Light of Imaging Studies: Brain Circuits and Treatment Strategies." *Neuropharmacology* 47, Supp. 1: 3–13.

Volkow, N. D., et al. (2011). "Addiction: Beyond Dopamine Reward Circuitry." *Proceedings of the National Academy of Sciences* 108: 15037–15042.

Volkow, N. D., et al. (2014). "Stimulant-Induced Dopamine Increases Are Markedly Blunted in Active Cocaine Abusers." *Molecular Psychiatry* 19: 1037–1043.

Volkow, N. D., et al. (2016a). "Neurobiologic Advances from the Brain Disease Model of Addiction." *New England Journal of Medicine* 374: 363–371.

Volkow, N. D., et al. (2016b). "The Risks of Marijuana Use During Pregnancy." *JAMA* 317: 129–130.

Volkow, N. D., et al. (2017). "Don't Worry, Be Happy: Endocannabinoids and Cannabis at the Intersection of Stress and Reward." *Annual Review of Pharmacology and Toxicology* 57: 285–308.

Volkow, N. D., et al. (2019a). "Prevention and Treatment of Opioid Misuse and Addiction: A Review." *JAMA Psychiatry* 76: 208–216.

Volkow, N. D., et al. (2019b). "The Neuro-science of Drug Reward and Addiction." *Physioloical Reviews* 99: 2115–2140.

Vonmoos, L. M., et al. (2014). "Cognitive Impairment in Cocaine Users Is Drug-Induced but Partially Reversible: Evidence from a Longitudinal Study." *Neuropsychopharmacology* 39: 2200–2210.

Vosahlikova, M., and Svoboda, P. (2016). "Lithium—Therapeutic Tool Endowed with Multiple Beneficiary Effects Caused by Multiple Mechanisms." *Acta Neurobiologica Experientalis* 75: 1–19.

Vossler, D. G., et al. (2016). "Long-Term Exposure and Safety of Lacosamide Monotherapy for the Treatment of Partial-Onset (focal) Seizures: Results from a Multicenter, Open-Label Trial." *Epilepsia* 57: 1625–1633.

Vyas, P., et al. (2020). "An Evaluation of Lumateperone Tosylate for the Treatment of Schizophrenia." *Expert Opinions in Pharmacotherapy* 21: 139–145.

Wade, A. G., et al. (2007). "Efficacy of Prolonged Release Melatonin in Insomnia Patients aged 55–80 Years: Quality of Sleep and next-Day Alertness Outcomes." *Current Medical Research Opinions* 23: 2597–2605.

Wade, A. G., et al. (2011). "Efficacy, Safety, and Tolerability of Escitalopram in Doses Up to 50 mg in Major Depressive Disorder (MDD): An Open-Label, Pilot Study." *BMC Psychiatry* 11: 42.

Wadehra, S. (2022, January/February). "COVID-Long Haulers and the New Chronic Pain Profile." *Practical Pain Management* 22(1).

Wadgave, U., and Nagesh, L. (2016). "Nicotine Replacement Therapy: An Overview." *International Journal of Health Sciences* 10: 425–435.

Walker, E. A., et al. (2021). "Antinociceptive and Discriminative Stimulus Effects of Six Novel Psychoactive Opioid Substances in Male Rats." *Journal of Pharmacology & Experimental Therapeutics* 379: 1–11.

Walkery, A., et al. (2021) "Review of Allopregnanolone Agonist Therapy for the Treatment of Depressive Disorders." *Drug Design, Development and Therapy* 15: 3017–3026.

Walkup, J. T., et al. (2008). "Cognitive Behavioral Therapy, Sertraline, or a Combination in Childhood Anxiety." *New England Journal of Medicine* 359: 2753–2766.

Walter, H. J., et al. (2020). "Clinical Practice Guideline for the Assessment and Treatment of Children and Adolescents with Anxiety Disorders." *Journal of the American Academy of Child and Adolescent Psychiatry* 59: 1107–1124.

Walton, M. A., et al. (2009). "Predictors of Violence Following Emergency Department Visit for Cocaine-Related Chest Pain." *Drug and Alcohol Dependence* 99: 79–88.

Wandner, L. D., et al. (2021). "NIH's Helping to End Addiction Long-term Initiative (NIH HEAL Initiative) Clinical Pain Management Common Date Element Program." *Journal of Pain*, in press.

Wang, G., et al. (2015). "Comparison of Vortioxetine Versus Venlafaxine XR in Adults in Asia with Major Depressive Disorder: A Randomized, Double-Blind Study." *Current Medical Research and Opinion* 31: 785–794.

Wang, J., et al. (2021). "Association of Aripiprazole with Reduced Hippocampal Atrophy During Maintenance Treatment of First-Episode Schizophrenia." *Journal of Clinical Psychopharmacology* 41: 244–249.

Wang, K. H., et al. (2015). "Neurotransmitter and Psychostimulant Recognition by the Dopamine Transporter." *Nature* 521: 322–327.

Wang, T. W., et al. (2021). "Characteristics of e-Cigarette Use Behaviors Among US Youth, 2020." *JAMA Network Open* 4: e2111336.

Ward, K., and Citrome, L. (2018). "Lisdexamfetamine: Chemistry, Pharmacodynamics, Pharmacokinetics, and Clinical Efficacy, Safety, and Tolerability in the Treatment of Binge Eating Disorder." *Expert Opinion on Drug Metabolism and Toxicology* 14: 229–238.

Ward, K., and Citrome, L. (2019). "Brexpiprazole for the Maintenance Treatment of Adults with Schizophrenia: An Evidence-Based Review and Place in Therapy." *Neuropsychiatric Disease Treatment* 15: 247–257.

Warden, S. J., and Fuchs, R. K. (2016). "Do Selective Serotonin Reuptake Inhibitors (SSRIs) Cause Fractures?" *Current Osteoporosis Reports* 14: 211–218.

Wasserman, D., et al. (2021). "Suicide Prevention in Childhood and Adolescence: A Narrative Review of Current Knowledge on Risk and Protective Factors and Effectiveness of Interventions." *Asia-Pacific Psychiatry* 13: e12452.

Watson, J. (2021). "More than Just a Hill of Beans; The Health Effects of Coffee." *Medscape.com*, Article 954638, July 12.

Waxmonsky, J. G., et al. (2014). "Does Pharmacological Treatment of ADHD in Adults Enhance Parenting Performance? Results of a Double-Blind Randomized Trial." *CNS Drugs* 28: 665–677.

Webster, L., et al. (2020). "Understanding Buprenorphine for Use in Chronic Pain: Expert Opinion." *Pain Medicine* 21: 714–723.

Wei, Y., et al. (2020). "A Historical Review of Antidepressant Effects of Ketamine and Its Enantiomers." *Pharmacology, Biochemistry and Behavior* 190: 172870.

Weimer, M. B., et al. (2021). "Removing One Barrier to Opioid Use Disorder Treatment: Is It Enough?" *JAMA* 325(12): 1147–1148.

Weinstein, S. M., et al. (2018). "Child- and Family-Focused Cognitive Behavioral Therapy for Pediatric Bipolar Disorder: Applications for Suicide Prevention." *Suicide and Life-Threatening Behavior* 48: 797–811.

Weintraub, M. J., et al. (2022). "Effects of Family Intervention on Psychosocial Functioning and Mood Symptoms of Youth at High Risk for Bipolar Disorder." *Journal of Consulting Clinical Psychology* 90: 161–171.

Weissman, M. M., et al. (2015). "Treatment of Maternal Depression in a Medication Clinical Trial and Its Effect on Children." *American Journal of Psychiatry* 172: 450–459.

Wen, X., et al. (2021). "Association of Gestational Opioid Exposure and Risk of Major and Minor Congenital Malformations." *JAMA Network Open* 4: e215708.

Wertlake, P. T., and Henson, M. D. (2016). "A Urinary Test Procedure for Identification of Cannabidiol in Patients Undergoing Medical Therapy with Marijuana." *Journal of Pain Research* 9: 81–85.

Wesseloo, R., et al. (2016). "Risk of Postpartum Relapse in Bipolar Disorder and Postpartum Psychosis: A Systematic Review and Meta-Analysis." *American Journal of Psychiatry* 173: 117–127.

Wetherill, R. R., et al. (2012a). "Acute Alcohol Effects on Contextual Memory BOLD Response: Differences Based on Fragmentary Blackout History." *Alcoholism: Clinical and Experimental Research* 36: 1108–1115.

White, A. M., and Hingson, R. (2014). "The Burden of Alcohol Use: Excessive Alcohol Consumption and Related Consequences Among College Students." *Alcohol Research* 35: 201–218.

White, A. M., et al. (2004). "Experiential Aspects of Alcohol-Induced Blackouts Among College Students." *American Journal of Drug and Alcohol Abuse* 30: 205–224.

White, A. M., et al. (2005). "College Students Lack Knowledge of Standard Drink Volumes: Implications for Definitions of Risky Drinking Based on Survey Data." *Alcoholism: Clinical and Experimental Research* 29: 631–638.

White, A. M., et al. (2022). "Alcohol-Related Deaths During the COVID-19 Pandemic." *JAMA* 327: 1704–1706.

White, C. M. (2018). "Pharmacologic and Medical Assessment of Kratom." *American Journal of Health System Pharmacy* 75: 261–267.

White, R. D., et al. (2013). "Attention Deficit Hyperactivity Disorder and Athletics." *Sports Health* 6: 149–156.

Whittington, M. D., et al. (2022). "Cost-Effectiveness and Value-Based Pricing of Aducanumab for Patients with Early Alzheimer's Disease." *Neurology* 98: e968–e977.

Wicinski, M., et al. (2021). "Cenobamate: Neuroprotective Potential of a New Antiepileptic Drug." *Neurochemical Research* 46: 439–446.

Wickham, K. A., and Spriet, L. (2018). "Administration of Caffeine in Alternate Forms." *Sports Medicine* 48 (Supplement 1): S79–S91.

Wiegmann, C., et al. (2020). "Alcohol and Dementia—What Is the Link? A Systematic Review." *Neuropsychiatric Disease & Treatment* 16: 87–99.

Wigal, S. B., et al. (2020a). "Diagnosis and Treatment Options for Preschoolers with Attention-Deficit/Hyperactivity Disorder." *Journal of Child and Adolescent Psychopharmacology* 30: 104–118.

Wigal, S. B., et al. (2020b). "Safety and Efficacy of Centanafadine Sustained-Release in Adults with Attention-Deficit Hyperactivity Disorder: Results of Phase 2 Studies." *Neuropsychiatric Disease and Treatment* 16: 1411–1426.

Wiggs, K. K. (2020). "Antiseizure Medication Use During Pregnancy and Risk of ASD and ADHD in Children." *Neurology* 95: e3232–3240.

Wightman, R. S., et al. (2021). "Opioid Overdose Deaths with Buprenorphine Detected in Postmortem Toxicology: A Retrospective Analysis." *Journal of Medical Toxicology* 17: 10–15.

Wilhelmus, M., et al. (2016). "Effects of a Single, Oral 60 Mg Caffeine Dose on Attention in Healthy Adult Subjects." *Journal of Psychopharmacology* 31: 222–232.

Williams, A. R., et al. (2020). "Acute Care, Prescription Opioid Use, and Overdose Following Discontinuation of Long-Term Buprenorphine Treatment for Opioid Use Disorder." *American Journal of Psychiatry* 177: 117–124.

Williams, S., et al. (2019). "Rational Deprescribing in the Elderly." *Annals of Clinical Psychiatry* 31: 144–152.

Williams, T., et al. (2022). "Pharmacotherapy for Post-Traumatic Stress Disorder." *Cochrane Database of Systematic Reviews* 3: CD002795.

Wilson, J. D., et al. (2021). "Trajectories of Opioid Use Following First Opioid Prescription in Opioid-Naïve Youths and Young Adults." *JAMA Network Open* 4: e21452.

Winhusen, T. M., et al. (2014). "A Randomized Trial of Concurrent Smoking Cessation and Substance Use Disorder Treatment in Stimulant Dependent Smokers." *Journal of Clinical Psychiatry* 75: 336–343.

Winslow, B. T., et al. (2007). "Methamphetamine Abuse." *American Family Physician* 76: 1169–1174.

Wise, R. A., and Koob, G. F. (2014). "The Development and Maintenance of Drug Addiction." *Neuropsychopharmacology* 39: 254–262.

Wisner, K. L., et al. (2020). "The Association Between Antidepressant Exposure and Birth Defects—Are We There Yet?" *JAMA Psychiatry*' 77: 1215–1216.

Witkin, J. M., et al. (2019). "Rapid-Acting Antidepressants." *Advances in Pharmacology* 86: 47–96.

Wohleb, E. S., et al. (2016). "Integrating Neuroimmune Systems in the Neurobiology of Depression." *Nature Reviews: Neuroscience* 17: 497–511.

Wolf, C. J. H., et al. (2021). "Characterization of the GHB Withdrawal Syndrome." *Journal of Clinical Medicine* 10: 2333.

Wolfschlag, M., and Hakansson, A. (2021). "Increased Risk for Developing Gambling Disorder Under the Treatment with Pramipexole, Ropinirole, and Aripiprazole: A Nationwide Register Study in Sweden." *PLoS One* 16: e0252516.

Wolraich, M. L., et al., and American Academy of Pediatrics Subcommittee on Children and Adolescents with Attention-Deficit/Hyperactivity Disorder. (2019). "Clinical Practice Guideline for the Diagnosis, Evaluation, and Treatment of Attention-Deficit/Hyperactivity Disorder in Children and Adolescents." *Pediatrics* 144: e20192528.

Wong, C. K., et al. (2017). "Spontaneous Adverse Event Reports Associated with Zolpidem in the United States 2003–2012." *Journal of Clinical Sleep Medicine* 13: 223–234.

Wong, S. S. C., et al. (2020). "Analgesic Effects of Cannabinoids for Chronic Non-Cancer Pain: A Systematic Review and Meta-Analysis with Meta-Regression." *Journal of Neuroimmune Pharmacology* 15: 801–829.

Worrell, D. S., and Gould, T. J. (2021). "Therapeutic Potential of Ketamine for Alcohol Use Disorder." *Neuroscience and Biobehavioral Reviews."* 126: 573–589.

Wright, J. D., et al. (2021). "Association of New Perioperative Benzodiazepine Use with Persistent Benzodiazepine Use." *JAMA Network Open* 4(6): e2112478.

Wright, J. H., et al. (2022). "Effect of Computer-Assisted Cognitive Behavior Therapy vs Usual Care on Depression Among Adults in Primary Care: A Randomized Clinical Trial." *JAMA Network Open* 5: e2146716.

Wu, L., et al. (2017). "Prevalence and Correlates of Treatment Utilization Among Adults with Cannabis Use Disorder in the United States." *Drug and Alcohol Dependence* 177: 153–162.

Wuo-Silva, R., et al. (2016). "Modafinil Induces Rapid-Onset Behavioral Sensitization and Cross-Sensitization with Cocaine in Mice: Implications for the Addictive Potential of Modafinil." *Frontiers in Pharmacology* 7: 420.

Xie, J., et al. (2021). "Association of Tramadol vs Codeine Prescription Dispensation with Mortality and Other Adverse Clinical Outcomes." *JAMA* 326: 1504–1515.

Xu, W., et al. (2015). "Link Between the SNCA Gene and Parkinsonism." *Neurobiology of Aging* 36: 1505–1518.

Yaden, D. B., et al. (2021). "Psychedelics in Psychiatry—Keeping the Renaissance from Going Off the Rails." *JAMA Psychiatry* 78: 469–470.

Yaffe, K., and Boustani, M. (2014). *"Benzodiazepines and Risk of Alzheimer's Disease." BMJ* 349: g5312.

Yan, H. D., et al. (2013). "Inhibitory Effects of Levetiracetam on the High-Voltage-Activated L-Type Ca(2+) Channels in Hippocampal CA3 Neurons of Spontaneously Epileptic Rat (SER)." *Brain Research Bulletin* 90: 142–148.

Yan, T., et al. (2020). "Health Care Cost in Patients with Schizophrenia Treated with Brexpiprazole Versus Other Oral Atypical Antipsychotic Therapy." *Clinical Therapeutics* 42: 77–93.

Yang, A., et al. (2010). "Genetics of Caffeine Consumption and Responses to Caffeine." *Psychopharmacology* 211: 245–257.

Yang, T., et al. (2020). "The Role of BDNF on Neural Plasticity in Depression." *Frontiers in Cellular Neuroscience* 14: 82.

Yashima, K., et al. (2021). "Evaluation of the Safety of Taking Lamotrigine During Lactation Period." *Breastfeeding Medicine* 16: 432–438.

Yaster, M., et al. (2020). "The Opioid Epidemic in Pediatrics: A 2020 Update." *Current Opinions in Anaesthesiology* 33: 327–334.

Yatham, L. N., et al. (2018). "Canadian Network for Mood and Anxiety Treatments (CANMAT) and International Society for Bipolar Disorders (ISBD) 2018 Guidelines for the Management of Patients with Bipolar Disorder." *Bipolar Disorders* 20: 97–170.

Yavi, M., et al. (2022). "Ketamine Treatment for Depression: A Review." *Discover Mental Health* 2: 9.

Yi, X., et al. (2018). "Trazodone for the Treatment of Insomnia: A Meta-analysis of Randomized Placebo-Controlled Trials." *Sleep Medicine* 45: 25–32.

Yilmaz, S., et al. (2022). "Do Psychological Interventions Reduce Symptoms of Depression for Patients with Bipolar I or II Disorder? A Meta-Analysis." *Journal of Affective Disorders* 301: 193–204.

Young, C. B. and E. C. Mormino (2022). "Prevalence Rates of Amyloid Positivity—Updates and Relevance." *JAMA Neurology* 79: 225–227.

Young, J. R., et al. (2021). "Pharmacotherapy for Preschool Children with Attention Deficit Hyperactivity Disorder (ADHD): Current Status and Future Directions." *CNS Drugs* 35: 403–424.

Young, S., and Woodhouse, E. (2021). "Assessment and Treatment of Substance Use in Adults with ADHD: A Psychological Approach." *Journal of Neural Transmission (Vienna)* 128: 1099–1108.

Young-Wolff, K. C., et al. (2021). "Rates of Prenatal Cannabis Use Among Pregnant Women Before and During the COVID-19 Pandemic." *JAMA* 326(17): 1745–1747.

Yu, S., et al. (2015). "Recent Advances in Methamphetamine Neurotoxicity Mechanisms and its Molecular Pathophysiology." *Behavioral Neurology,* Article 103969.

Yuen, W. S., et al. (2020). "Adolescent Alcohol Use Trajectories: Risk Factors and Adult Outcomes." *American Academy of Pediatrics* 146: e20200440.

Yunusa, I., and El Helou, M. L. (2020). "The Use of Risperidone in Behavioral and Psychological Symptoms of Dementia: A Review of Pharmacology, Clinical Evidence, Regulatory Approvals and Off-Label Use." *Frontiers in Pharmacology* 11: 3389.

Yunusa, I., et al. (2020). "Pimavanserin: A Novel Antipsychotic with Potentials to Address an Unmet Need of Older Adults with Dementia-Related Psychosis." *Frontiers in Pharmacology* 11: 87.

Yunusa, I., et al. (2022). "Risk of Opioid Overdose Associated with Concomitant Use of Oxycodone and Selective Serotonin Reuptake Inhibitors." *JAMA Network Open* 5: e220194.

Zaccara, G., and Prucca, E. (2014). "Interactions Between Antiepileptic Drugs, and Between Antiepileptic Drugs and Other Drugs." *Epileptic Disorders* 16: 409–431.

Zack, M., et al. (2015). "Differential Cardiovascular and Hypothalamic Pituitary Response to Amphetamine in Male Pathological Gamblers Versus Healthy Controls." *Journal of Psychopharmacology* 29: 971–982.

Zamani, N., et al. (2020). "Buprenorphine to Reverse Respiratory Depression from Methadone Overdose in Opioid-Dependent Patients: A Prospective Randomized Trial." *Critical Care* 24: 44.

Zantut, P. R. A., et al. (2020). "Effects of Cannabis and Its Components on the Retina: A Systematic Review." *Cutaneous and Ocular Toxicology* 39: 1–9.

Zarrabi, H., et al. (2016). "Clinical Features, Course and Treatment of Methamphetamine-Induced Psychosis in Psychiatric Inpatients." *BMC Psychiatry* 16: 44.

Zawilska, J. B., et al. (2021). "Carfentanil—from an Animal Anesthetic to a Deadly Illicit Drug." *Forensic Science International* 320: 110715.

Zeitzer, J. M., et al. (2020). "Effect of Suvorexant vs Placebo on Total Daytime Sleep Hours in Shift Workers: A Randomized Clinical Trial." *JAMA Network Open* 3: e206614.

Zhai, Y., et al. (2016). "Association Between Antipsychotic Drugs and Mortality in Older Persons with Alzheimer's Disease: A Systematic Review and Meta-Analysis." *Journal of Alzheimer's Disease* 52: 631–639.

Zhang, A., et al. (2017). "What Effects—If Any—Does Marijuana Use During Pregnancy Have on the Fetus or Child?" *The Journal of Family Practice* 66: 462–464.

Zhang, C., et al. (2014). "Alcohol Intake and Risk of Stroke: A Dose-Response Meta-Analysis of Prospective Studies." *International Journal of Cardiology* 174: 669–677.

Zhang, G., and Stackman Jr., R. W. (2015). "The Role of Serotonin 5-HT_{2A} Receptors in Memory and Cognition." *Frontiers in Pharmacology* 6: 225.

Zhang, L., et al. (2016). "Levetiracetam vs. Brivaracetam for Adults with Refractory Focal Seizures: A Meta-Analysis and Indirect Comparison." *Seizure* 39: 28–33.

Zhang, R., et al. (2020). "Association of Low to Moderate Alcohol Drinking with Cognitive Functions from Middle to Older Age Among US Adults." *JAMA Network Open* 3: e207922.

Zhang, T., et al. (2020). "Glutaminergic Neurons in the Prefrontal Cortex Mediate the Formation and Retrieval of Cocaine-Associated Memories in Mice." *Addiction Biology* 25: e12723.

Zhang, V. S., et al. (2019). "Opioid and Benzodiazepine Coprescribing in the United States Before and After US Food and Drug Administration Boxed Warning." *JAMA Psychiatry* 76: 1208–1210.

Zhang, Y., et al. (2016). "Is Coffee Consumption Associated with a Lower Risk of Hyperuricaemia or Gout? A Systematic Review and Meta-Analysis." *BMJ* 6: e009809.

Zhao, Q., et al. (2020). "Association of Heavy Drinking with Deviant Fiber Tract Development in Frontal Brain Systems in Adolescents." *JAMA Psychiatry* 12: 12–30.

Zheng, W., et al. (2019). "Brexanolone for Postpartum Depression: A Meta-Analysis of Randomized Controlled Studies." *Psychiatry Research* 279: 83–89.

Zheng, W., et al. (2020). "Adjunctive Intranasal Esketamine for Major Depressive Disorder; A Systematic Review of Randomized Double-Blind Controlled-Placebo Studies." *Journal of Affective Disorders* 265: 63–70.

Zhornitsky, S., and Potvin, S. (2012). "Cannabidiol in Humans: The Quest for Therapeutic Targets." *Pharmaceuticals* (Basel) 21: 529–552.

Zhou, M., et al. (2020). "Asenapine Transdermal Patch for the Management of Schizophrenia." *Psychopharmacology Bulletin* 50: 60–82.

Zhou, S., et al. (2016). "Secondhand Hookah Smoke: An Occupational Hazard for Hookah Bar Employees." *Tobacco Control* 0: 1–6.

Zhou, Z., et al. (2018). "Rational Incorporation of Molecular Adjuvants into a Hybrid Nanoparticle-Based Nicotine Vaccine for Immunotherapy Against Nicotine Addiction." *Biomaterials* 155: 165–175.

Zhu, L., et al. (2018). "Novel Opioid Receptor Agonists with Reduced Morphine-Like Side Effects." *Mini Review in Medicinal Chemistry* 18: 1603–1610.

Zigman, D., and Blier, P. (2012). "A Framework to Avoid Irrational Polypharmacy in Psychiatry." *Journal of Psychopharmacology* 26: 1507–1511.

Zimmermann, K. S., et al. (2020). "Esketamine as a Treatment for Pediatric Depression: Questions of Safety and Efficacy." *The Lancet Psychiatry* 7: 827–829.

Zorick, T., et al. (2019). "Effects of Citalopram on Cue-Induced Alcohol Craving and Thalamic $D_{2/3}$ Dopamine Receptor Availability." *International Journal of Neuropsychopharmacology* 22: 286–291.

Zou, R., et al. (2022). "Association of Maternal Tobacco Use During Pregnancy with Preadolescent Brain Morphology Among Offspring." *JAMA Network Open* 5: e2224701.

INDEX

Note: Page numbers followed by f indicate figures; those followed by t indicate tables; and those followed by n indicate footnotes.

A

B

E

M

N

P

S

T

U

V

W

X

Z